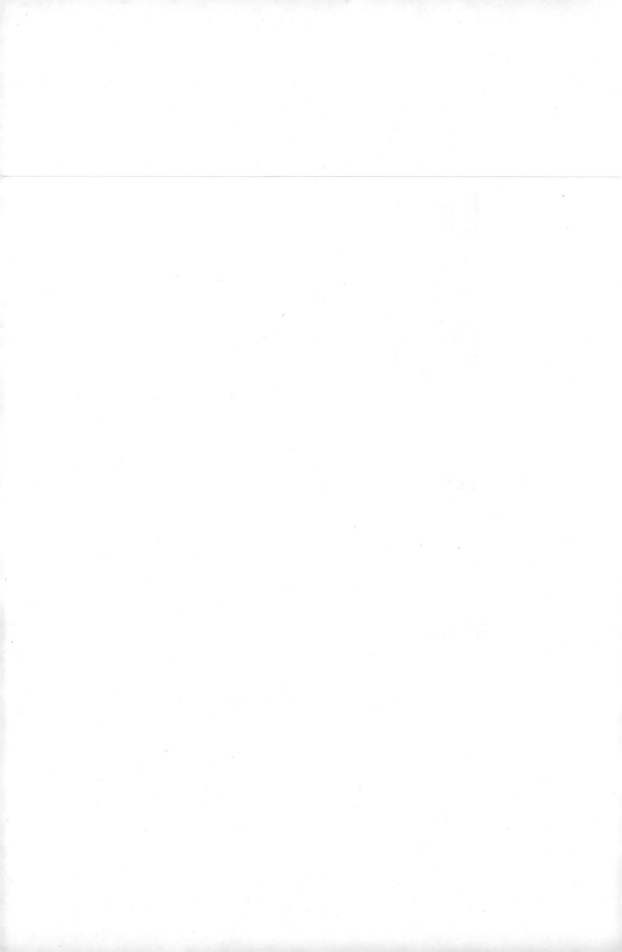

Therapeutic Exercise In Developmental Disabilities

THIRD EDITION

Barbara H. Connolly, EdD, PT, FAPTA
Professor and Chairman
Department of Physical Therapy
University of Tennessee Health Sciences Center
Memphis, Tennesee

Patricia C. Montgomery, PhD, PT, FAPTA
President
Therapeutic Intervention Programs, Inc
Minneapolis, Minnesota

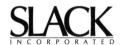

SLACK
INCORPORATED

An innovative information, education, and management company
6900 Grove Road • Thorofare, NJ 08086

www.slackbooks.com

ISBN: 978-155642-624-7

Published by: SLACK Incorporated
6900 Grove Road
Thorofare, NJ 08086 USA
Telephone: 856-848-1000
Fax: 856-853-5991
www.slackbooks.com

Contact SLACK Incorporated for more information about other books in this field or about the availability of our books from distributors outside the United States.

Therapeutic exercise in developmental disabilities / [edited by] Barbara H. Connolly, Patricia C. Montgomery.-- 3rd ed.
p. ; cm.
Includes bibliographical references and index.
ISBN 1-55642-624-0 (hardcover)
1. Developmental disabilities--Exercise therapy. 2. Physical therapy for children.
[DNLM: 1. Disabled Children--rehabilitation. 2. Physical Therapy Techniques--Child. 3. Physical Therapy Techniques--Infant. WS 368 T398 2004] I. Connolly, Barbara H. II. Montgomery, Patricia.

RJ506.D47T48 2004
615.8'2'083--dc22

2004017286

Printed in the United States of America.

Last digit is print number: 10   9   8   7   6   5   4   3

Dedication

This book is dedicated to children with developmental disabilities and the physical therapists and families who work together to manage their care and enrich their lives.

Contents

Acknowledgments

We would like to acknowledge the artwork of Sandy Lowrance that was initially prepared for the first edition of this text and has been reprinted in this edition. Our appreciation also goes out to the authors of the individual chapters for being so prompt and efficient in submitting their manuscripts. We wish to acknowledge our families for their support and patience during the many long hours we have spent away from them during the process of writing and editing this third edition.

About the Editors

Barbara H. Connolly, EdD, PT, FAPTA, received her BS degree in Physical Therapy from the University of Florida. She received a master's degree in Special Education with a minor in Speech Language Pathology, and a doctoral degree in Curriculum and Instruction from the University of Memphis. She is Professor and Chairman of the Department of Physical Therapy at the University of Tennessee Health Science Center. She also holds an adjunct academic appointment in the Graduate School of the University of Indianapolis and has served on the Board of Directors for the University of St. Augustine. She has served on the APTA Board of Directors, the APTA Pediatric Specialty Council, and the American Board of Physical Therapy Specialists. She is currently President of the Section on Pediatrics of the APTA. She also is past president of the Academic Administrators Special Interest Group for the Section on Education. She received the Golden Pen Award from the APTA as well as the Bud DeHaven Leadership Award, the Research Award, and the Jeanne Fischer Distinguished Mentorship Award from the Section on Pediatrics. She is the primary author of 17 publications in peer-reviewed journals, has written 18 book chapters, and has coauthored or edited seven textbooks for physical therapists. She has presented over 100 invited lectureships at the national and international level. She continues to remain active in providing professional development courses across the United States and is active in clinical practice through the UT faculty practice.

Patricia C. Montgomery, PhD, PT, FAPTA, received her BS degree in Physical Therapy from the University of Oklahoma, Norman, and her MA in Educational Psychology and PhD in Child Psychology from the University of Minnesota, Minneapolis. Dr. Montgomery has a private practice in pediatrics in the Minneapolis-St. Paul area and also provides continuing education courses for physical therapy clinicians. Dr. Montgomery has taught in physical therapy programs at several academic institutions and currently is an associate professor at the University of Tennessee Health Science Center. She has served on the APTA Board of Directors and as President of the Minnesota Chapter, APTA. Dr. Montgomery received the Pediatric Section, APTA Research Award; the Minnesota Chapter, APTA Outstanding Service Award; the APTA Dorothy Briggs Memorial Scientific Inquiry Award; and the APTA Lucy Blair Service Award. She also gave the inaugural Luise Lynch Lecture at the University of Oklahoma and the Third Annual John H. P. Maley Lecture at APTA Annual Conference. Dr. Montgomery is the first author of 16 publications in peer-reviewed journals and has coauthored several textbooks for physical therapists. She recently coauthored, with Barbara H. Connolly, PhD, PT, FAPTA, the text *Clinical Applications for Motor Control* (SLACK Incorporated, 2003). She also serves on the editorial board of *Pediatric Physical Therapy*.

Contributing Authors

Rona Alexander, PhD, CCC-SP, is a speech-language pathologist specializing in the assessment and treatment of oral-motor, feeding/swallowing, and respiratory-phonatory function in infants and children with neuromotor involvement. She maintains a private practice; provides consultation services; and conducts workshops on oral-motor, feeding/swallowing, and respiratory coordination development, assessment, and treatment. As a qualified speech instructor in Neurodevelopmental Treatment, Dr. Alexander teaches in basic pediatric 8-week and advanced NDT courses. She has contributed chapters on oral-motor, feeding/swallowing, and respiratory-phonatory function to numerous publications; is coauthor of the book entitled *Normal Development of Functional Motor Skills: The First Year of Life*; and is author of the ASHA CEU product *Pediatric Feeding and Swallowing: Assessment and Treatment Programming*. Dr. Alexander has served as a member of the Steering Committee for Special Interest Division 13: Swallowing and Swallowing Disorders.

Judith C. Bierman, PT, received her BS in Physical Therapy from the University of North Carolina. She has practiced in a wide variety of settings including hospitals, schools, infant programs, and residential centers. Her current practice in Augusta, Georgia spans ages from infancy to young adults. Ms. Bierman teaches extensively in continuing education courses, including the basic and advanced Neuro-Developmental Treatment courses, as well as other short courses aimed at advancing clinical skills for practitioners. She has held a variety of leadership roles in Neuro-Developmental Therapy Association and contributed significantly to the publication of a new book on NDT theory.

Regi Boehme, OTR/L, received her BS in Occupational Therapy from Western Michigan University and was a certified occupational therapy instructor in Neurodevelopmental Treatment. She was in private practice in the Milwaukee, Wisconsin area and served as a consultant to various pediatric facilities. Ms. Boehme lectured extensively throughout North America on topics related to treatment of children and adults with neurological impairments. Ms. Boehme passed away in July 2004 following a long illness.

Joanell A. Bohmert, MS, PT, received her BS degree and advanced MS degree in Physical Therapy from the University of Minnesota, Minneapolis. She is a full-time clinician with the Anoka-Hennepin school district with a focus on pediatrics and neurology. Ms. Bohmert was actively involved in the development and revision of the *Guide to Physical Therapist Practice* as a member of the project advisory group and liaison to the musculoskeletal panel for Part Two; member of the task force on development of Part Three; a project editor for the second edition, Parts One and Two; and currently is a member of the APTA board of directors oversight committee for the second edition. She has lectured extensively on the *Guide* and is an APTA Trainer for the *Guide*.

David D. Chapman PhD, PT, has devoted his professional career to working with infants and children who have developmental disabilities. He began in the public school setting after receiving his BS in Exercise Science at the University of Iowa and MS in Adapted Physical Education at Southern Illinois University-Carbondale. Following completion of his PhD in Kinesiology and Developmental Psychology at Indiana University, he joined the physical therapy program faculty at Indiana University at Indianapolis where he completed his BS in Physical Therapy. While there, Dr. Chapman taught biomechanics, human anatomy, and lifespan development; presented at numerous national and international conferences; and was instrumental in developing the present doctor of physical therapy curriculum. In 2003, Dr. Chapman received the Jeanne Hughes Award for the best manuscript published in *Pediatric Physical Therapy* adapted from a dissertation. Currently, Dr. Chapman practices full-time as a pediatric physical therapist at Bloomington Hospital's Children's Therapy Clinic in Bloomington, Indiana.

Susan K. Effgen, PhD, PT, holds the Joseph Hamburg Professorship in Rehabilitation Sciences in College of Health Sciences at the University of Kentucky where she also is the Director of the Rehabilitation Sciences Doctoral Program. She was formally the Director of Pediatric Physical Therapy at Hahnemann University. She received her BS degree in Physical Therapy from Boston University, her MMSc in pediatric physical therapy from Emory University, and her PhD in Special Education from Georgia State University. She has published numerous articles and has just completed a pediatric physical therapy textbook. Her research interests include service delivery and outcomes of early intervention and school-based therapy.

Meredith Hinds Harris, EdD, PT, is Associate Professor and Chair of the Department of Physical Therapy at Northeastern University. Dr. Harris was instrumental in the development of specialization in pediatrics for the APTA. She also served as the Chair of the first Specialty Council in Pediatrics for the APTA. Her experience in pediatrics includes employment at the Harlem Hospital NICU, the Kennedy Center for Developmental Disabilities at Albert Einstein College of Medicine, United Cerebral Palsy of NY State, and the Bobath Center in London, England. Her research activities have focused on developmental motor problems in children with HIV/AIDS and children with severe mental and physical disabilities.

Susan R. Harris, PhD, PT, FAPTA, is a Professor in the Division of Physical Therapy of the School of Rehabilitation Sciences and Associate Member in the Department of Pediatrics at the University of British Columbia in Vancouver. She also is Faculty Clinical Associate at Sunny Hill Health Centre for Children. Dr. Harris is currently Scientific Editor of *Physiotherapy Canada* and also serves on the editorial boards of *Infants and Young Children* and *Topics in Early Childhood Special Education*. Her pediatric research has focused on the early diagnosis of movement disorders in infants and the efficacy of early intervention for at-risk infants and children with neurodevelopmental disabilities. She is coauthor, with Dr. Marci Hanson, of the book *Teaching the Young Child with Motor Delays: A Guide for Parents and Professionals* (1986) and primary author of the soon-to-be-published manual for the Harris Infant Neuromotor Test (HINT).

Janet M. Wilson Howle, MACT, PT, is a clinician, teacher, author, physical therapy consultant, and founder/co-owner of Kaye Products, Inc. Ms. Howle received her BS and PT certificate from the University of Michigan and her MACT from the University of North Carolina, Chapel Hill. She trained in Neuro-Developmental Treatment with the Bobaths in 1971 to 1972 and finished her requirements as an NDT Coordinator-Instructor in Pediatrics with Mary Quinton in 1983. She currently teaches continuing education courses related to cerebral palsy and NDT in the United States and Europe. She was the recipient of the NeuroDevelopmental Treatment Association Award of Excellence in 2003 for her contributions to NDT. Ms. Howle has written and edited numerous articles and chapters in books and recently authored her first book, *Neuro-Developmental Treatment: Theoretical Foundations and Principles of Clinical Practice*.

Meg Barry Michaels, PhD, PT, is an Assistant Professor in the Graduate School of Physical Therapy at Slippery Rock University in Slippery Rock, Pennsylvania. She received a BA in Biology from MacMurray College, an MS in Community Health Education with an emphasis in physical therapy from Old Dominion University, and a PhD in Rehabilitation Sciences from the University of Pittsburgh. She has experience in a variety of clinical settings including clinical research, presented numerous continuing education programs, and is currently involved in clinical research with children with cerebral palsy.

Rebecca E. Porter, PhD, PT, is an Associate Professor in the Indiana University-Purdue University Indianapolis Department of Physical Therapy and an Associate Vice President for Enrollment Services, Indiana University. She received her BS in Physical Therapy, MS in Allied Health Education, and PhD in Medical Neurobiology from Indiana University. Dr. Porter has practiced in a variety of settings, presented continuing education workshops, lectured at several universities, and published in the area of neurological physical therapy. She is currently Treasurer of the Neurology Section, APTA. In 2003, she received the Anniversary Award from the Section on Pediatrics, APTA and the APTA Lucy Blair Service Award.

Janet Sternat, PT, received her BS degree in Physical Therapy from the University of Wisconsin-Madison in 1969. She is a Guild Certified Feldenkrais Practitioner and has training/certification in Neuro-Developmental Treatment, Sensory Integration, joint mobilization, and cranial-sacral techniques. Ms. Sternat has been a preceptor for physical therapy students at the University of Wisconsin-Madison, University of Wisconsin-Lacrosse, St. Scholastica-Duluth, and for physical therapist assistant students. She owned and operated a pediatric therapy practice in the River Falls, Wisconsin area for 20 years. During that time she founded Have-A-Heart, Inc, a nonprofit corporation that provides respite and home care services to children with disabilities. Ms. Sternat is currently working in the 0-3 programs serving children with disabilities in Wisconsin and providing professional development workshops for therapists and paraprofessionals serving pediatric clientele.

Ann F. VanSant, PhD, PT, is a Professor of Physical Therapy at Temple University, Philadelphia. She received her BS in Physical Therapy from Russell Sage College, an MS in Physical Therapy from Virginia Commonwealth University, and a PhD in Physical Education—Motor Development from the University of Wisconsin-Madison. Dr. VanSant is the Editor of *Pediatric Physical Therapy,* the official journal of the Section on Pediatrics of the APTA. Her research is designed to describe developmental differences in movement patterns used to perform functional tasks across the human lifespan.

Rebecca Welch, MSPT, PCS, graduated in 1992 with a BS in Physical Therapy from the University of Tennessee Health Science Center in Memphis. She received her MSPT in 2000 from the University of Tennessee and was certified as a pediatric clinical specialist in 2001. She is currently pursuing a PhD in Educational Psychology at the University of Memphis. Rebecca provided services in the NICU for 6 years at the University of Tennessee Medical Center in Knoxville. She is currently the Chief of Physical Therapy at the Boling Center for Developmental Disabilities at the University of Tennessee Health Science Center where she also serves as a consultant to the early intervention program at LeBonheur Children's Hospital and as part-time instructor for the Program in Physical Therapy.

Marilyn Woods, PT, has a BS degree from the Nebraska Wesleyan University, Lincoln, and a certificate in physical therapy from Mayo Clinic School of Physical Therapy. She is a member of the APTA-trained faculty for the *Guide to Physical Therapist Practice* and has given numerous workshops on the *Guide* to clinicians. Ms. Woods has been active in the Minnesota Chapter APTA quality assurance program for more than 20 years in both geriatric and pediatric subcommittees. Ms. Woods spent many years as a generalist in a small rural hospital in northern Minnesota. She recently retired from her position as supervisor of home care rehabilitation at Park-Nicollet Health System, Methodist Hospital in St. Louis Park, Minnesota, but continues to serve as a consultant to the Park-Nicollet Health System.

Preface

In this third edition of *Therapeutic Exercise in Developmental Disabilities*, the emphasis is on evidence-based practice. Although empirical evidence is only beginning to be accumulated, it is essential that physical therapists and other health care providers become aware of the scientific rationale that supports various intervention strategies and techniques. Therapists will need to continually review the scientific literature and revise their theoretical perspective as pertinent information is published. This text is designed to provide a framework for evaluation and intervention with children with developmental disabilities following the format provided in the *Guide to Physical Therapist Practice.* Case studies of five children representing typical developmental disabilities encountered by physical therapists were chosen as the mechanism for applying a problem-solving approach. The goal of physical therapy intervention is to promote optimal functional independence for children with integration into home, school, and community life. We hope that this text is valuable to students and clinicians and, in turn, to the children they treat.

Concepts of Neural Organization and Movement

Ann F. VanSant, PhD, PT

Introduction

Physical therapists apply principles derived from theories of motor control, motor learning, and motor development when designing intervention for children with motor disabilities. Motor control, motor learning, and motor development represent foundational sciences for physical therapy. Having studied these foundational sciences, therapists consciously or unconsciously subscribe to theories of how the nervous system is organized and how individuals learn and develop motor skills. Theories then are used clinically to:

1. Select tests and examinations that identify a child's impairments and functional abilities

2. Set objectives for intervention

3. Plan and sequence intervention activities

In this chapter, contemporary concepts of motor control and development are explored that currently affect the types of examinations, tests, and interventions that physical therapists use with children. Later, in Chapter 3, concepts of motor learning are explored and applied to the treatment of children.

In the best of worlds, sufficient research would guide the decision-making process and allow evidence-based practice across a wider range of functional limitations and impairments than is possible today. Where evidence of the reliability, validity, sensitivity, and specificity of clinical tests and examinations exists, those tools with strong credentials are the tools of choice; and, where there is evidence of treatment efficacy, that evidence must guide our practice. However, the current state of clinical science is such that the efficacy of many tests and interventions still is being examined and will continue to be examined over the course of our professional practice. As foundational sciences provide greater understanding, our clinical procedures will be refined and validated. We have a professional history of using theories in clinical practice with little evidence to support their utility. We now have reached a turning point in professional practice by recognizing the need to move toward evidence-based practice and by encouraging research into treatment efficacy. Yet, much of what we currently do still is not researched and we continue to rely on theoretical models for decision making. We must continue to assess our interventions. This chapter focuses on theory that addresses clinical practice and also addresses the need to develop and validate test instruments and contemporary interventions.

Motor Control

The term *motor control* refers to processes of the brain and spinal cord that govern posture and movement. Therapists traditionally gain their understanding of these control processes through courses in the neurosciences. Neuroscientists commonly focus their research on the neural processes underlying animal movement. Often their work focuses on the chemical or electrical activity of single nerve cells or nuclei in order to understand the organization of spinal motor mechanisms and mechanisms of higher control mediated by various brain structures. These control processes typically occur in extremely short time periods, often in fractions of seconds. It should be recognized that, although human posture and movement comprise behaviors that we can easily observe, the processes of motor control occurring within the central nervous system (CNS) cannot be observed directly. This is because the functions of the brain and spinal cord are, even in this world of high technology, relatively hidden from view. As therapists, we have a long history of observing human movement, and much of what is known about patients' motor control can be attributed to careful observation of posture and movement that was undertaken by neuroscientists,[1,2] physicians,[3-5] psychologists,[6] and therapists[7-9] in the last century.

Neuroscientists study the spatial (geographical) and temporal characteristics of CNS organization. They seek specifically to understand which brain structures are involved in controlling various postures and movements and how these structures contribute to motor control. Although the beginnings of neuroscience can be traced to traditional disciplines of neuroanatomy and neurophysiology, scientific interest in motor control has spread and now includes a broader range of disciplines, including behavioral scientists in psychology and kinesiology who, like physical therapists, observe motor behavior and then apply inductive reasoning to make conclusions about "central processes" that underlie motor activity. Their work rests on the premise that motor behavior is a reflection of CNS function.

Because postures and movements appear well-organized and have characteristic forms, such as those we observe in walking, running, or moving from sitting to standing, we know that processes of motor control are not random. In fact, postures and movements are comprised of well-defined patterns of action, and it is these action patterns that behavioral scientists and physical therapists observe and study to better understand the invisible internal control processes mediated by neural structures. The contributions of neurologists, whose past careful observations of motor behavior in patients with disorders of the brain, and contemporary behavioral scientists, who precisely studied the spatial and temporal characteristics of specific motor skills, have greatly added to and enriched our understanding of motor control.

Motor Development

In contrast to motor control, *motor development* refers to the processes of change in motor behavior that occur over relatively extended time periods. Typically, these extended time periods are measured in units that reflect age. The formal study of motor development originated in the behavioral sciences, specifically psychology and clinical medicine. Yet, these psychologists and physicians were influenced strongly by the biological scientists who studied how the CNS controlled movement, and, thus, there is affinity and overlap in classical thought about how the motor system develops and is controlled.[6]

Motor development, defined here as age-related change in motor behavior, results from internal and external influences and often has been attributed to processes such as matu-

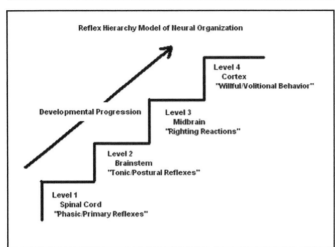

Figure 1-1. The reflex hierarchy represents a traditional model of neural organization and development. A staircase of levels of neuroanatomical structures and reflexive behaviors is surmounted with volitional behavior felt to be controlled in the cerebral cortex. Neuromotor development proceeds from Level 1 up to Level 4. The examination of reflexes and reactions helps the therapist determine the child's level of neuromotor development.

ration, growth, or learning. From our background in biological science we, as physical therapists, acquire respect for the influences of growth and maturation, which in medically-related disciplines are commonly thought to be biological processes. On the other hand, we know that developmental change in motor behavior can be affected by external influences from the environment, such as the teaching of specific skills or from cultural expectations. Controversies and debate over which changes in motor behavior are due to maturation and which are due to learning are as old as developmental science.

More recently, maturation-learning or nature-nurture controversies have led to the recognition that interactions between internal biological growth processes known as maturation and external influences cause developmental change. Debates over whether change in motor behavior is due to external influences, such as those brought about by a physical therapy program, or to maturational influences, such as brain development, will continue. These ongoing nature-nurture controversies are an important force that enables a greater understanding of motor development and of the intimate relationship of the individual to the world around him or her. Through debate and research designed to settle these arguments, the process of motor development further will be better delineated and therapists will know better how to affect positive change in children's motor abilities.

When working with infants and children, physical therapists observe motor behavior and use theories, models, and principles of motor control and development to help interpret their observations. Interventions then are designed based on a "model" or theoretical understanding of how the neuromotor system is organized and develops. Just as in studies of motor control, this process rests on the premise that motor behavior is a reflection of CNS function. The accuracy of observations of a child's behavior and the models of neuromotor organization and development that are used to interpret these observations are critical. Let's examine how a model of neural organization and development affects what therapists think and do.

If the CNS is envisioned in a traditional way, as a hierarchy consisting of levels of reflexive responses (Figure 1-1), which ultimately is controlled at the highest level by volitional activity, then examination procedures consistent with this model will include tests of reflexes to determine the level of CNS function. If neuromotor development is envisioned as moving from reflexive to volitional control, then our reflexive test also may be used to interpret how far up the developmental staircase a child has progressed. The hierarchy of reflexes, derived principally from classical research in the basic neurosciences, is one model that is used to understand neuromotor development. This model has been commonly used by physical therapists to examine and assess infants' and children's motor behavior in terms of "levels of neural organization and development."

The developmental reflex hierarchy also has been used to plan and sequence treatment. Having determined the level of neurodevelopmental function, the goal of intervention was to progress the child to higher levels where righting reactions and willful or volitional behaviors would prevail. Motor tasks representing these higher levels were used as treatment activities. This example is used here only as a means of understanding how models and concepts of neural organization and development affect what a physical therapist thinks and does. Models and theories are somewhat simplified abstract representations of some more complex process. They are neither right nor wrong, nor true or false; rather, theories and models should be judged by their usefulness in helping us: 1) understand how the CNS is organized and develops; 2) design effective testing and treatment procedures; and 3) predict how patients respond to treatment.

In the past, brain function was modeled as a telephone switchboard with an operator sitting in the brain making connections between one brain region and another. The telephone switchboard model now is virtually forgotten, and the computer serves as the model that helps us understand how the CNS functions. Because the variety of processes that can be represented, explained, and understood is greater when using a computer model of neural function than when using a telephone switchboard model, and because computers and their capabilities are relatively well-known to most individuals, the computer model of the brain currently is quite popular. It is important, however, to remember that models are not real. The brain is not a computer, but the computer model can be used to illustrate various aspects of brain function. Models are simply tools for understanding and only should be judged relative to their accuracy and usefulness for illustrating how the CNS functions and responds to different influences. In the sections that follow, some contemporary concepts and models of neuromotor organization and development are presented that hold promise for an even more thorough understanding of the motor behaviors observed in children.

Neural Organization and Development: The Active Organism Concept

The CNS traditionally has been viewed as a system of reflexes arranged in a hierarchy of complexity with volitional processes dominating or controlling the reflexive base.[10]

Because reflexes were studied in animals in situations that rendered them incapable of volitional movement, our understanding of reflexes is based in what is termed a *passive organism paradigm*. The parallel model of development portrays the infant as a passive, purely reflexive being, acting solely in response to the environment. Only when the cerebral cortex becomes mature and exerts its control over lower level reflexes is volitional behavior possible. This concept of the infant as a reflexive being can be considered a passive organism concept.

More recently there has been an increasing tendency to recognize the active role of the CNS in the creation and control of body actions. From the *active organism* perspective, the CNS is viewed as capable of anticipating the demands of the environment and planning ahead. We have regarded the CNS as the passive recipient of stimuli for so long, in accord with the reflex model of neural functioning, that we forgot the CNS is a living system and that activity is a primary characteristic of living things. The processes of planning, originating, and controlling motor acts require an active CNS. How can this active organism

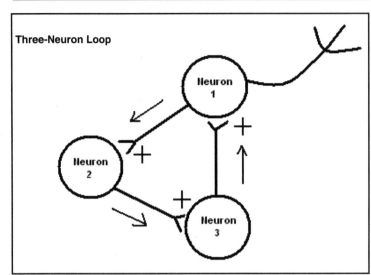

Three-Neuron Loop

Figure 1-2. These three neurons could, by virtue of their relationship to each other, generate a continuous, cyclic pattern of activity. Neuron 1, either through an external stimulus or through spontaneous activity, fires and activates Neuron 2. Neuron 2 in turn fires and activates Neuron 3, which fires and activates Neuron 1; this pattern of activity begins again, causing a repetitive cyclic pattern of neuronal activity that could continue indefinitely.

concept be modeled? This is where the computer and concepts of logical circuits can be helpful to portray neuromotor control processes. To understand how the CNS might be continuously active, consider the simple three-neuron loop portrayed in Figure 1-2. If three neurons are arranged in a circle or loop, continuous activity within the loop could be created either through an external stimulus or the spontaneous firing of a single neuron, be it accidental or not. An ongoing cyclic pattern of neural activity arises as an emergent property of the little system of three neurons. It is important to recognize that the cyclic activity is the property of the system of neurons, and not the property of any single neuron itself. Cyclic activity only results because of the relationship among the three neurons.

Computer programmers make use of such "loop" concepts to instruct computers to complete repetitive functions. Recently loops such as this one have been employed by neuroscientists in models used to illustrate rhythmic repetitive neuromotor functions, such as the gait cycle, the suck-swallow of infant feeding, and other motor phenomena that were previously regarded as a simple chaining together of reflexes.[11,12]

With neuroscientists offering a plausible explanation for continuous processes of activity within the CNS, the study of spontaneous behavior in infants has become of increasing interest for developmentalists.[13-15] Spontaneous, nonreflexive behaviors, previously ignored in scientific study, have become a focus for researchers interested in neurodevelopmental processes.

The active organism concept has caused therapists to question the traditional reflex hierarchy model. Physical therapists influenced by the view of the CNS as a passive mechanism developed models of evaluation and treatment consistent with this perspective. As our models are changing, so are our evaluation and treatment procedures. Therapists are relying less on reflex tests to determine developmental levels of neural organization and control and more often are documenting motor behaviors that are considered to be spontaneous or self-generated by the patients.[16-19]

The Concept of a Motor Pattern

In the past, the reflex was considered the fundamental unit of neuromotor behavior. That is, the reflex was regarded as the simplest form of movement and the foundation for all other forms of action. A reflex relies on an outside agent or force, called the stimulus, to generate motor behavior. Though easy to understand, the reflex is of limited usefulness in explaining movements that are not initiated by external stimuli. Neither volitional nor spontaneous movements are dependent on external agents for their initiation. For this reason the reflex is not a useful concept if we wish to explain either spontaneous or voluntary action.

Despite the insufficiency of reflex theory in explaining spontaneous and volitional movement, the reflex was useful in explaining stereotyped patterns of posture and movement that could be evoked with specific types of sensory stimulation. The reflex, by definition, encompasses a well-organized patterned motor response. Reflex responses involve consistent temporal and spatial relationships among muscle groups. For example, even in the simplest stretch reflex, muscles are controlled in relation to one another (agonists are activated, antagonists are inhibited) and produce observable behaviors. These stable relationships among muscle groups are termed *postural or movement patterns* (see Chapter 8).

The concept of patterns of posture and movement, the observable linkages between muscle groups, has been long accepted by therapists.[7,9,20] These postural and movement patterns, however, commonly have been linked to specific stimuli. Examples are the flexor withdrawal response pattern associated with a noxious stimulus applied to the sole of the foot and the tonic neck response patterns bound to specific postures of the neck.

The underlying neural representations of these observable response patterns dissociated or uncoupled from the stimuli that produce them are examples of motor patterns. A motor pattern is simply the neural representation of a posture or movement that underlies observable movement or postural patterns. The motor pattern specifies distinct temporal and spatial relationships between muscles. The concept of a motor pattern has a decided advantage over the concept of a reflex because the motor pattern is more versatile. The motor pattern need not be bound to a specific sensory stimulus. A motor pattern could be brought into action either by sensory stimuli or by internal processes within the CNS. If one considers the motor pattern, rather than the reflex, as the basic unit of neuromotor organization, it is possible to explain why, for example, there are so many different stimuli that can be used to evoke a specific movement pattern seen in an infant. This concept also explains why a child with hemiplegia demonstrates the same movement pattern during both volitional effort and in response to a variety of sensory stimuli.

The motor pattern has been offered as a concept that represents the CNS's solution to the problem of controlling a multitude of muscles and joints throughout the body.[21-23] From a biomechanical perspective, the human body can be modeled as a series of rigid segments (such as an arm or a forearm) connected by joint structures that both permit and restrict motion between the links. In determining possible movement combinations in the cardinal planes, beginning proximally at the shoulder girdle and moving distally to the terminal phalanx of a finger, it becomes obvious that the brain faces an enormous task to control so many possible combinations of movements at the joints. This is known as the *degrees of freedom* problem in motor control after the work of Bernstein.[12] By establishing functional linkages or motor patterns to define relationships between groups of muscles, motor control becomes simplified. The terms *motor patterns, motor synergies,* and *coordinative structures* have been used to refer to the functional units of neuromotor organization that ensure that the CNS need not control so many different combinations of action, but rather solves the degrees of freedom problem through an efficient system of muscle linkages.

Milani-Comparetti,[24] a physician and developmentalist, suggested that the motor pattern was the underlying neural basis for spontaneous action of fetuses observed through ultrasonography. When movements first were observed in the developing fetus, he was unable to identify stimuli that could be considered to trigger these actions. Fetal movements appeared spontaneous, being generated by the CNS. According to Milani-Comparetti, it was later in the course of prenatal development that links between sensory stimuli and the movements became evident. He termed the initial spontaneous actions *primary motor patterns* (PMPs). Later in fetal development, *primary automatisms* appeared. Primary automatisms linked sensory stimuli to PMPs and, in Milani-Comparetti's view, represented adaptations to the environment. Thus, the fetus was primarily active and secondarily responsive to the surrounding environment.

How are motor patterns formed? The traditional explanation has been that some motor patterns are "hard-wired" or preprogrammed genetically. Basic flexor and extensor motor patterns that are incorporated into the primary flexor and extensor reflex responses (flexor withdrawal and extensor thrust) traditionally have been considered inherent motor patterns. These flexor and extensor movement patterns seem, however, to be incorporated into reflexive responses to a variety of stimuli. In addition, spontaneous kicking movements of infants are in some ways similar to reflexive primary stepping movements.[25] As researchers who less rigidly interpret infant motor behavior as reflexive begin to study infants' motor behavior, motor patterns other than those characterized as reflexive responses have received increasing attention.

Milani-Comparetti believed that a full complement of movement patterns are available and used appropriately in functional contexts prior to birth.[24] He reported that the fetus demonstrates a great repertoire of motor behaviors in utero: changing position; reaching, grasping, moving, and releasing the umbilical cord when it brushes against the face; and moving into position in the birth canal in preparation for birth.

Why, then, do the motor abilities of the newborn seem so limited? Why should a fetus be considered so competent and a newborn appear so helpless? A plausible answer lies in the vast differences in the natural environments of the fetus and the newborn. Milani-Comparetti observed fetuses in utero, surrounded by amniotic fluid, and not experiencing the effects of gravity.[24] The prenatal and postnatal environments are drastically different. The newborn, who appears so fragile and incompetent, is experiencing the full force of gravity for the first time, yet the newborn infant is quite capable of breathing, sucking, and swallowing and, if Milani-Comparetti's views are correct, at the time of birth actively participates in the process of being born. Previous theories interpreted the behaviors of the newborn as purely reflexive, and more recently we have begun to appreciate the specific competence of the newborn. Therefore, we are less likely to view the infant as a passive organism dependent upon sensory stimuli to bring about action.

Feedback and Comparison of Intention and Result

Feedback is a very important and powerful concept when one considers issues of motor control and development. Feedback enables the process of comparing the result of one's action with the original intent of the act, allowing the individual to take corrective action. Feedback also calls into question the process of command and control in a motor system. Each of these two important aspects of feedback is discussed next.

Comparing the Results of Action With Intention and Its Effect on Motor Control

Feedback as an integral element of motor control provides the capacity to compare the intended and the actual result of neuromotor activity. Only through a process of comparison can unsuccessful actions be changed. Without feedback and comparison between intended and resultant actions, the CNS is destined to either repeat the same patterns without modification or to be totally dependent upon someone in the external environment to affect change in motor behavior. When the CNS is afforded the capacity to compare intention with outcome, an element of control is removed from the environment and the individual becomes less dependent on the external world for the correction of behavior. The individual need not wait for an external source to provide a correcting stimulus in order to change motor behavior. This awarding of control to the individual is having a profound influence on physical therapy. Therapists increasingly recognize the very active role patients must play in correcting their own behavior. They encourage children to form their own judgments about how well they performed and help them modify their motor behavior based on comparisons of self-generated feedback with the intended outcome. Children are capable of judging and correcting their actions and can be encouraged to do so. In the past, the traditional concept of infants as reflexive beings kept us from fully appreciating the infants' ability to initiate and to continue action until a goal is attained, be it fussing until fed or changed or swiping at an object until contacting it. Infants' capabilities rest on the use of feedback to judge the result of action. Thus, it appears that even young infants have the basic organizational elements of motor control. These include the ability to initiate action and feedback processes to modify and adapt motor patterns to function successfully in the world. With these basic elements of neuromotor organization in place, infants are quite ready to begin to meet the challenges of the environment.

Feedback and Its Effect on a Hierarchy of Motor Control

The newer concepts for understanding neuromotor function include motor patterns and the active organism that was modeled in Figure 1-2 using a simple circular arrangement of neurons. In the circular arrangement, feedback is a fundamental property of the small system of neurons. Information from Neurons 2 and 3 is fed back to Neuron 1 that served the function of initiating action. Feedback is a very important aspect of a circular system of neurons. Its importance in motor control is likely only superseded by its importance in motor learning (see Chapter 3). Motor acts must be adaptable if favorable outcomes are to occur, and feedback allows this adaptation. The process of modifying motor behavior to ensure a more successful outcome requires that the results of actions be relayed back to the CNS. *Lower centers* of the CNS provide feedback to *higher centers* with information needed to plan subsequent actions. Models of motor control have not always incorporated feedback. Models of neural organization without feedback loops are termed *open systems* and are characterized by a single direction of transfer of information, input to output (Figure 1-3).[26] *Closed systems*, on the other hand, are those that incorporate the concept of feedback and therefore provide the CNS control over actions that are to come. Feedback contributes to this control by providing the system with information regarding the results of action. Knowledge of the results of past action is needed in order to generate a modified action.

Although the idea of feedback is not new,[27] the effects of feedback loops on the traditional reflexive hierarchical model of neuromotor organization have not been fully recognized. Feedback loops, particularly those that link lower levels to the uppermost levels of

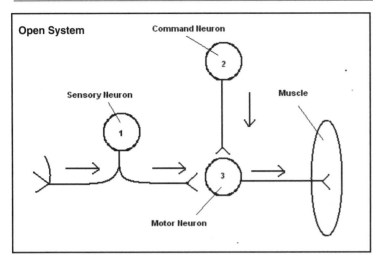

Figure 1-3. An open system is illustrated devoid of feedback. Information travels in only one direction. Neurons 1 and 2 conduct impulses toward Neuron 3, which in turn directs its activity toward the muscle.

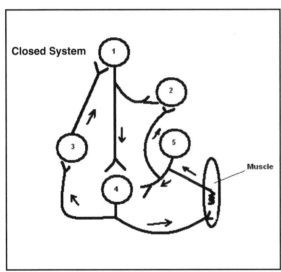

Figure 1-4. A closed-loop system with multiple feedback loops. Although Neuron 1 appears to be at the top of a hierarchy, and thus in command of the system, it is apparent on closer scrutiny that there is no hierarchy in this organizational arrangement of neurons. By inspecting Neurons 1 to 4, it is easy to see that each of these elements could conceivably be under the control of at least one other neuron: Neuron 1 receives information from Neurons 2 and 3, Neuron 2 receives information from Neurons 1 and 5, and so on. Only Neuron 5 appears to be outside the sphere of other neurons, yet Neuron 5 is indirectly affected by the activity of Neuron 4 as it activates the muscle and thus by way of sensory feedback influences Neuron 5.

a hierarchy, challenge the concept of hierarchical control. If information from lower levels is relayed to the top level of the control hierarchy (eg, the cerebral cortex), and, as a result of this feedback, actions are modified, then what level of the system is really in control (Figure 1-4)? Could it not be argued that the lower level centers control the higher levels? If an interneuron in the spinal cord provides information to the cortex concerning the state of a motor neuron and this information is used in modifying a subsequent motor act, then are not the interneuron and the motor neuron sharing in the control process? Can a model that provides feedback from the lowest to the highest level of control truly be hierarchical? Where does control reside in such a model? I would suggest that a "distributed control" model of neuromotor control can help resolve this dilemma.

The Concept of Distributed Control

Rather than envisioning a fixed hierarchy with a top level devoid of feedback controlling motor behavior, consider a less rigid model that enables sharing of the control function as an alternative.[28,29] Indeed, the CNS increasingly is being modeled as a flexible complex of systems and subsystems that share information in the process of controlling motor behavior.[30] This complex of systems is used to illustrate *distributed control*. In a distributed control model, the controller varies.[28] A subsystem with the most relevant information concerning the status of the individual in the context of the situation would assume control. The subsystem would be given control as a function of both the individual's state and the environmental situation in which the individual is functioning. With systems and subsystems in the CNS sharing information, consensus can be reached concerning which system might best serve as the primary controller at a specific point in time.

Memory

Another concept considered necessary for motor control is *memory*. Successful motor acts include elements of preplanning. For example, to be successful in a wheelchair transfer to a toilet, a child must position the chair in expectation of the activity that will follow, such as opening a door to a bathroom stall. The child must adjust the distance between his or her body and the door handle to successfully reach and pull the door open. The child needs to anticipate the arc of the door as it is opened. From where does this capacity to anticipate or predict the outcome of action arise? The ability to plan successful action is based in previous experiences. While practice usually is considered to be the reason for success, practice is more than just repeating an act over and over again. The key to the child's future motor success is the ability to use the results of one act to make the next motor act more successful. Key information related to the solution of the motor problem must be used in order to be successful in a situation not previously encountered. Commonly, the theoretical construct of memory is used to explain how an individual benefits from prior experience. It has been theorized that practice permits the formation of memory structures[31,32] that can be used in novel situations. Storing the exact solution for every problem encountered would not enable transfer of motor abilities to a novel situation. What has been proposed is that general rules or *schema*[32] that specify the relationships among the conditions surrounding performance, the intended action, and the results of the action are stored in memory. These schema enable the individual to solve novel motor problems.

In summary, integral elements of motor control include:

➤ The CNS as a fundamentally active agent with the capacity to generate action

➤ Motor patterns as the fundamental unit of neuromotor behavior

➤ The processes of feedback and comparison of intention and result that enable the modification of action

➤ A distributed control system that delegates the control of behavior to the most appropriate subsystem

➤ Memory structures, such as schema, that permit transfer of skills to new situations

Current Issues and Trends in Motor Control and Motor Development Theories

A recent trend in motor control and development theories is embodied in the emergence of *dynamical systems theories* of control and development.[33-36] These theories have arisen from systems theory, particularly dynamical systems that operate in accord with the laws of thermodynamics. A good introduction to the basic theory of dynamical systems can be obtained by reading the popular book *Chaos: Making a New Science.*[37] Two dynamical systems theories are discussed below: *Dynamical Pattern Theory*, a theory of motor control, and *Dynamical Action Theory*, a theory of motor development.

Dynamical Systems Theories

Dynamical Pattern Theory, developed by Kelso and his colleagues,[33,34] includes general principles of motor coordination that can be used to explain the motor behavior of a variety of animal forms, including man. The theory includes two main concepts: *order parameters* and *control parameters*. Order parameters are variables that represent the action of many subsystems and can be used to characterize coordinated behavior of the system. For example, the timing of action between the two limbs during walking could be considered an order parameter. One might plot the position of the right and left knee with respect to each other to characterize a coordinated walking pattern. In fact, plotting of common kinematic variables such as displacements, velocities, and accelerations across components of a coordinated system is common practice among dynamical system theory researchers. The convention of characterizing coordination through these so-called order parameters provides a quantitative measure of motor coordination. Such measures may be used in the future by therapists to evaluate their patients' coordination and to document the effect of therapy designed to change a patient's motor coordination.[38]

Variables that can initiate change in order parameters are termed control parameters. For example, there is a variety of movement patterns that are used to rise to standing from the floor.[39,40] Dehadrai[41] demonstrated that adding extra weight to individuals caused the movement patterns to change. King[42] has shown that constraints to ankle motion provided by ankle foot orthoses also trigger movement pattern changes. The change in an order parameter (the movement patterns used to rise) results when some critical value of a control parameter (in these examples weight or ankle motion) is reached.

Thelen[36,43] has extended dynamical systems theory to motor development. A basic assumption of Thelen's theory is that biological organisms are complex multidimensional systems. No single subsystem is more important in determining behavior than any other subsystem. In classical theories of motor development, the CNS held a preeminent role in the determination of behavior. According to dynamical systems theory of motor development, organized behavior is an emergent property of the complex set of subsystems that constitute the individual, the environments surrounding the individual, and the task to be performed. Behavioral patterns represent a compression of the many degrees of freedom and infinite number of possible forms of action.

Thelen and her coworkers[44] have studied the development of stepping and kicking in infants while exploring the components of dynamical systems theory. According to reflexive theory, primary stepping behavior of infants disappears as a result of cortical maturation, which enables inhibitory influences to be exerted over the spinal level stepping reflex. Thelen and her colleagues in an elegant series of studies demonstrated that rather than cortical maturation, increasing weight of the lower limbs might be one reason why babies stop stepping.[43]

Some behavioral patterns are more common than others. In dynamical systems terms these patterns are called attractors.[45] Attractors are preferred patterns of the system. Attractors are further described as having deep or shallow attractor wells. Deep attractor wells can be used to portray behavior that is quite stable and relatively difficult to change. Shallow attractor wells are characteristic of behaviors that are easily changed (Figure 1-5).[46,47]

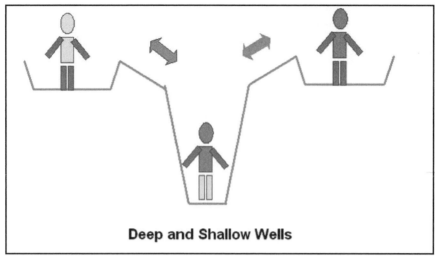

Deep and Shallow Wells

Figure 1-5. This portrayal of deep and shallow wells illustrates the number of times a child demonstrated specific sets of movement patterns during performance of the task of rising. The child was asked to rise from a supine position on a floor mat 10 consecutive times. The shallow well to the left represents performance of two of 10 trials of rising from the floor. The center deep well is reflective of six of 10 trials that were performed using a movement strategy that differed from the shallow well strategy in both head and trunk and lower limb patterns. The movement pattern strategy represented by the deep well could also be called an attractor pattern. The shallow well on the right illustrates another two of the 10 trials were performed with upper limb and head and trunk patterns the same as the deep well strategy, only lower limb patterns differed. An interpretation of this mapping of one child's preferred patterns of rising illustrate a deep well strategy that is commonly performed and two shallow well strategies that are less commonly observed.

Developmental change is brought about by control parameters reaching critical values that bring the system to a period of instability. During developmental transitions from one stable attractor state to another, individuals are particularly sensitive to control variables. During phase transitions, very small influences can have very large effects on behavior. Transitions from one phase to another have been likened to a ball being balanced at the top of a hill—just a slight puff of wind might determine the outcome. A large effect that results from such a small change in a control parameter is a characteristic of nonlinear dynamical systems. It is suggested that therapists be sensitive to phase transitions in their patients and try to discover the control parameter that is driving the system to new forms of behavior.

Previously, therapists tended to look for all explanations of developmental change in the CNS. Dynamical systems theory makes us aware of the role of many elements of the complex system of the child, the child's environment, and the motor tasks the child is required to perform. In dynamical systems theory terminology, the CNS was the control parameter. Thelen's discovery that movement patterns of infants may vary as a function of the child's weight brings a whole host of interesting concepts to the forefront. As physical therapists, we know that postural and movement patterns vary with age across childhood. One explanation for this observation is that the physical size of the body is changing with age and, therefore, motor patterns may reflect an appropriate, but temporary, solution in the face of changing body dimensions. Thus, motor patterns used to accomplish a task, such as rising to stand, might vary not only as a result of practice, but also as a result of the relative size of different body segments. As the child grows and changes in relative body proportions, different motor patterns may serve as the most appropriate solution to the same task. As an example, envision a small 3- or 4-year-old child who, when asked to sit on the bed, must first climb up on the mattress using both arms and legs to accomplish the task. That same child grown to adolescence may sit on the bed directly from standing. Given that the bed has remained an unchanging object in the environment of the child, why have the movement patterns changed? It is difficult to deny that the older child by virtue of size alone is able to sit directly on the bed. The younger child, although he may have a motor pattern for sitting down, is confronted with a mattress at a height that does not allow sitting directly from standing. Variability in motor patterns may be brought about through changes in the relative size of an individual with respect to fixed features of the environment. Yet, variability in motor patterns is not due solely to the physical growth of an individual.

Children who are developing normally appear to vary their motor patterns for the sheer joy of the experience and to learn about their bodies and their environments. Given that a child is able to throw an object, he experiments with throwing far, accurately, and as hard as possible. He throws not only balls, but anything that is throwable: books, food, a stool, and so forth. As a result of all this throwing, he learns of his body and his world. He learns about books, their weight, how they tend to open when thrown, and why books are not to be thrown. Food, although throwable, spatters about and is also not supposed to be thrown. Should he attempt to throw a stool, he discovers stools are not throwable, at least not when you are small. Several things result from all this throwing. The child learns to vary the throwing pattern to accommodate the objects; learns of the size, weight, and consistency of the objects; and learns socially acceptable behaviors, such as "Don't throw in the house!" Young children also learn about their environment and their motor abilities by using an object to accomplish a variety of tasks.

For example, a large ball can be used to sit on, lie on, push, kick, roll, hug, and even stand on. Thus, an object can be used for purposes not necessarily in the mind of the inventor. The most popular toys are those that can be put to a variety of uses, and the most boring are those that can be used for but one activity. Think of the versatility of something as simple as a cooking pot. The young child plays for hours with containers or things that serve as containers, such as boxes, pots, bags, and purses. Things get put in, dumped, poured, thrown, and kicked into and out of these containers. Again, the child learns of the world about him and of his motor abilities in that world. This is where the rules relating the child's body to the environment are acquired. The young child initiates and varies the task out of curiosity and joy in seeing the effect of his actions on the world around him.

We must recognize that different phases in the human lifespan are characterized by different motor behaviors, different environments, and different demands on the neuromotor system. Infancy seems to be a period when fundamental laws about the body and the physical world are discovered. Early childhood is a time for expansion of motor abilities within the environment. Various forms of locomotion are acquired, such as running, hopping, skipping, jumping, riding tricycles, skating, and riding bicycles.

In addition, some degree of accuracy in fine motor tasks is demanded of children when they begin school. They must manage their clothes, draw, cut, paste, and begin to print letters and numbers. Children of school age begin to participate in games with other children that require the application of fundamental movements such as throwing, running, and catching. Children begin to acquire fine motor skills, particularly those that require control of small objects or tools, such as pencils, rulers, screwdrivers, needles, and thread. Through motor abilities, children come to know their unique competencies. As children grow and develop, they participate in team or individual sports, select hobbies that enable achievement, and develop pride in their physical abilities. During this period, the ability to discriminate kinesthetic and visual cues and to modify behaviors becomes more discrete. The generalizability of motor activity appears to decrease. In late childhood, individuals tend to learn what they practice and attempt to improve. Spending hours in front of a video screen with a mouse or joystick will likely result in improved performance only in tasks that require speed and accuracy in control of a visual blip by means of a mouse or joystick. Eye-hand coordination will not improve in general. The videogame addict will not become a better pitcher or catcher in softball as a result of hours in front of the television. The motor patterns used for the latter tasks are entirely different than those required by the videogame.

Having learned the rules of using the eyes to direct and control the path of the upper extremity during late infancy and early childhood, later childhood seems the time for taking pride in the degree of discrimination and subsequent control over very specific movement patterns. Over the course of infancy, childhood, and adolescence, sensory and motor subsystems develop at different rates and share in the control of motor behavior at different times. Likewise, the environments in which children function are changing with time. The relatively protected environments of infancy provided by the home or infant day care facility gradually are replaced by the nursery and school that require increasing responsibility and independence of children.

Application of the Newer Concepts of Motor Control and Motor Development to the Evaluation and Treatment of Children

Having presented newer concepts of neuromotor control and development, the logical next step is to indicate how these ideas can be applied to examination, evaluation, and intervention for the child with motor dysfunction. Examination of the child should incorporate the concepts presented in the first part of this chapter. We need to select tests and measures that can be used to assess motor patterns, the child's spontaneous motor activity, and activity evoked by sensory stimuli or objects in the environment. We need to examine and assess the child's ability to modify his or her motor behavior based on both external and internal feedback. We need to test and assess the child's ability to remember the rules for solving a motor problem. Finally, we should test and assess the environment, or environments, in which the child is expected to function. A recent example of an attempt to create a functional environment in which to examine a child's motor behavior has been reported by Rosenberg.[48]

As is frequently the case, concepts arising in foundational sciences gradually lead to changes in clinical practice. As we explore the usefulness of the information embodied in these new models and ideas, clinical concepts are being refined, and standard testing procedures and interventions are being developed. Yet, at this time, progress is being measured against a stricter standard. Our profession requires full exploration of the psychometric properties of new tests, including reliability, validity, sensitivity, specificity, and, ultimately, the predictive validity of the measure. Further, our interventions must be examined in rigorous studies designed to determine their effectiveness. We have worked for generations without strong evidence on which to base our practice. New paradigms of motor control, as appealing as they may be, do not replace the need for research data to support our interventions.

As a physical therapist, I attempt to help the child become motorically independent, capable of controlling and caring for his or her own body. I encourage the child to develop those processes that enable adaptation to changing environments. As we wait for this evidence, I would recommend that therapists teach not just motor skills, but how to learn motor skills. Be careful not to overly structure therapy sessions so that you are totally directing and controlling the child's actions. Try not to enforce adult standards of performance on children and do not unnecessarily restrict the tasks and objects to which motor patterns are applied. Resist viewing the infant or child as passively waiting for your stimulation and instruction to develop and learn. Look for the inherent ability of each child to produce motor patterns spontaneously, as well as in response to manipulations. Examine the child's environment for control parameters that might be influencing behavior. Try to foster in each child self-control as well as responsiveness to external demands.

Look for variability in the child's actions. It has been argued that variability in motor patterns is the essence of normalcy. Indeed, stereotypic motor behavior is a well-recognized sign of pathology. For the child with cerebral palsy, one of the most significant findings of motor pathology is the lack of variability in motor behavior. That is, the same motor patterns are used repeatedly across a great variety of tasks. Variability in the child's motor behaviors needs to be fostered in therapy. To do this we need to be less prescriptive about which specific movement patterns the child uses to accomplish a motor task. No single "right" or "normal" way to move generalizes to all situations. Encouraging the child to explore movement options within a specific task enables the formation of rules that can be applied in future situations. Persuade the child to explore objects in the environment and how they can be used. Stairs can be used for so many different tasks, such as climbing, sitting, jumping, and sliding. Within each of these tasks, stairs afford a multitude of movement patterns, including climbing on hands and knees, climbing on hands and feet, standing on two feet, sitting with feet on the step below, or sitting sideways on the stair with legs extended. The child will explore these options if given the opportunity and encouragement.

Having recognized that different motor abilities are exhibited at different ages, do not forget to focus on age-appropriate tasks. Remember that, by school age, children are expected to have acquired independence in mobility and basic elements of self-care. Do your best to see that these expectations are met. Encourage school-aged children to select tasks they determine to be of interest and importance and encourage the children to share in the responsibility for improving motor performance and caring for their bodies.

Keep in mind that each child may be influenced by your attitude about the child's motor abilities. If a child's motor performance is judged against your standard of normalcy, and if that performance never meets your standard, the child may infer failure through your feedback. The child may eventually become totally dependent on external standards for judging his or her motor performance and, as a result, lose the desire and ability to acquire skills on his own. The child may, therefore, never seek the experience of setting ever-increasing demands for the sheer pleasure of working to meet those demands. Encourage the school-aged child to participate in setting goals for treatment so that he or she might increasingly become active, responsible, and competent. And, above all, remember that our role as physical therapists is to promote independent function. It is no longer sufficient to focus on remediation of impairments without regard for functional gains. Improvements in coordination, balance, strength, or range of motion may or may not effect a functional change. It is our duty as therapists to never lose sight of our role in promoting independence for each child who seeks our care.

References

1. Sherrington CS. *The Integrative Action of the Nervous System.* New Haven, Conn: Yale University Press; 1906.

2. Magnus R. Some results of studies in the physiology of posture. *Lancet.* 1926;585:531-535.

3. Twitchell TE. The restoration of motor function following hemiplegia in man. *Brain.* 1951; 74:443-480.

4. Paine RS, Brazelton TB, Donovan DE, et al. Evolution of postural reflexes in normal infants and in the presence of chronic brain syndromes. *Neurology.* 1964;14:1036-1048.

5. Schaltenbrand G. The development of human motility and motor disturbances. *Archives of Neurology and Psychiatry.* 1928;20:720-730.

6. McGraw MB. *The Neuromuscular Maturation of the Human Infant.* New York, NY: Hafner Publishing; 1966.

7. Bobath B. *Abnormal Postural Reflex Activity Caused by Brain Lesions.* 3rd ed. Rockville, Md: Aspen Systems; 1985.

8. Brunnstrom S. *Movement Therapy in Hemiplegia: A Neurophysiological Approach.* New York, NY: Harper & Row; 1970.

9. Knott M, Voss DE. *Proprioceptive Neuromuscular Facilitation: Patterns and Techniques.* 2nd ed. New York, NY: Harper & Row; 1968.

10. Wyke B. The neurologic basis of movement: a developmental review. In: Holt KS, ed. *Clinics in Developmental Medicine: Movement and Child Development.* Philadelphia, Pa: JB Lippincott; 1975;55:19-33.

11. Delcomyn F. Neural basis of rhythmic behavior in animals. *Science.* 1980;210:492-498.

12. Grillner S, Wallen P. Central pattern generators for locomotion, with special reference to vertebrates. *Ann Rev Neurosci.* 1985;8:233-261.

13. Connolly KJ. Maturation and ontogeny of motor skills. In: Connolly KJ, Prechtl HFR, eds. *Clinics in Developmental Medicine: Maturation and Development: Biological and Psychological Perspectives.* Philadelphia, Pa: JB Lippincott; 1981:77/78;216-230.

14. Prechtl HFR. The study of neural development as a perspective of clinical problems. In: Connolly KJ, Prechtl HFR, eds. *Clinics in Developmental Medicine: Maturation and Development: Biological and Psychological Perspectives.* Philadelphia, Pa: JB Lippincott; 1981:77/78;198-215.

15. Thelen E. Rhythmical stereotypes in normal human infants. *Animal Behavior.* 1979;27:699-715.

16. Campbell SK, Osten ET, Kolobe THA, et al. Development of the Test of Infant Motor Performance. *Phys Med Rehabil Clin N Am.* 1993;4:541-550.

17. Campbell SK, Kolobe THA, Osten E, et al. Construct validity of the Test of Infant Motor Performance. *Phys Ther.* 1995;75:585-596.

18. Piper MC, Darrah J. *Motor Assessment of the Developing Infant.* Philadelphia, Pa: WB Saunders; 1994.

19. Piper MC, Pinnell LE, Darrah J, et al. Construction and validation of the Alberta Infant Motor Scale (AIMS). *Canadian Journal of Public Health.* 1992;83:S46-S50.

20. Stockmeyer SA. An interpretation of the approach of Rood to the treatment of neuromuscular dysfunction. *Am J Phys Med.* 1967;46:900-956.

21. Bernstein N. *The Coordination and Regulation of Movement.* New York, NY: Pergamon Press; 1967.

22. Easton TA. On the normal use of reflexes. *Am Sci.* 1972;60:591-599.

23. Kelso JAS, ed. *Human Motor Behavior: An Introduction.* Hillsdale, NJ: Lawrence Erlbaum Associates; 1982.

24. Milani-Comparetti A. The neurophysiologic and clinical implications of studies on fetal motor behavior. *Sem Perinat.* 1981;5:183-189.

25. Kamm K, Thelen E, Jensen J. A dynamical systems approach to motor development. *Phys Ther.* 1990;70:763-775.

26. Stelmach GE. Motor control and motor learning: the closed-loop perspective. In: Kelso JAS, ed. *Human Motor Behavior: An Introduction.* Hillsdale, NJ: Lawrence Erlbaum Associates; 1982: 93-115.

27. Smith KU. Cybernetic foundations for rehabilitation. *Am J Phys Med.* 1967;46:379-467.

28. Davis WJ. Organizational concepts in the central motor networks of invertebrates. In: Herman RL, Grillner S, Stein P, Stuart G, et al, eds. *Advances in Behavioral Biology: Neural Control of Locomotion.* New York, NY: Plenum Press; 1976; 18: 265-292.

29. Kilmer WL, McCollough WS, Blum J. A model of the vertebrate central command system. *Int J Man-Machine Studies.* 1969;1:279-309.

30. Brooks VB. *The Neural Basis of Motor Control.* New York, NY: Oxford University Press; 1986: 18-37.

31. Adams JA. A closed loop theory of motor learning. *J Motor Beh.* 1971;3:111-150.

32. Schmidt RA. A schema theory of discrete motor skill learning. *Psy Rev.* 1975;82:225-260.

33. Kelso JAS, Tuller B. A dynamical basis for action systems. In: Gazzaniga MS, ed. *Handbook of Cognitive Neuroscience.* New York, NY: Plenum Press; 1984:321-356.

34. Kugler PN, Turley MT. *Information, Natural Law, and the Self-Assembly of Rhythmic Movements.* Hillsdale, NJ: Lawrence Erlbaum Associates; 1987.

35. Schoner G, Kelso JAS. Dynamic pattern generation in behavioral and neural systems. *Science.* 1988;239:1513-1520.

36. Thelen E, Kelso JAS, Fogel A. Self-organizing systems and infant motor development. *Dev Rev.* 1987;7:39-65.

37. Gleick G. *Chaos: Making a New Science.* New York, NY: Penguin Press; 1987.

38. Scholtz JP. Dynamic pattern theory—some implications for therapeutics. *Phys Ther.* 1990; 70:827-843.

39. VanSant AF. Rising from a supine position to erect stance: description of adult movement and a developmental hypothesis. *Phys Ther.* 1988;68:185-192.

40. VanSant AF. Children's body action in righting from supine to erect stance: pre-longitudinal screening of developmental sequences. *Phys Ther.* 1988;68:1330-1338.

41. Dehadrai LB. *The Effect of Three Levels of Weight on the Movement Patterns Used to Rise From Supine to Standing* [master's thesis]. Philadelphia, Pa: Temple University; 1991.

42. King LA, VanSant AF. The effect of solid ankle foot orthoses on movement patterns used to rise from supine to stand. *Phys Ther.* 1995;75:952-964.

43. Thelen E. Dynamical approaches to the development of behavior. In: Kelso JAS, Mandell AJ, Schelsinger ME, eds. *Dynamical Patterns in Complex Systems.* Singapore: World Scientific Publishing; 1989:348-362.

44. Thelen E, Fisher DM. Newborn stepping: an explanation for a disappearing reflex. *Dev Psy.* 1982;18:760-775.

45. Heriza C. Motor development: traditional and contemporary theories. In: Lister MJ, ed. *Contemporary Management of Motor Control Problems: Proceedings of the II Step Conference.* Alexandria, Va: Foundation for Physical Therapy; 1991:99-126.

46. Brown E, Burns J, Choy M, et al. Variability of movement profiles among adolescents rising from bed: a developmental analysis. Poster presentation at: American Physical Therapy Association Combined Sections Meeting; February 14, 2003; Tampa, Fla.

47. Miller TH, King, LA, VanSant AF. Deep and shallow well attractors. Platform presentation at:. Mid East Motor Development Consortium Annual Meeting; October 2, 1999; Madison, Wisc.

48. Weber DA. Easley-Rosenberg A. Creating an interactive environment for pediatric assessment. *Ped Phys Ther.* 2001;13:77-84.

Suggested Reading

Anokhin PD. Systemogenesis as a general regulator of brain development. *Prog Br Res*. 1964;9:54-86.

Arbib MA. *The Metaphorical Brain: An Introduction to Cybernetics as Artificial Intelligence and Brain Theory*. New York, NY: Wiley-Interscience; 1972.

Bruner JS. Organization of early skilled action. *Child Dev*. 1973;44:1-11.

Eckert HM. A concept of force-energy in human development. *Phys Ther*. 1965;45:213-218.

Frank LK. The cultural patterning of child development. In: Falkner F, ed. *Human Development*. Philadelphia, Pa: WB Saunders; 1966:411-432.

Holt K, ed. *Movement and Child Development, Clinics in Developmental Medicine*. Philadelphia, Pa: JB Lippincott; 1975:55.

Hunt JMcV: Environmental programming to foster competence and prevent mental retardation in infancy. In: Walsh RN, Greenough WT, eds. *Advances in Behavioral Biology: Environments as Therapy for Brain Dysfunction*. New York, NY: Plenum Press; 1976:201-255.

Ianniruberto A, Tajani E. Ultrasonographic study of fetal movements. *Sem Perinat*. 1981;5:175-181.

Kugler PN, Kelso JAS, Turvey MT. On the control and coordination of naturally developing systems. In: Kelso JAS, Clarke JE, eds. *The Development of Movement Control and Coordination*. New York, NY: John Wiley & Sons; 1982:5-78.

Oppenheim RW. Ontogenetic adaptations and retrogressive processes in the development of the nervous system and behaviour: a neuroembryological perspective. In: Connolly KJ, Prechtl HFR, eds. *Clinics in Developmental Medicine: Maturation and Development: Biological and Psychological Perspectives*. Philadelphia, Pa: JB Lippincott; 1981:73-109.

Prechtl HFR, ed. *Clinics in Developmental Medicine: Continuity of Neural Function from Prenatal to Postnatal Life*. Philadelphia, Pa: JB Lippincott; 1984:94.

Roberton MA, Halverson LE. *Developing Children—Their Changing Movement: A Guide for Teachers*. Philadelphia, Pa: Lea & Febiger; 1984.

Shephard RJ. *Physical Activity and Growth*. Chicago, Ill: Yearbook Medical Publishers; 1982.

Young JZ. *Programs of the Brain*. New York, NY: Oxford University Press; 1978.

CHAPTER 2

EXAMINATION AND EVALUATION: TESTS AND ADMINISTRATION

Barbara H. Connolly, EdD, PT, FAPTA

The use of standardized norm-referenced and criterion-referenced tests as a part of the examination process has become an integral part of the developmental therapist's practice. Using the patient/client management process as described in the *Guide to Physical Therapist Practice*,[1] the physical therapist selects specific tests and measures as a means of gathering data about the patient. These tests and measures are used to identify impairments and functional limitations in the child; then to help establish a diagnosis, prognosis, and plan of care; and finally, to select appropriate interventions. Tests and measures that are used as a part of the initial examination allow the therapist to confirm or reject hypotheses about the factors that may contribute to the child's current level of functioning. Additionally, the tests and measures may be used to support the therapist's clinical judgments about necessary interventions, appropriate goals, and expected outcomes for the child.

The information obtained through tests and measures is used in the dynamic process of evaluation in which the therapist makes clinical judgments based on data gathered during the examination. Additional data may be gathered during the examination process by the therapist obtaining a history, performing a systems review, and obtaining information about the child's family and environment. Therefore, the use of standardized tests and measures is but a small part of the larger processes of examination and evaluation. Assessment of a child involves more than merely the administration of a test and is qualitative as well as quantitative.

Tests and measures also are used after the initial examination and evaluation to indicate achievement of the outcomes that are indicated at specific points of care (eg, short- and long-term goal attainment) or at the end of an episode of care. *Reexamination* as defined in the *Guide to Physical Therapist Practice* is "the process of performing selected tests and measures after the initial examination to evaluate progress and to modify or redirect interventions."[1] With the pediatric population, reexamination may occur at the end of short periods of time (eg, 1 month) or at the end of an academic school year. Some standardized tests and measures perform the function of guiding interventions by stating functional goals that can be placed directly into the child's plan of care. One example is the School Function Assessment (SFA) which identifies those functional skills needed in a school-based program for children between the ages of 5 and 12 years.[2] The Gross Motor Function Measure[3] also allows for the placement of test items directly into the child's individualized family service plan (IFSP) or the individualized educational plan (IEP). The authors of the SFA stated that the use of specific skills from the test can appropriately be used in the child's IEP. However, other tests and measures, such as the Bruininks-Oseretsky Test of Motor Proficiency (BOTMP),[4] should not have items from the examination used in the child's IEP since these items represent novel and new tasks for children and not functional activities.

When a child is being assessed, the therapist must consider more than just the passing or failing of an item on a test or measurement. The therapist should consider the child's ability to perform a variety of tasks in a variety of settings or contexts, the meaning of the child's performance in terms of total functioning, and the likely explanation for those performances. Using this level of analysis, the therapist must consider other factors that might influence the child's performance at any given time. These factors include current life circumstances, health history, developmental history, cultural influences, and extra personal interactions. Current life circumstances relate to the child's current health, the day-to-day functioning of the family unit, as well as the family's living arrangements. For example, if the child is not feeling well during the examination, the therapist may not get an accurate picture of the child's abilities. If the family is in crisis due to illness of family members, transient living arrangements, or disruptions in the day-to-day life of the family, the child may have been unable to adjust to these changes. This may affect how the child performs during an examination, particularly if the child's sleep cycles or eating habits have been disrupted.

The child's health history is an important factor in the acquisition of certain motor skills. The child who has had poor health or nutrition is apt to be delayed in the acquisition of skills such as sitting, creeping, and walking. Delays in overall development may be seen if the child has a history of repeated hospitalizations. Additional musculoskeletal problems may be noted, such as torticollis, if the child has been unable to lie on the stomach and remained in a supine position for extended periods of time. These musculoskeletal problems may interfere with the attainment of certain developmental skills, such as holding the head in midline or bringing the hands to midline.

Examination of the child's developmental history is important in determining the child's past rate of achievement of developmental milestones and in deciding what performance might be expected in the future. Even with the best intervention, the child who progressed only 2 months in gross motor skills during a 12-month period may not progress 12 additional months during the next 12-month period. The developmental history also allows the therapist to identify events that might have had profound effects on the child, either physically or psychologically.

Therapists, as well as other professionals, are becoming more aware of ethnicity influences on development in infancy and early childhood. *Ethnicity* encompasses the individual's cultural background, religion, language, and nationality. Ethnicity differs from race since ethnicity refers to social characteristics, while race designates a group of individuals with specific physical characteristics. However, race is never independent of environmental and cultural contexts. Typically, Hispanic Americans, Asian Americans, Native Americans, and African Americans are considered as both racial and ethnic categories while Italian Americans, Irish Americans, and Polish Americans, for example, are referred to as ethnic groups. In examining ethnicity, the examiner must consider the environment in which the child is developing, which includes values, birth order, employment status of the parent(s), and family unit in which the child (with or without siblings) is being raised. The family composition, a single mother or father, grandparents serving as parents, or foster parents, also must be taken into consideration. For example, Hopkins and Westra[5] found that Jamaican, English, and Indian mothers differed in their expectations of motor skills development in their infants. The Jamaican mothers expected their infants to sit and to walk significantly earlier than did the Indian and English mothers. In fact, the Jamaican mothers made their infant practice stepping early in infancy. Another study showed that infants raised in Côte d'Ivoire, Africa developed motor skills at an earlier age than infants reared in France.[6] Thus, if the examiner is unaware of the attitudes and values of the child's immediate family, an inaccurate picture may be obtained. The family who values excellence in gross motor performance is more likely to have a child involved in motor activities than the family who values excellence in fine motor activities. More recently, researchers using the Peabody Developmental Gross Motor Scales (PDMS) found that the gross motor maturation of children of Hispanic descent was similar to that of children of Caucasian descent.[7] However, these authors concluded that children of African American descent consistently achieved gross motor skills at an earlier age than the normative sample of children from the PDMS. Thus, if these ethnicity differences were not taken into consideration when using the PDMS, the outcome of the tests might indicate that the child of African American descent was performing gross motor skills at an age-appropriate level, when in fact, the child actually had a delay when compared to his peers. The use of culturally sensitive standardized tests and measures would most likely control for these variables when the therapist attempts to identify "typical" and "atypical" development.

The acculturation of the child also plays a major role in the assessment. Children who have limited exposure to toys may respond differently than the described "standard" response on a certain test. If the child has never seen a yellow tennis ball, but has seen yellow apples, he is apt to try to eat the ball rather than toss it.

Extrapersonal interactions to be considered during the assessment include the reaction of the child to the examiner and the conditions under which the child is observed. Gender "mismatches" may affect the outcome of the testing. For example, if the only men that a child has been exposed to in the home environment were abusive, then the child's response to a male therapist might be affected. In other situations, a male therapist might be a great role model for a young boy in therapy and the interaction would be strikingly different from the first scenario. Likewise, young boys who do not like girls because they have "cooties" might not respond appropriately to a female therapist. A child may not perform well because he or she refuses to cooperate with the examiner or refuses to separate from the parent. Another child may participate well under all circumstances and with any examiner, while another child might only participate in a familiar surrounding. Communication problems with the parents also may interfere with obtaining adequate information about the child during the examination. Identification of ethnicity issues that might interfere with the establishment of rapport with the parent would be crucial prior to the examination if the test relies heavily on a parental questionnaire (eg, Infant/Toddler Sensory Profile[8]). The interpretation of the child's performance must be tentative particularly if these extrapersonal interactions are operating. The child may actually be able to function at a higher level than what was formally assessed.

Purposes of Tests and Measures

Tests and measures may be performed for the purposes of discrimination or placement, for assessment of progress, or for predicting outcomes. They may also be used to discriminate immature or atypical behavior from "typical" behaviors. Very often these tests and measures are used for screening children to determine if therapy services are necessary. Norm-referenced tests, those standardized on groups of individuals, must be used in this discrimination process to determine if a child's performance is typical of a child of a similar age. Norm-referenced tests also should be used when using assessment as a means of determining the appropriate placement of the child in a special service. These also allow the examiner to determine the developmental age of the child and to compare the child's performance to typically developing children. Tests such as the Peabody Developmental Motor Scales, Second Edition (PDMS-2)[9] or the Bruininks-Oseretsky Test of Motor Proficiency[4] may be administered to children to determine which children need placement into intervention programs based on the developmental scores obtained. These norm-referenced tests also may be used for program placement, an important aspect of managing the child with a disability. The therapist must assess the level of the child's current functioning and then plan activities that will help the child progress in his or her abilities. A criterion-referenced test, one that measures a child's development of particular skills in terms of absolute levels of mastery, also may be appropriate for such program planning. Items on the criterion-referenced tests may be linked directly to specific instructional objectives and therefore facilitate the writing of behavioral objectives for the child. Examples of criterion-referenced tests that serve this function are the Gross Motor Function Measure[3] and the SFA.[2] The use of selective items from a norm-referenced test to develop behavioral objectives should be discouraged since this may lead to "teaching the test" and developing splinter skills. Assessment of the child's progress using the same criterion-referenced test used for program planning is appropriate since the examiner wishes to determine if the child has achieved mastery of certain skills. Norm-referenced tests may be used but the tests should be used only once or twice yearly so that "teaching the test" does not occur. Overall program evaluation may be an important purpose of assessment. If one is comparing a new method of teaching gross or fine motor skills with a current method, assessment of the children in each group using a norm-referenced test would be imperative. The therapist would need to be able to compare the overall performance of each group with their peers as established by the norm-referenced tests.

Few tests used in physical therapy allow for prediction of outcomes based upon a predictive index that classifies individuals based on what is believed or expected will be their future status. However, the Movement Assessment of Infants (MAI)[10] is an example of a test that can be used for this purpose. Scores for each item on the MAI have been designated as normal or questionable for a 4-month-old infant. When an infant receives a questionable score, a high-risk point is given. High-risk points then are totaled for each of the four sections and combined for a high-risk score.[10] Seventeen items on the MAI were shown to be significant predictors of cerebral palsy.

Norm-Referenced vs Criterion-Referenced Tests

The purposes of norm-referenced and criterion-referenced tests were described briefly in the preceding section. More delineation, however, needs to be made between the two types of tests. As previously stated, norm-referenced tests have standards or reference points which represent average performances derived from a representative group. Criterion-referenced tests have reference points which may not be dependent on a reference group. In other words, with criterion-referenced tests, the child is competing against him- or herself, not a reference group. Norm-referenced tests may not overlap with actual objectives of instruction, whereas criterion-referenced tests are directly referenced to the objectives of instruction. Therefore, norm-referenced tests may not be as sensitive to the effects of instruction as criterion-referenced tests. Table 2-1 presents a comparison of norm-referenced and criterion-referenced tests in more detail.

Psychometric Characteristics of Tests

Norm-referenced tests must meet minimal standards of reliability and validity before being widely accepted. As with other tests, tests of motor abilities should be both reliable and valid. *Reliability* refers to the consistency between measures in a series. Types of test reliability include alternate forms, interrater, split-half (internal consistency), and

Table 2-1
Comparison of Norm-Referenced and Criterion-Referenced Measurements

Norm-Referenced	Criterion-Referenced
Standard or reference points are average, relative points derived from the performance of a group	Reference points are fixed at specified cutoff points and do not depend on reference points
Evaluates individual performance in comparison to a group of persons; child competing against others	Evaluates individual performance in relation to a fixed standard; child competing against self
May or may not have a relationship to a specific instructional content	Is content specific
Tests may have a low degree of overlap with actual goals and objectives	Tests are directly referenced to the goals and objectives of instruction
Does not indicate when individuals have mastered a segment of the spectrum of goals and objectives	Identifies the goals and objectives that the individual has mastered
Designed to maximize variability and produce scores that are normally distributed	Variability of scores is not desired; a large number of perfect or near-perfect scores is desired
Designed to maximize differences among individuals	Designed to discriminate between successive performances of one individual
Requires good diagnostic skills	Geared to provide information for use in planning instruction
Tests not sensitive to effects of the instruction	Tests are very sensitive to the effects of instruction
Is generally not concerned with task analysis	Depends on task analysis
Is more summative (used at the end of instruction) than formative or is strictly diagnostic	Is more formative (used at various points during instruction) than summative although it can be used both ways

test-retest. Alternate forms reliability assesses the relationship of scores by an individual on two parallel forms of the test. The Miller Analogy Tests are a good example of alternate form reliability in which scores obtained by the same individual on the two forms of the test are highly correlated. Interrater reliability examines the relationship between items passed and failed between two independent observers. Split-half reliability is the measure of internal consistency of a test. The test is split into two halves and the scores obtained on the two halves by the individual are correlated. Test-retest reliability refers to the relationship of an individual's score on the first administration of the test to his score on the second administration. Test-retest reliability scores may be adversely affected by practice or memory. Scores for reliability often are expressed as percent agreement or correlational values obtained through statistical tests such as Spear Rho, Pearson Product Moment, Intraclass Correlation (ICC), or Kappa.

Validity is the extent to which a test measures what it purports to measure. For example, the PDMS-2 is valid for measuring gross and fine motor proficiency, but not developmental reflexes or muscle tone. Another example would be the MAI which is valid for assessment of muscle tone but not fine motor development. Three types of validity—construct, content, and criterion—are used to assess the viability of a test. Construct validity examines the theory or hypothetical constructs underlying the test. For example, the Pediatric Evaluation of Disability Inventory (PEDI)[11] is based on the theory that children with functional limitations can be identified using the scales. Content validity refers to test appropriateness, or how well the content of the test samples the subject matter or behaviors about which conclusions are to be drawn. The specific items on the test must be representative of the behaviors to be assessed. Construct and content validity are not determined using single measures of correlation but are determined by examining the results of the tests. Criterion-related validity is measured by examining concurrent validity and predictive validity. Concurrent validity represents the relationship of the performance on the test with performance on another well-reputed test. Predictive validity examines the relationship of the test to some actual behavior of which the test is supposed to be predictive. For example, high-risk scores on the MAI should be predictive of a later diagnosis of cerebral palsy.

Accuracy refers to the ability of a test to provide either positive predictive validity or negative predictive validity. *Sensitivity* indicates the ability of a measurement to detect dysfunction/abnormality (ie, to identify those individuals with a positive finding who already have or will have a particular characteristic or outcome).[12] *Specificity* indicates the ability of a measurement to detect normality (ie, the proportion of people who have a negative finding on a test and who do not exhibit a certain particular characteristic). Newer tests often will provide this information for the clinician. For example, the sensitivity of the DeGangi-Berk Test of Sensory Integration (TSI)[13] ranges from 0.66 for reflex integration to 0.84 for bilateral motor integration. The specificity of the TSI ranges from 0.64 for bilateral motor integration to 0.85 for the total test.

Standardized Tests and Measurements Used in Pediatric Physical Therapy

Standardized refers to tests which are commercially available to physical therapists and which include directions for administration. These directions for administration allow the tests to be given in a standard format by a variety of individuals. Standardized tests may be norm referenced or criterion referenced. Standardized tests also may include only a test manual or a test manual as well as test materials. The following section presents a description of selected tests and measurements used in pediatric physical therapy. The section is not all encompassing but presents those tests and measurements that are frequently used for the purposes of examination and evaluation.

Newborn Developmental and Screening Assessments

Neurological Assessment of the Preterm and Full-Term Infant[14]
1981
Lilly Dubowitz and Victor Dubowitz

Purpose:	To provide information relative to neurological maturation and changes in infants. The test documents deviations in neurological signs and their eventual resolution.
Ages:	Full-term infants up to the third day of life. Preterm infants up to term gestational age beginning when infant can tolerate handling and is medically stable.
Time:	10 to 15 minutes for testing and scoring.
User Qualifications:	Medical professions who have knowledge of neonatal neurology.
Test Kit:	Consists of manual and score sheets.
Test Areas:	Test items are drawn from the assessment tools of Saint-Anne Dargassies,[15] Prechtl,[16] Parmelee,[17] and Brazelton.[18] Areas assessed are habituation, movement and tone, reflexes, and neurobehavioral.
Administration:	Infant assessed two-thirds of the way between feedings. Scoring of the items is done on a five-point ordinal scale. All of the items do not have to be administered with each infant and no single total score is achieved. The pattern of responses, however, is examined and compared with case histories described in the test manual. Infants are categorized as normal, abnormal, or borderline depending on tone, head control, or number of deviant signs noted during the examination.
Psychometric Characteristics:	**Criterion-referenced** measurement. No **reliability** information is reported on the scale by the authors. **Concurrent validity** was determined by comparing the results on the scale with ultrasound scans used to detect intraventricular bleeds. The results revealed that 24 of 31 infants born at less than 36 weeks gestation with ultrasound evidence of a bleed had three or more abnormal clinical signs out of six items administered, as compared with only two of 37 infants of the same gestational age without evidence of intraventricular bleeds.[14] Of the 37 infants without evidence of intraventricular bleeds, 21 had no abnormal clinical signs as compared with only one of the 31 infants with documented bleeds. No studies on **predictive abilities** of this test are available. **Sensitivity**: 0.65 **Specificity**: 0.91

Neonatal Behavioral Assessment Scale (NBAS)[18,19]
1984
T. Berry Brazelton

Purpose: To provide a behavioral scale for infants from birth to the approximate post-term age of 2 months. To describe an infant's interaction with the caregiver. The NBAS is not considered a neurological assessment, although it contains some neurological items as outlined by Prechtl.[20]

Ages: Full-term neonates, 37 to 48 weeks postconceptual age. Additional items are given for infants born before 37 weeks.

Time: 30 to 35 minutes to administer. An additional 10 to 15 minutes required for scoring.

User
Qualifications: A training program is recommended for examiners to become reliable in administration.

Test Kit: Consists of manual and score sheets.

Test Areas: Includes assessment of the infant's state of consciousness and use of state to maintain control of his reactions to environmental and internal stimuli. Thought to be an important mechanism reflecting the infant's potential for organization of sensory input. For each of the behavioral items, the appropriate state of consciousness for testing is indicated.

Areas tested include:
➤ Ability to organize states of consciousness
➤ Habituation of reactions to disturbing events
➤ Attention to and processing of simple and complex environmental events
➤ Control of motor activity and postural tone
➤ Performance of integrated motor acts
Nine supplementary items are used for preterm or fragile infants and address the quality of alert responsiveness, cost of attention, examiner persistence, general irritability of the neonate, robustness and endurance, regulatory capacity, state regulation, balance of muscle tone, and reinforcement value of the infant's behavior.

Administration: The initial test is done ideally on the third day after birth (since the infant may be disorganized during the first 48 hours) and done between feedings. Each of the biobehavioral items is scored individually according to the criteria given in the test manual. The mean score for each item is based on the behavior exhibited by an average full-term (7 pounds), normal, infant with an APGAR of no less than 7 at 1 minute and 8 at 5 minutes and whose mother did not have more than 100 mg of barbiturates for pain or 50 mg of other sedative drugs as premedication in the 4 hours prior to delivery. The infant is scored on his best, not his average, performance. Seven total cluster scores for the infant are obtained.

continued

Psychometric
Characteristics: **Criterion-referenced** measurement.

Construct and content validity demonstrated by Tronick and Brazelton [21] showed that NBAS was superior to a standard neurological examination given during the neonatal period.

Predictive validity demonstrated through prediction of mental and motor scores on the Bayley Scales of Infant Behavior with correlation scores of 0.67 to 0.80.[19] Bakow et al reported good correlations between the NBAS items of alertness, motor maturity, tremulousness, habituation, and self-quieting with infant temperament at 4 months.[22]

Interrater reliability is stated to be at 0.90 if one completes training at one of the six training sites.

Test-retest reliability: Sameroff[23] found low test-retest relationships between days 2 and 3 in a group of full-term infants. Test-retest reliabilities, however, may be affected by changes in the infant's chronological age, behavioral state, and internal physiological state.

Infant Neurobiological International Battery (INFANIB)[24]
1994
Patricia H. Ellison

Purpose: To discriminate between infants with normal neurological function and abnormal neurological function.

Ages: Infants and toddlers between 1 to 18 months of age. Can be used with preterm infants.

Time: 20 to 30 minutes.

User
Qualifications: Clinicians who evaluate neonates.

Test Kit: Consists of manual and score sheets. Manual contains photographs, descriptions, and examples of infants performing the items.

Test Areas: Areas assessed include:
➤ Spasticity
➤ Vestibular function
➤ Head and trunk control
➤ French angles
➤ Legs

continued

Administration: Items individually administered to infant. Scoring procedures are in test manual and on score sheet. Performance of infant is compared with criteria for infant's corrected age. Four age groups are used for assessment using cut scores identified for each of the age groups. Scores are summed for each subscale and total test. The total scores are compared to the cut scores that identify the infant as "abnormal," "transient," or "normal."

Psychometric
Characteristics: **Criterion-referenced** measurement.
Predictive validity demonstrated through high prediction of cerebral palsy at 12 months of age using spasticity (86.8%) and trunk (87.1%) subscales at 6 months of age.
Internal consistency: Alpha for total score=0.88 for infants younger than 8 months, 0.43 for infants older than 8 months, and 0.91 for total group.
Interrater reliability found to be 0.97 for total test score in a study of 65 infants with seven evaluators.[25]
Test-retest reliability shown to be 0.95 in infants used for the above study on interrater reliability.[25]

Test of Infant Motor Performance (TIMP)[26]
2001 – Fifth Version
Suzanne Campbell

Purpose: Comprehensive assessment of developing head and trunk control as well as selective control of arms and legs. Test is currently in its fifth version.

Ages: 32 weeks postconceptional age to 4 months post-term in premature infants; 4 months chronologic age in term-born infants. Age-related standards based upon performance of white (non-Hispanic), black (African and African American), and Latino (Mexican and Puerto Rican) infants from the Chicago metropolitan area.

Time: Average of 30 minutes to administer and score.

User
Qualifications: Physical therapists and occupational therapists.

Test Kit: Consists of test manual and score sheets. Need rattle, squeaky toy, bright red ball, and soft cloth.

continued

Test Areas: The TIMP has two sections: 1) Observed Scale of 28 dichotomously scored items used to examine spontaneous movements such as head centering and individual finger, ankle, and wrist movements, and 2) Elicited Scale of 31 items scored on five-, six-, or seven-point scales which assesses the infant's responses to placement in various positions and to sights and sounds.

Administration: All observations and test procedures should be done with infants in state 3, 4, or 5 as defined by Brazelton in the Neonatal Behavioral Assessment Scale. Verbal and/or visual prompts may be used. No more than three trials allowed for each item. If infant fails to meet full criterion, the behavior is scored at the next lower response level. Based upon the infant's outcome on the test, he or she is described as average, low average, below average, or far below average.

Psychometric
Characteristics: **Content validity**: Expert review of items by experienced pediatric physical therapists, occupational therapists, and psychologists. Item analysis funded by the Foundation for Physical Therapy (APTA).
Construct validity: TIMP has been found to be sensitive to age changes with scores being highly correlated with age (r=0.83).[27] Discriminative validity supported by cross-sectional studies using TIMP that demonstrated that children with many medical complications have significantly lower scores than healthier children.
Concurrent validity: Correlation between raw scores on the TIMP and on the Alberta Infant Motor Scales (AIMS)[28] was r=0.64.[29] The correlation between the TIMP raw scores and the AIMS percentile ranks was r=0.60 (P=0.0001). The TIMP score also was found to identify 80% of infants at the same level as the AIMS.
Test-retest reliability was assessed over a 3-day period on 106 infants (white, black, and Latino). The subjects ranged in age from 32 weeks postconceptional age to 16 weeks past term. Reliability was found to be r=0.89 (P<.0001) with 54% of the scores varying less than eight points out of a possible 170 points.[30]
Interrater reliability of r=0.949 if the therapists are trained. The test developers recommend that rate agreement of 90% on item ratings with experienced testers should be obtained when training new TIMP users.

Screening Instruments

Denver II[31]
1990
William K. Frankenburg, Josiah Dodds, Phillip Archer, Beverly Bresnick, Patrick Maschka, Norman Edleman, and Howard Shapiro

Purpose:	Originally developed in 1967 to identify developmental delays in infants and young children. Current edition is revision of the Denver Developmental Screening Test[32] and the Revised Denver Developmental Screening Test.[33]
	The test also can be used to monitor children who are at-risk for developmental problems.
Ages:	1 week to 6 years, 6 months.
Time:	15 minutes.
User Qualifications:	Nurses, physical therapists, occupational therapists, early childhood educators, and psychologists.
Test Kit:	The materials needed for testing are included in the test kit and are used to ensure that the test remains standardized. A skein of red wool, box of raisins, rattle with a narrow handle, small bottle with a 5/8-inch opening, bell, tennis ball, and eight 1-inch cubical colored counting blocks are included in the test materials. The screening manual contains instructions for test administration and interpretation as well as recommendations for follow-up (Figure 2-1).
Test Areas:	Consists of 125 items which are arranged on the test form in four sectors to screen the following areas of function: ➤ Personal—social ➤ Fine motor—adaptive ➤ Language ➤ Gross motor
Administration:	Test items are individually administered using the materials supplied in the test kit. Scoring procedures are explained in the test manual and the total score is based on the number of items passed or failed in relation to the age of the child. The score is further categorized as "normal," "suspect," or "untestable."
Psychometric Characteristics:	**Norm-referenced measurement:** Norms for the Denver II are based on a study of 2096 children from all regions of Colorado. Controlled variables within age groups included maternal education, residence, and ethnicity. The goal of the sampling procedure was to provide norms that would be representative of children in the United States.[34]

continued

However, questions have been raised about the appropriateness of the test for different ethnic groups, and research on potential false-positive results from the Denver II has been conducted.[35] Kerfeld et al[36] found that the Denver II should be used with caution when screening for developmental delay in Alaska Native children and raised the issue of appropriate utilization of the instrument with other ethnic groups not included in the norming.

Interrater reliability: Mean percent agreement for all items stated to be 0.99 (±0.016).[30]

Test-retest reliability for the same items was 0.90 (±0.12).[31]

Sensitivity of test stated to be 0.83.

Specificity of test stated to be 0.43.

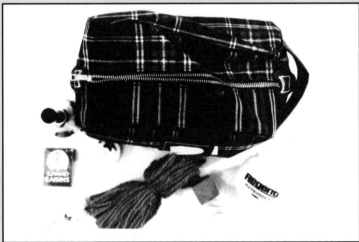

Figure 2-1. Testing kit for the Denver II.

Milani-Comparetti Motor Development Screening Test, Third Edition[37]
1992
A. Milani-Comparetti and E.A. Gidoni
(Wayne Stuberg for revised edition)

Purpose: Originally developed by two Italian child neurologists, Milani-Comparetti and Gidoni, and published in 1967,[38] the test was further adapted by Meyer's Children's Rehabilitation Institute and published in a slightly different format in 1978 and in 1992.[37,39]
Purpose is to evaluate motor development in relation to the emergence and disappearance of primitive reflexes and the sequential development of higher patterns of movement and postural control.

Ages: Birth to 2 years.

Time: 10 to 15 minutes to administer and score.

User
Qualifications: Physical therapists and physicians.

Test Kit: The test manual has complete instructions for standardization of administration. The graphic scoring chart allows ease of understanding at a glance if the child is scoring above or below his age line. No special equipment is needed for the testing except for a tilt board. A regular table and mat are needed.

Test Areas: **Spontaneous motor behaviors** (locomotion, sitting, and standing) and **evoked responses** (primitive reflexes, righting reactions, protective extension reactions, and equilibrium reactions).

Administration: The child is observed for spontaneous motor behaviors and is manipulated by the examiner for the evoked responses. The score sheet provides drawings and the test manual provides a description of the performance expected. The individual test items are to be graded pass (either by direct observation or by parental report if the child is uncooperative) or fail. A total score is not obtained.

Psychometric
Characteristics: **Norm-referenced measurement**: Norming for the third edition was performed on 312 children between 1 and 16 months of age living in Omaha, Nebraska. The original Milani-Comparetti screening tool was developed based on clinical observations of normally and abnormally developing babies over a 5-year period. Certain motor behaviors that were considered to be interrelated and which had a relationship between functional motor achievement and underlying structures of motor behaviors were included in the test. Limited validity and reliability studies were available for the first two editions of the test.[40-42]

continued

Interrater reliability for the current edition has been shown to be between 0.89 and 0.95 for percent agreement. Item interrater reliability varied from 0.79 (standing) to 0.98 (hand grasp, body lying supine). Limited data are available for the reliability levels when using the tool for children with varying degrees of developmental disabilities.

Test-retest reliability was found to be between 0.82 to 1.0 for percent agreement. Item test-retest reliability varied from 0.80 (body supine lying) to 1.0 (Moro, backward protective reaction, pull to sit, standing up from supine, and locomotion).

Specificity of the test has been found to be between 0.78 and 0.89.
Sensitivity of the test has been found to be between 0.44 and 0.67.

Movement Assessment of Infants (MAI)[10]
1975
Lynette S. Chandler, Mary S. Andrews, and Marcia W. Swanson

Purpose:	Created out of a need for a uniform approach to the evaluation of high-risk infants. Purpose is to provide a detailed and systematic appraisal of motor behaviors during the first year of life and to allow monitoring of the effects of physical therapy on infants whose motor behaviors are at or below 1 year of age.
Ages:	Birth to 12 months.
Time:	45 to 90 minutes for administration and scoring.
User Qualifications:	Physical therapists.
Test Kit:	A test manual and score sheets are included.
Test Areas:	Evaluates muscle tone, primitive reflexes, automatic reactions, and volitional movements and yields a record of the infant's observed behavior.
Administration:	Items are individually administered by the examiner. Handling of the infant is required. Scores for each item on the MAI have been designated as normal or questionable for a 4-month-old infant. When an infant receives a questionable score, a high-risk point is given. High-risk points then are totaled for each of the four sections and combined for a high-risk score. Scores for asymmetries and distribution variations also are included when determining the final score. The ratings of normal and questionable were determined by the authors on the basis of educational experience, review of the literature, and clinical pediatric experience.
Psychometric Characteristics:	**Criterion-referenced measurement:** Profiles for normal motor behavior of 4- and 8-month-old infants have been developed. For the 4-months profile, however, children used in establishing the profile were Caucasian with only a few exceptions (Asian). Apparently no children of African American descent were included.

continued

Construct validity was demonstrated through the ability of the test to discriminate between infants born at <32 weeks gestation from those born between 32 and 36 weeks gestation at 4-months corrected age.[42] However, Schneider, Lee, and Chasnoff[43] expressed concerns about the use of the MAI with healthy 4-month-old infants. In a sample of 50 4-month-old infants, 30% of the infants were found to have total risk scores greater than seven which differed significantly from the 15% of infants used in the original MAI profile. Based on these findings, these researchers suggested that the current MAI profile may not reflect accurately normal motor behavior of healthy 4-month-old infants.

Predictive validity has been extensively studied. The MAI at 4 months was shown to correctly identify 73.5% of children with cerebral palsy at 3 to 8 years of age and 62.7% of those who did not have cerebral palsy. Seventeen items were shown to be significant predictors of cerebral palsy.[10]

Interrater reliability has been documented as being r=0.72.[44] However, Haley et al[45] using percent agreement and the Kappa statistic found 2% of the items had Kappa coefficients with excellent interrater reliability and 58% had fair to good interrater reliability. Forty percent of the items had poor interrater reliability. Ten percent of the items had excellent intrarater reliability, 42% had fair to good intrarater reliability, and 48% of the items had poor intrarater reliability.

Test-retest reliability has been documented as being r=0.76[43] when infants were tested 1 week apart.

Specificity noted to be 0.78 at 4 months and 0.64 at 8 months.[46]

Sensitivity noted to be 0.83 at 4 months and 0.96 at 8 months.[46]

Bruininks-Oseretsky Test of Motor Proficiency

The short form of the BOTMP can be used for screening purposes, such as early identification of motor problems. Discussion on the use of the BOTMP will be included in the section on comprehensive developmental testing.

Motor Development and Motor Control Tests

Alberta Infant Motor Scales (AIMS)[28]
1994
M. C. Piper and J. Darrah

Purpose:	The AIMS was developed to be used in the identification of motor delay (discrimination), the evaluation of change in motor performance over time resulting from maturation or intervention, and the provision of use full information for treatment planning.
Ages:	Birth to 18 months.
Time:	20 to 30 minutes to administer and score.
User Qualifications:	Physical therapists.
Test Kit:	A test manual and score sheets are included. No specific toys, prompts, or conditions are used.
Test Areas:	The infant is tested in four positions (supine, prone, sitting, and standing). A total of 58 gross motor skill items are included. Three aspects of motor performance are observed: weight-bearing, posture, and anti-gravity movement.
Administration:	The test can be done in the clinic or the home. The infant should be unclothed and allowed to set the pace and momentum of the test. Minimal handling should be done by the therapist. Each item on the test is scored as "observed" or "not observed." For each of the four positions, the sum of the observed items is a positional score. The sum of the positional scores is the total score, which is then converted to a percentile rank (Figure 2-2).
Psychometric Characteristics:	**Norm-referenced measurement**: Normative sample consisted of 2202 infants from Alberta, Canada, who were chosen based on age and gender. However, no information was provided regarding race or ethnicity of children used in the norming. Questions regarding the use of the AIMS with children from different races or ethnicity have been raised.[47] **Construct validity** was determined by comparing scores from infants who were identified as at-risk or with known motor delays against the norms that had been established.[48] The authors stated that using the scores allowed the identification of infants as "abnormal," "at-risk," or "normal."[49] For **concurrent validity**, the total scores on the AIMS of 103 typically developing infants and 68 abnormal or at-risk infants were correlated with the Peabody Developmental Motor Scales gross motor raw scores and with the motor scales of the Bayley Scales of Infant Development. Correlation coefficients between 0.84 and 0.99 were determined for the typically developing infants and between 0.93 and 0.95 with the abnormal and at-risk infants.[47]

continued

Interrater reliability was assessed using two therapists on 253 typically developing infants. Using the Pearson Product Moment Correlation Coefficient, r values ranged from 0.96 to 0.99.

Test-retest reliability was assessed using the same 253 infants. Using the Pearson Product Moment Coefficient, r values ranged from 0.86 to 0.99 when the same assessor scored the AIMS on both testing days. However, the r values ranged from 0.82 to 0.94 if a different assessor performed the test-retest. The lowest reliability scores were noted in the infants who were 0 to 3 months of age.

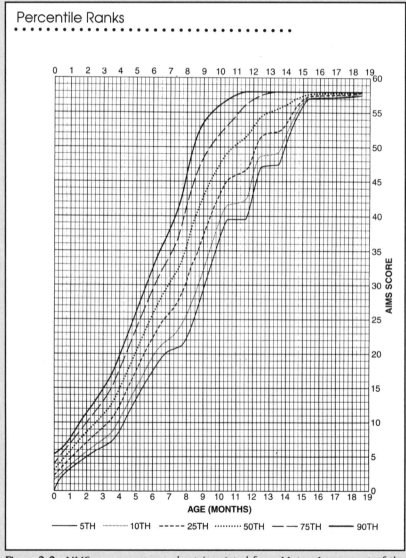

Figure 2-2. AIMS summary score sheet (reprinted from *Motor Assessment of the Developing Infant,* Piper MC and Darrah J, copyright 1994, with permission from Elsevier).

Toddler and Infant Motor Evaluation (TIME)[50]
1994
Lucy Jane Miller and Gale H. Roid

Purpose:	The TIME has three specific purposes: 1) to identify those children who are suspected to have motor delays or deviations, 2) to develop appropriate interventions, and 3) to conduct treatment efficacy research.
Ages:	4 months to 3 years, 6 months.
Time:	Administration time for entire assessment ranges from 10 to 20 minutes for young children and 20 to 40 minutes for older children. Scoring takes additional time, and amount of time depends on examiner's familiarity with the test. The functional performance subtest interview requires an additional 15 minutes.
User Qualifications:	Occupational therapists and physical therapists.
Test Kit:	The test manual and score sheets are very thorough. Written descriptions and line drawings are given for each item. The child is engaged in play in a familiar environment with a varying sequence of task presentation.
Test Areas:	Five primary subtests include: mobility, motor organization, stability, functional performance, and social/emotional abilities. Three optional subtests are recommended to be used by advanced clinicians and researchers. These include component analysis, quality rating, and atypical positions.
Administration:	The test has a specific order of administration with the subtests given in the following order: social/emotional, mobility, motor organization, stability, and functional performance. The social/emotional abilities subtest is completed before and after the test session and addresses state/activity level, attention, and emotions/reactions. The mobility and motor organization subtests are scored during observations of the parent(s) playing with the child. The items are grouped into four developmental levels and are scored on a pass/fail scale. Stability is assessed and scored based on observations of the child during the mobility and motor organization subtests. The functional performance subtest is administered by the examiner through an interview with the parents. The subtest includes questions related to self-care, self-management/mastery, relationships/interactions, and function in the community. The five primary subtests yield scaled scores.
Psychometric Characteristics:	**Norm-referenced** for the five primary subtests; the optional subtests are not norm referenced. Norming occurred on a sample of 731 children from across the United States who did not have motor delays or deviations. The sample was stratified by age, race/ethnicity, gender, and socioeconomic status. Children with biological or environmental risk for developmental delays were not included in the sample.

continued

Construct validity was determined by analyzing children with and without motor delays using the test. A standardized mean difference between groups with and without delays averaged 1.5 standard deviations. Age trend analysis also showed that with increasing age, children perform an increasing number of items and master increasingly more difficult items.[49]

Interrater reliability of the test has been found to range from r=0.88 for motor organization to r=0.99 for mobility when using the Pearson Product Moment Correlation Coefficient. [49]

Test-retest reliability using the same examiner is reported to range from r=0.96 for mobility to r=0.99 for motor organization and atypical positions.[49]

Specificity scores have been reported for mobility (92.6%), stability (96.9%), and atypical positions (98.6%).

Sensitivity scores have been reported for mobility (88.2%), stability (80.6%), and atypical positions (97.2%).

Bayley Scales of Infant Development (BSID II)[51]
1993
Nancy Bailey

Purpose: The primary purpose is to identify developmental delay and to monitor a child's developmental progress.

Ages: 1 to 42 months.

Time: 25 minutes to 1 hour dependent on the child's age.

User Qualifications: Psychologists, physical therapists, and occupational therapists.

Test Kit: The test manual for the BSID II provides in-depth explanations of how the test is to be administered. All materials needed, except for facial tissues, stairs, walking board, and stop watch are included.

Test Areas: The Mental Scale of the BSID II is designed to assess the following: sensory-perceptual acuities, discriminations, and the ability to respond to these; the early acquisition of "object constancy" and memory, learning and problem-solving ability; vocalizations and the beginnings of verbal communication; and the early evidence of the ability to form generalizations and classifications. All of these are thought to be the basis of abstract thinking. The Motor Scale is designed to measure degree of control of the body, coordination of the large muscles, and finer manipulatory skills of the hands and fingers.

continued

In addition to the Mental and Motor Scales, the BSID II contains an Infant Behavior Record which is to be completed after the other scales have been administered. The Infant Behavior Record helps assess the nature of the child's social and objective orientations toward his environment as expressed in attitudes, interests, emotional energy, activity, and tendencies to approach or withdraw from stimulation.

Administration: The test is individually administered with scoring according to the test manual. A binary scoring system of pass/fail is used. Scoring of the Mental Scale yields a Mental Development Index (MDI) for the child. Information from the motor scale is expressed as a Psychomotor Development Index (PDI). The mean standard score for each of the indexes for all age ranges is 100 with a standard deviation of 15 points. The indexes derived from the mental and motor scales have limited value in the prediction of later abilities, as the rates of development for any given child may be highly variable. The primary value of the scores is to provide a basis for establishing the child's current status and for instituting early corrective measures.

Psychometric
Characteristics: **Norm-referenced measurement:** The BSID II is the product of years of revisions, renorming, and expansions. The 1958 to 1960 version of the test drew heavily from three previous scales: the California First Year Mental Scale, the California Preschool Mental Scale, and the California Infant Scale of Motor Development. A second version was published in 1960 followed by a third revision published in 1969. The current version was published in 1993 and was normed on 1700 children. The normative sample was selected based upon age, gender, race/ethnicity, geographic region, and parent education and was representative of these characteristics as identified on the 1988 US census.

Concurrent validity has been demonstrated with the McCarthy Scales of Children's Abilities with r values for the MDI ranging from 0.57 to 0.77 and r values for the PDI ranging from 0.18 to 0.59. Correlation with the Wechsler Preschool and Primary Scale of Intelligence – Revised (WPPSI-R) revealed r values ranging from 0.21 to 0.73 for the MDI and from 0.14 to 0.41 for the PDI. The mental scale appears to relate higher than the motor scale with tests that assess general cognitive abilities.

Interrater reliability for the motor scale is r=0.75 and 0.96 for the mental scale.

Test-retest reliability also is higher for the mental scale than for the motor scale with r=0.87 for the MDI and r=0.78 for the PDI. However, both values indicate high correlations.

Peabody Developmental Motor Scales, Second Edition (PDMS-2)[9]
2000
M. Rhonda Folio and Rebecca R. Fewell

Purpose:	The PDMS-2 was designed to: 1) estimate a child's motor competence, 2) compare gross and fine motor disparity, 3) provide qualitative and quantitative aspects of individual skills, 4) evaluate a child's progress, and 5) provide a research tool.
Ages:	Birth to 6 years.
Time:	Total test requires 45 to 60 minutes. Each section requires 20 to 30 minutes to administer.
User Qualifications:	Physical therapists, occupational therapists, diagnosticians, early intervention specialists, adapted physical educators, and psychologists.
Test Kit:	The PDMS-2 kit includes the examiner's manual, profile/summary form (Figure 2-3), examiner record booklet, guide to item administration, motor activities program, Peabody Motor Development Chart, manipulatives, and optional computerized scoring program.
Test Areas:	The six subtests that comprise the PDMS-2 are:

➤ Reflexes (gross motor, birth to 11 months)
➤ Stationary (gross motor)
➤ Locomotion (gross motor)
➤ Object manipulation (gross motor, 12 months to 6 years)
➤ Grasping (fine motor)
➤ Visual-motor integration (fine motor)

Administration:	The Guide to Item Administration provides detailed descriptions of each item. Each item description includes: 1) the age at which 50% of the children in normative sample mastered the item, 2) the testing position, 3) the stimulus (if needed), 4) the procedure to be used to test the item, 5) the criteria for scoring the item, and 6) an illustration of a child performing the item.
	The testing environment may be in a room, hallway, or even outdoors. The child should wear nonslippery shoes or go barefoot. For seated items, the child's feet should touch the floor. If necessary, the parent or caregiver may remain during the testing.
	Items are scored on a three-point scale. Raw scores convert to age equivalent (AE), percentiles, and standard scores. Standard scores convert to three indexes of motor performance: gross motor, fine motor, and total motor.
Psychometric Characteristics:	**Norm-referenced measurement**
	Norming took place on a sample of 2003 children residing in 46 states and one Canadian province during Winter 1979 and Spring 1998. The demographics used for the norming mirrored the 1997 US Bureau of the Census data.

continued

PDMS-2

Profile/Summary Form

Peabody Developmental Motor Scales   Second Edition

Section I. Identifying Information

Child's Name ELIZABETH S.   Female ☒ Male ☐

	Year	Month	Day	
Date Tested	02	05	09	Examiner's Name
Date of Birth	00	07	08	Examiner's Title ___
Chronological Age	01	10	01	
Prematurity Adjustment	−	−		
Corrected Age				
Age in Months				

Section II. Record of Scores

PDMS-2	Raw Score	Age Equivalent	%ile	Standard Scores	
Reflexes					
Stationary	36	11 months	4	7	
Locomotion	50	15 months	2	4	
Object Manipulation	6	13 months	5	5	
Grasping					
Visual–Motor Integration					

Sum of Standard Scores 16

	GMQ	FMQ	TMQ
Quotients	70		
Percentiles	2%		

Section III. Profile of Scores

Standard Scores	Reflexes	Stationary	Locomotion	Object Manipulation	Grasping	Visual–Motor Integration	Standard Scores	Quotients	Gross Motor	Fine Motor	Total Motor	Quotients
20	.	.	.	.	.	.	20	150	.	.	.	150
19	.	.	.	.	.	.	19	145	.	.	.	145
18	.	.	.	.	.	.	18	140	.	.	.	140
17	.	.	.	.	.	.	17	135	.	.	.	135
16	.	.	.	.	.	.	16	130	.	.	.	130
15	.	.	.	.	.	.	15	125	.	.	.	125
14	.	.	.	.	.	.	14	120	.	.	.	120
13	.	.	.	.	.	.	13	115	.	.	.	115
12	.	.	.	.	.	.	12	110	.	.	.	110
11	.	.	.	.	.	.	11	105	.	.	.	105
10	—	.	.	.	.	.	10	100	—	—	—	100
9	.	.	.	.	.	.	9	95	.	.	.	95
8	.	.	.	.	.	.	8	90	.	.	.	90
7	.	.	.	.	.	.	7	85	.	.	.	85
6	.	.	.	.	.	.	6	80	.	.	.	80
5	.	.	.	.	.	.	5	75	.	.	.	75
4	.	.	.	.	.	.	4	70	.	.	.	70
3	.	.	.	.	.	.	3	65	.	.	.	65
2	.	.	.	.	.	.	2	60	.	.	.	60
1	.	.	.	.	.	.	1	55	.	.	.	55

Figure 2-3. PDMS-2 profile/summary form (reprinted with permission from Folio MR, Fewell RR. *Peabody Developmental Motor Scales-2.* Pro-Ed: Austin, Tex; 2000).

Content validity was used to determine if the test content covered a representative sample of the behavior domain to be measured. The PDMS-2 items were based upon a developmental framework and a Taxonomy of Psychomotor Domain which shows hierarchical sequencing.[52] Content validity also was assessed through item analysis and item response theory modeling.

continued

Criterion-predictive validity studies compared the scores on the PDMS -2 with the original PDMS and with the Mullen Scales of Early Learning (MSEL:A). Correlation values between the PDMS-2 and the PDMS were r=0.84 for the gross motor quotient and r=0.91 for the fine motor quotient. Correlation values between the PDMS-2 and the MSEL:A were r=0.86 for the gross motor scores and 0.80 for the fine motor scores.[9]

Interrater reliability was assessed using two examiners who reviewed 30 completed protocols for 3- to 11-month-old infants and 30 completed protocols for 15- to 36-month-old children. Interscorer reliability values ranged from r=0.96 (total motor scores) to 0.99 (locomotion).[9]

Test-retest reliability testing was performed on children in the two age groups of 2 to 11 months and 12 to 17 months. The Pearson Product Moment Correlations were found to range from r=0.73 (fine motor quotient in 2- to 11-month-old infants) to r=0.96 (total motor quotient for 12- to 17-month-old infants).

Test of Gross Motor Development-2 (TGMD-2)[53]
2000
Dale Ulrich

Purpose:	Test was developed to assess gross motor functioning in children. The author states that the test is to be used for: identification and screening, instructional programming, assessment of individual progress, program evaluation, and as a research tool.
Ages:	3 to 10 years.
Time:	15 to 20 minutes to administer and score.
User Qualifications:	Physical therapists.
Test Kit:	Test manual and score sheets (Figure 2-4) included in test kit. Examiner must supply materials which are described in the manual.
Test Areas:	Locomotor, object control.
Administration:	Items are individually administered to the child. The test conditions should be arranged prior to testing to facilitate ease of administration. Children should wear rubber-soled shoes or be barefoot during the testing.

Each item on the test contains three to four specific performance components which indicate mastery of the skill.

Each of the performance components is scored as 1 if observed for two of three trials and 0 if not observed two of three trials. Practice and three test trials are given for each component. Raw scores are converted to percentiles, standard scores, age-equivalent scores for the two areas (locomotor and object control), and a total gross motor quotient.

continued

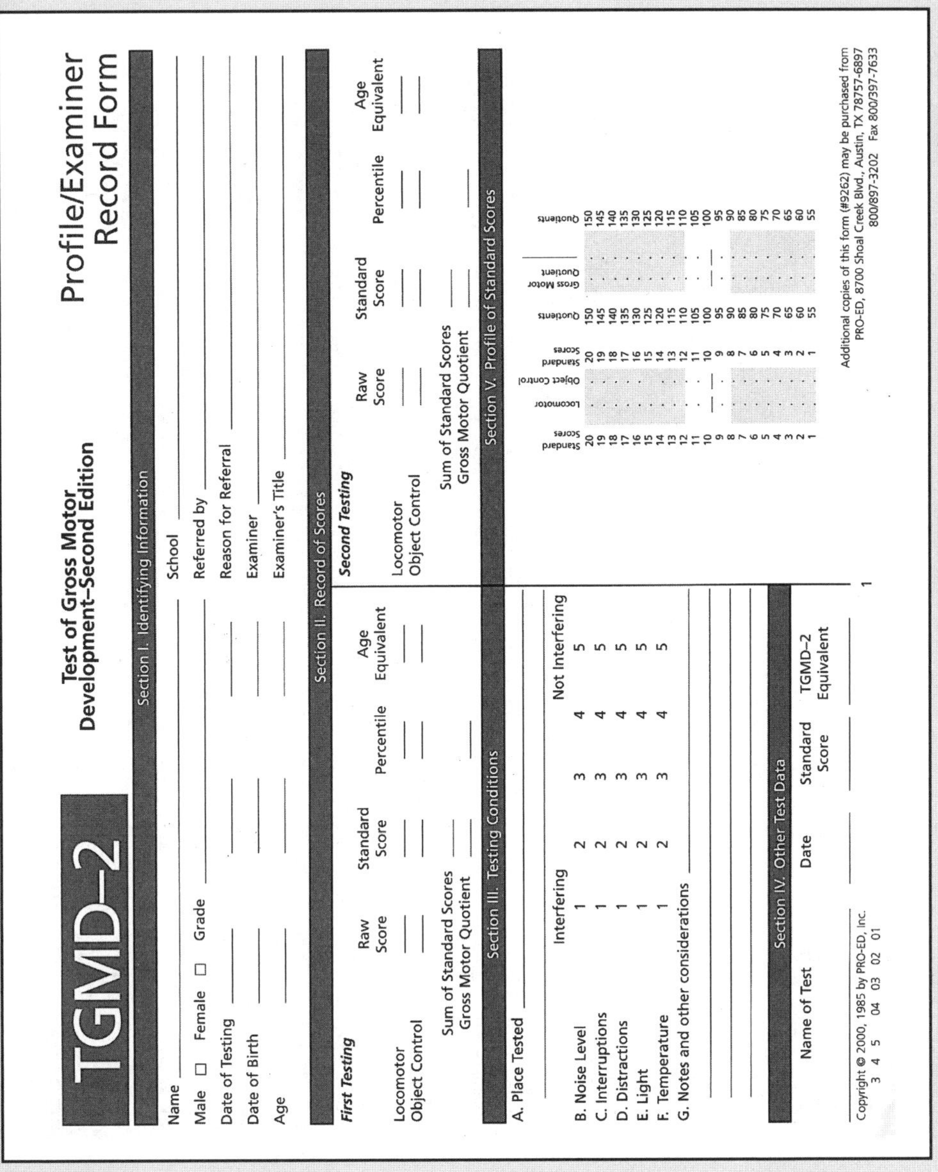

TGMD–2

Test of Gross Motor Development–Second Edition

Profile/Examiner Record Form

Section I. Identifying Information

Name ______ School ______

Male ☐ Female ☐ Grade ______ Referred by ______

Date of Testing ______ Reason for Referral ______

Date of Birth ______ Examiner ______

Age ______ Examiner's Title ______

Section II. Record of Scores

First Testing

	Raw Score	Standard Score	Percentile	Age Equivalent
Locomotor	___	___	___	___
Object Control	___	___	___	___

Sum of Standard Scores ___
Gross Motor Quotient ___ ___

Second Testing

	Raw Score	Standard Score	Percentile	Age Equivalent
Locomotor	___	___	___	___
Object Control	___	___	___	___

Sum of Standard Scores ___
Gross Motor Quotient ___ ___

Section III. Testing Conditions

A. Place Tested ______

	Interfering				Not Interfering
B. Noise Level	1	2	3	4	5
C. Interruptions	1	2	3	4	5
D. Distractions	1	2	3	4	5
E. Light	1	2	3	4	5
F. Temperature	1	2	3	4	5

G. Notes and other considerations ______

Section IV. Other Test Data

Name of Test	Date	Standard Score	TGMD–2 Equivalent

Section V. Profile of Standard Scores

Standard Scores	Locomotor	Object Control	Standard Scores	Quotients	Gross Motor Quotient	Quotients
20			20	150		150
19			19	145		145
18			18	140		140
17			17	135		135
16			16	130		130
15			15	125		125
14			14	120		120
13			13	115		115
12			12	110		110
11			11	105		105
10			10	100		100
9			9	95		95
8			8	90		90
7			7	85		85
6			6	80		80
5			5	75		75
4			4	70		70
3			3	65		65
2			2	60		60
1			1	55		55

Copyright © 2000, 1985 by PRO-ED, Inc.
3 4 5 04 03 02 01

1

Additional copies of this form (#9262) may be purchased from
PRO-ED, 8700 Shoal Creek Blvd., Austin, TX 78757-6897
800/897-3202 Fax 800/397-7633

Figure 2-4. TGMD-2 profile/examiner record form (reprinted with permission from Ulrich D. *Test of Gross Motor Development-2*. PRO-Ed: Austin, Tex; 2000).

Psychometric Characteristics: **Norm-referenced measurement.**

Ulrich used the 1997 census to make sure that the normative sample represented the nation as a whole using geographic area, gender, race, residence, educational attainment of parents, disability status, and age as the stratification criteria. Twelve hundred eight children from 10 states were used in the normative sampling.[52]

continued

Content validity was based on discriminative powers of test which identified children who were significantly behind their peers.

Criterion-predictive validity study revealed that scores on the TGMD-2 compared to scores on the Comprehensive Scales of Student Abilities. When the tests were administered 2 weeks apart, a moderate correlation of r=0.63 was found.[52]

Content sampling was done to assess internal consistency. R values ranged from 0.76 to 0.94.[52]

Interrater reliability on the test was found to be very high with correlational values of r=0.98 found for locomotor, object control, and the gross motor quotient.[52]

Test-retest reliability scores for a sample of children between 3 to 10 years of age ranged from 0.88 to 0.96.[52]

Bruininks-Oseretsky Test of Motor Proficiency (BOTMP)[4]
1978
Robert H. Bruininks

Purpose: The purpose of the test is to assess gross and fine motor skills in children and to assist in decision making about appropriate educational and therapeutic placement. The short form of the test can be used for screening for special purposes, such as early identification of developmental problems.

Ages: 4.5 to 14.5 years.

Time: The complete battery typically takes 45 to 60 minutes to administer, while the short form can be administered in 15 to 20 minutes.

User
Qualifications: Physical therapist, occupational therapists, and physical educators.

Test Kit: The test manual has instructions that are written clearly and, although some instructions may be complex, substitutions of words that the individual child may understand are allowed. Certain items on the tests are identified for use as a short form and can be administered for screening. Most equipment for the test is included in the test kit.

Test Areas: The specific motor areas assessed by the subtests of the BOTMP are running speed and agility, balance, bilateral coordination, strength, upper limb coordination, response speed, visual motor control, and upper limb speed and dexterity.

Administration: Items are individually administered to the child. All items on the test are to be administered although some items may be difficult for younger children. Raw scores from each of the areas of assessment can be converted into point scores which may be further converted to standard scores. From the standard scores, one can calculate composite scores for gross and fine motor tasks. In addition, one can determine age levels of functioning in each of the specific areas.

continued

Psychometric
Characteristics: **Norm-referenced measurement**

The BOTMP was developed through a series of analytical studies. The original test was developed in 1973 with the test items being administered to 75 children. Following analysis of the results on this initial test, a second version was administered to 250 children between 5 to 14 years of age in the St. Paul-Minneapolis area. The children were selected randomly from schools that represented central city and suburbia and various socioeconomic and ethnic groups. The final version was written after analyzing the results of this second field test. The final items on the test were selected based on item difficulty, item discrimination, correlation between performance on an item and chronological age, and intercorrelations among items in the same content area. Standardization of the final version was done on 765 subjects who were representative of the 1970 US census according to geographic region, community size, gender, and race. At least 38 children were assessed at each of the age levels of the test.

Validity: The manual reports that validity of the BOTMP is based on how well it assesses the constructs of motor development or proficiency. **Construct validity** is stated to be present due to the statistical characteristics of the test. Scores of each subtest were found to be correlated significantly with the chronological age of the children in the standardization group with correlations ranging from 0.57 to 0.86 with a median of 0.78. Validity was assessed by comparing the scores of normal children with the scores of children with either mental retardation or learning disabilities.

Interrater reliability was determined using the eight items of the visual motor control subtest. For two separate groups of raters, the interrater reliability coefficients were found to be 0.98 and 0.90.[4]

Test-retest reliability was assessed on 63 second graders and 63 sixth graders with the retest being given 7 to 12 days after the first test. The reliability coefficient for the Battery Composite was 0.89 for the second graders and 0.86 for the sixth graders.[4]

Standard error of measurement (SEM) for the composites and for the subtests. In general, the SEM for the composites were four or five standard score points and the SEM for the subtests were two to three standard score points.

Gross Motor Function Measure (GMFM)[54]
2002
D. J. Russell, P. L. Rosenbaum, L. M. Avery, and M. Lane

Purpose:
The purpose of the observational instrument is to measure change in gross motor function over time. Therapists have indicated that the test also is useful for 1) describing the child's current level of motor function, 2) determining treatment goals, and 3) providing easy explanations to parents concerning their child's progress.

Ages:
All items on the GMFM can be completed by a 5-year-old child with normal gross motor ability.

Time:
45 to 60 minutes. An additional session can be scheduled for a child that tires before completing the entire test. However, the second session should be held within 1 week, and any item completed during the first session should not be retested.

User
Qualifications: Physical therapists.

Test Kit:
Test materials required to administer the GMFM generally are found in the physical therapy department. The test manual is essential for scoring of the test forms.

Test Areas:
Eighty-eight items are used to assess activities of motor function in five dimensions: 1) lying and rolling; 2) sitting; 3) crawling and kneeling; 4) standing; and 5) walking, running, and jumping.

Administration: The test items are individually administered with a demonstration and three trials for each item. A generic scoring system is present, based on how much of each activity the child can complete. Each item is scored on a four-point rating scale. In addition to a total score, a score may be obtained for each of the five dimensions. Each dimension score and the total score are converted to a percentage of the maximum score for that dimension (Figure 2-5).

Psychometric
Characteristics: **Criterion-referenced measurement**
The test has been validated on children between 5 months and 16 years. The total validation sample included 111 children with cerebral palsy, 25 with head injury, and 34 preschoolers with no known physical disabilities.[53] Of the 111 children with CP, 88 had spastic-type CP and 23 had nonspastic-type CP. Russell et al also have shown that the GMFM is a valid measure of change in gross motor function in children with cerebral palsy.[55] The total GMFM score was correlated with parents' judgments of change in motor function (r=0.54) and therapists judgments (r=0.65). Additionally, Trahan and Malouin found that the GMFM was sensitive to changes over an 8-month period in gross motor performance in a group of children with different types of cerebral palsy.[56] Russell et al have shown that the GMFM is a valid measure of change for children with Down syndrome and is responsive to differences in potential for change among children with Down syndrome.[57]

continued

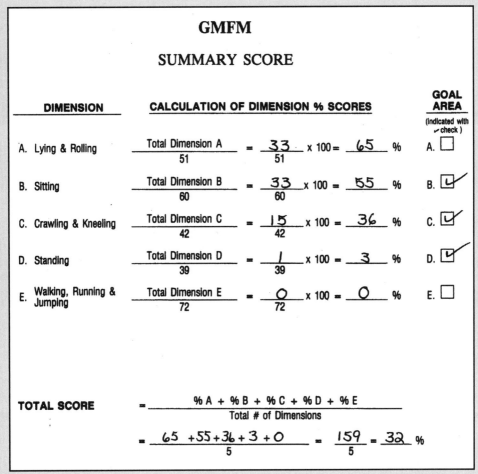

GMFM

SUMMARY SCORE

DIMENSION	CALCULATION OF DIMENSION % SCORES	GOAL AREA (Indicated with ✓ check)
A. Lying & Rolling	$\dfrac{\text{Total Dimension A}}{51} = \dfrac{33}{51}$ x 100 = 65 %	A. ☐
B. Sitting	$\dfrac{\text{Total Dimension B}}{60} = \dfrac{33}{60}$ x 100 = 55 %	B. ☑
C. Crawling & Kneeling	$\dfrac{\text{Total Dimension C}}{42} = \dfrac{15}{42}$ x 100 = 36 %	C. ☑
D. Standing	$\dfrac{\text{Total Dimension D}}{39} = \dfrac{1}{39}$ x 100 = 3 %	D. ☑
E. Walking, Running & Jumping	$\dfrac{\text{Total Dimension E}}{72} = \dfrac{0}{72}$ x 100 = 0 %	E. ☐

$$\text{TOTAL SCORE} = \frac{\% A + \% B + \% C + \% D + \% E}{\text{Total \# of Dimensions}}$$

$$= \frac{65 + 55 + 36 + 3 + 0}{5} = \frac{159}{5} = 32 \%$$

Figure 2-5. GMFM summary score sheet (reprinted with permission from Russell DJ, Rosenbaum PL, Avery LM, Lane M. *Gross Motor Function Measure [GMFM 66 and GMFM-88] User's Manual.* London, England: McKeith Press; 2002).

Interrater reliability intraclass correlation coefficients (ICCs) for children with CP range from 0.87 (lying and rolling) to 0.99 (standing, walking, running, and jumping; total).[53] Ruck-Gibis et al found the ICCs for interrater reliability to be 0.98 for the lying and rolling dimension and 0.99 for the other dimensions and total score when testing children diagnosed with osteogenesis imperfecta.[58] In children with Down syndrome, ICCs for interrater reliability has been reported as ranging from 0.73 (lying and rolling) to 0.98 (standing).[56]

Intrarater reliability ICCs computed for children with cerebral palsy range from 0.92 for standing to 0.99 for all other dimensions as well as the total score.[53] The intrarater reliability ICCs for children with osteogenesis imperfecta were calculated to be 0.99 for all five dimensions and the total score.[57]

continued

Test-retest reliability has been assessed with children with Down syndrome and found to be very high. The ICCs were found to range from 0.87 (crawling and kneeling) to 0.99 (standing).[57] The high test-retest reliability indicates that the GMFM is stable over a short period of time when no real change in the child's function is expected to occur.

Sensorimotor Tests

Infant/Toddler Sensory Profile[59]
2002
Winnie Dunn

Purpose:	The purpose of the test is: 1) to help professionals evaluate the possible contributions of sensory processing to the infant/toddler's daily performance patterns, 2) to provide information about the infant/toddler's tendencies to respond to stimuli, and 3) to identify which sensory systems are likely to be contributing to or creating barriers to functional performance.
Ages:	Birth to 36 months.
Time:	15 minutes to administer and 10 minutes to score.
User Qualifications:	Occupational therapists, physical therapists, psychologists, and speech-language pathologists.
Test Kit:	Test manual, caregiver questionnaire, and summary score sheet comprise the test.
Test Areas:	The areas assessed are: ➤ General processing ➤ Auditory processing ➤ Visual processing ➤ Tactile processing ➤ Vestibular processing ➤ Oral sensory processing Five quadrant scores which reflect the child's responsiveness to sensory experiences are obtained and are based on Dunn's Model of Sensory Processing. Sensation seeking and Low Registration indicate high threshold responses, while Sensory Sensitivity and Sensation Avoiding reflect low threshold responses. A Low Threshold Quadrant score is obtained by combining the Sensory Sensitivity and Sensory Avoiding quadrant scores.
Administration:	Administered in three general ways: 1) the Caregiver Questionnaire can be sent to the caregiver with a cover letter explaining the purpose of the instrument, 2) the caregiver can complete the form while the therapist is evaluating the infant/toddler, or 3) the therapist can help the caregiver fill out the form.

continued

Each item is scored on a scale that corresponds to the frequency with which the caregiver(s) sees the behavior in the infant/toddler. The following scale is used:

➤ Almost always (90%)=1 point
➤ Frequently (75%)=2 points
➤ Occasionally (50%)=3 points
➤ Seldom (25%)=4 points
➤ Almost never (10% or less)=5 points

Raw scores obtained in each of the areas then are compared to cut scores for infants/toddlers.

Based upon the infant/toddler's scores, the child's performance in each of the areas may be described as "typical performance," "less than others," or "more than others." In the "less than others" and "more than others" categories, the child may be further described as having a probable difference or definite difference.

Psychometric
Characteristics: **Criterion-referenced measurement**

Norming took place from 1998 to 2000 and included evaluations of 401 infants and toddlers without disabilities between birth and 36 months of age. The sample was 51.1% boys and 48.9% girls. Children were selected from four different regions of the United States (West 21%, North Central 35%, South 13%, and Northeast 30%). The majority of the children were Caucasian (84.5%) and were from suburban communities (58.4%).

Construct validity and content validity were addressed through the use of five focus groups and expert panels at the University of Kansas School of Allied Health. Items for the test were selected based upon the panelists' decisions about which area each item represented. A pilot study on a sample of 401 infants and toddlers was done using 68 occupational therapists. Analyses on the data from this study yielded information about items that were inappropriate for particular age groups and to identify patterns in the data.

Test-retest reliability was measured by having a subsample (n=32) from the standardization sample rate their child 2 to 3 weeks after the initial rating. The test-retest correlation coefficient was found to be r=0.86 for the sensory-processing section scores and r=0.74 for the quadrant scores.

Sensory Profile[60]
1999
Winnie Dunn

Purpose:	The purposes of the test are to: 1) capture information about child's sensory processing, 2) link sensory processing to daily life performance, 3) provide information for theory-based decision making, and 4) include caregivers as members of the team.
Ages:	5 to 10 years of age (can be used with caution with 3- to 4-year-old children).
Time:	30 minutes to administer and 20 minutes to score.
User Qualifications:	Occupational therapists, physical therapists, psychologists, speech-language pathologists, teachers, and physicians.
Test Kit:	Test manual, caregiver questionnaire, and summary score sheet comprise the test.
Test Areas:	The Sensory Profile consists of 125 items groups into three main sections: Sensory Processing, Modulation, and Behavioral and Emotional Responses.
	The Sensory Processing section indicates the child's responses to the basic sensory systems (auditory, visual, vestibular, touch, multisensory, and oral sensory processing).
	The Modulation section reflects the child's regulation of neural message through facilitation or inhibition of various types of responses. Areas of sensory modulation assessed are: sensory processing related to endurance/tone; modulation related to body position and movement; modulation of movement affecting activity level; modulation of sensory input affecting emotional responses; and modulation of visual input affecting emotional responses and activity level.
	The Behavior and Emotional Responses section reflects the child's behavioral outcomes of sensory processing and is expressed as emotional/social responses, behavioral outcomes of sensory processing, and items indicating thresholds for response.
Administration:	Caregivers complete a questionnaire that describes children's responses to daily sensory experiences. The caregiver completes the form by indicating the frequency of the child's responses.
	Each item is scored on a scale that corresponds to the frequency with which the caregiver(s) sees the behavior in the infant/toddlers. The following scale is used:

➤ Always (100%)=1 point
➤ Frequently (75%)=2 points
➤ Occasionally (50%)=3 points
➤ Seldom (25%)=4 points
➤ Never (0%)=5 points

continued

Raw scores obtained in each of the areas then are compared to cut scores which were determined for each area. Based upon the scores obtained, the child's performance in each of the areas may be described as "typical performance" (relates to scores at or above the point 1 SD below the mean), "probable difference" (relates to scores at or above the point 2 SD below the mean), or "definite difference" (relates to scores below the point 2 SD below the mean).

Psychometric
Characteristics: **Criterion-referenced measurement**
Norming took place from 1993 to 1999 and included evaluations of 1200 children with and without disabilities between the ages of 3 and 14 years. The sample of children without disabilities was between the ages of 3 and 10 years and was equally representative of boys and girls. Children were selected from four different regions of the United States (West 15%, North Central 30%, South 25%, and Northeast 29%). The majority of the children were Caucasian (91.4%) and were from suburban communities (60.9%).

Construct validity and content validity were addressed through the use of literature review, expert review, and category analysis. **Convergence (concurrent)** and **discriminant validity** were assessed by comparing scores from the Sensory Profile with scores from the School Function Assessment (SFA). Correlational values of r=0.68 to 0.72 were found between the fine motor/perceptual area of the Sensory Profile and the three sections of the SFA. However, low correlations were found between the more detailed performance items on the SFA and the items on the Sensory Profile. The author suggested that the Sensory Profile taps more global sensory processing and is not related to specific tasks, such as those included on the SFA.

Internal consistency (reliability) was assessed using the Cronbach's alpha. The values for alpha for the various sections ranged from 0.47 to 0.91.

The **Standard Error of Measurement** (SEM), an index of the degree to which obtained scores differ from true scores, is provided for each possible quadrant raw score total for each cut-score group. The more reliable a test is, the smaller the SEM. SEM values for the Profile ranged from 0.92 to 2.89.[60]

Sensory Profile for Adolescents/Adults[61]
2002
Catana E. Brown and Winnie Dunn

Purpose:	The purpose of the test is to: 1) capture information about an individual's sensory processing, 2) link sensory processing with everyday experiences, 3) provide information for theory-based decision making, and 4) include the individual in his or her assessment and intervention process.
Ages:	11 to 65+ years.
Time:	10 to 15 minutes to complete and 20 minutes to score.
User Qualifications:	Occupational therapists, physical therapists, adult education teachers, psychologists, social workers, vocational counselors, and physicians.
Test Kit:	The profile consists of a user's manual, a self-questionnaire, and a summary score sheet.

Test Areas: Areas of assessment are:
➤ Taste/smell processing
➤ Movement processing
➤ Visual processing
➤ Touch processing
➤ Activity level
➤ Auditory processing

Administration: Administered in four general ways: 1) the self-questionnaire can be sent to the individual with a cover letter explaining the purpose of the instrument, 2) the individual can complete the form while the therapist is present, 3) the therapist can administer the instrument by reading and recording the individual's responses to each item, or 4) the questionnaire can be completed in a group setting with the therapist present and available to answer questions.

Each item is scored on a scale that corresponds to the frequency with which the individual responds in the manner described. The following scale is used:
➤ Almost always (100%)=5 points
➤ Frequently (75%)=4 points
➤ Occasionally (50%)=3 points
➤ Seldom (25%)=2 points
➤ Almost never (5%)=1 point

Raw scores obtained in each of the areas then are compared to cut scores that were determined for each area. Based upon the scores obtained, the individual's performance in each of the areas may be described as much less than most people, less than most people, similar to most people, more than most people, or much more than most people.

continued

Psychometric
Characteristics: **Criterion-referenced measurement**
Norming included a sample of 950 adolescents and adults without disabilities. The majority of the sample were Caucasian and from the midwestern region of the United States (92%). The sample was divided into three age groups: adolescent, adult, and older adult.
Construct validity and content validity were addressed through the use of literature review, expert review, and examination of the relationship of test scores to external variables. Convergence (concurrent) and discriminant validity were assessed by comparing scores from the Adolescent/Adult Sensory Profile with scores obtained on the New York Longitudinal Scales (NYLS) Adult Temperament Questionnaire.[62] This study revealed moderate correlations between the Profile and the following areas on the NYLS: approach/withdrawal, adaptability, mood, and sensory threshold.
Internal consistency (reliability) was assessed using the coefficient alpha. The values for alpha for the various sections ranged from 0.639 to 0.775.
The **Standard Error of Measurement** (SEM), an index of the degree to which obtained scores differ from true scores, is provided for each possible quadrant raw score total for each cut-score group. The more reliable a test is, the smaller the SEM. SEM values for the Profile ranged from 3.58 to 4.51.[61]

Test of Sensory Functions in Infants (TSFI)[63]
1989
Georgia A. DeGangi and Stanley I. Greenspan

Purpose: The TSFI was designed to measure sensory processing and reactivity in infants. The TSFI is intended as both a research and a clinical tool for infants with regulatory disorders (eg, difficult temperament, irritability) and developmental delays and infants who are at-risk for later learning and sensory processing disorders. The TSFI may be used in combination with other standardized developmental motor, neuromotor, and cognitive tests to determine the infant's developmental functioning.

Ages: 4 to 18 months of age.

Time: 25 minutes to administer and score.

User
Qualifications: Occupational therapists, physical therapists, pediatricians, psychologists, and infant educators.

Test Kit: All materials needed for the test are included in the test kit. The test manual is comprehensive with scoring easy to follow (Figure 2-6). Illustrations also are provided in the test manual.

continued

Test of Sensory Functions in Infants (TSFI)

Administration and Scoring Form

Georgia A. DeGangi, Ph.D., O.T.R., and Stanley I. Greenspan, M.D.

Published by
WPS WESTERN PSYCHOLOGICAL SERVICES
12031 Wilshire Blvd., Los Angeles, CA 90025-1251
Publishers and Distributors

Name of Infant: _A A_

Birth Date: _____ Date of Testing: _____

Age (in months): _9 mos_   Sex: ☐ M ☒ F

Reason for Referral: _Hyper responsive to movement_

Directions

Administer the test according to the instructions presented in the Manual (WPS Catalog No. W-262C). During administration, score the items and record the item scores on the other side of this form. Each item is scored using a numerical rating scale. The criteria for scoring are summarized on the back of this form and detailed in the Manual. Determine the infant's score on each item according to these criteria and enter the number on the right.

After administration, add the item scores for each subtest and enter

the total next to the subtest name. Add the five subtest scores to obtain the Total Test Score and enter that number on the bottom right of the page. Then transfer the subtest scores and the Total Test Score to the profile form below by entering the scores in the appropriate boxes under the column heading "Score."

To use the profile form, place an "X" in the box that includes the infant's score on each subtest and the Total Test. Complete the profile by connecting the X's.

Profile Form

Subtest	Score	4-6 months Normal	4-6 months At Risk	4-6 months Deficient	7-9 months Normal	7-9 months At Risk	7-9 months Deficient	10-12 months Normal	10-12 months At Risk	10-12 months Deficient	13-18 months Normal	13-18 months At Risk	13-18 months Deficient
Reactivity to Tactile Deep Pressure	10	9-10	8	0-7	(9-10)	8	0-7	9-10	8	0-7	9-10	8	0-7
Adaptive Motor Functions	13	7-15	6	0-5	(11-15)	10	0-9	14-15	13	0-12	15	14	0-13
Visual-Tactile Integration	8	4-10	3	0-2	9-10	(7-8)	0-6	9-10	7-8	0-6	9-10	7-8	0-6
Ocular-Motor Control	2	1-2		0	(2)	1	0	2	1	0	2	1	0
Reactivity to Vestibular Stimulation	7	10-12	9	0-8	10-12	9	(0-8)	10-12	9	0-8	11-12	10	0-9
Total Test	40	33-40	30-32	0-29	41-49	(38-40)	0-37	44-49	41-43	0-40	44-49	41-43	0-40

Figure 2-6. TSFI administration and scoring form (Material from the TSFI copyright ©1983 Western Psychological Services. Reprinted by permission of the publisher, Western Psychological Services, 12031 Wilshire Blvd, Los Angeles, Calif, 90025, USA, www.wpspublish.com. Not to be reprinted in whole or in part for any additional purpose without the expressed, written permission of the publisher. All rights reserved).

Test Areas: The TSFI is a 24-item test that consists of five subtests which assess five areas of sensory function: 1) reactivity to tactile deep pressure, 2) visual-tactile integration, 3) adaptive motor responses, 4) ocular-motor control, and 5) reactivity to vestibular stimulation.

Administration: Individually administered to infant who may sit on the caregiver's lap for all except the vestibular subtest. Test results classify an infant as normal, at-risk, or deficient for the total test and in each of the five subtests. Cut scores are provided for four age groups: 4 to 6 months, 7 to 9 months, 10 to 12 months, and 13 to 18 months (see Figure 2-7).

continued

Psychometric
Characteristics: **Criterion-referenced measurement**

Content validity was assessed by using a two-stage judgmental review with a panel of eight infant assessment experts examining item-behavior congruence and representativeness. The judges used ratings of high, moderate, or poor for each item. Seventy-five percent to 85% of the ratings of item-behavior congruence were high for all items on the TSFI. Eighty-seven percent of the ratings of representativeness were high for all the subtests except Reactivity to Vestibular Stimulation, which was rated high 75% of the time. The panel concluded that: 1) the test items measured the behaviors they were intended to measure, and 2) the groups of items which constituted the individual subtests were representative of their respective domains. The content validity was stated to be moderate to high for the total test.

Construct validity was assessed through use of an analysis of item discrimination indexes, the estimation of classification decision accuracy, and the interrelationships of different subtests. The TSFI was found to be most accurate for diagnostic purposes in identifying normal infants 4 to 18 months old and infants with sensory dysfunction age 10 to 18 months old.[63] A false normal rate for the total test score was found to be 14% to 45%; a false delayed rate for the total test score was 11% to 19%.

Criterion validity was found to be low when compared to the Bayley Scales of Infant Development,[64] the Bates Infant Characteristics Questionnaire,[65] and the Fagan Test of Infant Intelligence.[66] However, the authors stated that this signifies the specific nature of the areas of behavior stimulated by the TSFI.

Interrater reliability was determined by using an occupational therapist and a physical therapist who scored the same test behaviors on the same children at the same time. Using intraclass correlations, coefficients from 0.88 to 0.99 were found for each of the five subtests and the total test scores. Interrater reliability of the TSFI has been evaluated with babies exposed to cocaine in utero.[67] Results showed the total test score to be highly reliable (r=0.92). However, the Ocular-Motor Control and Reactivity to Tactile Deep Pressure subtests were found to have lower interrater reliabilities (r=0.25 and r=0.67, respectively).

Decision-consistency reliability, as well as **test-retest reliability**, were examined. High levels of classification consistency were found throughout the test (81% to 96%). Pearson Product Moment correlation coefficients between test-retest scores were measured to assess stability of separate scores. Stability of the total test was good (r=0.81). There was also good stability determined for the Visual-Tactile Integration subtest (r=0.84) and the Ocular-Motor Control subtest (r=0.96). Stability was fair for the Reactivity to Tactile Deep Pressure subtest (r=0.77). Although test-retest reliability coefficients for vestibular and adaptive motor functioning domains were low (r=0.26 and r=0.64, respectively), DeGangi and Greenspan stated that subtest results may still be incorporated into the total test score due to its reliability. Similar results were found on a test-retest reliability study conducted by Jirikowic and colleagues for infants with developmental delays.[68]

DeGangi-Berk Test of Sensory Integration[69]
1983
Georgia A. DeGangi and Ronald A. Berk

Purpose:	To capture information about child's sensory processing for those for whom Sensory Integration and Praxis Test clinical observations are not appropriate. The tool is designed for early identification of sensory integrative dysfunction in preschool children.
Ages:	3 to 5 years.
Time:	30 minutes to administer and 20 minutes to score.
User Qualifications:	Occupational therapists and physical therapists.
Test Kit:	All materials needed for the test are included in the test kit except for a rolling pin, a scooter board, and a hula-hoop. The test manual is comprehensive with illustration and scoring instructions.

Test Areas: 36 scores on 13 separate items in three areas which are:
➤ Postural control—Assesses antigravity postures necessary for stabilization of the neck, trunk, and upper extremities as well as muscle cocontraction of the neck and upper extremities.
➤ Bilateral motor integration—Emphasizes bilateral motor coordination. Components of laterality include trunk rotation, crossing midline, rapid unilateral and bilateral hand movements, stability of upper/lower extremities in bilateral symmetrical postures, and dissociation of trunk and arm movements.
➤ Reflex integration—Assesses asymmetrical tonic reflexes, symmetrical tonic neck reflexes, and associated reactions.

Administration: Each of the individual test items are weighted with point values ranging from 0 to 1 to 0 to 4. Criteria for the assigning of a point value are described in the test manual. Scores for Postural Control, Bilateral Motor Integration, and the Total Test are obtained from administration of the entire battery. These scores are then compared against "normed" scores for children between 3 to 4 years of age or 5 years of age. Based on these "normed" scores, an individual child's score may be interpreted as normal, at-risk, or deficient. The authors stated that these results can be used for either screening or diagnosis, depending upon the needs of the child and examiner.

Psychometric Characteristics: **Criterion-Referenced Measurement**
Construct validity of the test was assessed by using two criterion groups of normal and delayed children. A total of 139 children, 101 normal and 38 delayed, representing ages 3 to 5 years, and three ethnic groups (eg, black, Hispanic, and white) were used. Results from administration of the original 73 items to these groups of children aided in determining item validity, decision validity, and test structure. The authors found that the total test scores could be used for screening decisions with better

continued

DeGangi-Berk Test of Sensory Integration Protocol Booklet

Georgia A. DeGangi, Ph.D., OTR and Ronald A. Berk, Ph.D.

Published by

WPS WESTERN PSYCHOLOGICAL SERVICES
12031 Wilshire Blvd., Los Angeles, CA 90025-1251
Publishers and distributors

Name: BJ   Sex: Ⓜ F   Test Date: ___ year ___ month ___ day

Address: ___   Birthdate: ___ year ___ month ___ day

School: ___   Grade: 3   Age: 3 year 1 month 29 day   Examiner: BC

Referred by: Teacher – Preschool

Reason for Referral: Poor coordination; ? gravitational insecurit

DIRECTIONS: Administer the test according to the instructions presented in the Manual. During administration, score the items and record the item scores in this booklet. Each item is scored using a numerical rating scale. The criteria for scoring are summarized in this booklet and detailed in the Manual. Determine the child's score on each item according to these criteria, and circle the corresponding number on the right. After administration, add the item scores in each column across all pages. Enter the subtest scores in the boxes at the bottom of the columns on page 4. Then transfer the subtest scores to the boxes below, and add them to obtain the Total Test Score.
To use the profile for Postural Control, Bilateral Motor Integration, and the total test, place an "X" in the box which includes the child's score on each. Complete the profile by connecting the X's.

10	+	13	+	4	=	27
Postural Control Score		Bilateral Motor Integration Score		Reflex Integration Score		Total Test Score

PROFILE

Functioning Level	Postural Control		Bilateral Motor Integration		Total Test Score	
	Ages 3-4	Age 5	Ages 3-4	Age 5	Ages 3-4	Age 5
Normal	20-30	20-30	30-42	30-42	52-88	52-88
At Risk	17-19		26-29		47-51	
Deficient	0-16	0-19	0-25	0-29	0-46	0-51

Note: The Reflex Integration score should be used only to determine the Total Test Score.

W-190C

Item Number	Description	Scoring Criterion	Item Score — Postural Control	Item Score — Bilateral Motor Integration	Item Score — Reflex Integration
1	**MONKEY TASK** Ability to hold position	Unable to hold .... 0 / Loses grip .... 1 / Head 6" below .... 2 / Head 2-6" below 3			
2	Number of seconds held	0 seconds .... 0 / 1-5 seconds .... 1 / 6-10 seconds .... 2 / 11-15 seconds .... 3 / 16 or more seconds 4			
3	**SIDE-SIT COCONTRACTION** Amount of resistance	None .... 0 / Slight .... 1 / Moderate to maximum 2			
4	Number of seconds held	0 seconds .... 0 / 1-5 seconds .... 1 / 6-10 seconds .... 2 / 11 or more seconds 3			
5	**ROLLING PIN ACTIVITY** Ability to maintain grasp Left Side / Right Side	Loses grasp .... 0 / Maintains grasp .... 1 // Loses grasp .... 0 / Maintains grasp 1			
6	Crosses midline, left — Point A / Point B / Point C	Does not cross .... 0 / Crosses .... 1 (each)			
7	Crosses midline, right — Point D / Point E / Point F	Does not cross .... 0 / Crosses .... 1 (each)			
8	**PRONE ON ELBOWS** Amount of resistance	None .... 0 / 1-2" head movement .... 1 / No head movement 2			
9	**WHEELBARROW WALK** Elbow position	Slight to moderate flexion .... 0 / Extends arm 1			
10	Distance	0-1 foot .... 0 / 2-4 feet .... 1 / 5-8 feet .... 2 / 9-10 feet 3			
11	**AIRPLANE** Placement of support	Shoulder .... 0 / Mid-chest .... 1 / Waist .... 2 / Hips 3			

Figure 2-7. Sample of completed TSI score sheet (Material from the TSFI copyright ©1983 Western Psychological Services. Reprinted by permission of the publisher, Western Psychological Services, 12031 Wilshire Blvd, Los Angeles, California, 90025, USA, www.wpspublish.com. Not to be reprinted in whole or in part for any additional purpose without the expressed, written permission of the publisher. All rights reserved.)

continued

than 80% accuracy and a 9% false normal error rate. The subtests of Postural Control and Bilateral Motor Integration were very accurate with false normal error rates below 7%. Based on the cutoff score used in the decision validity study, the test was found to be more effective in excluding normal children from a delayed population than excluding delayed children in a normal population.

Interrater reliability was assessed by using three different therapists and two independent samples of children which included a total of 33 children (26 normal and 7 delayed). Interrater reliabilities of 0.80 to 0.88 were found for the Postural Control and Bilateral Motor Integration subtests. The reliability scores for the Reflex Integration subtest varied from 0.24 to 0.66. Therefore, the authors cautioned against using the Reflex Integration subtest alone in making diagnoses.

Decision consistency reliability was determined by using a sample of 29 children, 23 normal and 6 delayed, who were tested twice during a 1-week retest interval. Three observers conducted the testing. High levels of classification consistency were found for all three subtests and for the total test with reliability scores ranging from 0.79 to 0.93.

Test-retest reliability information was obtained from the study on decision consistency reliability. The test-retest reliability coefficients ranged from 0.85 to 0.96 when each subtest, as well as the total test, was considered.

Sensitivity: 0.66 (reflex integration) to 0.84 (bilateral motor integration).
Specificity: 0.64 (bilateral motor integration) to 0.85 (total test).

Miller Assessment of Preschoolers (MAP)[70]
1982
Lucy Jane Miller

Purpose: The MAP was designed to identify children who exhibit mild to moderate developmental delays. The MAP was developed primarily for two purposes: 1) to develop a short screening tool to identify those children who need further evaluation, and 2) to provide a comprehensive, clinical framework that would be useful in identifying the child's strengths and weaknesses as a basis for further intervention.

Ages: 2 years, 9 months to 5 years, 8 months.

Time: 20 to 30 minutes to administer and score.

User Qualifications: Occupational therapists and physical therapists.

Test Kit: Manual, scores sheets, and materials needed for the test are included.

Test Areas: The 27 test items are divided into five performance indices: foundations, coordination, verbal, nonverbal, and complex tasks.

continued

Administration: The test is individually administered using the materials included in the test kit. Most of the items are novel and presented in a game-like fashion. A profile of the individual child's performance is derived by comparing the final scores to a table of Final Percentile Scores and a graphic profile of the child's abilities is obtained.

Psychometric
Characteristics: **Norm-referenced measurement**
The test was normed on a nationally randomly selected stratified sample of 600 normal preschool children and on a select sample of 60 children with preacademic problems. No children with physical or other identified disabilities were used in the sampling. The test edition used in the normative study contained 530 items; however, only 27 items and a series of structured observations were used in the final edition. The final edition of the test was standardized in all nine of the US Census Bureau regions on a randomly selected sample of 1200 preschoolers with appropriate ratios according to sex, age, race, size of residential community, and socioeconomic factors.

Construct validity was assessed by examining how many children who were previously identified as functionally delayed would be identified by the MAP. Seventy-five percent of the children were correctly identified in the study.

Content validity assessed through a correlational analysis of each item and index revealed that the test items contributed to the total test significantly ($P<0.01$); each index was found to be fairly equal (0.64 to 0.77). Interrater reliability coefficient of 0.98 was obtained in a study involving 40 children and two examiners.[70]

Test-retest reliability on a sample of 90 children showed that the final score category of 81% of the children remained stable over two testing sessions 1 to 4 weeks apart. The coefficient of internal consistency on the total sample was 0.79.

Sensory Integration and Praxis Tests (SIPT)[71]
1989
A. Jean Ayres

Purpose: The tests were developed to measure the sensory integration processes that underlie learning and behavior.

Ages: 4 to 8 years, 11 months.

Time: The entire test battery takes approximately 2 hours to administer. An additional 45 minutes to an hour is needed for scoring and an additional hour for interpretation after the profile is developed.

User
Qualifications: Certification in administration and interpretation of these tests is necessary for use of the test as a diagnostic tool. Occupational therapists and physical therapists are eligible for certification.

Test Kit: The SIPT test materials and score sheets are included in the test kit.

Test Areas: The 17 subtests of the SIPT are categorized into four overlapping groups: Tactile, Vestibular, and Proprioceptive Sensory Processing Tests; Form and Space Perception and Visuomotor Coordination Tests; Praxis Tests; and Bilateral Integration and Sequencing Tests. Table 2-2 identifies the subtests that comprise the four groupings.

Administration: The SIPT is individually administered. The tests are then computer scored based on completed computer score sheets which are sent to Western Psychological Services for weighting of scores and determination of standard scores based on available norms. Scoring also can be done by the examiner if a computer scoring disk is purchased.

Psychometric
Characteristics: **Norm-referenced measurement**
                    The SIPT represents an evolution of the Southern California Sensory Integration Tests (SCSIT)[72] and the Southern California Postrotary Nystagmus Test (SCPNT).[73] Ayres, during the 1960s and 1970s, performed numerous factor analyses on the subtests of the SCSIT.[74-77] Based on these factor analyses, several of the subtests from the SCSIT were not included on the new SIPT either due to their lack of clinical usefulness, the difficulty in administrating the subtest, or poor reliability in measurement of the function.
                    In the development of the new subtests for the SIPT and in the revision of the SCSIT, field and pilot studies were done during the early 1980s. In these pilot studies, three criteria were used in the selection of the final tests and individual test items: the capability of each item to distinguish between dysfunctional and normal children, evidence of a logical association between items and functions under assessment, and interrater/test-retest reliability. Based on these pilot studies, the final version of the SIPT was comprised of tests designed to assess sensory perception and the processing of tactile, proprioceptive, vestibular, and visual input as well as several aspects of praxis.

continued

Table 2-2
SIPT Subtests

Tactile and Vestibular Proprioceptive Sensory Processing

Kinesthesia
Finger identification
Graphesthesia
Localization of tactile stimuli
Postrotary nystagmus
Standing and walking balance

Form and Space Perception and Visuomotor Coordination

Space visualization
Figure-ground perception
Manual form perception
Motor accuracy
Design copy

Praxis

Design copying
Constructional praxis
Postural praxis
Praxis on verbal command
Sequencing praxis
Oral praxis

Bilateral Integration and Sequencing

Oral praxis
Sequencing praxis
Graphesthesia
Standing and walking balance
Bilateral motor coordination
Space visualization contralateral use
Space visualization preferred hand use

The SIPT was normed using the 1980 US Census to determine the appropriate representation of the US population in the normative sample. The variables considered in selecting the sample were age, sex, ethnicity, type of community, and geographic location. The final normative sample was comprised of approximately 2000 children, between the ages of 4 years, 0 months to 8 years, 11 months with an almost equal number of boys and girls. Children in the sample were evaluated by selected examiners who were trained on the administration and scoring of the SIPT and who were tested on their administration skills at workshops held around the United States. Preliminary analyses of the normative sample revealed significant age and sex differences on the SIPT tests. Therefore, separate norms were established for boys and girls in 12 age groups. Additionally, means and standard deviations were computed for each of the normative subgroups. Most of the individual tests of the SIPT also yielded subscores for time and accuracy.

continued

Content validity was established according to Ayres through the work that led to the development of the SCSIT, the refinement of the SCSIT, and through consultation with experts in the area of sensory integration. **Construct validity** was examined through the use of numerous factor analyses conducted by Ayres and reported in the SIPT manual. Additionally, multiple discriminant analyses were used by Ayres with a matched sample of 352 children without dysfunction and children with sensory integrative problems. The weights for time and accuracy scores that adequately discriminated between the two groups of children were used in the final version of the test. In preliminary studies using the SIPT in various populations, each of the subtests of the SIPT discriminated between children without dysfunction and those with dysfunction at a statistically significant level (P<0.01).[72] Construct validity has been further supported by Murray, Cermak, and O'Brien who studied 21 children with learning disabilities and 18 children without learning disabilities, aged 5 to 8 years, to determine the relationship between form and space perception, constructional abilities, and clumsiness.[78] The children with learning disabilities in the study were further divided into two groups, clumsy and nonclumsy, based on their scores on a test of motor behaviors. All children in the study were assessed using six of the SIPT subtests that measure form and space perception and visual construction. Results indicated that both groups of learning disabled children scored lower than the nonlearning disabled children on four of the six SIPT subtests (space visualization, motor accuracy, design copying, and constructional praxis) at a significant level. Within the two learning disabled groups, the clumsy and nonclumsy children differed significantly from each other only on the Motor Accuracy and Design Copying subtests. The degree of clumsiness in the 12 children who were identified as clumsy was correlated significantly with three of the six subtests (Space Visualization, Motor Accuracy, and Design Copying).

Test-retest reliability coefficients for the 17 subtests of the SIPT were reported by Ayres as ranging from 0.48 to 0.93.[38] The praxis tests had the highest test-retest reliability, but reliabilities for most of the other tests were acceptable. Four of the tests had reliability coefficients below 0.70: Postrotary Nystagmus, Kinesthesia, Localization of Tactile Stimuli, and Figure-Ground Perception. Ayres reported that the small sample size and the predominance of children with dysfunction in the test-retest reliability study, and the nature of the assessed neural functions in the SIPT may have affected the test-retest reliability of these subtests.[72]

Interrater reliability studies for the SIPT revealed correlation coefficients for all of the major SIPT scores to be between 0.94 and 0.99 when trained examiners were used.[72]

Clinical Observations of Motor and Postural Skills (COMPS)[79]
2000
Brenda Wilson, Nancy Pollock, Bonnie Kaplan, and Mary Law

Purpose: To screen children for the presence or absence of motor problems with a postural component.

Ages: 5 to 16 years.

Time: 15 to 20 minutes to administer.

User Qualifications: Occupational therapists and physical therapists.

Test Kit: The test kit is comprised of a test manual, two asymmetrical tonic neck reflex measurement tools, and a score sheet.

Test Areas: The COMPS is made up of six items :
➤ Slow movements
➤ Rapid forearm rotation
➤ Finger-nose touching
➤ Prone extension posture
➤ Asymmetrical tonic neck reflex
➤ Supine flexion posture

Administration: The test should be administered in the sequence of the six items as outlined in the test manual. It is most important that the last three items be given in the order listed. Stretch to the flexors muscles is stated to have a facilitation effect on these muscles and thus the administration of the Supine Flexion item immediately following the Prone Extension could result in an exaggerated performance. The tool is not designed nor recommended to be used for children with known neurological or neuromotor problems.

Psychometric Characteristics: **Criterion-referenced measurement**
The test was originally developed for children between the ages of 5 to 9 years. The authors later tested 261 children between the ages of 10 to 16 years to develop standards for older children.
Interater reliability intraclass correlation coefficients (ICCs) were found to be 0.57 between occupational therapists with pediatric experience and those without, with children with developmental coordination disorder (DCD). The ICC for occupational therapists with pediatric experience with this group of children was 0.76. When evaluating children without DCD, the ICC between occupational therapists with experience and those without, was found to be 0.81. The ICCs between occupational therapists with pediatric experience in the group of children without DCD was higher at 0.90.
Test-retest reliability using the ICC was found to be 0.87 for children with DCD and 0.76 for the non-DCD group.

continued

The Cronbach's coefficient alpha was used to assess **internal consisten-cy**. The alpha coefficient for the total test with younger children was 0.77. The internal consistency for the older children was at 0.69. Both of these values were at an acceptable level of internal consistency.

Construct validity was assessed by the examination of the discriminant values of the test. The analysis showed that the COMPS discriminated between those children who had DCD and those who were non-DCD.

Concurrent validity was assessed by comparing scores on the COMPS with test performance of the younger DCD group and the non-DCD group on six measures other than the COMPS (balance subtest from the Bruininks-Oseretsky Test of Motor Proficiency, the Motor Accuracy tests from the Sensory Integration and Praxis Tests dominant and nondomi-nant hand, the VMI, and tests of Standing Balance eyes open and eyes closed). Scores ranged from 0.40 on the motor accuracy test to 0.48 on the VMI when using the Pearson r.

Sensitivity was found to be 82% to 100% for the younger children (5 to 9 years) and 23% to 59% for the older children (10 to 12 years and older).

Specificity was found to be 63% to 90% for the younger children and 88% to 98% for the older children.

Sensory Integration Inventory for Individuals With Developmental Disabilities—Revised (SII-R)[80]
1992
Judith E. Reisman and Bonnie Hanschu

Purpose: To screen for clients who might benefit from a sensory integration treat-ment approach.

Ages: Any age child or adult with developmental disabilities.

Time: 20 to 30 minutes to administer and score.

User
Qualifications: Occupational therapists and physical therapists.

Test Kit: The test is comprised of a test manual and a score sheet (Figure 2-8).

Test Areas: The SII-R addresses the areas of tactile, vestibular, and proprioceptive processing as well as general reactions to sensory input. The individual's responses to these sensory inputs are linked to the following:
➤ Tactile—Dressing, activities of daily living, personal space, social, self-stimulatory behaviors, and self-injurious behaviors.
➤ Vestibular—Muscle tone, equilibrium responses, posture and move-ment, bilateral coordination, spatial perception, emotional expres-sion, and self-stimulatory behaviors.
➤ Proprioception—Muscle tone, motor skills (planning and body image), self-stimulatory behaviors, and self-injurious behaviors.

continued

SENSORY INTEGRATION INVENTORY-REVISED
FOR INDIVIDUALS WITH DEVELOPMENTAL DISABILITIES

CLIENT INFORMATION

Name of client.

Date of birth.

Living unit.   Day program

Diagnoses:

Medications:

Does this client have a seizure disorder?
If yes, is it controlled?   Last seizure ___ / ___ / ___

Visual impairment?   Hearing impairment?
Wears glasses?   Wears hearing aid?

Targeted maladaptive behaviors:
☐ Cyclical   ☐ Non-cyclical

Person(s) interviewed:

Inventory completed by: _____ Title _____ On ___ / ___ / ___

Results interpreted by: _____ Title _____ On ___ / ___ / ___

Conclusion:
☐ Sensory integrative dysfunction may be present. Further evaluation is needed.
☐ Sensory integrative dysfunction may be ruled out.

Reisman, Hanschu, 1992

SENSORY INTEGRATION INVENTORY-REVISED
FOR INDIVIDUALS WITH DEVELOPMENTAL DISABILITIES

TACTILE

Dressing
Y N ?
___ T1. Layers clothing
___ T2. Pushes up pant legs, sleeves, shirts
___ T3. Strips off clothing
___ T4. Refuses to undress
___ T5. Frequently adjusts clothing as if it binds or is uncomfortable
___ T6. Wraps self in clothing or bedding
___ T7. Insists on something wrapped around wrist, arm, finger
___ T8. Avoids/irritated by certain clothing textures
___ T9. Indicates distress when barefoot
___ T10. Insists on being barefoot
Comments:

Other Activities of Daily Living
___ T11. Spits out/rejects certain food textures
___ T12. Resists grooming (circle which)
   a. face washing   e. toothbrushing
   b. shaving   f. nail trimming
   c. hair combing   g. bathing
   d. hair cutting   h. hair washing
Comments:

Personal Space
___ T13. Insists on large personal space
___ T14. Prefers to be in corner, under table, behind furniture
Comments:

Social
___ T15. Looks fearful, angry, or uncomfortable when approached, or touched
___ T16. Withdraws or hits when peers reach toward client or are nearby
___ T17. Withdraws or hits when staff reach toward client, or are nearby
___ T18. Rubs spot after being touched
___ T19. Exhibits clingy behavior
___ T20. Tries to handle or touch everything/everyone
___ T21. Avoids palm/hand contact with objects or people
Comments:

Self-stimulatory Behaviors
___ T22. Engages in persistent hand to mouth activity
___ T23. Mouths objects or clothing
___ T24. Rubs or plays with spit
___ T25. Persistently has hand in pants or pants pocket
___ T26. Sits on hands/feet
___ T27. Pushes or rubs body against objects/walls/people
___ T28. Insists on holding an object in hand(s)
___ T29. Rubs finger(s) against hand or other fingers
Comments:

Self-injurious Behaviors
___ T30. Scratches
___ T31. Pinches
___ T32. Rubs
___ T33. Hits/slaps
___ T34. Pulls hair
___ T35. Bites hand/wrist/arm
Comments:

Copyright 1992. Do not reproduce. If not printed in blue ink, this form has been illegally reproduced.

Reisman, Hanschu, 1992

Figure 2-8. Sample score sheet (tactile) (reprinted with permission from Reisman JE, Hanschu B. *Sensory Integration Inventory for Individuals With Developmental Disabilities—Revised*. Stillwater, Minn: PDP Press; 1992).

continued

Administration: The Inventory can be used in two ways. The first is by the therapy staff who are familiar with the individual and who can complete the questionnaire. The second is as a semistructured interview of those who are most familiar with the individual. The individual questions on the Inventory are scored as yes or no. The item is scored as "yes" if the behavior is typical and has been observed, reported, or can be elicited through testing. The item is scored as "no" if the behavior if not typical or characteristic of the individual. A question mark can be used if the tester is unsure if the behavior is typical even though it has been observed. There are no set numbers of questions that must be marked yes before an individual is considered to have sensory integrative dysfunction. The Inventory is best used as a means of explaining an individual's behavior in his day-to-day environment.

Psychometric
Characteristics: **Criterion-referenced measurement**
The test was originally developed at the Cambridge Regional Human Service Center (CRHSC) which provided services for approximately 300 adults with mental retardation. The pilot for the tools was used to screen clients at the CRHSC. After the publication of the first edition of the Inventory, therapists reported that the Inventory was useful in assessing individuals who could not cooperate fully in a testing situation. These included children with autism and pervasive developmental disorders and adults with schizophrenia, Alzheimer's disease, and other psychogeriatric conditions.[80]
No psychometric characteristics are reported in the test manual.

Sensorimotor Performance Analysis (SPA)[81]
1989
Eileen W. Richter and Patricia C. Montgomery

Purpose: To provide a qualitative record of an individual's performance on selected motor tasks.

Ages: 5 to 21 years.

Time: 30 to 45 minutes to administer and score.

User
Qualifications: Physical therapists and occupational therapists with experience in pediatrics.

Test Kit: The test is comprised of a test manual and a score sheet (Figure 2-9). Minimal equipment is necessary for the administration: tape, tilt board, suspended tether ball, pencils, large paper, table and chairs, scissors, pellets, small bottle, and a drawing of a "+" and an "o."

continued

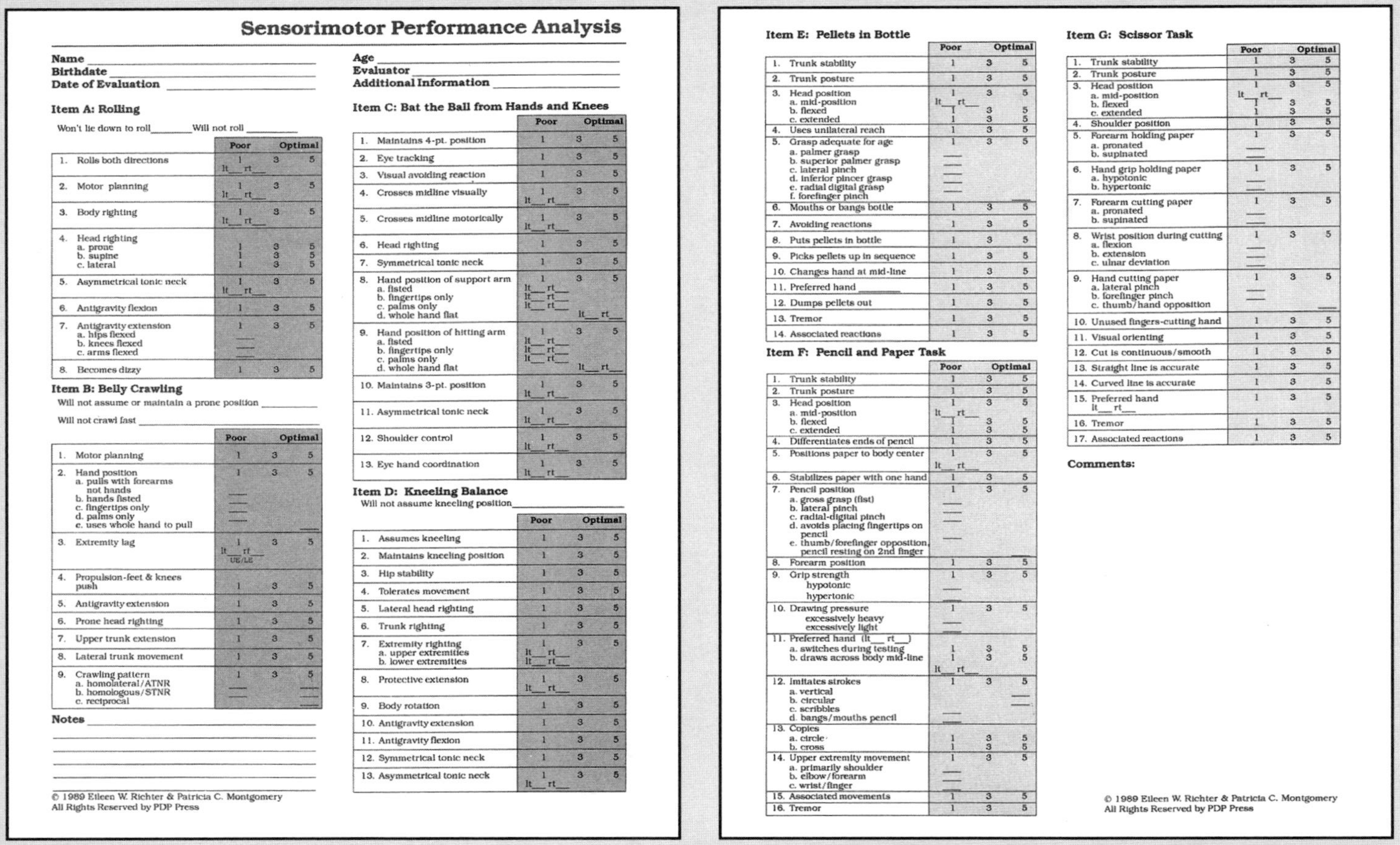

Sensorimotor Performance Analysis

Name ___ Age ___
Birthdate ___ Evaluator ___
Date of Evaluation ___ Additional Information ___

Item A: Rolling

Won't lie down to roll___ Will not roll___

	Poor		Optimal
1. Rolls both directions	1 lt__rt__	3	5
2. Motor planning	1 lt__rt__	3	5
3. Body righting	1 lt__rt__	3	5
4. Head righting			
a. prone	1	3	5
b. supine	1	3	5
c. lateral	1	3	5
5. Asymmetrical tonic neck	1 lt__rt__	3	5
6. Antigravity flexion	1	3	5
7. Antigravity extension	1	3	5
a. hips flexed	___		
b. knees flexed	___		
c. arms flexed	___		
8. Becomes dizzy	1	3	5

Item B: Belly Crawling

Will not assume or maintain a prone position ___

Will not crawl fast ___

	Poor		Optimal
1. Motor planning	1	3	5
2. Hand position	1	3	5
a. pulls with forearms not hands	___		
b. hands fisted	___		
c. fingertips only	___		
d. palms only	___		
e. uses whole hand to pull			___
3. Extremity lag	1 lt__rt__ UE/LE	3	5
4. Propulsion-feet & knees push	1	3	5
5. Antigravity extension	1	3	5
6. Prone head righting	1	3	5
7. Upper trunk extension	1	3	5
8. Lateral trunk movement	1	3	5
9. Crawling pattern	1	3	5
a. homolateral/ATNR	___		___
b. homologous/STNR	___		___
c. reciprocal			___

Notes ___

Item C: Bat the Ball from Hands and Knees

	Poor		Optimal
1. Maintains 4-pt. position	1	3	5
2. Eye tracking	1	3	5
3. Visual avoiding reaction	1	3	5
4. Crosses midline visually	1 lt__rt__	3	5
5. Crosses midline motorically	1 lt__rt__	3	5
6. Head righting	1	3	5
7. Symmetrical tonic neck	1	3	5
8. Hand position of support arm	1	3	5
a. fisted	lt__rt__		
b. fingertips only	lt__rt__		
c. palms only	lt__rt__		
d. whole hand flat			lt__rt__
9. Hand position of hitting arm	1	3	5
a. fisted	lt__rt__		
b. fingertips only	lt__rt__		
c. palms only	lt__rt__		
d. whole hand flat			lt__rt__
10. Maintains 3-pt. position	1 lt__rt__	3	5
11. Asymmetrical tonic neck	1 lt__rt__	3	5
12. Shoulder control	1 lt__rt__	3	5
13. Eye hand coordination	1 lt__rt__	3	5

Item D: Kneeling Balance

Will not assume kneeling position___

	Poor		Optimal
1. Assumes kneeling	1	3	5
2. Maintains kneeling position	1	3	5
3. Hip stability	1	3	5
4. Tolerates movement	1	3	5
5. Lateral head righting	1	3	5
6. Trunk righting	1	3	5
7. Extremity righting	1	3	5
a. upper extremities	lt__rt__		
b. lower extremities	lt__rt__		
8. Protective extension	1 lt__rt__	3	5
9. Body rotation	1	3	5
10. Antigravity extension	1	3	5
11. Antigravity flexion	1	3	5
12. Symmetrical tonic neck	1	3	5
13. Asymmetrical tonic neck	1 lt__rt__	3	5

Item E: Pellets in Bottle

	Poor		Optimal
1. Trunk stability	1	3	5
2. Trunk posture	1	3	5
3. Head position	1	3	5
a. mid-position	lt__rt__		
b. flexed	1	3	5
c. extended	1	3	5
4. Uses unilateral reach	1	3	5
5. Grasp adequate for age	1	3	5
a. palmer grasp	___		
b. superior palmer grasp	___		
c. lateral pinch	___		
d. inferior pincer grasp	___		
e. radial digital grasp	___		
f. forefinger pinch			___
6. Mouths or bangs bottle	1	3	5
7. Avoiding reactions	1	3	5
8. Puts pellets in bottle	1	3	5
9. Picks pellets up in sequence	1	3	5
10. Changes hand at mid-line	1	3	5
11. Preferred hand ___	1	3	5
12. Dumps pellets out	1	3	5
13. Tremor	1	3	5
14. Associated reactions	1	3	5

Item F: Pencil and Paper Task

	Poor		Optimal
1. Trunk stability	1	3	5
2. Trunk posture	1	3	5
3. Head position	1	3	5
a. mid-position	lt__rt__		
b. flexed	1	3	5
c. extended	1	3	5
4. Differentiates ends of pencil	1	3	5
5. Positions paper to body center	1 lt__rt__	3	5
6. Stabilizes paper with one hand	1	3	5
7. Pencil position	1	3	5
a. gross grasp (fist)	___		
b. lateral pinch	___		
c. radial-digital pinch	___		
d. avoids placing fingertips on pencil	___		
e. thumb/forefinger opposition, pencil resting on 2nd finger			___
8. Forearm position	1	3	5
9. Grip strength	1	3	5
hypotonic	___		
hypertonic	___		
10. Drawing pressure	1	3	5
excessively heavy	___		
excessively light	___		
11. Preferred hand (lt__ rt__)			
a. switches during testing	1	3	5
b. draws across body mid-line	1 lt__rt__	3	5
12. Imitates strokes	1	3	5
a. vertical			___
b. circular			___
c. scribbles	___		
d. bangs/mouths pencil	___		
13. Copies			
a. circle	1	3	5
b. cross	1	3	5
14. Upper extremity movement	1	3	5
a. primarily shoulder	___		
b. elbow/forearm	___		
c. wrist/finger	___		
15. Associated movements	1	3	5
16. Tremor	1	3	5

Item G: Scissor Task

	Poor		Optimal
1. Trunk stability	1	3	5
2. Trunk posture	1	3	5
3. Head position	1	3	5
a. mid-position	lt__rt__		
b. flexed	1	3	5
c. extended	1	3	5
4. Shoulder position	1	3	5
5. Forearm holding paper	1	3	5
a. pronated	___		
b. supinated	___		
6. Hand grip holding paper	1	3	5
a. hypotonic	___		
b. hypertonic	___		
7. Forearm cutting paper	1	3	5
a. pronated	___		
b. supinated	___		
8. Wrist position during cutting	1	3	5
a. flexion	___		
b. extension	___		
c. ulnar deviation	___		
9. Hand cutting paper	1	3	5
a. lateral pinch	___		
b. forefinger pinch	___		
c. thumb/hand opposition			___
10. Unused fingers-cutting hand	1	3	5
11. Visual orienting	1	3	5
12. Cut is continuous/smooth	1	3	5
13. Straight line is accurate	1	3	5
14. Curved line is accurate	1	3	5
15. Preferred hand	1 lt__rt__	3	5
16. Tremor	1	3	5
17. Associated reactions	1	3	5

Comments:

Figure 2-9. Sample score sheet (reprinted with permission from Richter EW, Montgomery PC. *The Sensorimotor Performance Analysis.* Hugo, Minn: PDP Press; 1989).

continued

Test Areas:	The SPA tasks are:

➤ Rolling
➤ Belly crawling
➤ Bat the ball from three point
➤ Kneeling balance
➤ Pellets in a bottle
➤ Paper and pencil task
➤ Scissor task

Administration: The SPA is individually administered to the child and the criterion for each task is on the test form. The criterion is scored on a continuum from 1 to 5. Poor performance is represented by 1, inadequate by 3, and optimal by 5. Operational definitions for the scores for each item are presented in the test manual. Sixteen sensorimotor components are analyzed during each task on the test. These sensorimotor components include: asymmetrical tonic neck reflex (ATNR), symmetrical tonic neck reflex (STNR), antigravity extension, antigravity flexion, body righting, head righting, equilibrium/righting reactions, vestibular function, tactile processing, visual processing, bilateral integration, motor planning, tone/strength, stability/mobility, neurological status, and developmental level.

Psychometric
Characteristics: **Criterion-referenced measurement**

Concurrent validity: The test was originally developed for use with children with mental challenges. No specific sensorimotor tests were appropriate at the time of development of the SPA for examining concurrent validity.

Test-retest reliability was assessed in a study with 10 children who were mentally challenged (IQ between 50 to 80) who did not have accompanying physical disabilities such as neuromotor disorders. The subjects' performance on the SPA was compared to their performance 1 week later. Test-retest reliability coefficients ranged from 0.89 to 0.97.

Interrater reliability was determined using the same children as those used for test-retest reliability. Using the first test session, a second observer simultaneously assessed and scored the children. Correlation coefficients ranged from 0.15 to 0.91. There was poor agreement between raters for the ATNR (r=0.21), STNR (r=0.15), and tactile processing (r=0.31). If these three scores were eliminated, an interrater reliability score of 0.76 was obtained.

Functional Assessments

STANDARDIZED ASSESSMENT OF INSTRUMENTAL DAILY LIVING SKILLS

Pediatric Evaluation of Disability Inventory (PEDI)[11]
1992
Stephen M. Haley, Wendy J. Coster, Larry H. Ludlow, Jane T. Haltiwanger, and Peter J. Anrellos

Purpose:	To sample key functional capabilities and performance in children, to identify the level of independence in performance of activities, to determine the extent of modifications needed to perform the task, to monitor progress in functional capabilities, and to assist with intervention planning.
Ages:	6 months to 7.5 years.
Time:	45 to 60 minutes to administer and score. The time necessary is dependent on a number of factors, including the parent's degree of comfort with the examiner, the complexity of the child's disability, and the parent's ability to provide the information requested.
User Qualifications:	Physical therapists, occupational therapists, speech-language pathologists, nurses, and educators.
Test Kit:	The test is comprised of a test manual and a score sheet (Figure 2-10). The test manual is detailed and has operational definitions for scores for each part of the PEDI.
Test Areas:	The PEDI contains three measurement sections. Part I, Functional Skills, is a checklist record of the child's abilities in functional skills. The Functional Skills Scale is divided into three sections: self-care, mobility, and social function. Part II, Caregiver Assistance, assesses the amount of assistance needed by the child during complex functional activities. Part III, Modifications Scale, identifies the modifications needed by the child during the completion of the functional skills.
Administration:	The PEDI depends on parental report. The checklist may be given to parents for independent completion or it may be completed by an examiner during an interview. If the parents fill out the checklist independently, the examiner should review the answers with the parents after completion.
	Items in Part I, Functional Skills Scale, are scored as "capable" (1) or "unable" (0). At the end of each section of Part I, the scores are added up to obtain a domain score. In Parts II and III, each of the 20 items requires one score for Caregiver Assistance and one for Modifications. At the end of each content domain, the scores are added up for the Caregiver Assistance item scores and a list of frequencies for each of the Modifications Scale levels is obtained. The summary scores from each Part of the PEDI can be transposed into a Composite Score and further into normative standard scores and scaled scores.

continued

CHAPTER 10: PEDI CASE STUDIES

Pediatric Evaluation of Disability Inventory

VERSION 1.0

Name _CASE 3 (MARK)_   Test Date _____ Age _11_

ID# _____   Respondent/Interviewer _____

SCORE SUMMARY

Composite Scores

DOMAIN		RAW SCORE	NORMATIVE STANDARD SCORE	STANDARD ERROR	SCALED SCORE	STANDARD ERROR	FIT SCORE*
Self-Care	Functional Skills	29			48.2	1.7	
Mobility	Functional Skills	18			40.3	2.3	
Social Function	Functional Skills	59			59.9	1.3	
Self-Care	Caregiver Assistance	15			49.8	3.7	
Mobility	Caregiver Assistance	10			42.7	4.3	
Social Function	Caregiver Assistance	21			75.3	5.6	

*Obtainable only through use of software program

MODIFICATION FREQUENCIES

SELF-CARE (8 ITEMS)				MOBILITY (7 ITEMS)				SOCIAL FUNCTION (5 ITEMS)			
None	Child	Rehab	Extensive	None	Child	Rehab	Extensive	None	Child	Rehab	Extensive
3	2	3	0	2	0	1	4	5	0	0	0

Score Profile

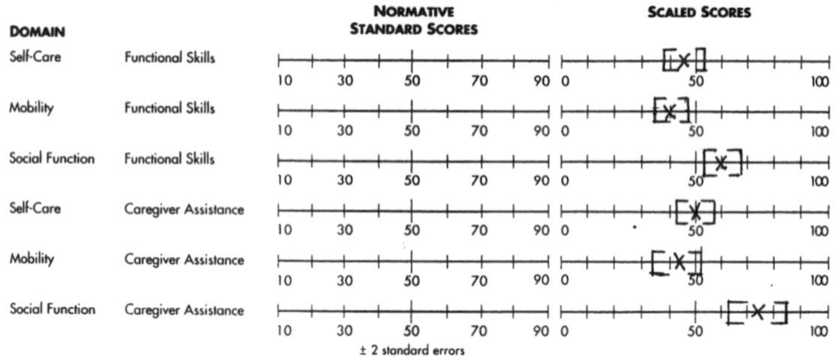

± 2 standard errors

© 1992 New England Medical Center and PEDI Research Group. Reproduction of this form without prior written permission is prohibited.

Figure 2-10. Sample score sheet (reprinted with permission from Haley SM, Coster WJ, Ludlow LH, et al. *Pediatric Evaluation of Disability Inventory [PEDI].* Boston, Mass: Trustees of Boston University, Center for Rehabilitation Effectiveness; 1992).

Psychometric
Characteristics: **Norm-referenced measurement**

Standardization of the PEDI was conducted on a regional sample of nondisabled children (n=412) who were selected via a stratified quota sampling strategy according to demographic data based upon the 1980 US census. Normative data were collected between May 1990 and June 1991. Three small samples of children with disabilities were used as clinical validation samples. The samples included children with:

continued

1) relatively minor injuries but seen at a tertiary pediatric trauma center, 2) severe disabilities enrolled in a hospital-based school program, and 3) children with cerebral palsy, developmental delay, and traumatic brain injury and enrolled in a hospital-based day school program.

Concurrent validity: During the pilot development of the PEDI, scores on the PEDI for a sample of children with disabilities were compared to scores on the Battelle Developmental Inventory Screening Test (BDIST).[82] The overall correlations between the two instruments were moderate (r=0.70 to 0.73).[83] An additional study using more severely involved children compared scores on the PEDI, the BDIST, and the Functional Independence Measure for Children (WeeFim).[84] Strong correlations were found between the PEDI and these two instruments (r=0.80 to 0.97).

Discriminant validity studies revealed that the PEDI could predict accurately a child's group (nondisabled or clinical) except for a few scores (social function and mobility) in the children ages 6 months to 2 years.[11]

Internal consistency of all six scales was determined using the Cronbach's coefficient alpha. These correlations were found to range between 0.95 to 0.99.

Interrater reliability using the ICC was calculated for a normative sample of children. Scores ranged from 0.96 to 0.99 for the Caregiver Assistance Scales. The scores for Modifications ranged from 0.79 to 1.00. ICCs for a clinical sample of children were found to range from 0.84 to 1.00 for both the Caregiver Assistance and the Modifications scales.

School Function Assessment (SFA)[2]
1998
Wendy Coster, Theresa Deeney, Jane Haltiwanger, and Stephen Haley

Purpose:	To measure a student's performance of functional tasks that support participation in the academic and social aspects of the educational environment between grades K to 6. An additional purpose was to facilitate collaborative program planning for students with varying disabling conditions.
Ages:	Children in kindergarten through sixth grade.
Time:	New users of the SFA should allow a minimum of 1.5 to 2 hours to complete the assessment. Once familiar with the test, the time to administer either individual parts or the entire scale should decrease. Typically, the assessment is not completed within a single day. However, the assessment period should not extend longer than 2 to 3 weeks.
User Qualifications:	Physical therapists, occupational therapists, speech-language pathologists, psychologists, and educators.

continued

Test Kit:	The test is comprised of a user's manual, a ratings scale guide, and a record form (Figure 2-11). The test manual is detailed and has operational definitions for scores for each part of the SFA.
Test Areas:	The SFA is divided into three parts. Each part has one or more scales. Part I, Participation, allows for assessment of the student's participation in six major school-related activity settings. Part II, Task Supports, is comprised of four scales. Two types of support, assistance and adaptations are rated for physical and cognitive/ behavioral tasks. Part III, Activity Performance, is comprised of 21 separate scales: Travel, Maintaining and Changing Positions, Recreational Movement, Manipulation with Movement, Using Materials, Setup and Cleanup, Eating and Drinking, Hygiene, Clothing Management, Up/Down Stairs, Written Work, Computer and Equipment Use, Functional Communication, Memory and Understanding, Following Social Conventions, Compliance with Adult Directives and School Rules, Task Behavior/Completion, Positive Interaction, Behavior Regulation, Personal Care Awareness, and Safety.
Administration:	The SFA is a judgment-based questionnaire that is completed by one or more school professionals who know the student well. The ratings from Part I are summed to yield a Participation total raw score. In Part II, Task Supports, a total raw score for each of the following scales is generated: Physical Tasks Assistance, Physical Tasks Adaptation, Cognitive/ Behavioral Tasks Assistance, and Cognitive/Behavioral Tasks Adaptations. A total raw score is generated for each of the 21 separate scales in Part III, Activity Performance. The raw scores obtained are converted to a criterion score using tables in the test manual. A standard error value (SEM) also is obtained for each criterion score. Two criterion cutoff scores are provided for each scale, one for grades K to 3 and one for grades 4 to 6. By using the criterion scores, the examiner can create a functional profile for the student by plotting the student's score for each scale on the profile graph.
Psychometric Characteristics:	**Criterion-referenced measurement** A sample of 363 students with disabilities participated in the standardization of the SFA. The children were drawn from 112 different sites in 40 states. Fifty-seven percent of the students were in regular classrooms and 43% were in special education but with some degree of mainstreaming. More boys (66%) than girls (34%) were represented in the standardization. Three-hundred-fifteen children who were in regular education comprised the remainder of the sample. Forty-seven percent of the students in regular education were male and 53% were female. The sample of special needs and regular education students mirrored the race/ethnicity percentages of children in the 1990 US Census. Two **content validity** studies were conducted during the development of the SFA using panels of experts.

continued

Adaptations Checklist (continued)

Cognitive
- [ ] alternative curriculum
- [ ] alternative/modified materials
- [ ] adjusted expectations/objectives
- [ ] additional repetition or practice
- [ ] alternative/modified directions
- [ ] alternative/modified form of evaluation
- [ ] multisensory approach
- [ ] change in pace or sequence of activities
- [ ] extended time
- [ ] use of notebooks or lists
- [ ] peer involvement
- [ ] other (describe below)

Comments/Descriptions: _____

Communication
- [ ] signal system
- [ ] communication board
- [ ] communication book
- [ ] speech output device
- [ ] mouthstick
- [ ] headwand
- [ ] choice program
- [ ] hearing aids
- [ ] microphone
- [ ] interpreter
- [ ] Braille
- [ ] other (describe below)

Comments/Descriptions: _____

Computer
- [ ] specialized software
- [ ] control switches
- [ ] modified hardware/keyboard
- [ ] calculator
- [ ] environmental controls
- [ ] other (describe below)

Comments/Descriptions: _____

Seating/Mobility/Transportation
- [ ] cane
- [ ] crutches
- [ ] walker
- [ ] manual wheelchair
- [ ] electric wheelchair
- [ ] stroller
- [ ] positioning chair/system
- [ ] seating supports
- [ ] cushion
- [ ] wheelchair accessories
- [ ] orthotics
- [ ] prosthetics
- [ ] specially equipped vehicle
- [ ] car seat
- [ ] adapted bus/van
- [ ] other (describe below)

Comments/Descriptions: _____

Other Adaptations
- [ ] one-to-one aide
- [ ] peer assistance program

Comments/Descriptions: _____

School Function Assessment Summary Score Form

Name: _____   Date: _____

	Total Raw Score	Criterion Score	Criterion Standard Error	Criterion Cut-off Score K-3	Criterion Cut-off Score 4-6
Part I Participation					
Regular Classroom + S Settings				100	100
Special Education Classroom + S Settings				100	100
Part II Task Supports					
Physical Tasks—Assistance				100	100
Physical Tasks—Adaptations				100	100
Cognitive/Behavioral Tasks—Assistance				77	92
Cognitive/Behavioral Tasks—Adaptations				91	100
Optional Tasks					
Up/Down Stairs—Assistance					
Up/Down Stairs—Adaptations					
Written Work—Assistance					
Written Work—Adaptations					
Computer and Equipment Use—Assistance					
Computer and Equipment Use—Adaptations					

Functional Profile

Setting	Rating	Classroom Reg. Spec.	Playground/ Recess	Transportation	Bathroom/ Toileting	Transitions	Mealtime/ Snack Time

(Scale: 0 10 20 30 40 50 60 70 80 90 100)

	Criterion Cut-off Score
Part III Activity Performance	
Physical Tasks	
Travel	100
Maintaining and Changing Positions	100
Recreational Movement	83
Manipulation With Movement	93
Using Materials	83
Setup and Cleanup	87
Eating and Drinking	100
Hygiene	92
Clothing Management	93
Up/Down Stairs	100
Written Work	73
Computer and Equipment Use	65
Cognitive/Behavioral Tasks	
Functional Communication	91
Memory and Understanding	79
Following Social Conventions	73
Compliance With Adult Directives and School Rules	76
Task Behavior/Completion	72
Positive Interaction	81
Behavior Regulation	74
Personal Care Awareness	92
Safety	91

Figure 2-11. Summary score form (reprinted from Coster W, Deeney T, Haltiwanger J, Haley S. *School Function Assessment.* Copyright ©1998 by The Psychological Corporation, a Harcourt Assessment Company. Reproduced by permission. All rights reserved.).

continued

Concurrent validity and **internal consistency** of the SFA was examined using the Cronbach's coefficient alpha. These correlations were found to range between 0.92 to 0.98. A second method used was the consideration of fit statistics of each item within a scale. Analyses of the scales confirmed the coherence of the items within each scale.

Test-retest reliability was assessed on a convenience sample of 23 students who were examined twice over a 2- to 3-week period of time. The reliability coefficient scores between the test and retest were between 0.82 and 0.98. Approximately 40% of the sample had been identified as having a motor impairment. A second test-retest study on another sample of children with a variety of disabilities using the ICC-2 revealed correlation coefficients ranging from 0.80 to 0.97 on Part II of the SFA. The correlation coefficients were higher for Part III, Activity Performance, with scores ranging from 0.90 to 0.98.

Summary

This overview of selected standardized criterion-referenced and norm-referenced tests should supply the developmental therapist with an understanding of the components of an acceptable test. The information provided for each of the tests also should assist the therapist in the selection of the appropriate test for a given child in a given situation. The developmental therapist should be aware of other components of an examination of a child in addition to the administration of a test and should use the information gathered from other parts of the examination in the total evaluation of the child.

References

1. American Physical Therapy Association. Guide to physical therapist practice. 2nd ed. *Phys Ther.* 2001;81:42-48.
2. Coster W, Deeney T, Haltiwanger J, Haley S. *School Function Assessment.* San Antonio, Tex: The Psychological Corporation; 1998.
3. Russell D, Rosenbaum P, Gowland C, et al. *Gross Motor Function Measure.* Toronto, Canada: Gross Motor Measures Group; 1993.
4. Bruininks RH. *Bruininks-Oseretsky Test of Motor Proficiency. Examiner's Manual.* Circle Pines, Minn: American Guidance Service; 1978.
5. Hopkins B, Westra T. Maternal expectations of their infants' development: an intracultural study. *Genetic Psychology Monographs.* 1989;114:377-420.
6. Dasen P, Inhelder B, Lavalee M, et al. *Naissance de l'intelligence chex l'enfant Baoule de Côte d'Ivoire.* Bern, Switzerland: Hans Huber; 1978.
7. Cohen E, Boettcher K, Maher T, et al. Evaluation of the Peabody Developmental Gross Motor Scales for young children of African American and Hispanic ethnic backgrounds. *Pediatr Phys Ther.* 1999;1:191-197.
8. Dunn W. *Infant/Toddler Sensory Profile.* San Antonio, Tex: The Psychological Corporation; 2000.
9. Folio MR, Fewell RR. *Peabody Developmental Motor Scales. Examiner's Manual.* 2nd ed. Austin, Tex: Pro-Ed; 2000.
10. Chandler L, Andrews M, Swanson M. *The Movement Assessment of Infants: A Manual.* Rolling Bay, Wash: Infant Movement Research; 1980.

11. Haley SM, Coster WJ, Ludlow LH, Haltiwanger JT, Anrellos PJ. *Pediatric Evaluation of Disability Inventory.* Boston, Mass: New England Medical Center Hospitals; 1992.

12. Sackett DL, Strauss SE, Richardson WS, et al. *Evidence-Based Medicine: How to Practice and Teach EBM.* 2nd ed. New York, NY: Churchill Livingstone; 2000.

13. Berk RA, DeGangi GA. *DeGangi-Berk Test of Sensory Integration.* Los Angeles, Calif: Western Psychological Services; 1983.

14. Dubowitz L, Dubowitz V. The neurological examination of the full term newborn infant. *Clinics in Developmental Medicine.* No. 79. Philadelphia, Pa: JB Lippincott; 1981.

15. Saint-Anne Dargassies S. *Neurological Development in the Full Term and Premature Neonate.* London, England: Excerta Medica; 1977.

16. Prechtl HFR. The neurological examination of the full term newborn infant. *Clinics in Developmental Medicine.* No. 63. Philadelphia, Pa: JB Lippincott; 1977.

17. Parmelee AH, Michaelis R. Neurological examination of the newborn. In: Hellmuth J, ed. *Exceptional Infant. Vol. 2: Studies in Abnormalities.* London, England: Butterworths; 1971.

18. Brazelton TB. *Neonatal Behavioral Assessment Scale.* Philadelphia, Pa: JB Lippincott; 1973.

19. Brazelton TB. *Neonatal Behavioral Assessment Scale.* 2nd ed. Philadelphia, Pa: JB Lippincott; 1984.

20. Prechtl HFR. Assessment methods for the newborn infant: a critical evaluation. In: Stratton P, Chichest J, eds. *Psychobiology of the Human Newborn.* New York, NY: Wiley; 1982.

21. Tronick E, Brazelton TB. Clinical uses of the Brazelton Neonatal Behavior Assessment. In: Friedlander BZ, Sterritt BM, Kirk GE, eds. *Exceptional Infant: Assessment and Intervention.* Vol. 3. New York, NY: Brunner/Mazel; 1975.

22. Bakow H, Samaroff A, Kelly P, et al. Relation between newborn and mother-child interactions at four months. Paper presented at: Biennial Meeting of the Society for Research in Child Development; 1973; Philadelphia, Pa.

23. Sameroff AJ. Organization and stability of newborn behavior: a commentary on the Brazelton Neonatal Behavioral Assessment Scale. *Monographs of the Society of Research in Child Development.* 1978;43:56.

24. Ellison PH. *Infant Neurobiological International Battery.* Tucson, Ariz: Therapy Skill Builders; 1994.

25. Castro AV, de Sanchez IE, Landinez NS. Reliability of the infant neurological international battery (INFANIB) for the assessment of neurological integrity in infancy to high risk Colombian infants. Unpublished thesis. Bogota, Colombia: Instituto Materno. Infantil of Bogota; 1985.

26. Campbell S. *Test of Infant Motor Performance.* Chicago, Ill: Test of Infant Motor Performance, LLC; 2001.

27. Campbell SK, Kolobe THA, Osten ET, et al. Construct validity of the Test of Infant Motor Performance. *Phys Ther.* 1995;75:585-596.

28. Piper MC, Darrah J. *Motor Assessment of the Developing Infant.* Philadelphia, Pa: WB Saunders; 1994.

29. Campbell SK, Kolobe THA. Concurrent validity of the Test of Infant Motor Performance with the Alberta Infant Motor Scale. *Pediatr Phys Ther.* 2000;12:2-9.

30. Campbell SK. Test-retest reliability of the Test of Infant Motor Performance. *Pediatr Phys Ther.* 1999;11:60-66.

31. Frankenburg WK, Dodds J, Archer P, et al. *Denver II Technical Manual.* Denver, Colo: Denver Developmental Materials; 1990.

32. Frankenburg WK, Dodds JB, Fandal AW, et al. *Denver Developmental Screening Test: Reference Manual.* Denver, Colo: University of Colorado Medical Center; 1975.

33. Frankenburg WK, Fandal AW, Sciarillo W, Burgess D. The newly abbreviated and revised Denver Developmental Screening Test. *Journal of Pediatrics.* 1981;99:995-999.

34. Frankenburg WK, Dodds J, Archer P, et al. The Denver II: a major revision and restandardization of the Denver Developmental Screening Tool. *Pediatrics.* 1992;89:91-97.

35. Glascoe FP, Bryne KE, Ashford LF, et al. Accuracy of the Denver II in developmental screening. *Pediatrics.* 1992;89:1221-1225.

36. Kerfeld CI, Guthrie MR, Stewart KB. Evaluation of the Denver II as applied to Alaska Native children. *Pediatr Phys Ther.* 1997;9:23-31.

37. Stuberg W, et al. *The Milani-Comparetti Motor Development Screening Test.* 3rd ed. rev. Omaha, Neb: University of Nebraska Medical Center; 1992.

38. Milani-Comparetti A, Gidoni EA. Routine developmental examination in normal and retarded children. *Dev Med Child Neurol.* 1967;9:631-638.

39. Trembath J. *The Milani-Comparetti Motor Development Screening Test.* Omaha, Neb: University of Nebraska Medical Center Print Shop; 1978.

40. Vander Linden D. Ability of the Milani-Comparetti Developmental Examination to predict motor outcome. *Phys Occup Ther Pediatr.* 1985;5:27-38.

41. Stuberg WA, White PJ, Miedaner JA, Dehne PR. Item reliability of the Milani-Comparetti Motor Development. Screening Test. *Phys Ther.* 1989;69:328-335.

42. Darrah J, Piper MC, Byrne PJ, Warren S. The utilization of the movement assessment of infants risk profile with preterm infants. *Phys Occup Ther Pediatr.* 1991;11:1-12.

43. Schneider JW, Lee W, Chasnoff IJ. Field testing of the movement assessment of infants. *Phys Ther.* 1988;68:321-327.

44. Harris SR, Haley SM, Tada WL, Swanson MW. Reliability of observational measures of the Movement Assessment of Infants. *Phys Ther.* 1984;64:471-475.

45. Haley SM, Harris SR, Tada WL, Swanson MW. Item reliability of the movement assessment of infants. *Phys Occup Ther Pediatr.* 1986;6:21-39.

46. Swanson MW, Bennett FC, Shy KK, Whitfield MF. Identification of neurodevelopmental abnormality at four and eight months by the movement assessment of infants. *Dev Med Child Neurol.* 1992;34:321-337.

47. Coster W. Critiques of the Alberta Infant Motor Scale (AIMS). *Phys Occup Ther Pediatr.* 1995; 15:53-64.

48. Piper MC, Pinnell LE, Darrah J, et al. Construction and validation of the Alberta Infant Motor Scale. *Can J Public Health.* 1992;83:546-550.

49. Piper MC, Darrah J, Pinnell L, et al. Discriminative validity of the Alberta Infant Motor Scale. *Dev Med Child Neurol.* 1992;66:55-56.

50. Miller LJ, Roid GH. *Toddler and Infant Motor Evaluation: A Standardized Assessment.* Tucson, Ariz: Therapy Skill Builders; 1994.

51. Bayley N. *Bayley Scales of Infant Development.* 2nd ed. San Antonio, Tex: The Psychological Corporation; 1993.

52. Harrow AJ. *A Taxonomy of the Psychomotor Domain: A Guide for Developing Behavioral Objectives.* New York, NY: David McKay; 1972.

53. Ulrich D. *Test of Gross Motor Development–2.* Austin, Tex: Pro-Ed; 2000.

54. Russell DJ, Rosenbaum PL, Avery LM, Lane M. *Gross Motor Function Measure (GMFM–66 and GMFM-88) User's Manual.* London, England: McKeith Press; 2002.

55. Russell D, Rosenbaum PL, Cadman DT, et al. The Gross Motor Function Measure: a means to evaluate the effects of physical therapy. *Dev Med Child Neurol.* 1989;31:341-352.

56. Trahan J, Malouin F. Changes in the Gross Motor Function Measure in children with different types of cerebral palsy: an eight-month follow-up study. *Pediatr Phys Ther.* 1999;11:12-17.

57. Russell D, Palisano R, Walker S, et al. Evaluating motor function in children with Down syndrome: validity of the GMFM. *Dev Med Child Neuro.* 1998;40:693-701.

58. Ruck-Gibis J, Plotkin H, Hanley J, et al. Reliability of the Gross Motor Function Measure for children with osteogenesis imperfecta. *Pediatr Phys Ther.* 2001;13:10-17.

59. Dunn W. *Infant/Toddler Sensory Profile.* San Antonio, Tex: The Psychological Corporation; 2002.

60. Dunn W. *Sensory Profile*. San Antonio, Tex: The Psychological Corporation; 1999.

61. Brown CE, Dunn W. *Sensory Profile for Adolescents/Adults*. San Antonio, Tex: The Psychological Corporation; 2002.

62. Chess S, Thomas A. *The New York Longitudinal Scales Adult Temperament Questionnaire Test Manual*. Scottsdale, Ariz: Behavioral Developmental Initiatives; 1998.

63. DeGangi GA, Greenspan SI. *Test of Sensory Functions in Infants (TSFI)*. Los Angeles, Calif: Western Psychological Services; 1989.

64. Bayley N. *Bayley Scales of Infant Development*. New York, NY: The Psychological Corporation; 1969.

65. Bates JE. *Infant Characteristics Questionnaire, Revised*. Bloomington, Ind: Indiana University; 1984.

66. Fagan JF. New evidence of the prediction of intelligence from infancy. *Infant Mental Health Journal*. 1982;3(4):219-228.

67. Benson AM, Lane SJ. Interrater reliability of the Test of Sensory Functions in Infants as used with infants exposed to cocaine in utero. *Occup Ther J Res*. 1994;14:170-177.

68. Jirikowic TL, Engel JM, Deitz JC. The Test of Sensory Functions in Infants: test-retest reliability for infants with developmental delays. *Am J Occup Ther*. 1997;51:733-738.

69. DeGangi GA, Berk RA. *DeGangi-Berk Test of Sensory Integration*. Los Angeles, Calif: Western Psychological Services; 1983.

70. Miller LJ. *Miller Assessment of Preschoolers*. Littleton, Colo: Foundation for Knowledge in Development: 1982.

71. Ayres AJ. *Sensory Integration and Praxis Tests*. Los Angeles, Calif: Western Psychological Services; 1989.

72. Ayres AJ. *Southern California Sensory Integration Tests*. Rev. ed. Los Angeles, Calif: Western Psychological Services; 1980.

73. Ayres AJ. *Southern California Postrotary Nystagmus Test Manual*. Los Angeles, Calif: Western Psychological Services; 1975.

74. Ayres AJ. Patterns of perceptual motor dysfunctions in children: a factor analysis study. *Perceptual and Motor Skills*. 1965;20:335-368.

75. Ayres AJ. Deficits in sensory integration in educationally handicapped children. *J Learn Disabil*. 1969;2:160-168.

76. Ayres AJ. Types of sensory integrative dysfunction among disabled learners. *AJOT*. 1972;26:13-18.

77. Ayres AJ. Cluster analyses of measures of sensory integration. *AJOT*. 1977;31:362-366.

78. Murray EA, Cermak SA, O'Brien A. The relationship between form and space perception, constructional abilities, and clumsiness in children. *AJOT*. 1990;44:623-628.

79. Wilson BN, Pollock N, Kaplan BJ, Law M. *Clinical Observations of Motor and Postural Skills*. 2nd ed. Framingham, Mass: Therapro; 2000.

80. Reisman JE, Hanschu B. *Sensory Integration Inventory for Individuals with Developmental Disorders-Revised*. Hugo, Minn: PDP Press; 1992.

81. Richter EW, Montgomery PC. *The Sensorimotor Performance Analysis*. Hugo, Minn: PDP Press; 1989.

82. Newborg J, Stock JR, Wnek L. Battelle Development Inventory. Allen, Tex: DLM Teaching Resources; 1984.

83. Feldman AB, Haley SM, Coryell J. Concurrent and construct validity of the Pediatric Evaluation of Disability Inventory. *Phys Ther*. 1990;70:602-610.

84. Uniform Data System, State University of New York at Buffalo. *Guide for the Functional Independence Measure for Children (Wee-FIM)*. Version 1.5. Buffalo, NY: Center for Functional Assessment Research; 1991.

CHAPTER 3

ESTABLISHING FUNCTIONAL OUTCOMES AND ORGANIZING INTERVENTION

Patricia C. Montgomery, PhD, PT, FAPTA

When providing pediatric services, physical therapists are responsible for determining the treatment techniques to be used, when to use them, and how long intervention should continue. Making the transition between didactic information and theoretical frameworks to actual "hands-on" intervention can be a long, frustrating, and anxiety-producing experience for both therapists and children. If the academic focus is on techniques, physical therapists may not develop strategies for planning and sequencing treatment. One purpose of this chapter is to identify some of the variables that influence treatment planning. A method for selecting appropriate treatment techniques and sequence of application is suggested by working backwards from the establishment of behavioral functional outcomes. A second purpose of this chapter is to discuss principles of motor learning that are applicable to planning and administering treatment.

The information presented in this chapter is intended to serve as one possible process for developing a strategy for organizing treatment. Such a framework involves a number of therapist and patient variables that will alter its applicability in different situations. In addition, many experienced clinicians have no difficulty determining the content of individual treatment sessions in relation to therapeutic goals. These clinicians, however, may not be able to describe the cognitive processes they use to make such determinations.

Therefore, a specific strategy for treatment planning and sequencing may be useful to many physical therapists, particularly the student and new graduate, who have little clinical experience. Evaluation of patient progress in relation to intervention is essential in clinical as well as research settings. The approach of goal setting and use of measurable behavioral objectives in relation to treatment outcome presented in this chapter usually is mandated by third-party payers.

Variables Influencing Treatment Planning

The theoretical framework a physical therapist uses to plan intervention will be affected by the understanding of and degree of agreement with specific theories of motor control, motor learning, and motor development. Although physical therapy curricula contain similar content in therapeutic exercise, there will be differences in which theories are emphasized and which therapeutic techniques are taught depending on physical therapy faculty, and, in turn, their training and clinical experiences. In my opinion, this is not a negative, but a positive phenomenon as it provides the physical therapist with several approaches to treatment that eventually can be validated or invalidated by clinical research. Although we may be criticized for not having a singular approach to therapeutic exercise that has been validated through research, our profession is no different than many other health professions. For example, the oncologist may not know what causes a certain form of cancer and may not have a proven cure, but the patient is treated based on information available at that time, while research studies are in progress that may lead to more effective treatment in the future. The analogy of the physical therapist using current state-of-the-art information in therapeutic exercise with pediatric patients is clear.

A second variable affecting treatment planning is the physical therapist's ability to integrate general evaluation and intervention strategies taught in the basic curriculum with specific techniques used in the treatment of the pediatric population. For example, techniques for improving strength, endurance, and flexibility are essential in the treatment of many children. Orthopedic and cardiovascular considerations in relation to exercise, weight-bearing, various positions, and the use of adaptive devices are important, but may be neglected if the emphasis is on normalizing movement patterns and developing age-appropriate motor skills through the use of specific neurophysiological techniques.

A third variable is the selection of examination tools. Norm-referenced tests are designed primarily to detect whether or not a child has a motor delay in relation to a same-age non-disabled peer group.[1] Criterion-referenced tests measure a child's performance against set criteria or his own previous performance, therefore providing information on the most appropriate focus of treatment. Generally, the more physically and mentally challenged the child is, the more difficult it is to determine current abilities and potential for change and fewer standardized examination tools are available. An in-depth discussion of tests currently used in pediatrics was provided in the preceding chapter.

Physical therapists rely on clinical observations or qualitative assessments of sensory and motor abilities to supplement the results of formal examinations. These clinical observations also may be used as a substitute for unavailable or inappropriate examination tools. The applicability of qualitative clinical evaluations in relation to choosing specific treatment techniques is documented in subsequent chapters.

Another variable affecting the process of treatment planning is clinical experience in determining functional outcomes and observing change resulting in attainment or failure to accomplish specific objectives. For example, motor milestones, such as rolling, sitting, and crawling, may be used as functional outcomes. The physical therapist working with the child with severe disabilities, however, may discover that these outcomes must be broken down into smaller units to effectively measure progress over specified periods of time.

Developing a Strategy for Planning Treatment

The first step in developing a strategy for planning individual treatment is to assess your level of knowledge. What has your academic and clinical training provided to prepare you for working with children? A basic prerequisite is a thorough understanding of normal motor development that is necessary for optimal examination, evaluation, and intervention. What areas of knowledge do you need to supplement with additional information or training? If your caseload consists of children with learning disabilities who demonstrate subtle motor problems, for example, additional study of pertinent resource material may be necessary. The physical therapist must assume the responsibility of being adequately prepared to plan intervention for specific children.

The second step is to identify various intervention approaches that can be used. A systems perspective suggests that numerous variables interact to determine outcome. Some of these variables are intrinsic (eg, degree of pathology to the central nervous system

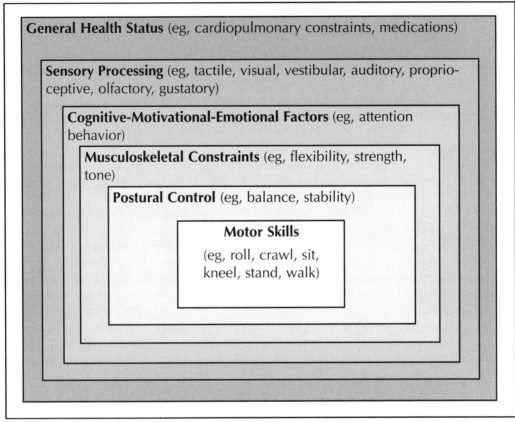

Figure 3-1. Intrinsic variables that interact in the development of motor skills. Extrinsic variables include cultural and environmental factors.

[CNS], cognitive status) while others are extrinsic (eg, cultural influences, environmental factors). Figure 3-1 illustrates some of the intrinsic factors that should be considered in pediatric examination, evaluation, and intervention. Each physical therapist will address the mental organization of these variables differently, but will, hopefully, create a framework useful in evaluating and treating children in a holistic manner.

The third step in planning treatment is to choose appropriate examination tools. Most normative tests provide information as to whether the child is performing below, at, or above expectations as compared to a non-disabled child of the same age. Few tests will provide information regarding what to do to improve the child's performance. Normative and criterion-referenced tests, however, may reveal areas of deficits and test results can be used for monitoring developmental change (see Chapter 2).

During the evaluation process, summarize what the child can and cannot do. Make a list of the sensory tasks or motor activities he should be accomplishing. Emphasis should be on the functional movements and tasks the child needs to perform optimally in his natural environment(s) (eg, home, preschool, school, community). The most difficult aspect of the evaluation process is to determine why he cannot do the tasks or movements. The examination and evaluation procedures throughout this text are intended to assist the physical therapist in delineating specific problem areas.

The next step is to determine if it is reasonable to project long-term outcomes for the child in relation to normal or typical skills. For the high-risk preterm infant who is mildly delayed in motor skills at an adjusted age of 6 months, it may be appropriate to use typical developmental skills, such as rolling, crawling, and walking. For the 5-year-old child with severe spastic quadriplegia, who will not attain typical motor skills, goals that reflect improved independence or obtainment of specific functional skills are more appropriate. For example, a long-term outcome may be "to improve voluntary use of one upper extremity so the child can independently punch the keys on a computer." The issue of "quality" of movement is controversial. One opinion is that the best strategy is to strive for normal quality of movement. There are many children, however, who do not have the capability of normal movement and valuable time may be lost working toward unattainable goals when the major objective of the physical therapist should be to improve the child's functional abilities.

Finally, treatment planning is done within a general framework of appropriate intervention for children. Pellegrino[2] reviewed the disablement model in relation to a basic paradigm shift that has occurred in the past 25 years in how intervention for individuals with developmental disabilities is viewed. In the old paradigm "optimizing development" meant getting to the next developmental milestone, and individual treatment plans in rehabilitation for children were organized with milestones as goals. Pelligrino suggested that over-emphasis on the individual steps of development may result in an unbalanced, and perhaps fundamentally flawed, view of the process of development. In the current paradigm, development is defined as "participation" and the "goal of intervention then becomes to increase and improve participation in a larger number and wider variety of societal settings."[2]

Functional Outcomes

One of the most important responsibilities of the physical therapist is to determine therapeutic goals and functional outcomes for the child. Although therapists may know what "improving postural control" is, various therapists may use different observational data to support the conclusion that this therapeutic goal has been met. It is our responsibility, then, to describe the behavior or set of behaviors that allows other observers (eg, therapists, physicians, parents, teachers) to arrive at the same conclusion regarding the child's level of function. Precise, unambiguous specifications regarding a behavior also decrease the amount of subjectivity in the evaluation process. For example, the objective "the child will ambulate independently with a walker" does not tell us if there are any constraints on the child's abilities. If we state "the child will ambulate independently with a reverse walker in all environments during daily activities," we clarify the behavioral objective and the desired functional outcome.

Behavioral objectives consist of a behavior that can be observed and measured. Specific criteria describing the behavior may include the conditions under which the behavior will occur. Using successful completion of a minimum number of trials or performance of a behavior during a percentage of a set time period would be examples of specified conditions.

Functional limitations identified in a child are related to theoretical perspectives. If a child cannot maintain an upright head position and sitting balance, for example, we can hypothesize that there are deficits in postural control, deficient strength in the neck and trunk muscles, deficits in cognitive and motivational functions, or a combination of factors. We can be accurate in our description of the child's posture and movement, but we only can hypothesize about underlying causes or impairments.

Physical therapy goals and functional outcomes for the child also depend on the theoretical framework of the physical therapist. In hierarchical models, goals often related to altering muscle tone, decreasing reflex patterns of movement, achieving developmental motor milestones, and improving sensory processing. In more contemporary models, goals relate to initiation, speed, and variability of movement and to variables described in a systems approach.[3] Traditional goals of physical therapy intervention, such as those addressing strength, endurance, and flexibility, also are used in pediatrics. The terms *goals, objectives,* and *outcomes* may have different or similar definitions depending on the framework in which they are used. The *Guide to Physical Therapist Practice*[4] uses anticipated goals and expected outcomes in the plan of care stating that both should be measurable and time limited. In this text, we have chosen to use the term "goal" to specify general physical therapy strategies (eg, increase, strength, improve balance) and the term "functional outcome" to specify the measurable, functional objective that would be linked to the general goal. General goals can be written in measurable, time-specific terms as well. For example, a strengthening goal can be expressed as the number of times an individual can lift a specified weight. Goals in various frameworks may overlap. The essential element that ties them together is the use of measurable functional outcomes.

We may agree with the goal of improving postural control in the child with spastic quadriplegia, but how do we measure the success of our intervention? The disablement model[4] suggests that the first step is to identify functional limitations, in this case, related to postural control. Then the underlying impairments that contribute to the functional limitations can be hypothesized and therapeutic goals determined. Finally, specific, measurable functional outcomes within a specific time frame are used to measure progress.

The following section provides examples of functional limitations in:

➤ Mobility skills (assuming specific positions, making transitions of movement from one position to another, moving through the environment)

➤ Upper extremity skills

➤ Sensory-perceptual skills

➤ Cognitive skills

The functional limitation is identified first, followed by general impairments hypothesized to contribute to the functional limitation. Examples of therapeutic goals are listed, followed by specific functional outcomes to be achieved with intervention.

Establishing Functional Outcomes

Limitations in Mobility Skills

EXAMPLE 1

➤ *Functional limitations*: In prone, child does not lift his head off the floor, but only can slide it from side to side to clear his airway

➤ *Impairments*: Deficits in motor control that limit ability to control head position, weakness in trunk and neck muscles, limited tolerance for prone position

➤ *Goals*: Improve head control in prone position, increase strength in trunk and neck extensors

➤ *Functional outcomes*: In prone, child will lift head 45 to 90 degrees, two out of three trials, and maintain this position for 10 seconds to view an object or toy

EXAMPLE 2

➤ *Functional limitations*: In prone position, child cannot maintain prone on elbows. As child turns his head, shoulder girdle support decreases in the extremity on the skull side and he collapses

➤ *Impairments*: Deficits in motor control that interfere with coordination of head, trunk, and upper extremities for support in prone; decreased upper extremity and trunk strength; reliance on asymmetrical tonic neck movement pattern (see Chapter 8)

➤ *Goals*: Improve motor control and coordination of upper extremities, head, and upper trunk; improve bilateral use of upper extremities for support in prone; increase upper extremity and trunk strength

➤ *Functional outcomes*: In prone, child will be able to achieve and maintain prone on elbows for 20 to 30 seconds as he turns his head to either side to watch a moving toy.

EXAMPLE 3

➤ *Functional limitations*: Child is able to transition from prone to sitting only by pushing up on extended arms, pulling legs underneath trunk, and "W" sitting

➤ *Impairments*: Deficits in motor control, poor motor planning, limited trunk rotation

➤ *Goals*: Increase variety of movement transitions from prone to sitting, increase trunk flexibility

➤ *Functional outcomes*: When placed on the floor in prone, child will use more than one movement pattern to transition into sitting during five trials. Child will assume at least two different sitting positions over a 5-minute observation period of free play

EXAMPLE 4

➤ *Functional limitations*: In sitting, child hyperextends his head and supports head with elevated shoulders. Child does not consistently reposition head upright when tilted more than 10 degrees in any direction

➤ *Impairments*: Deficits in motor control, weakness in neck muscles, poor trunk balance/stability, deficits in sensory processing (eg, visual, somatosensory, vestibular)

➤ *Goals*: Improve head control in sitting, increase trunk and neck strength, improve sitting balance

➤ *Functional outcomes*: In sitting, child will tuck chin and maintain an erect head position 50% of the time in an observation period of 5 minutes. Child will maintain head in midline when tilted 20 degrees in any direction from the upright in sitting

EXAMPLE 5

➤ *Functional limitations*: When child loses balance in sitting, he does not attempt to catch himself with his arms

➤ *Impairments*: Deficits in motor control, poor sitting balance, slow or inadequate processing of sensory information regarding position in space

➤ *Goals*: Improve motor control and sitting balance, improve reaction time to sensory input, improve protective responses to loss of balance

➤ *Functional outcomes*: When placed in sitting, child will prop on extended arms for 1 minute without collapsing. In sitting, child will successfully catch himself two of three trials when slowly pushed off balance in a lateral direction

EXAMPLE 6

➤ *Functional limitations*: Child is ambulatory but must wear a helmet because he does not protect himself adequately when he falls

➤ *Impairments*: Deficits in motor control, slow or inadequate processing of sensory information regarding position in space, weakness of upper extremities

➤ *Goals*: Improve motor control, increase response time to sensory input, increase strength of upper extremities

➤ *Functional outcomes*: Child will be able to deliberately fall forward and sideways from a standing position and catch himself with his arms. Child will be able to deliberately fall backwards from a standing position and "sit down" with protective reactions of the arms. In walking during the school day, child will not hit his head on the floor if he falls

EXAMPLE 7

➤ *Functional limitations*: Child tends to use both legs together. For example, when sitting the child cannot shift weight onto one hip and flex opposite hip and knee to put on a sock

➤ *Impairments*: Deficits in motor control with poor lower extremity dissociation and poor postural control, lower extremity and trunk weakness, deficits in motor planning

➤ *Goals*: Improve lower extremity control of isolated movements, increase general lower extremity and trunk strength, improve balance; improve motor planning

➤ *Functional outcomes*: In sitting on the floor, child will shift weight and leave one leg extended while flexing opposite leg to put on socks or pants. Child will crawl on hands and knees with a reciprocal lower extremity pattern with verbal reminders. Child will independently ride a tricycle for a distance of 6 feet

EXAMPLE 8

➤ *Functional limitations*: In ambulation using a reverse walker, child walks too slowly to keep up with peers in the hallways at school

➤ *Impairments*: Deficits in motor control, poor motor planning, decreased strength and endurance, poor balance

➤ *Goals*: Increase speed of ambulation with walker

➤ *Functional outcomes*: Child will march in time (20 steps/minute or faster) to fast music while standing with a walker. Child will ambulate independently with walker 20 feet in 10 seconds in the classroom. Child will keep up with peers while walking with his or her walker for a distance of 50 feet

Limitations in Upper Extremity Skills

EXAMPLE 9

➤ *Functional limitations*: In supine, child cannot bring hands to mouth or hands together at midline of body

➤ *Impairments*: Deficits in motor control—unable to coordinate upper extremities for functional movements, decreased strength in upper extremities

➤ *Goals*: Improve ability to volitionally control upper extremity movements in supine position

➤ *Functional outcomes*: In supine, child will be able to bring either hand to mouth. In supine, child will be able to bring together at midline for hand-to-hand contact and to manipulate objects (eg, toys)

EXAMPLE 10

➤ *Functional limitations*: Child uses gross grasp and release and cannot move objects to the radial side of the hand or orient the hand to get objects or food to the mouth

➤ *Impairments*: Deficits in fine motor control, limited control over individual fingers

➤ *Goals*: Improve hand skills and isolated use of fingers

➤ *Functional outcomes*: Five out of 10 attempts, child will grasp small objects with radial portion of hand. Child will grasp bread stick and bring it to the mouth independently. In one of five trials, child will use a three-finger pinch to pick up a small object (eg, a piece of cereal). Child will isolate index finger to point at pictures in a book

EXAMPLE 11

➤ *Functional limitations*: Child only reaches with forearm pronation and cannot bring the forearm to neutral to grasp objects that have a vertical orientation

➤ *Impairments*: Deficits in upper extremity motor control, poor motor planning, decreased upper extremity range of motion

➤ *Goals*: Improve ability of child to bring forearm to neutral and into some degree of supination

➤ *Functional outcomes*: Child will orient the forearm to neutral two of three trials to grasp a vertical baton. Child will bring both forearms to neutral to grasp a large ball. Child will use slight supination of both forearms to hold a large box

EXAMPLE 12

➤ *Functional limitations*: Child does not use right upper extremity during play or when large toys requiring bilateral upper extremity are presented for him to hold

➤ *Impairments*: Deficits in motor control, impaired somatosensory processing from right upper extremity

➤ *Goals*: Increase frequency of attempts at independent movement with right upper extremity

➤ *Functional outcomes*: In ring sitting, child will use his right arm, with verbal reminders, to pick up three of five puzzle pieces placed to his right. Child will use his right hand spontaneously to clap in a game of patty-cake, imitating the therapist on five of 10 attempts. Child will use both hands to hold a 12-inch diameter ball, three of five trials

EXAMPLE 13

➤ *Functional limitation*: Child sits with a stiff trunk position and does not cross the midline of the body in upper extremity tasks. He usually turns his whole body to manipulate objects on either side

➤ *Impairments*: Deficits in motor control, poor trunk rotation, limited flexibility of trunk

➤ *Goals*: Improve flexibility of trunk and active rotational movements

➤ *Functional outcomes*: Child will roll using trunk rotation (ie, observed separation between shoulders and pelvis) rather than "log-rolling." In tailor sitting, child will be able to rotate trunk two of three trials to view an object behind him without moving base of support ([BOS] ie, legs and pelvis). In two of three trials, child will cross midline of body with arm to reach for an object (rather than turning entire body to avoid crossing midline). In standing, child will be able to independently perform "windmills" (ie, touching left foot with right hand, then right foot with left hand)

Limitations in Sensory/Perceptual Skills

EXAMPLE 14

➤ *Functional limitations*: Child does not enjoy or tolerate movement activities. He will not attempt to play on moveable equipment/toys. He avoids interacting with peers during gross motor activities

➤ *Impairments*: Hypersensitivity to vestibular stimulation, "postural insecurity" (ie, deficient postural control)

➤ *Goals*: Decrease sensitivity to vestibular stimulation, improve balance, increase confidence in participating in gross motor activities

➤ *Functional outcomes*: Child will tolerate swinging slowly on playground swing for 3 minutes. Child will participate in scooter board games with his peers

EXAMPLE 15

➤ *Functional limitations*: Child is sensitive to tactile input. He does not like to be touched, wear new clothes, or have his face or hair washed. He does not use his hands to explore or play in various textured mediums

➤ *Impairments*: Hypersensitivity to tactile stimulation

➤ *Goals*: Decrease tactile hypersensitivity

➤ *Functional outcomes*: Child will seek out hugs from adults. Child will not cry or scream when his hair is washed. Child will play independently for 5 minutes to complete a finger painting project

EXAMPLE 16

➤ *Functional limitations*: Child does not consistently look at objects placed in his visual field and does not maintain eye contact with adults or peers for more than 1 to 2 seconds

➤ *Impairments*: Deficits in visual focus and tracking, possible cognitive/emotional deficits (eg, autism), poor head control, poor eye-head coordination

➤ *Goals*: Improve visual focus and tracking, improve eye-head coordination, increase interest in environmental objects and people

➤ *Functional outcomes*: Child will orient two of three trials to an object lit by a flashlight. Child will maintain visual focus on a specific toy for 10 seconds. Child will turn eyes and head two of three trials to follow a moving object. Child will maintain eye contact with an adult 50% of the time during a 1-minute social interaction

EXAMPLE 17

➤ *Functional limitations*: Child tends to neglect the left side of his body and space during motor activities, usually orienting to his right and demonstrating difficulty with bilateral activities

➤ *Impairments*: Deficits in somatosensory processing from the left side of the body, deficits in visual perception, deficits in motor control

➤ *Goals*: Improve somatosensory and visual awareness of left side of the body and left side of space, increase spontaneous use of left side of body, increase frequency of orientation to the left side

➤ *Functional outcomes*: Child will actively remove sticky tape or stickers placed on right arm (using his left hand). Child will "twirl" to the left and right when "dancing" to music

Limitations in Cognitive Skills

EXAMPLE 18

➤ *Functional limitations*: Child is slow to move in response to verbal requests. As a result, siblings and others assist the child, decreasing opportunities for the child to practice motor skills and to increase his independence

➤ *Impairments*: Deficits in motor control, sensory processing deficits, cognitive/motivational deficits

➤ *Goals*: Improve speed in initiation of movement

➤ *Functional outcomes*: In sitting, child will initiate reaching for a toy less than 5 seconds after a verbal request to "get the toy." In prone, child will belly crawl toward a toy within 5 seconds after toy is placed near him on floor

EXAMPLE 19

➤ *Functional limitations*: Child moves very slowly when feeding himself and takes more than 45 minutes to finish a meal

➤ *Impairments*: Poor oral-motor skills, attention deficit (ie, increased distractibility)

➤ *Goals*: Improve oral-motor skills and attention during mealtime

➤ *Functional outcomes*: Child will feed himself and complete a meal within 30 minutes with only verbal reminders from adult

EXAMPLE 20

➤ *Functional limitations*: Child cannot walk independently from the classroom to the gym because he is distracted by other children

➤ *Impairments*: Cognitive and motivational deficits

➤ *Goals*: Improve selective attention for gross motor tasks

➤ *Functional outcomes*: Child will walk independently from classroom to gym within 5 minutes, 100% of time when no other children are present in hallway. Child will walk independently from classroom to gym within 10 minutes, 100% of time when other children are present in hallway

EXAMPLE 21

➤ *Functional limitations*: Child independently controls electric wheelchair, but runs into objects, walls, and people

➤ *Impairments*: Deficits in motor control, cognitive deficits, poor motor planning

➤ *Goals*: Improve fine motor control and general motor planning

➤ *Functional outcomes*: Child will successfully complete a 20-foot obstacle course two of three trials without hitting walls or two of three obstacles. When using a rear-view mirror mounted on the wheelchair, the child will successfully back up 3 feet. Child will be able to turn the wheelchair around in a 4-foot-square space in the class-room

Establishing Short-
and Long-Term Functional Outcomes

One example of a long-term outcome is that "the child will ambulate independently with a walker in the home." The therapist analyzes this task and develops short-term outcomes that are appropriate for eventually reaching the long-term outcome. Examples of short-term outcomes for this functional skill might include:

➤ The child will pull to stand at furniture two of three trials when a toy is placed out of reach on the furniture

➤ The child will cruise to the left or right a distance of 3 feet at furniture to obtain toys

➤ When placed, the child will maintain balance in upright with the walker for 5 minutes

➤ The child will make forward progress with the walker on a smooth surface for a distance of 10 feet

➤ The child will make forward progress with the walker on a carpeted surface for a distance of 10 feet

➤ The child will demonstrate the ability to motor plan a distance of 15 feet and turn the walker to avoid two obstacles in his path

➤ The child will demonstrate protective reactions each time he falls or attempts to lower himself from the walker

➤ The child will be able to lower himself independently from the walker to the floor or to a chair, two of three attempts

➤ The child will be able to get into his walker from the floor or a chair independently, two of three attempts

After determining long- and short-term functional outcomes, the therapist then selects appropriate treatment techniques to enable the child to achieve each outcome (refer to subsequent chapters). During treatment, the therapist continually evaluates the effectiveness of treatment techniques, adding, omitting, or revising intervention as necessary for the child's success. As the child makes progress, long- and short-term outcomes may be altered or new outcomes may be instated and the process begins again (Figure 3-2).

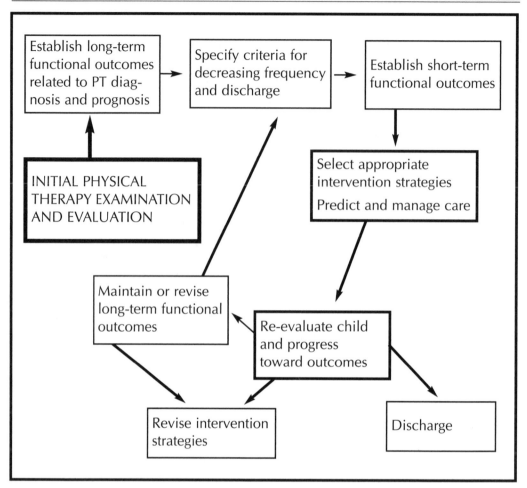

Figure 3-2. Treatment planning: the process.

Discharge Plan

As part of the physical therapy diagnosis and prognosis, the plan of care should include criteria for decreasing frequency of physical therapy intervention and discharge from physical therapy. Beginning with the initial evaluation, discharge planning should be a component of documentation. Early discussion of criteria for decreasing frequency of intervention and eventual discharge from physical therapy will educate the child's care-givers about the focus of physical therapy (eg, improving function and independence) and possible strategies for motor intervention for the child with life-long disabilities (eg, transitioning from private to school physical therapy services, transitioning from direct to indirect physical therapy services, transitioning from physical therapy to adaptive physical education or community-based motor activities, transitioning to activities with emphasis on lifelong fitness).

The concept of "episodic care" can be introduced through discharge planning so care-givers can be reassured that discharge may not be final, but that reevaluation and intervention can occur if new problems are identified. The discharge plan also is helpful for payers to provide an idea of the anticipated frequency and duration of therapy services. Several examples of discharge planning follow.

Sample Discharge Plans

Example 1

➤ *Child*: Angela—4 months old—Birth asphyxia (not yet demonstrating a significant delay, prognosis is poor and therapist anticipates increasing frequency)

➤ *Discharge plan*: Due to Angela's young age, it is difficult to anticipate the duration of physical therapy services. She is at risk for cerebral palsy and developmental delay due to her birth history. Her progress will be reevaluated every 2 to 3 months and based on achievement of developmental motor skills, rate of progress, and school services, recommendations for frequency of intervention will be made. Bimonthly visits are recommended at this time with a possible increase to weekly when Angela begins to work on gross motor skills such as rolling, crawling, and sitting

Example 2

➤ *Child*: Devin—8 months old—Cerebral palsy (mild impairments, currently attempting to pull to stand, prognosis good for independent ambulation)

➤ *Discharge plan*: Frequency of home-based physical therapy services will be decreased when Devin begins to pull to stand and cruise around furniture. He will be discharged from physical therapy when he begins to walk independently. In the meantime, weekly physical therapy sessions will be coordinated with his school program where he receives home visits from an occupational therapist

Example 3

➤ *Child*: Brittany—3 years, 2 months—Developmental delay (child is demonstrating very slow progress toward independent ambulation—has been cruising at furniture for 12 months, therapist is trying to decrease frequency of intervention and family is resisting any decrease in services)

➤ *Discharge plan*: It is anticipated that Brittany will need physical therapy services until she reaches her full potential for independent ambulation. Her motor skills and progress toward goals are reevaluated every 3 months with recommendations made for frequency of physical therapy services. If Brittany continues to work on her upright mobility skills (ie, cruising and walking with assistance) for longer periods of time, frequency of physical therapy can be decreased from weekly to 2 times/month. If Brittany's motor skills plateau over a 3- to 6-month period, frequency of physical therapy can be decreased further to periodic monitoring of her program

Example 4

➤ *Child*: Billy—2 years, 3 months—Cerebral palsy/visual impairment (child is now walking independently, although balance is poor, private therapist anticipates that his needs can be met by the school physical therapist who will see him 2 times/month and is planning on discharge)

➤ *Discharge plan*: Billy is currently being followed every other week for private physical therapy. His program has been coordinated with his school physical therapist.

Now that Billy has met his long-term goal of walking independently, his needs can be met by the school physical therapist and he will be discharged from private physical therapy services at the end of this month

Example 5

➤ *Child*: Hannah—4 years, 6 months—L 2, 3 Myelomenigocele (child appears to be functioning at the highest level possible within the constraints of her impairments, therapist would like to discharge her from private services and resume therapy at some future point if she has surgery or her needs change [ie, "episodic care"])

➤ *Discharge plan*: At this time, it appears that Hannah is performing to the best of her capability within the limits of her disability. It is recommended that physical therapy sessions be decreased to twice per month for the next month, then once a month until her school program is established. She will be eligible for motor services in her special education program. At that point, it will be appropriate to discharge Hannah from private physical therapy services. Should any new problems develop or medical interventions (eg, surgery) occur, Hannah's physical therapy needs could be reevaluated

Example 6

➤ *Child*: Jeremy—5 years—Cerebral palsy, spastic diplegia (child is walking independently for short distances with potential for independent community ambulation, child is receiving private physical therapy services during the summer months when school therapy services are not provided)

➤ *Discharge plan*: Jeremy will be followed for six to eight visits over the summer to work on specific goals related to independent ambulation. One visit in September will be used to make a joint visit with staff at his new school program. School staff will be updated on his progress and motor status. Motor-related services in his educational program will be coordinated between his school physical therapist and adapted physical education teacher. Jeremy then will be discharged from private physical therapy

Criteria for Termination of Physical Therapy Services

According to the *Guide to Physical Therapist Practice*[4] discharge is the process of ending physical therapy services following a single episode of care. Discharge occurs when anticipated goals and expected outcomes have been achieved. Discontinuation is the process of ending physical therapy services when the patient or caregiver declines further intervention, the patient is unable to continue progress toward outcomes because of medical or other complications or because financial/insurance resources have been expended, or the physical therapist determines that the patient will no longer benefit from intervention. Children with life-long disabilities may require multiple episodes of care following changes in physical status (due to growth or surgical interventions), caregivers, environments, or task demands. In each episode of care, the physical therapist plans for discharge or discontinuation of services.

Motor Learning

The clinical approach of physical therapists to children with pathology of the CNS generally has concentrated on issues of motor control. In the 1950s and 1960s physical and occupational therapists proposed a variety of "neurophysiologic" theories (eg, Neurodevelopmental Treatment [NDT], Proprioceptive Neuromuscular Facilitation [PNF], Sensory Integration [SI]) to address motor control problems.[5] More recently, systems theories have been incorporated in therapeutic approaches. Although the focus on motor control has been consistent, physical therapists traditionally have been less influenced by research in the field of motor learning.

Movement can be categorized into two general classes.[6] One class of movements, such as control of our limbs and walking, appears to be determined primarily by genetic make-up and/or through growth and development. These movements are fairly stereotyped across members of the same species. What CNS structures are involved and how the CNS organizes individual and coordinated movements of the limbs and body are basic questions in the study of motor control. Attempting to classify the relative contributions of genetics and experience, however, always results in a "nature vs nurture" debate (see Chapter 8).

A second class of movements, such as riding a bicycle, writing, or performing a somersault, can be considered *learned*. These movements do not appear to be genetic and require varying (usually long) periods of practice and experience to master. How movements are produced as the result of practice or experience is the major question in the study of motor learning.

Although issues of motor control and motor learning in relation to movement (genetic or practiced) may be somewhat differentiated in normal individuals, the distinction becomes very blurred in the child (and adult) with pathology of the CNS. If a child has damage to CNS structures that produce a specific movement pattern, such as components of the gait cycle, he may have to practice or adapt the movements he is able to produce in order to develop ambulation. In this case, ambulation could be considered a "skill" and is perhaps a better example of motor learning than motor control.

Because most of the functional tasks we want children with disabilities to perform require a combination of motor control and motor learning, applying principles of motor learning to physical therapy intervention is essential. There are few motor learning studies of children with specific disabilities to guide our intervention sessions, however, so we rely on information from studies of typically developing children and adults without disabilities. We should remain cautious in application of principles of motor learning until research studies validate their use with populations of children with disabilities.

Selected motor learning issues and their application to pediatrics are described briefly in the following sections. The reader should refer to publications by Schmidt[6-8] and Winstein[9,10] for more detailed discussions of principles of motor learning.

Performance vs Learning

Motor learning is not directly observable. It is defined as "a set of processes associated with practice or experience leading to relatively permanent changes in the capability for movement."[6] A common example of motor learning that most of us can relate to is learning how to ride a bicycle. It is a motor task that required repeated practice with an adult or sibling assisting with balance or the use of training wheels. Then, there was that magical moment when we rode the bicycle independently (without training wheels) for a few feet, gradually increasing the distance we were able to ride before stopping or crashing. Most of us became skilled at riding a bicycle. As we age, we may not ride a bicycle for many years, but if the opportunity occurs, we can get on a bike and ride away. This is an example of a skill that took many months (perhaps years) to perfect, but resulted in a relatively permanent change in our ability to perform the skill.

When a physical therapist facilitates movement through manual guidance (eg, handling), such as assisting the child with shoulder protraction during reaching, the child's "performance" at that moment is affected. The child's performance can be observed visually or kinesthetically. It only would be evident that the child had "learned" a skill if he consistently and appropriately used protraction of the shoulder over a period of time without intervention. Another example of performance vs learning is the common intervention strategy of facilitating hip abduction and weight shifting during gait training through manual guidance of the pelvis of the child with cerebral palsy. If the child demonstrates this gait pattern only during treatment sessions with manual facilitation and reverts to "scissoring" when attempting ambulation on his own, only performance during the treatment session has changed. The child has not acquired a skill that can be generalized to other settings. In most instances, physical therapists use handling and facilitation or inhibition techniques to assist the child initially to perform a more efficient or coordinated movement. This is an attempt to provide the child with kinesthetic information (ie, feedback) on how this movement feels and to give him an idea of the movement(s) the therapist wants the child to attempt. Handling becomes less frequent as the child is able to produce some aspects of the movement independently. When the child is able to perform the entire movement independently and consistently, not only has he improved his performance, but he also has acquired a skill. Physical therapy that has as its end result only changes in performance is not cost-effective and is of limited value to the child. The goal in physical therapy is for the child to acquire motor skills that will increase his independence in a variety of environments and decrease his dependence on the physical therapist or others.

Transfer of Learning

Transfer of learning refers to a gain (or loss) in the capability for producing a movement or performing a task as the result of practice or experience of another movement or task. According to Schmidt,[6] in research on transfer of learning, two major points emerge. One point is that the amount of transfer between tasks appears to be quite small. The second point is that the amount of transfer depends on the similarity of the tasks; the more similar the tasks, the more likely transfer will occur.

One assumption made in traditional neurophysiologic approaches was that a motor skill learned in one position would provide positive transfer to a skill in another position. For example, it was assumed that having a child practice trunk extension in prone would assist with trunk extension in sitting and standing. Another example is the hypothesis that facilitating balance reactions while the child sits on a therapy ball will improve the child's balance while he sits on the floor.

In the first example, prone extension is a different task for the CNS to organize than trunk extension in sitting and standing where the biomechanical constraints and pull of gravity vary (Figure 3-3). In the second example, responses to externally produced perturbations present different control issues for the CNS than those for achieving and maintaining sitting balance through a feed-forward mechanism (see Chapter 8). The biomechanical aspects of the two sitting positions also vary. In a study that required typically

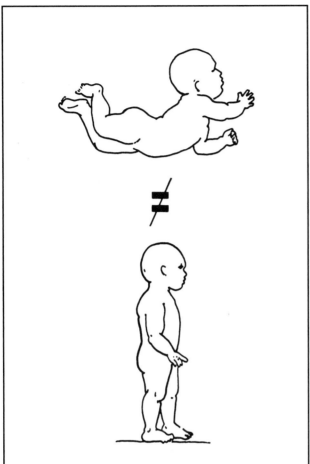

Figure 3-3. Trunk extension in upright position may have different requirements of motor control than extension in prone. (reprinted with permission from Montgomery PC, Connolly B. *Clinical Applications for Motor Control.* Thorofare, NJ: SLACK Incorporated; 2003.)

developing infants to crawl up and down slopes, then eventually to walk up and down slopes, Adolph demonstrated there was no transition of learning from crawling to walking.[11] Instead, infants who had become competent at crawling up and down slopes had to learn, all over again, how to cope with slopes when in an upright position.

Until research studies offer a clearer understanding of the positive transfer of practice between specific movements and skills in children with various impairments, physical therapists can ensure a comprehensive approach to treatment by having children practice the specific target movements or tasks, in addition to those prerequisite movements or tasks assumed to provide positive transfer. This means that, in addition to practicing trunk extension in prone, children will practice trunk extension in sitting and standing; and, in addition to facilitating balance reactions while sitting on a therapy ball, children are provided with ample opportunities to practice independent floor sitting.

Part-Whole Transfer

Another technique used by physical therapists is to have children practice components of a motor task before attempting to practice the entire task (ie, part-whole transfer). For example, children may work in a standing position on balance and lower extremity control, such as kicking a ball, before walking. According to Schmidt, the problem may be that "practice on a part in isolation may so change the motor programming of the part that for all practical purposes it is no longer the same as it is in the context of the total skill."[6]

Research suggests that the effectiveness of part-whole transfer depends on the nature of the task. When tasks are strictly serial in nature, as in an assembly line, practice of parts transfers highly to the whole task. Motor tasks are, however, seldom strictly serial in nature. For example, when reaching for an object from a standing position, milliseconds prior to lifting the arm to reach, the leg and trunk muscles must contract to provide stability and prevent a weight shift forward and possible fall. In walking, there are precise temporal and spatial relationships among and between the muscles of each leg. Schmidt[6] stated that part to whole transfer also might depend on the extent to which the movement is governed by a single motor program. Generally, if a movement is fast, it probably is governed by a single program and should be practiced as a whole. Throwing a ball is an example of a ballistic-type feed-forward movement that is better practiced as a whole. Multi-limb movements occurring simultaneously may be governed by a single program. There is, however, little research to guide physical therapists in determining which movements and tasks may benefit from part to whole transfer. Winstein stated that "natural breaks in the resultant velocity profile of a multi-segmental movement could reflect the end of one subunit and the beginning of the next."[9] In summary, the assumption that breaking down a task for practice always will improve performance on the whole task can be challenged. Physical therapists should include practice on the whole task as well as practice of component parts in treatment.

Variable (Random) vs Constant (Blocked) Practice

The amount of variability within a practice session may affect motor learning. Children, in particular, perform better on a novel task when earlier practice is variable as opposed to constant.[6,12] This suggests that providing variations of tasks and varying practice among tasks during treatment may be more beneficial for motor learning than having children perform a large number of repetitions of a single movement or task. One hypothesis is that each time a component of a task or the task itself is varied, children must concentrate anew and problem solve in relation to the required movements or task. With numerous repetitions, movement becomes automatic and children may concentrate less and not be required to actively problem solve regarding the motor requirements.

Repetition is an essential element in improving motor control. Undoubtedly, there must be a sufficient number of repetitions to receive feedback about movements or success in accomplishing a task and to engage in trial and error learning. The therapist must look for cues that children are performing movement in a rote fashion with little attention to the task, and, at that point, vary the task requirements. Treatment sessions should be structured to accommodate differences in attention level and activities should be motivating. A practical example would be to have children change positions and practice various skills several times within a 45-minute treatment session, dictated by their attention spans and the difficulty of the tasks. This would be preferable to predetermining the structure of a treatment session, for example, spending 15 minutes working on prone extension, 15 minutes working on sitting balance, and 15 minutes working on gait. Schmidt stated that "blocked (constant) practice and drills are highly ineffective ways to generate learning and should almost never be used."[7] The exception would be very early practice when children initially are acquiring a movement or basic skill. Schmidt suggested that once a movement can be performed, practice should be randomized. A related point is that practice needs to be somewhat difficult and require effort on the part of the children. The challenge for the physical therapist is to find activities that entice children to attempt and repeat movements that require effort and concentration.

Feedback/Knowledge of Results

One of the most important variables enhancing motor learning is feedback or information that is provided to the child about his performance as he attempts to move or accomplish a task. Intrinsic feedback refers to information obtained through sensory systems (eg, visual, somatosensory, vestibular) as movement is attempted or produced. Extrinsic feedback refers primarily to verbal information (eg, from a physical therapist) related to performance. Extrinsic feedback also can be provided through nonverbal means, such as a switch device that activates a musical toy each time the child lifts his head to an upright position in sitting.

Knowledge of Performance vs Knowledge of Results

Gentile[13] distinguished between knowledge of performance (KP—feedback about the movement itself) and knowledge of results (KR—feedback about the outcome of the movement). Providing the child information on how effectively the back muscles are contracting (KP) vs providing information on how effectively he is maintaining an upright sitting posture (KR) is a specific example. Most research to date has focused on information regarding movement outcome (KR) and the current assumption is that the mechanisms of KR and KP are similar.[6]

Thorpe and Valvano[14] examined the effects of presenting KP and KP augmented by a cognitive strategy to 13 children with cerebral palsy during practice of a novel skill (ie, moving a Pedalo/standing therapeutic exercise equipment). Results suggested that some of the children benefited greatly from KP and the use of cognitive strategies as they practiced the task.

Traditional vs Contemporary View

The traditional view of feedback (prior to the 1980s) was that feedback that was more frequent, more immediate, more accurate, or produced more information had the most positive effect on learning.[6,7] More recent research caused a reexamination of how feedback enhances learning. It appears that while frequent feedback may enhance motor performance, it actually may be detrimental to motor learning. This sometimes is a startling notion to physical therapists if the role of feedback has been viewed in a traditional manner. One hypothesis is that feedback that is provided too frequently interferes with the child's ability to learn to detect and correct errors. Less frequent feedback or fading feedback appears to be more beneficial for motor learning.[6-10] In practical terms this means physical therapists should avoid providing feedback after every trial or attempt at movement. Schmidt[6] stated that more guidance may be needed in complex tasks, whereas less guidance may be needed in simple motor tasks.

Various schedules of feedback have been examined experimentally and have been reviewed elsewhere.[6-8] An alternative to constant feedback would be to provide feedback in summary form after several trials. Another alternative is "bandwidth KR" where feedback is given only if the movement or performance is outside a given error range. The absence of KR informs the child that his movement is acceptable. A practical example would be monitoring the child's tendency to "W-sit" during a treatment session. The

Figure 3-4. "W-sitting" with internally rotated and buttocks flat on floor.

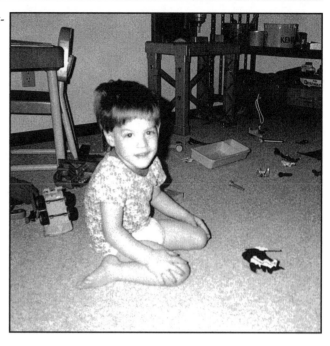

child can be instructed that kneel-sitting on the feet is acceptable, but kneel-sitting while internally rotating the hips with the feet out to the side of the body with the buttocks on the floor is unacceptable (Figures 3-4 and 3-5). The therapist decides to call the child's attention to his "W-sitting" position whenever the child sits in this position for more than 30 seconds. The absence of feedback at other times informs the child that his sitting posture is acceptable. Another example would be calling the child's attention to foot placement only when the foot is placed outside of an area where it could serve as a BOS during a series of attempts to move from half-kneeling to standing at a sofa. Although the child may vary his foot placement from trial to trial, as long as he could shift his weight adequately to push to stand, he would receive no feedback. Bandwidth KR can be used to allow more variability of movement, prevent too frequent feedback (after every trial), and allow the child to concentrate on intrinsic feedback to monitor his movements.

Application to Pediatrics

Several principles of KR have special applicability in the treatment of children. When KR is provided, it is provided during or immediately after a movement or task is completed. The interval between completion of a movement and feedback from the therapist should be "empty." In other words, children should not be asked to perform other movements or be distracted by the therapist or environment. It is hypothesized that children may be retaining in short-term memory kinesthetic information regarding the movement and that this process should proceed without distractions. Therapists should be cautious about distracting children unnecessarily by talking or calling attention to toys or other objects in the environment.

In research with children, it has been determined that performance is disrupted when shortening the period of time following KR and when a subsequent attempt is made to repeat the movement or task.[6] The assumption is that new solutions to motor problems are being processed and a certain amount of time is necessary for this to occur. Children

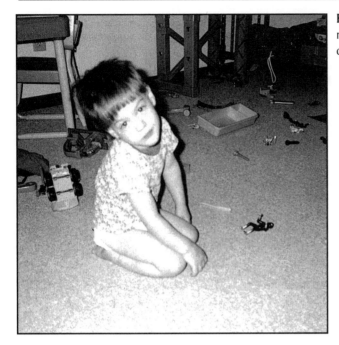

Figure 3-5. "Heel-sitting" with hips in neutral alignment and buttocks resting on feet.

should be allowed to initiate repetitions of movements and tasks at self-determined speeds.

One limitation in applying motor learning principles to physical therapy is that we do not know how applicable various concepts are to infants and children with impaired cognition. Seeger[15] summarized studies of adults with disabilities demonstrating that cognitive processes may compete with processes for postural control. Hsiang and coworkers[16] investigated the influence of three different concurrent cognitive tasks on gait characteristics in typically developing 5- to 7-year-old children. Gait speed was lower under the three dual tasks conditions than when walking alone. Cadance and step length also decreased under some of the dual-task conditions. Results of this study indicated that it may be difficult for children to maintain motor performance while simultaneously processing cognitive information. Additional research related to cognitive interference in typically developing children and children with disabilities is necessary to determine clinical implications.

Guidance

Guidance refers to a number of procedures ranging from physically assisting movement (facilitation/handling) to verbally talking the child through a task.[6] In general, guidance tends to prevent the child from making errors. One hypothesis in support of facilitation and handling (guidance) is that improved quality of movement will be produced and the child will be less apt to learn incorrect movements and, therefore, will not repeat or learn these less desirable movements. In an opposite view, motor learning appears to be most effective in trial and error situations. The child must learn which internal commands lead to effective or ineffective outcomes, and the only way to learn this is to make and try to correct errors.

Although research is limited, it appears that guidance is most effective in early practice of new, unfamiliar tasks. Guidance also may be more effective for slow movements where feedback may be used for control and monitoring.

Physical guidance may be beneficial in showing the child what to do and perhaps in reducing fear when having the child attempt new motor skills. The physical therapist initially assists the child in producing a response or movement that can be improved with practice; less guidance is used as the child takes more responsibility for producing the movement.

Too much guidance, however, may act as a "crutch," preventing the child from experiencing errors and learning from his own attempts at movement. In the presence of a damaged CNS, it may be idealistic to assume that we can facilitate normal movement. The goal of physical therapy should be for the child to produce the most efficient and effective movements to accomplish functional tasks. The physical therapist must decide when facilitation designed to improve quality of movement should be discarded and emphasis placed on alternative strategies for accomplishing a motor task.

Motor-Learning Summary

Feedback appears to be essential for motor learning. Providing feedback less frequently, however, may be more beneficial for learning than immediate feedback following each attempt at movement. The use of less frequent verbal feedback and less manual facilitation of movement may be frustrating for the physical therapist because the child's performance may actually deteriorate during the treatment session. Schmidt[7] suggested that the goal of physical therapy is not necessarily to produce the best performance during therapy, but to organize practice to maximize retention (eg, learning).

Organizing Treatment

Context

In Gibson's[17] theoretical model for understanding human behavior, called *ecological psychology*, the child and the environment are linked. Objects in the environment are described in terms of affordances or what they offer the child for perceptual exploration and movement. For example, while observing a 7-month-old child belly crawling on the floor, a toy is placed on an 18-inch high sofa (Figure 3-6). The child sees the toy and appears interested in it, but does not attempt to reach the toy. If the sofa cushion (6 inches in height) is placed on the floor and the toy is placed on top of the cushion, the child reaches up to the sofa cushion, pulls himself up on his knees, and reaches for the toy (Figure 3-7). The top of the sofa was too high for the child to reach from a prone position and, therefore, did not afford the child a surface to pull up on. The sofa cushion on the floor, however, was of an appropriate height and afforded the child the opportunity to pull up into a kneeling position to obtain the toy.

Physical therapists working with children construct "affordances" in the environment to elicit functional movements.[18] The importance of practicing skills in various environments (eg, home, school, community) that relate to long-term functional goals also is recognized. Physical therapists want children to be able to perform specific skills, such as ambulation, in a variety of environments (ie, different contexts). Being able to walk safely in a therapy room with a tile floor and few obstacles or distractions does not ensure that

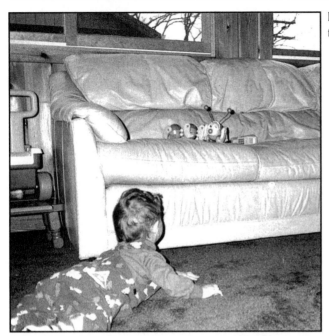

Figure 3-6. From prone, child is unable to pull to kneeling at a sofa.

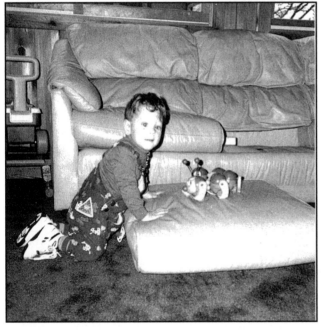

Figure 3-7. From prone, child is able to pull to kneeling at a sofa cushion.

children will be able to walk safely on carpet in a cluttered, noisy, and visually distracting classroom or in a variety of community settings.

To ensure use of the same skill in varied contexts, the physical therapist has children practice the skill in each environment and makes modifications or alters training as necessary. This often is a difficult concept for some third-party payers, who prefer to reimburse physical therapy services that are delivered on an outpatient basis in a hospital or medically related facility. Medicare guidelines for home-based services have been inappropriately applied to children and some payers only will allow home-based services for children who are medically fragile and unable to leave the home environment. This is an outdated practice that should be discarded. Environments in which it is important for children to function include the home, school, neighborhood, and community settings including church, shopping mall, and playground. Several physical therapy sessions spent on the neighborhood playground may appear frivolous to a third party payer. This is the best context, however, in which children can learn skills that will enable them to effectively and safely move and interact with peers in a playground setting. It also may be more efficient to design home programs for children in their own environments, using the furniture and natural affordances available (eg, stairs, specific bathroom layout). Physical therapists in outpatient settings have to make a concentrated effort to provide caregivers with appropriate suggestions for carry-over in home, school, or community environments. There are instances, however, when outpatient physical therapy may be the most efficient setting for providing pediatric services. For example, when specific equipment is needed (eg, whirlpool, treadmill) or when children do not perform well in the home environment and are more cooperative in an outpatient setting. Hopefully, third-party payers will become more flexible in allowing physical therapy services to be provided in the settings in which therapy will be most effective in achieving improved functional independence.

The Normal Developmental Sequence

Physical therapists traditionally have used normal development as a guide for evaluating and treating children with pathology of the CNS. Normal development has been considered the "gold standard" for movement and all of the traditional neurophysiologic theorists used the "normal developmental sequence" as a basic principle in their approaches. However, research has shown that a single normal developmental sequence of motor skills does not exist. Bottos and coworkers[19] completed a prospective study of 424 children (270 infants cared for in a neonatal intensive care unit and 154 infants without perinatal complications who served as a control group) and documented the locomotor strategies used before the acquisition of independent walking. There were a variety of sequences used by both the preterm and full-term children. For example, 9% of the children never crawled on hands and knees, but moved by shuffling on their bottoms (ie, hitching) and 12% just stood up and walked. There were, therefore, more typical and less typical sequences of motor development documented. Follow-up data until the children were 5 years of age demonstrated that the children who chose alternative patterns such as bottom shuffling or "just walking" did not demonstrate intellectual or language delays any more frequently than infants who belly crawled or crawled on hands and knees before walking. Studies by Adolph[11,20,21] also confirmed that motor development does not adhere to a strict progression of obligatory, discrete stages.

Early motor skills (eg, rolling, belly crawling, sitting, all-fours creeping, pulling to stand, cruising, walking) provide physical therapists with information regarding components of movements and patterns used by typically developing children. These developmental motor milestones are important functional goals. However, they do not have to be achieved in a specific sequence. Karel and Berta Bobath[22] recognized this many years ago, stating in 1984:

> *"However, we soon found that it was not enough—indeed, it was wrong—to try to follow the normal developmental sequence too closely. We had made the child rigidly go through the stage of rolling over, before going on to sitting, side-sitting, kneeling, kneel-standing, half-kneeling, crawling, and then finally stand-*

ing; one stage after the other. But that sequence is not followed faithfully by normal children…. normal children develop many activities simultaneously, which reinforce each other to culminate in a 'milestone'."

The developmental sequence of skill acquisition has been demonstrated to be variable in both in typically developing children and children with disabilities.[19-24] This variability is a compelling argument for not using the developmental sequence as a rigid, prescriptive model for treatment. In traditional hierarchical models the child would be discouraged from practicing "higher" skills before "lower" skills were mastered. For example, practice of ambulation would be delayed until sitting balance was established. Arguments for and against using the developmental sequence as a model in the treatment of children and adults have been discussed previously.[25-28]

An alternative approach to using a developmental sequence is to have the child practice a variety of age-appropriate functional tasks that he might reasonably be expected to accomplish. A child 2 years of age with spastic diplegia, for example, may have difficulty maintaining floor sitting due to increased muscle activity or tightness of the hamstrings, yet he may be able to control his balance in upright using a walker. This child may never master the task of independent floor sitting and, if the developmental sequence were followed prescriptively, he would not be allowed to practice ambulation skills. The child with spastic hemiplegia might never crawl on hands and knees because his involved upper extremity will not support his weight. Research studies have shown that most, if not all, children with spastic hemiplegia become ambulatory.[29,30] It would be illogical to prevent the child with hemiplegia from ambulating until he could crawl on hands and knees. The alternative approach is to work on a variety of skills simultaneously, allowing the child to progress with the acquisition of skills at varying rates as allowed by neurological, biomechanical, cognitive, and other factors (eg, a systems approach).

How basic motor skills are accomplished does not need to mirror "normal." Consider the child with arthrogryposis who is limited in how he moves because of lack of specific muscles and certain joint limitations. This child will not be able to produce "normal" movement using the same muscles and joint range of motion of nondisabled peers. Yet, by using the muscles and joint range of motion available, the child with arthrogryposis may be able to accomplish the motor skills necessary to function independently. Do we conclude that the quality of his movements is poor because they do not look like the movements produced by a typically developing peer?

Latash and Anson[31] questioned current assumptions regarding movement patterns in individuals with movement disorders. They stated that current assumptions include: "1) patterns of voluntary movements seen in the general population are the only correct ones, 2) deviations from 'normal' movement patterns reflect a failure of the CNS to behave 'correctly,' and 3) we know more about motor control than the CNS does."

These authors suggested that an alternative hypothesis be considered, specifically that under certain conditions, as in children with motor impairments, the CNS may reconsider its priorities. Perhaps the changed motor patterns that result should not be considered pathological, but rather adaptive to a primary disorder and may even be viewed as optimal for a given state. For each particular motor task, Latash and Anson suggested that the main criterion is functional success. Perhaps movements should be judged primarily by their effectiveness in accomplishing a task. For example, rather than evaluating gait in terms of heel-strike, stance, toe-off, and swing-through or examining the specific muscles involved in each phase, gait should be evaluated in terms of its major functional components. Functional components would include support and propulsion in stance, clearance of the foot during swing, and a transfer of momentum in swing.[32]

If children with developmental disabilities are able to accomplish the functional components of ambulation perhaps the quality of their movements should be considered good, regardless of how closely they approximate typical movement patterns. Moore and coworkers[33] found, for example, that oxygen cost was higher for reciprocal walking than for a swing-through gait in adolescents with low lumbar myelomeningocele. The authors suggested that a swing-through gait was the more efficient walking pattern for this group of subjects. Energy consumption is a critical variable to consider during motor tasks. Franks, Palisano, and Darbee[34] demonstrated that the high energy cost of walking (compared to using a wheelchair) may have adversely affected certain aspects of school performance in three (9, 10, and 15 years old) students with myelomeningocele.

Another important issue in evaluating the quality of movement is to determine the potential for the development of secondary problems.[35] For example, "W-sitting" when used excessively may contribute to decreased range of motion in hip external rotation, knee instability, and excessive ankle eversion, resulting in a poor BOS in standing. Reaching only with the forearm in a pronated position will limit active forearm supination and muscle tightness may result. Prolonged wearing of ankle-foot orthoses may result in decreased ankle plantarflexion range of motion that will make floor mobility (eg, crawling on all fours, tall kneeling) and dressing and undressing the lower extremities more difficult. The child and family must be informed about the risk of secondary problems and, together with the therapist, make decisions about which patterns of movements and positions should be promoted.

Sequencing Treatment

Usually several impairments occur simultaneously in children with developmental disabilities. For example, children may demonstrate deficits in sensory processing, motor control, strength, and attention. In organizing treatment and attempting to address various problem areas simultaneously, there are two general treatment sequences to consider. The first is the overall sequence of treatment over an extended period of time, for example, a 3-month period or a school year. Careful formulation of long- and short-term functional objectives will aid the therapist in obtaining a mental overview of the necessary emphasis in treatment. The second consideration is sequencing treatment within an individual treatment session which may vary from a half-hour to an hour or longer.

Variables to be considered when determining the content of an individual treatment session are the cognitive abilities of the child, motivation, age, and endurance. A *play* vs a *work* approach can be varied depending on the age, personality, and interests of the child. Toys can be used quite effectively to motivate the young child and infant and to maintain interest during therapy. If a child resists or fatigues during certain activities, such as abdominal strengthening, three or four treatment techniques designed to strengthen the abdominal muscles can be interspersed during an individual session.

Techniques for behavior management can be employed to assist in specific sensory or motor tasks and also as a way to modify negative behavior during therapy. Checklists of exercises, which when completed yield a reward, often are helpful to motivate the child and to help the child be more organized during therapy. A small kitchen timer can be used to designate specific *work* (15 minutes) vs *play* (3 minutes) sessions, or specific rewards can be given for each 15-minute "crying-free" period of time.

A final, but perhaps the most important, consideration is the availability of caregivers for carryover of treatment. Whenever possible, the physical therapist should involve the family, school personnel, and other caregivers in the child's therapy program. Clearly defined behavioral objectives will assist in this process and the therapist can facilitate the child's progress by training others in the child's environment(s) in related therapeutic activities, and, when necessary, the use of adaptive equipment. Byl[36] reviewed animal and human research that documented the importance of repetition, attention, and positive feedback in motor learning and motor control. Maximum neural adaptation occurs in individuals committed to learning. Therefore, providing motivation for the child and caregivers to "practice, practice, practice" is essential.

Documenting Progress

Physical therapists are responsible not only for determining functional outcomes for the child, but also for determining whether the objectives have been met. Various methods for charting progress have been described.[37] An important component is to differentiate motor performance from motor learning. One method used to determine whether functional objectives have been learned is to observe the child at the beginning of the treatment session to document his performance before treatment begins. Another method is to have the parent or teacher chart specific movements or tasks (eg, number of times the child assumes all fours independently per day) between treatment sessions. Reference materials, including *Standards of Practice for Physical Therapy* and *Guidelines for Documentation*, are available through the American Physical Therapy Association and provide comprehensive information regarding appropriate components of documentation.

Summary

Developing a strategy for planning and sequencing treatment requires physical therapists to impose organization on the many variables affecting this process. Although individual therapists will have differing theoretical frameworks, the use of well-defined, long- and short-term functional outcomes will improve communication among professionals, parents, other caregivers, and third party payers about the child's current functioning, physical therapy intervention, and progress.

References

1. Montgomery PC, Connolly BH. Norm-referenced and criterion-referenced tests: use in pediatrics and application to task analysis of motor skills. *Phys Ther.* 1987;67:1873-1876.
2. Pellegrino L. Cerebral palsy: a paradigm for developmental disabilities. *Dev Med Child Neurol.* 1995;37:834-838.
3. Horak FB. Assumptions underlying motor control for neurologic rehabilitation. In: Foundation of Physical Therapy. *Contemporary Management of Motor Control Problems: Proceedings of the II STEP Conference.* Alexandria, Va: American Physical Therapy Association; 1991:85-87.
4. American Physical Therapy Association. *Guide to Physical Therapist Practice.* Alexandria, Va: Author; 2001.
5. Connolly BH, Montgomery PC. Framework for examination, evaluation, and intervention. In: Montgomery PC, Connolly BH, eds. *Clinical Applications for Motor Control.* Thorofare, NJ: SLACK Incorporated; 2003:1-23.
6. Schmidt RA, Lee TD. *Motor Control and Learning. A Behavioral Emphasis.* 3rd ed. Champaign, Ill: Human Kinetics; 1999.

7. Schmidt RA. Motor learning principles for physical therapy. In: Foundation for Physical Therapy. *Contemporary Management of Motor Control Problems: Proceedings of the II STEP Conference.* Alexandria, Va: American Physical Therapy Association; 1991:49-64.

8. Schmidt RA, Wrisberg CA. *Motor Learning and Performance.* 2nd ed. Champaign, Ill: Human Kinetics Publisher, Inc; 2000.

9. Winstein CJ. Designing practice for motor learning: clinical implications. In: Foundation for Physical Therapy. *Contemporary Management of Motor Control Problems: Proceedings of the II STEP Conference.* Alexandria, Va: American Physical Therapy Association; 1991:65-76.

10. Winstein CJ. Knowledge of results and motor-learning—implications for physical therapy. *Phys Ther.* 1991;71:140-149.

11. Adolph KE. Learning in the development of infant locomotion. *Monogr Soc Res Child Dev.* 1997;62:1-158.

12. Shapiro DC, Schmidt RA. The schema theory: recent evidence and developmental implications. In: Kelso JAS, Clark JE, eds. *Development of Movement Control and Coordination.* New York, NY: Wiley; 1981.

13. Gentile AM. A working model of skill acquisition with application to teaching. *Quest.* 1972;17:3-23.

14. Thorpe DE, Valvano J. The effects of knowledge of performance and cognitive strategies on motor skill learning in children with cerebral palsy. *Pediatr Phys Ther.* 2002;14:2-15.

15. Seeger MA. Balance deficits: examination, evaluation, and intervention. In: Montgomery PC, Connolly BH (eds). *Clinical Applications for Motor Control.* Thorofare, NJ: SLACK Incorporated; 2003:271-306.

16. Hsiang H-J, Mercer VS, Thorpe DE. Effects of different concurrent cognitive tasks on temporal-distance gait variables in children. *Pediatr Phys Ther.* 2003;15:105-113.

17. Gibson JJ. *The Ecological Approach to Visual Perception.* Boston, Mass: Houghton Mifflin Company; 1979.

18. Fetters L. Cerebral palsy: contemporary treatment concepts. In: Foundation for Physical Therapy. *Contemporary Management of Motor Control Problems: Proceedings of II STEP Conference.* Alexandria, Va: American Physical Therapy Association; 1991:219-224.

19. Bottos M, Dalla Barba B, Stefani D. Locomotor strategies preceding independent walking: prospective study of neurological and language development in 424 cases. *Dev Med Child Neurol.* 1989;31:25-34.

20. Adolph KE, VereiJken B, Denny MA. Learning to crawl. *Child Dev.* 1998;69:1299-1312.

21. Adolph KE. Specificity of learning: why infants fall over a veritable cliff. *Psychol Sci.* 2000;11:290-295.

22. Bobath B, Bobath K. The neuro-developmental treatment. In: Scrutton D, ed. *Management of the Motor Disorders in Cerebral Palsy. Clinics in Developmental Medicine #90.* London, England; 1984:6-18.

23. Bottos M, Puato ML, Viancello A, et al. Locomotion patterns in cerebral palsy syndromes. *Dev Med Child Neurol.* 1995;37:883-899.

24. Cintas H. Cross cultural variation in motor development. *Phys Occup Ther Pediatr.* 1988;8:1-20.

25. VanSant A. Motor control, motor learning, and motor development. In: Montgomery PC, Connolly BH, eds. *Clinical Applications for Motor Control.* Thorofare, NJ: SLACK Incorporated; 2003:25-50.

26. Attermeier S. Should the normal motor developmental sequence be used as a theoretical model in patient treatment? In: Foundation for Physical Therapy. *Contemporary Management of Motor Control Problems: Proceedings of the II STEP Conference.* Alexandria, Va: American Physical Therapy Association; 1991:85-87.

27. Atwater SW. Should the normal developmental sequence be used as a theoretical model in pediatric physical therapy? In: Foundation for Physical Therapy. *Contemporary Management of Motor Control Problems: Proceedings of the II STEP Conference.* Alexandria, Va: American Physical Therapy Association; 1991:89-93.

28. VanSant AF. Should the normal developmental sequence be used as a theoretical model to progress adult patients? In: Foundation for Physical Therapy. *Contemporary Management of Motor Control Problems: Proceedings of the II STEP Conference.* Alexandria, Va: American Physical Therapy Association; 1991:95-97.

29. Bleck EE. Locomotor prognosis in cerebral palsy. *Dev Med Child Neurol.* 1975;17:18-25.

30. Molnar GE, Gordon SU. Cerebral palsy: predictive value of selected clinical signs for early prognostication of motor function. *Arch Phys Med Rehabil.* 1976;57:153-158.

31. Latash ML, Anson JG. What are "normal" movements in atypical populations? *Behav Brain Sci.* 1996;19:55-106.

32. Oatis CA. Perspectives on examination, evaluation, and intervention for disorders of gait. In: Montgomery PC, Connolly BH, eds. *Clinical Applications for Motor Control.* Thorofare, NJ: SLACK Incorporated; 2003:335-363.

33. Moore CA, Nejad B, Novak RA, et al. Energy cost of walking in low lumbar myelomeningocele. *J Pediatr Orthop.* 2001;21:388-391.

34. Franks CA, Palisano RJ, Darbee JC. The effect of walking with an assistive device and using a wheelchair on school performance in students with myelomeningocele. *Phys Ther.* 1991;71:570-577.

35. Gudjonsdottir B, Mercer VS. Hip and spine in children with cerebral palsy: musculoskeletal development and clinical implications. *Pediatr Phys Ther.* 1997;9:179-185.

36. Byl NN. Neuroplasticity: applications to motor control. In: Montgomery PC, Connolly BH, eds. *Clinical Applications for Motor Control.* Thorofare, New Jersey: SLACK Incorporated; 2003:79-106.

37. Effgen S. Systematic delivery and recording of intervention assistance. *Pediatr Phys Ther.* 1991;3:63-68.

THE CHILDREN: HISTORY AND SYSTEMS REVIEW

Barbara H. Connolly, EdD, PT, FAPTA
Patricia C. Montgomery, PhD, PT, FAPTA

One of the major problems experienced by the student, new graduate, or clinician inexperienced in pediatric developmental therapy is integrating theory with practice. A problem-solving approach can be helpful for developing skill in the practical application of examination, evaluation, and intervention strategies. To facilitate a problem-solving approach, we have selected five case studies that represent typical issues encountered by the clinician. Contributing authors were asked to address impairments and functional limitations observed in five children with varying developmental problems and to suggest appropriate intervention strategies from a variety of perspectives. In general, the disablement model used in the *Guide to Physical Therapist Practice* (Chapter 5) is stressed. An alternative framework, the enablement model, from the Word Health Organization is also presented (Chapters 11 and 13). Composite history and systems reviews are presented in this chapter for each of the children and should be reviewed briefly before proceeding to the subsequent chapters.

Case Study #1: Jason

➤ Practice pattern 5C: Impaired Motor Function and Sensory Integrity Associated With Nonprogressive Disorders of the Central Nervous System—Congenital Origin or Acquired in Infancy or Childhood

➤ Medical diagnosis: Cerebral palsy, right hemiparesis

➤ Age: 24 months

Examination

HISTORY

Jason was the first born of nonidentical twins with a birthweight of 1660 grams. His Apgars were 7 at 1 minute and 9 at 5 minutes. He did not require mechanical ventilation and was discharged from the neonatal intensive care unit (NICU) after 40 days on caffeine-citrate due to bradycardia with feedings. Initial follow-up at 2 months of gestational age was nonremarkable. At his follow-up visit at 6 months of age definite asymmetries in stretch reflexes and voluntary use of his extremities were noted. Jason was referred for early intervention services. He currently receives home-based services consisting of weekly visits from his local school district (alternating between teacher and occupational therapist) and once per week visits from a private speech therapist and a private physical therapist. Jason is not on any medication and has not had any surgical procedures.

Systems Review

➤ *Anthropometric characteristics*: Jason is noted to have a slightly smaller right upper extremity (only noticeable in the upper arm) as compared to the left. He is of average height and weight for his age.

➤ *Arousal, attention, and cognition*: Testing indicates that Jason's IQ falls within the average range. He has delayed expressive language and relies more on gestures for communication than other children his age. Tactile stimulation generally results in an increased activity level.

➤ *Assistive and adaptive devices*: None.

➤ *Gait, locomotion, and balance*: Jason began walking at 15 months of age. His gait is characterized by a short swing phase on the right, short stride length with retraction of the pelvis on the right, minimal right knee and ankle flexion at mid-swing, short stance phase on the right with genu recurvatum, and a valgus position of the right foot at mid-stance. He initiates walking with the left side and turns and changes direction from the left side only. He falls frequently during the day.

➤ *Integumentary integrity*: Normal.

➤ *Joint integrity and mobility*: Within normal range to passive movement.

➤ *Motor function (motor control and motor learning)*: Jason is able to follow directions and attempts to imitate motor skills, although he has generally poor coordination of his right extremities. He has slow and often ineffective protective reactions on the right side. Isolated control of right forearm and finger movements is difficult.

➤ *Muscle performance*: Weakness is evident in the right upper extremity, particularly in the triceps and supinators of the forearm. He also has generalized weakness in the right lower extremity.

➤ *Neuromotor development and sensory integration*: Jason has good head control in all positions. He can assume an all-fours position and bear partial weight on his right upper extremity. He can crawl but occasionally collapses on the right arm. He can get into standing independently from the middle of the floor by assuming a bear stance and rising. He uses a gross grasp with the right hand for most fine motor tasks. He attempts to run, but is clumsy and usually falls. Gross motor skills range between 12 to 15 months.

➤ *Orthotics*: None.

➤ *Posture*: In standing, Jason demonstrates an asymmetrical posture with a slight anterior tilt of the pelvis and pelvic retraction on the right. He has an observable asymmetry in the rib cage. The right upper extremity usually is held in a position of shoulder retraction with elbow, wrist, and finger flexion.

➤ *Range of motion*: Active reach of the right arm is limited to 90 degrees of humeral abduction. Jason also demonstrates tightness to passive stretch in the hip muscles and lateral trunk flexors on the right with limitation in trunk rotation.

➤ *Reflex integrity*: Hyperactive stretch reflexes are present to tendon tap at the ankle (plantarflexors), knee (quadriceps), and elbow (biceps) on the right. Normal stretch reflexes are evident on the left side of the body.

➤ *School/play, community, and leisure integration*: Jason enjoys age-appropriate play activities and demonstrates typical behaviors for a 24-month-old child when his sibling or other children are present.

➤ *Self-care (ADL)*: Jason drools occasionally, especially when concentrating on an activity. He is a "messy" eater, often losing food out of his mouth. He does not seem to notice when food escapes from his mouth. He is just beginning to assist with dressing and undressing activities. He also is beginning to show some interest in toilet-training.

➤ *Sensory integrity*: General neglect of the right side of the body, especially the right upper extremity, is noted. Tactile defensive behaviors occasionally are observed.

➤ *Ventilation and respiration*: Breathiness is noted during speech and consonants are limited in quantity and quality. He often gasps for breath after drinking.

Case Study #2: Jill

➤ Practice pattern 5C: Impaired Motor Function and Sensory Integrity Associated With Nonprogressive Disorders of the Central Nervous System—Congenital Origin or Acquired in Infancy or Childhood

➤ Medical diagnosis: Cerebral palsy, spastic quadriparesis, microcephaly, mental retardation, seizure disorder

➤ Age: 7 years

Examination

HISTORY

Jill was born full-term following a normal pregnancy. Her APGAR scores were 5 at 1 minute and 8 at 5 minutes. Jill had seizures during the neonatal period and had an abnormal electroencephalogram (EEG). She was on mechanical ventilation for several days and initially had feeding difficulties. She was discharged from the NICU on anti-seizure medication. At the time of discharge, she was drinking well from a bottle. At a 4-month follow-up visit with her pediatrician, decreased head growth was noted. She had a normal eye exam and BAER (brainstem auditory evoked response). Jill has continued to have occasional seizures. She had orthopedic surgery (heelcord and adductor releases) at 5 years of age. Jill received weekly intervention services (occupational, speech, and physical therapy) through a private agency from the time of her discharge from the NICU until she entered a public school program full days at 6 years of age. Jill is in an educational setting where she is in a special education classroom. She is mainstreamed with other children for part of each day. She receives occupational, speech, and physical therapy services (30 minutes per week each) on an indirect basis. Programming is carried out in the classroom with the help of a classroom aide.

Systems Review

➤ *Anthropometric characteristics*: Jill has a small head (microcephaly) and is below the 10th percentile in height and weight for her age.

➤ *Arousal, attention, and cognition*: Testing indicates that Jill's IQ is below 50 (severe mental retardation). She often is lethargic, which appears to be related to her seizure medication. When she is alert, she is easily distracted and has poor selective attention. She is a sociable child, however, and is easily motivated. Jill has few words and communicates through variations in vocalization patterns.

➤ *Assistive and adaptive devices*: Jill has an adapted manual wheelchair. She has a prone stander at school and at home.

➤ *Gait, locomotion, and balance*: Jill is nonambulatory and has poor potential for assisted ambulation. She is unable to maintain her balance in any position (eg, sitting, kneeling, all fours, standing).

➤ *Integumentary integrity*: Skin integrity is normal, but Jill is at risk for skin irritation due to lack of active movement and prolonged positioning in sitting.

➤ *Joint integrity and mobility*: Rib cage and shoulder girdle immobility are noted.

➤ *Motor function (motor control and motor learning)*: Motor control is very limited. Jill has poor head control in all positions. She attempts to grasp, but her hand often closes involuntarily prior to obtaining an object. Voluntary release is difficult and she is unable to manipulate objects with her fingers. She has limited voluntary movement of her extremities. She also has poor ocular control and lacks downward gaze.

➤ *Muscle performance*: Jill has generalized weakness due to her limited motor control and paucity of active movement. Poor muscle development/bulk is noted throughout her extremities.

➤ *Neuromotor development and sensory integration*: Gross motor skills are at approximately a 3-month level. Jill can lift her head momentarily in prone, but not in supine. She maintains her head in neutral when held vertically, but generally has poor head control. She is not able to sit without support. She can roll to side-lying from supine, but does not roll over. She has no independent floor mobility. Protective and equilibrium responses to movement are absent. Movement through space results in autonomic distress. She demonstrates hypersensitivity in the oral area with increased lip retraction and head extension.

➤ *Orthotics*: Jill has static ankle ankle-foot orthoses (AFOs) that she uses when she stands in her stander.

➤ *Posture*: A kyphotic posture is noted in the upper back with her head and neck often in hyperextension. She has a mild scoliosis and an indented sternum.

➤ *Range of motion*: Tightness is noted in capital extensors, pectorals, shoulder girdle muscles, hip flexors, and lumbar extensors. Active reach is 60 degrees of humeral abduction and passive range is limited to 90 degrees.

➤ *Reflex integrity*: Hyperactive tendon reflexes are noted in upper and lower extremities (+3 to +4). Jill demonstrates increased resistance (stiffness) to passive movements of her extremities and trunk.

➤ *School/play, community, and leisure integration*: Jill needs adult assistance to participate in play and classroom activities. She enjoys watching videos and children's television programs, but needs assistance or positioning for head control. She is participating in a community-sponsored adaptive swimming class and therapeutic horseback riding (hippotherapy).

➤ *Self-care (ADL)*: Oral-motor skills are poor and Jill has difficulty eating and drinking. She demonstrates severe cheek/lip retraction and jaw thrusting. Her tongue is thick in contour and often retracted. Coordination with respiration during feeding is poor with much coughing and choking. Jill occasionally will assist in dressing by pushing her arms through sleeves and can assist in standing-pivot transfers, otherwise she is totally dependent on caregivers for self-cares. She is not toilet trained.

➤ *Sensory integrity*: Vision is normal, although she has poor ocular-motor control. Hearing also is within the normal range. Jill demonstrates hypersensitivity to movement (vestibular stimulation) and to tactile stimulation in and around the mouth.

➤ *Ventilation and respiration*: Jill's rib cage generally is immobile and she demonstrates an asynchronous respiratory pattern. She is susceptible to upper respiratory infections.

Case Study #3: Taylor

➤ Practice pattern 5C: Impaired Motor Function and Sensory Integrity Associated With Nonprogressive Disorders of the Central Nervous System—Congenital Origin or Acquired in Infancy or Childhood

➤ Medical diagnosis: Myelomeningocele, repaired L1-2

➤ Age: 4 years

Examination

HISTORY

Taylor was a full-term infant, born by Cesarean section due to fetal distress and breech presentation. At birth a large myelomeningocele was noted and was closed surgically. A ventricular-peritoneal shunt was surgically inserted on day 5. Taylor had increased apnea and was on a respirator. He had questionable seizures, but his EEG was normal. He had a suspected Arnold-Chiari malformation that was treated by surgical release of the posterior fossa. He had equinovarus deformities and underwent serial casting beginning at 2 weeks of age. Following a 4-month hospital stay Taylor was discharged home on a cardiorespiratory monitor due to continued apnea. He was referred for physical therapy services at discharge. He subsequently had surgery to correct bilaterally dislocated hips. Taylor attends a preschool program 3 mornings a week. He receives occupational therapy once each week and physical therapy twice each week in his preschool program. The school district is considering placement for Taylor in a regular kindergarten classroom next year.

Systems Review

➤ *Anthropometric characteristics:* Taylor's lower extremities are small in proportion to his upper extremities and trunk. His head is slightly larger (95th percentile) in proportion to his body due to hydrocephalus.

➤ *Arousal, attention, and cognition*: Taylor has visual perceptual problems, which has made cognitive testing difficult. His performance suggests that his cognitive skills are in the low normal range. He has good attention skills and usually is cooperative and motivated in the classroom.

➤ *Assistive and adaptive devices*: Taylor currently uses an anterior walker and a free-standing orthosis (parapodium). He self-propels in a manual wheelchair.

➤ *Gait, locomotion, and balance*: External support is necessary for standing. Taylor ambulates with a swing-to gait using a parapodium and a walker, but is ready for long leg braces and crutches. Balance reactions are slow in sitting and standing. He has good protective reactions in sitting, but not in standing.

➤ *Integumentary integrity*: Taylor has had frequent skin breakdowns in the sacral area and in his feet/ankles.

➤ *Joint integrity and mobility*: Mobility is limited in his feet, but his ankles can be positioned at 90 degrees of dorsiflexion for standing activities.

➤ *Motor function (motor control and motor learning)*: Taylor has loss of motor function in his lower extremities. He has poor active trunk extension. He has good head control in all positions and normal upper extremity coordination.

➤ *Muscle performance*: Generalized weakness is noted in upper extremities and trunk, especially in abdominal muscles.

➤ *Neuromotor development and sensory integration*: Taylor rolls with poor leg dissociation. He can get in and out of sitting and into all fours independently. He attempts to pull to kneeling. In sitting and all fours he "hangs on his ligaments" rather than using muscle activity. He has normal grasp, manipulation, and release. He has visual acuity problems and wears glasses. He has particular difficulty with figure-ground discrimination and bending his head to look at the floor disturbs his balance. He has a mean sentence length of three to four words and sounds produced are within normal limits. He is being evaluated for speech and language services.

➤ *Orthotics*: Taylor uses articulating ankle AFOs for standing activities but is being fit for long leg braces.

➤ *Posture*: In all fours, Taylor demonstrates a lordotic posture and "hangs" on his shoulder girdle. In sitting, he slumps rather than using muscle activity to sit upright.

➤ *Range of motion*: Taylor's range of motion is within functional limits. He has slightly tight hip flexors and hip adductors.

➤ *Reflex integrity*: Tendon reflexes are absent in the lower extremities, normal in upper extremities.

➤ *School/play, community, and leisure integration*: Taylor is a sociable child who is interested in age-appropriate play and leisure activities. He is most interested in peer interaction in his home and in his classroom as he cannot keep up with peers outside or on the playground. He is enrolled in a Saturday karate class in the community that includes children who are nondisabled and disabled.

➤ *Self-care (ADL)*: Taylor can put on and take off T-shirts. He needs assistance for lower body dressing. Oral motor skills are normal and there are no feeding problems. He needs assistance with other self-cares such as toileting.

➤ *Sensory integrity*: Taylor demonstrates loss of cutaneous and proprioceptive sensation below T12.

➤ *Ventilation and respiration*: Taylor tends to hold his breath when using his upper extremities for weight-bearing or strenuous tasks. He has inadequate abdominal strength to support sustained exhalation. Overall endurance for physical activity is decreased compared to peers.

Case Study #4: Ashley

➤ Practice pattern 5B: Impaired Neuromotor Development

➤ Medical diagnosis: Down syndrome

➤ Age: 15 months

Examination

HISTORY

Ashley was a full-term infant born to a 26-year-old primipara mother who had experienced an uncomplicated pregnancy. Ashley was diagnosed with Down syndrome shortly after birth. She had esophageal atresia and primary repair was not possible. A gastrostomy was present for the first 6 months of age. She had a ventricular-septal defect that was surgically repaired at 8 months. Ashley has a history of chronic otitis media with mild conductive hearing loss. Pressure equalizing tubes were placed at 12 months. Although her parents were encouraged to contact local early intervention programs when Ashley was discharged from the hospital, they did not seek services until she was 10 months old. Ashley and her mother attend a parent/caregiver-infant early intervention program twice weekly with consultative physical therapy, occupational therapy, and speech therapy services available at each session. The family has declined home-based services.

Systems Review

➤ *Anthropometric characteristics*: Ashley's height and weight are within the normal range for children her age with Down syndrome. Facial features are characteristic of children with Down syndrome.

➤ *Arousal, attention, and cognition*: Formal IQ testing has not been completed on Ashley, although she has mild mental retardation associated with her medical diagnosis. She is a passive child, needing encouragement and stimulation to attend to motor and cognitive tasks. She has several words that she uses singly rather than in combination (eg, "more," "mama," "dada").

➤ *Assistive and adaptive devices*: None.

➤ *Gait, locomotion, and balance*: Ashley pulls to stand but is not yet attempting to cruise at furniture. She will walk with maximal assistance with two hands held. She has slow and usually ineffective protective and equilibrium reactions in sitting, all fours, and standing.

➤ *Integumentary integrity*: Normal.

➤ *Joint integrity and mobility*: Hypermobility is noted in all upper and lower extremity proximal and distal joints.

➤ *Motor function (motor control and motor learning)*: Although Ashley appears to have a typical variety of movement patterns, her movements are very slow. Postural reactions are delayed. Ashley needs multiple repetitions of cognitive and motor tasks for skill achievement and retention.

➤ *Muscle performance*: Ashley has poor muscle definition throughout her body, particularly noticeable in the shoulders and hips. She tends to lock her elbows into extension and externally rotate her arms when making movement transitions. She has poor stability in weight-bearing positions (eg, all fours, kneeling).

➤ *Neuromotor development and sensory integration*: Ashley has good head control in all positions. She rolls independently, transitions in and out of sitting and in and out of a hands and knees position. She also pulls to kneeling and pulls to stand at furniture. She tends to use straight plane movements without using trunk rotation. She does not appear hypersensitive to tactile input. She generally is apprehensive about movement activities. She grasps objects but cannot release them with control. She cannot pick up pellet-sized objects.

➤ *Orthotics*: None.

➤ *Posture*: In standing, Ashley has a wide base of support with lumbar lordosis, knee hyperextension, and foot pronation. Her trunk posture is kyphotic in sitting, but lordotic in quadruped.

➤ *Range of motion*: Hypermobility is noted in both proximal and distal joints of the extremities. She tends to keep her shoulders elevated with shortened capital extensor muscles.

➤ *Reflex integrity*: Decreased tendon reflexes (hypotonia) are present throughout upper and lower extremities. Low muscle tone also is noted throughout the face and trunk.

➤ *School/play, community, and leisure integration*: Ashley observes other children but does not interact with them. She tends to fling objects or toys to dispose of them. Play is seldom goal directed.

➤ *Self-care (ADL)*: Ashley has poor oral-motor skills. She uses a suckle pattern in feeding. Her tongue is thick in contour and protrudes from her mouth. She drinks from a cup only at snack time. Solids are inconsistently presented. She tends to lose food from her mouth. She does not assist in any other self-cares.

➤ *Sensory integrity*: Vision is normal. Mild conductive hearing loss has been noted. Ashley tends to avoid movement-based activities.

➤ *Ventilation and respiration*: Ashley has decreased respiratory-phonotory functioning. She is a mouth breather and occasionally drools.

Case Study #5: John

➤ Practice pattern 5B: Impaired Neuromotor Development
➤ Medical diagnosis: Attention deficit hyperactivity disorder, developmental coordination disorder
➤ Age: 5 years

Examination

HISTORY

John was a premature infant who spent a short time in the NICU before being discharged to home. He was noted to have slightly delayed motor milestones (sat at 9 months of age, walked at 18 months). He has always been considered to be a very active child. He is easily frustrated with motor tasks and temper tantrums are frequent. He is noted to be "clumsy" and is unable to perform gross and fine motor tasks as well as his peers (eg, cannot ride a bike without training wheels, has poor handwriting/printing). He recently was evaluated by a developmental pediatrician and neuropsychologist and received dual diagnoses of ADHD and DCD. He has been placed on Ritalin. John is in a half-day kindergarten program but does not qualify for special education services. He is receiving occupational and physical therapy (each two times/month) through a private agency.

Systems Review

➤ *Anthropometric characteristics*: Average height and weight for his age

➤ *Arousal, attention, and cognition*: John's attention span has improved since he began taking medication. He still has difficulty with selective attention and often has to be redirected to task. Formal IQ testing on the Stanford-Binet suggests above average intelligence. John has an expressive language delay, often omitting consonants in words and words in sentences

➤ *Assistive and adaptive devices:* None

➤ *Gait, locomotion, and balance*: John walks independently, but occasionally walks on his toes. He can walk with a heel-toe gait when reminded. He tends to walk too quickly with poor balance, often bumping into environmental objects or other people. He cannot walk a 4-inch balance beam without falling off and only can maintain his balance on one foot for 1 to 2 seconds

➤ *Integumentary integrity*: Normal

➤ *Joint integrity and mobility*: Normal.

➤ *Motor function (motor control and motor learning)*: John does not have an abnormal neurological examination that would indicate impaired motor control, although he is consistently characterized as being "clumsy." He has difficulty varying the speed of movement and coordinating upper and lower extremities, such as required when performing "jumping jacks." He has motor planning problems and has difficulty learning new motor tasks. He requires more practice than his peers to master each motor skill. Skills do not generalize easily

➤ *Muscle performance*: Upper extremity strength is decreased for his age. For example, he has difficulty supporting his weight on his arms to "wheelbarrow." Endurance for age-appropriate activities, such as soccer, is decreased compared to his peers.

➤ *Neuromotor development and sensory integration*: John ambulates independently. He can run, although he does so in a poorly coordinated pattern. He cannot skip but gallops instead. He has difficulty with ball skills (eg, catching, throwing, dribbling) and eye-hand coordination. He uses a modified lateral pinch for coloring and printing. He occasionally demonstrates signs of tactile defensiveness

➤ *Orthotics*: None

➤ *Posture*: John tends to walk with stiff legs and a decreased arm swing. He often leans forward as he walks

➤ *Range of motion*: Range of motion is within normal limits

➤ *Reflex integrity*: Normal

➤ *School/play, community, and leisure integration*: John prefers videogames to gross motor play. He avoids physical activity and group sports. His parents have been encouraged to explore community resources for John (eg, swimming, karate classes, T-ball, soccer) and to encourage his participation

➤ *Self-care (ADL)*: John has difficulty using utensils during meals and prefers finger foods. He is independent in dressing, but has difficulty with buttons, snaps, and zippers. He prefers Velcro closures, T-shirts, and sweatpants. He is independent in toileting, but needs to be monitored to do an adequate job bathing and tooth brushing

➤ *Sensory integrity*: Vision and hearing are normal. Testing indicates problems with tactile discrimination, kinesthesia, and stereognosis

➤ *Ventilation and respiration*: Normal.

Conclusion

The preceding case descriptions can be used as references for information in the remaining chapters. Each chapter is designed to present a specific perspective for evaluation and intervention of children with developmental disabilities. Chapter 15 presents a comprehensive review of various proposed strategies in relation to each child in the five case studies. In addition, considerations relevant to case management for each child will be discussed.

CHAPTER 5

APPLYING THE *GUIDE TO PHYSICAL THERAPIST PRACTICE*

Joanell A. Bohmert, MS, PT
Marilyn Woods, PT

The purpose of this chapter is to apply the *Guide to Physical Therapist Practice, Second Edition (Guide)* to clinical practice.[1] The *Guide* is the primary resource document that describes the practice of the physical therapist. The *Guide* provides the concepts and framework with which physical therapists organize practice.

Development of the *Guide*

The *Guide* was developed by the American Physical Therapy Association (APTA) based on the needs of members to justify physical therapy practice to state legislators. This process began in 1992 with a Board-appointed task force and culminated in the publication of *Guide to Physical Therapist Practice, Volume I: A Description of Patient Management* in the August 1995 issue of *Physical Therapy*.[2] The process was refined with adoption of the conceptual framework of Volume I and passage of RC 32-95 by the APTA House of Delegates, which provided for the process to develop Volume II.

Volume II was designed to describe the preferred patterns of practice for patient/client groupings commonly referred for physical therapy. The process for completion of Volume II was by expert consensus and included a Project Advisory Group, a Board Oversight Committee, and four Panels. Volume II also was intended to reflect current APTA standards, policies, and guidelines. Membership review was provided throughout the development with over 600 individual field reviewers and general input at various APTA sponsored forums.[1] In 1997, Volume I and Volume II became Part One and Part Two of the *Guide*. Part One was refined to reflect information obtained in the development of Part Two with the House of Delegates approving the conceptual framework of Part Two in June 1997. The first edition of the *Guide* was published in the November 1997 issue of *Physical Therapy*.[3]

The *Guide* was developed with the understanding that it is an evolving document that will need to be updated to reflect changes that occur in the base of knowledge for physical therapists.[3] Since publication in November 1997, the *Guide* has been formally revised two times to reflect membership input and changes in APTA policies by the House of Delegates.[4,5] In addition, the *Guide* is evolving through further description of practice. In 1998, APTA initiated Part Three and Part Four of the *Guide* to catalog the specific tests and measures used by physical therapists in four systems areas and the areas of outcomes, health-related quality of life, and patient/client (this term is used throughout this chapter to conform with the specifications of the *Guide*) satisfaction. An additional goal was to develop standardized documentation forms that incorporated the patient/client management process. This further development of the *Guide* also involved expert task force members, field reviews, and membership input at APTA forums. Documentation templates for inpatient and outpatient settings were developed and are published in Appendix 6 of the *Guide*.[1] During this time, APTA also developed a patient/client satisfaction instrument which is available as Appendix 7 of the *Guide*.[1]

During 1999 to 2001, work continued on reviewing tests and measures. Part Four was incorporated into Part Three with the result being a listing of tests and measures, which were used in Chapter 2 of the *Guide*. Part Three contains reference literature describing the tests and provides available data regarding each test's reliability and validity. Part Three is available only on CD-ROM. This part is searchable and linked to Chapter 2, as well as to specific patterns. The CD-ROM includes the entire *Guide* (ie, Parts One through Three). During 1999 and 2000, the *Guide* was revised further to reflect input from membership, leadership, Part Three revisions, and changes in House policies. This revision resulted in the publication of the *Guide to Physical Therapist Practice, Second Edition* in the January 2001 issue of *Physical Therapy*.[1]

The *Guide* is intended to describe the practice of the physical therapist to those within the physical therapy community and to those outside physical therapy, including policy makers, regulators, payers, administrators, and other professionals. The *Guide* does this through a general description of physical therapist practice that is based on:

➤ The disablement model

➤ A description of the physical therapist's roles in prevention, health/wellness and fitness, and in primary, secondary, and tertiary care

➤ Standardization of terminology

➤ Delineation of tests and measures and interventions

➤ Delineation of preferred practice patterns[1]

The *Guide* also states what it is not intended to do:

➤ The *Guide* does not provide specific protocols for treatments, nor are the practice patterns contained in the *Guide* intended to serve as clinical guidelines

➤ The *Guide* is not intended to set forth the standard of care for which a physical therapist may be legally responsible in any specific case[1]

Organization of the *Guide*

The *Guide* is available in print format (which does not include Part Three) and CD-ROM (which includes all Parts). The *Guide* is organized in three parts with an Introduction, appendices, and indices. The Introduction addresses the concepts, development, and content overview of the *Guide*.

Part One: A Description of Patient/Client Management

Part One provides the foundation for practice. Chapter 1 is an overview of who physical therapists are and what they do and includes a description of the five elements of patient/client management. Chapter 2 is a description of the 24 tests and measures categories. Chapter 3 is a description of the 11 intervention categories.

Part Two: Preferred Practice Patterns

Part Two contains four chapters of practice patterns, which describe the patient/client management process grouped by body system. These systems are:

➤ Chapter 4: Musculoskeletal
➤ Chapter 5: Neuromuscular
➤ Chapter 6: Cardiovascular/Pulmonary
➤ Chapter 7: Integumentary

Part Three

Part Three is a catalog of specific tests and measures used by physical therapists with citations of related literature on the reliability and validity of each tool.[6] The specific tests and measures are linked through Chapter 2 and through the Patterns.

Appendices

➤ A glossary of terms used in the *Guide*
➤ APTA Standards of Practice, Ethics documents, and Documentation Guidelines
➤ APTA Documentation Template for Inpatient and Outpatient Settings
➤ Patient/Client Satisfaction Questionnaire
The Indices include a numerical and alphabetical index to ICD-9-CM Codes.

Concepts of the *Guide*

The *Guide* has three key concepts on which it is based. These concepts include the disablement model, a continuum of service that goes across all settings, and the five elements of patient/client management.

Disablement Model

The first concept is the disablement model that serves as the basis for physical therapist practice. The disablement model provides a structure for physical therapist practice. Disablement is a process that addresses the consequences of the pathology/pathophysiology on the person and the role the person has in society.

Several models of disablement have been developed.[7-9] The concept was first proposed by Nagi,[7,10,11] a sociologist, then by the World Health Organization (WHO),[8,12] and, finally, by the National Center for Medical Rehabilitation and Research (NCMRR).[9] The models all vary in the terminology used to describe the process of disablement, however, the concepts of the process are consistent. The *Guide* provides an overview and comparison of these models on pages S19-S21.[1] The *Guide* uses the terminology based on Nagi's model, and the concepts of the disablement process serve as the basis for physical therapy practice (Table 5-1).

The disablement process incorporates four components: pathology, impairment, functional limitation, and disability (Figure 5-1). Disablement is not unidirectional. It cannot be assumed that pathology leads to impairments, that impairments lead to functional limitations, or that functional limitations lead to disability. There are many factors that can impact the process and change the relationship of the four components. These factors include those of the individual and those of the environment. Individual factors include:

➤ Those inherent to the individual (eg, biological and demographic)
➤ Those in which the individual makes choices (eg, health habits, personal behaviors, lifestyles)

Table 5-1
Definitions Used in the *Guide*

Pathology/Pathophysiology (Disease, Disorder, Condition)

An abnormality characterized by a particular cluster of signs and symptoms and recognized by either the patient/client or practitioner as "abnormal." It is primarily identified at the cellular level.

Impairment

A loss or abnormality of anatomical, physiological, mental, or psychological structure or function.

Functional Limitation

The restriction of the ability to perform, at the level of the whole person, a physical action, task, or activity in an efficient, typically expected, or competent manner.

Disability

The inability to perform or a limitation in the performance of actions, tasks, and activities usually expected in specific social roles that are customary for the individual or expected for the person's status or role in a specific sociocultural context and physical environment. In the *Guide*, the categories of roles are self-care, home management, work (job/school/play), and community/leisure.

Adapted from American Physical Therapy Association. Appendix 1: glossary. Guide to physical therapist practice. 2nd ed. *Phys Ther.* 2001;81:S677-683.

➤ The psychological attributes of the individual (eg, motivation, coping, social support)

➤ The individual's social support (social interactions and relationships)

Environmental factors include:

➤ Available health-care

➤ Physical therapy services

➤ Medications

➤ Other therapies

➤ The physical and social environment[1]

The Institute of Medicine (IOM) introduced the concept of prevention being a factor that could impact the disablement model in 1991.[13] In this model of disablement, prevention is the act of providing intervention, before or within the disablement process, at the level of the components (ie, pathology, impairment, functional limitation, disability), or at the level of risk factors to positively impact the individual. This concept of impacting the process of disablement was expanded further by IOM in 1997 to include rehabilitation as a method of preventing disability, thereby resulting in "enabling" the individual and removing disability from the process.[14]

The disablement model is the model the physical therapist uses to view how an individual interacts with the environment and how that impacts the individual's sense of well-being or health-related quality of life.[15-30] As a primary resource for physical therapist practice, the *Guide* incorporates the concepts of disablement through:

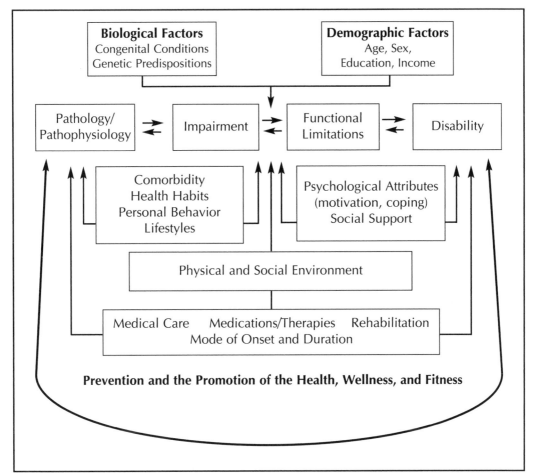

Figure 5-1. An expanded disablement model, showing interactions among individuals and environmental factors, prevention, and the promotion of health, wellness, and fitness (reprinted with permission from the American Physical Therapy Association. Guide to physical therapist practice. 2nd ed. *Phys Ther.* 2001;81:S24, as adapted from Guccione AA. Arthritis and the process of disablement. *Phys Ther.* 1994;74;410).

1. The four main components of the disablement process: pathology/pathophysiology, impairment, functional limitation, and disability
2. Individual factors: risk reduction/prevention; health, wellness, and fitness; and patient/client satisfaction
3. Environmental factors: societal resources

These factors are addressed throughout the continuum of service within the patient/client management model, concluding in the global outcomes.

Continuum of Service

The second concept of the *Guide* is that "physical therapist practice addresses the needs of both patients and clients through a continuum of service across all delivery settings."[1] The continuum of service requires that the physical therapist address the health-related quality of life for all patients and clients. This is done by addressing the four components of disablement and all the factors (individual and environmental) that impact these components. These factors include:

➤ Risk reduction/prevention (primary, secondary, tertiary)
➤ Promotion of health, wellness, and fitness
➤ Acute care
➤ Habilitation
➤ Rehabilitation
➤ Chronic care
➤ Specialized maintenance

The delivery setting is the location in which the patient/client is present, for example in the home/residence, community/leisure setting, or at work (job/school/play).

The *Guide* incorporates the continuum of service in the wide range of patient/client diagnostic classifications of the preferred practice patterns (primary prevention) and within the preferred practice patterns throughout the patient/client management process.

Five Elements of Patient/Client Management

The third concept is that physical therapist practice includes the patient/client management model. This model includes the five essential elements of examination, evaluation, diagnosis, prognosis, and intervention that result in optimal outcomes. Figure 5-2 illustrates the patient/client management process with a brief explanation of the five elements. The patient/client management process is dynamic and allows the physical therapist to progress the patient/client in the process, return to an earlier element for further analysis, or exit the patient/client from the process when the needs of the patient/client cannot be addressed by the physical therapist.

The patient/client management process incorporates the disablement model throughout the five elements and outcomes and is to be used throughout the continuum of service in all settings. This is the physical therapist's clinical decision-making model.

The *Guide* provides a description of the elements of patient/client management in Part One, Chapter 1. The preferred practice patterns in Part Two are organized by the five elements of patient/client management. Appendix 6 of the *Guide* is the documentation template of the patient/client management for inpatient and outpatient settings developed by APTA.[1]

Application of the *Guide* to Clinical Practice

The *Guide* can be applied in a number of ways. We will explain an application of the *Guide*, Second Edition, by looking at the structure of the preferred patterns in Part Two. You will need the *Guide*, Second Edition to follow the examples. We will show you how the patient/client management process and the disablement model are incorporated into Parts One, Two, and Three. We will then show you specific applications of the *Guide* for the case studies described in Chapter 4.

For a more detailed explanation of the *Guide*, the reader is encouraged to read the *Guide, Second Edition* and related articles.[1,6,31]

For the purpose of application we will use, as an example, Chapter 5: Neuromuscular, Table of Contents, (p S305), and Pattern 5C: Impaired Motor Function and Sensory Integrity Associated With Nonprogressive Disorders of the Central Nervous System—Congenital Origin or Acquired in Infancy or Childhood (pp S339-S356).

DIAGNOSIS

Both the process and the end result of evaluating examination data, which the physical therapist organizes into defined clusters, syndromes, or categories to help determine the prognosis (including the plan of care) and the most appropriate intervention strategies.

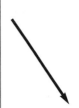

EVALUATION

A dynamic process in which the physical therapist makes clinical judgments based on data gathered during the examination. This process also may identify possible problems that require consultation with or referral to another provider.

PROGNOSIS

Determination of the level of optimal improvement that may be attained through intervention and the amount of time required to reach that level. The plan of care specifies the interventions to be used and their timing and frequency.

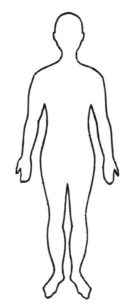

EXAMINATION

The process of obtaining a history, performing a systems review, and selecting and administering tests and measures to gather data about the patient/client. The initial examination is a comprehensive screening and specific testing process that leads to a diagnosis classification. The examination process also may identify possible problems that require consultation with or referral to another provider.

INTERVENTION

Purposeful and skilled interaction of the physical therapist with the patient and, if appropriate, with other individuals involved in care of the patient, using various physical therapy methods and techniques to produce changes in the condition that are consistent with the diagnosis and prognosis. The physical therapist conducts a reexamination to determine changes in patient status and to modify or redirect intervention. The decision to reexamine may be based on new clinical findings or on lack of patient progress. The process of reexamination also may identify the need for consultation with or referral to another provider.

OUTCOMES

Results of patient management, which include the impact of physical therapy interventions in the following domains: pathology/pathophysiology (disease, disorder, or condition); impairments, functional limitations, and disabilities; risk reduction/prevention; health, wellness, and fitness; societal resources; and patient satisfaction.

Figure 5-2. The elements of patient management leading to optimal outcomes (reprinted with permission from the American Physical Therapy Association. Guide to physical therapist practice. 2nd ed. *Phys Ther.* 2001;81:S35).

Table of Contents

This page, S305, identifies the patterns included in this chapter on the neuromuscular system. While the patterns are grouped by four body systems, the physical therapist will need to address the "whole" patient/client to determine the system in which the primary impairment(s) that drive the intervention are located. The physical therapist should not assume that the patient/client automatically will be classified in the system of their associated pathology or condition. For example, in a patient/client with a pathology diagnosis of cardiovascular accident, the system of origin of the pathology is the cardiovascular system. The system of primary impact of the pathology is the neuromuscular system. The system of secondary or tertiary impact may be the musculoskeletal, cardiovascular/pulmonary, or integumentary system.

Likewise, the physical therapist should not assume that the patient/client will be automatically classified in the system of the most frequently seen impairments associated with the identified pathology or condition. Using the above example, the system of the primary impairment(s) that drive the intervention for this specific patient/client may be cardiovascular/pulmonary (aerobic capacity), neuromuscular (motor control), musculoskeletal (muscle performance), or integumentary (primary prevention/risk reduction for integumentary). Only through examination, evaluation, and diagnosis is the physical therapist able to identify the primary impairment(s) for a specific patient/client that will drive the interventions for this episode of care. Once the physical therapist has identified the primary impairments that are impacting the patient's/client's functional abilities the physical therapist can then classify the patient/client in the appropriate pattern.

Title Page

The title page (p S339) identifies the title and the patient/client diagnostic classification characteristics for this specific pattern. The title is the diagnostic classification or the diagnosis by the physical therapist for patients/clients grouped in this pattern. The titles are based on the impairment or group of impairments that drive the intervention for that patient/client grouping. Patterns may or may not have a condition or pathology/pathophysiology associated with them. When there is only an impairment(s) listed in the title, the patient/client can be included with or without an associated condition or pathology/pathophysiology. It is up to the physical therapist to decide if the condition or pathology/pathophysiology significantly alters the patient/client management from that described in the pattern and whether to make the decision to include the patient/client. In the *Guide*, physical therapists need to classify/diagnose the patient/client by the impairment(s) that is driving the intervention, not the associated condition or pathology/pathophysiology. This concept is important to remember when classifying pediatric patients/clients as many of them have pathologies/conditions that are life-long conditions but the pathology/condition, in and of itself, is not the reason for the need for physical therapy.

The title also may specify an age-range. If an age is not specified, the pattern applies to all ages. In the *Guide*, there are two patterns that apply only to pediatric patients/clients: they are pattern 5C: Impaired Motor Function and Sensory Integrity Associated With Nonprogressive Disorders of the Central Nervous System—Congenital Origin or Acquired in Infancy or Childhood and pattern 6G: Impaired Ventilation, Respiration/Gas Exchange, and Aerobic Capacity/Endurance Associated With Respiratory Failure in the Neonate. There is one pattern that begins in adolescence, Pattern 5D: Impaired Motor Function and Sensory Integrity Associated With Nonprogressive Disorders of the Central

Nervous System—Acquired in Adolescence or Adulthood. The remaining 29 patterns of the *Guide* are not age specific but are available for consideration when classifying pediatric patients/clients.

Patient/Client Diagnostic Classification

This section (p S339) is a description of examination findings that may support the inclusion, exclusion, or classification in multiple patterns. The "inclusion" findings are organized into two categories:

➤ Risk Factors or Consequences of Pathology/Pathophysiology (Disease, Disorder, or Condition)

➤ Impairments, Functional Limitations, or Disabilities

The *Exclusion or Multiple-Pattern Classification* findings are organized into two different categories:

➤ Findings that may require classification in a different pattern

➤ Findings that may require classification in additional patterns

All patterns include a "note" which addresses risk factors or consequences of pathology/pathophysiology that may require modification of the pattern or exclusion of the patient/client. The examples listed in the pattern are specific to that pattern.

ICD-9-CM Codes

This section (p S340) is provided as an example of codes that relate to the patient/client diagnostic grouping for the pattern. This is not an inclusive or exclusive list. Patients/clients may be placed in the pattern if their primary impairments are consistent with the pattern, regardless if their assigned ICD-9-CM code is or is not listed.

For example, a patient/client with a pathology of cerebral palsy has an assigned ICD-9-CM code of 343 infantile cerebral palsy. The physical therapist has determined that the primary impairment that is impacting the patient's/client's functional abilities is muscle performance and classifies the patient/client into pattern 4C Impaired Muscle Performance. However, ICD-9-CM 343 infantile cerebral palsy is not listed for pattern 4C (p S162). The patient/client still is appropriate for pattern 4C as the primary impairment for this episode of care is impaired muscle performance.

Examination

The examination (p S341) is required for all patients/clients and is performed prior to the initial intervention. The three components of the examination are delineated in each pattern. *Patient/Client History* (p S341), a complete list of the types of data that may be generated from the patient/client history, is found in every pattern. It also is found on page S36, in Chapter 1. *The System Review* (p S342) contains a complete list of what the system review may include. The components of the system review are listed in every pattern and also can be found on pages S34 to 35 of Chapter 1. Pages S342 to S344 identify the *Tests and Measures* categories and bullets that are specific to the pattern. Chapter 2 describes the tests and measures categories in detail including:

➤ A general definition and purpose

➤ Clinical indications

➤ Tests and measures methods and techniques

➤ Tools used for gathering data

➤ The data generated

The clinical indications provided in each test and measure are examples of specific findings of the history and system review which may indicate the need for use of that specific tests and measures category (p S48). Clinical indications are provided in the following disablement areas: pathology/pathophysiology (disease, disorder, or condition); impairments; functional limitations; disability; risk factors; and health, wellness, and fitness. Part Three of the *Guide* provides a catalog of specific tests and measures with citations to related literature on the psychometric properties of each tool. You will be able to access the information on a specific test multiple ways. The tests are linked from the bullets listed under the Tests and Measures category (page S49) in each of the 24 categories. This will give you an entire list of tests and measures appropriate for that test category. The tests also are linked in the patterns through the tests and measures bullets, however, these tests are specific to that pattern. By clicking through Part Three, you will be able to locate specific tests and the literature that relates to that tool. Thus, a tool that is appropriate to your specific patient/client can be selected. (Note: The tests and measures and literature are only accurate and current as of the date stated in the CD-ROM.)

It should be noted that with pediatric patients/clients or any patient/client that cannot appropriately respond for themselves, the *Guide* assumes that the parent/guardian or caregiver would be the responsible party to respond on behalf of the child or patient/client. It also should be noted that it is appropriate to assess the parent's/guardian's or caregiver's abilities to manage the child. If in the process of examining the caregiver's abilities you determine the caregiver has issues that may require their own episode of care, you should recommend a separate examination of the caregiver.

Evaluation, Diagnosis, and Prognosis (Including the Plan of Care)

These sections (p S345) are grouped together on one page in each pattern. The page includes an explanation of the evaluation and diagnostic process and the factors that may impact the process. During the *evaluation*, examination data are analyzed, taking into consideration the patient's/client's expectations and patient's/client's potential for remediation or accommodation. Begin by looking for a clustering of impairments that appear to be impacting the functional limitations; disabilities; and health, wellness, and prevention needs of the patient/client. Most pediatric patients/clients will have conditions/pathologies that are life-long conditions. As a result, they always will have impairments; functional limitations; disabilities; and health, wellness, and prevention needs. The key to evaluation, is to determine which impairments are the ones that are impacting the functional limitations, disabilities; and health, wellness, and prevention for this episode of care.

The patient's/client's *diagnosis* is determined at this point in the patient/client management process. The pattern title is the diagnostic classification for the pattern. You need to determine your specific patient's/client's diagnosis, identifying the primary impairments that will drive the interventions. Remember, the diagnosis is not the pathology, it is the impairment(s) you have identified that are impacting the patient's/client's functional abilities. You then determine if your patient/client can be managed in this pattern with or without modifications, if another pattern is needed in addition to this pattern, or if a different pattern is more appropriate.

Page S345, includes a *prognosis* statement that identifies the optimal level of improvement in impairments and functional abilities as well as the amount of time needed. For patterns that include patient's/client's with life-long conditions, the prognosis statement provides for improvement "within the context of the impairments, functional limitations, and disabilities"[1] as the patient/client always will have some level of impairment that may impact the level of function. The prognosis also includes a column identifying the expected range of number of visits per episode of care. The range is based on following the patient/client throughout the continuum of service across all settings. It is anticipated that 20% of patients/clients who are appropriate for this pattern will be outside this range for each episode of care. The column "Factors That May Require New Episode of Care or That May Modify Frequency of Visits/Duration of Care"[1] provides a listing of individual and environmental factors that are specific to that pattern. The prognosis also has a "note" section in patterns where the patient/client may require multiple episodes of care. This section also lists factors that, in addition to those in the factor column, may impact this pattern. These factors, whether they are of the individual or of the environment, may increase or decrease the frequency or expected range of visits.

Intervention

The three components of *intervention* are delineated in each pattern. The first two: *coordination, communication, and documentation* and *patient/client-related instruction* are required for all patients/clients. The third component; the nine *procedural intervention* categories, is selected for the specific pattern.

Pages S346 to 355 list the intervention categories, bullets, and anticipated goals and expected outcomes specific for the pattern. Chapter 3 describes the interventions categories in detail including general definitions, clinical considerations, interventions, and anticipated goals and expected outcomes. For coordination, communication, and documentation and patient/client-related instruction, the examples of the clinical considerations that may direct that intervention and the anticipated goals and expected outcomes related to that intervention are listed, but are not grouped by disablement areas. For the nine procedural intervention categories, the clinical considerations provided in intervention are examples of "examination findings that direct the type and specificity of"[1] that intervention and are grouped in the following disablement areas:

➤ Pathology/pathophysiology (disease, disorder, or condition)

➤ History of medical/surgical conditions or signs and symptoms

➤ Impairments

➤ Functional limitations

➤ Disability

➤ Risk reduction/prevention

➤ Health, wellness, and fitness needs (see p S104)

Examples of anticipated goals and expected outcomes related to that intervention are grouped in the following disablement areas: pathology/pathophysiology; impairment; functional limitation; disability; risk reduction/prevention; health, wellness, and fitness; societal resources; and patient/client satisfaction. You can use the examples provided within the pattern to assist you in determining if the patient/client can be managed in this pattern and to assist you in selecting the anticipated goals and expected outcomes.

Reexamination, Global Outcomes for Patients/Clients in This Pattern, and Criteria for Termination of Physical Therapy Services

The final page of this pattern, page S356, groups these sections together. *Reexamination* can be performed at any time, after the initial examination, in the episode of care. It may result in:

➤ Modification of the anticipated goals, expected outcomes, frequency, or duration of care

➤ Reclassification of the patient/client to a different pattern, addition of another pattern, or termination of the physical therapy service

Global outcomes for patients/clients in this pattern are measured at the end of the episode of care and measure the impact of physical therapy service in the domains of:

➤ Pathology/pathophysiology

➤ Impairment

➤ Functional limitation

➤ Disability

➤ Risk reduction/prevention

➤ Health, wellness, and fitness

➤ Societal resources

➤ Patient/client satisfaction

These are the same domains for the anticipated goals and expected outcomes identified in the interventions. The *Guide* defines anticipated goals and expected outcomes as the "intended results of patient/client management and indicate changes in impairments, functional limitations, and disabilities and the changes in health, wellness, and fitness needs that are expected as the result of implementing the plan of care."[1] Goals and outcomes need to be meaningful to the patient/client, measurable, and time specific.

The two processes of *termination of physical therapy service* are discharge and discontinuation. Discharge occurs when the anticipated goals and expected outcomes have been achieved. Discontinuation occurs when services are ended but the anticipated goals and expected outcomes have not been met. This may occur at the request of the patient/client or guardian. In other instances, the patient/client is unable to make progress toward outcomes due to individual or environmental/economical factors, or the physical therapist determines the patient/client will no longer benefit from the current episode of care.[1]

Case Study #1: Jason

➤ Practice pattern: 5C: Impaired Motor Function and Sensory Integrity Associated With Nonprogressive Disorders of the Central Nervous System—Congenital Origin or Acquired in Infancy or Childhood

➤ Medical diagnosis: Cerebral palsy, right hemiparesis

➤ Age: 24 months

How does the patient/client management model help you determine what is wrong with Jason and what you need to do? During the examination how did you know which specific tests and measures to use? How did you know to place Jason in Practice Pattern 5C? This case is an example of how to use all of the elements in the Patient/Client Management in the *Guide*.

Examination

HISTORY

The first information you received about Jason is from his history. You received his previous medical information, physical therapy chart/notes, and information provided to you from his parents. You interview Jason's mother and father to complete the information from the history section of the examination. Based on the information in his history, you began to form a picture of what his parents' concerns are and what impairments may be impacting Jason's ability to do what he wants to do. You now have an overview of his medical status and how that may impact your examination today as well as how it may impact Jason's prognosis and plan of care.

➤ General demographics: Jason is a 24-month-old male who is English speaking

➤ Social history: Jason lives with his mother and father who are the primary care givers. He has a brother who is a non-identical twin

➤ Employment/work (job/school/play): Jason enjoys age-appropriate play activities

➤ Growth and development: At 6 months of age there were definite asymmetries in stretch reflexes and voluntary use of his extremities

➤ Living environment: He lives in a split-level home. There is a small play area in the back yard and a community park two blocks away

➤ General health status (self-report, family report, caregiver report)
  • General health perception: Jason has been healthy other than the usual childhood illnesses, such as colds and flu
  • Physical function: Jason began walking at 15 months, and sleeping through the night
  • Psychological function: Jason is a happy, healthy 2-year-old
  • Role function: Son, brother, grandchild
  • Social function: Jason enjoys age-appropriate play but becomes frustrated that he cannot keep up with or make himself understood to his brother or peers

➤ Social/health habits (Past and Current): No members of immediate family smoke

➤ Family history: Noncontributory

➤ Medical/surgical history: Jason was first born of nonidentical twins with a birth weight of 1660 g. His Apgars were 7 at 1 minute and 9 at 5 minutes. He did not require mechanical ventilation and was discharged from the neonatal intensive care unit (NICU) after 40 days on caffeine-citrate due to bradycardia with feedings. Initial follow-up at two months of chronological age was nonremarkable. At his follow up at 6 months of chronological age definite asymmetries in stretch reflexes and voluntary use of his extremities were noted. Jason was referred for early intervention services. Jason is not on any medication and has not had any surgical procedures

➤ Current conditions/chief complaint: Parents are concerned about general developmental delay and lack of use of his right side for play and self-care. Currently he is receiving home-based services consisting of weekly visits from the local school district alternating between teacher and occupational therapist. Parents would like to see him walk without falling, keep up with his brother, and be able to communicate with others

➤ Functional status and activity level: Parents report Jason is just beginning to assist with dressing and undressing activities. He also is beginning to show some interest in toilet training. He is a "messy" eater. He is very active but has difficulty keeping up with his brother. Family is very active in the community and enjoys outdoor activities

➤ Medications: None

➤ Other clinical tests: Jason is on an individual family service plan (IFSP)—*you will need to review the IFSP to address potential overlap in goals and objectives* (see Chapter 14).

Systems Review

You next complete a review of Jason's systems by observing and taking measurements for:

➤ Anatomical and physiological status
➤ Cardiovascular
   A. Blood pressure: 75/130
   B. Edema: None observed
   C. Heart rate: 100 bpm
   D. Respiratory rate: 25 bpm
➤ Integumentary
   • Presence of scar formation: None
   • Skin color: Good
   • Skin integrity: Good
➤ Musculoskeletal (gross range of motion; within normal limits on left, some limitation on right)
   • Gross strength: Decreased on the right
   • Gross symmetry: Asymmetrical posture and positioning of right side
➤ Neuromuscular (Gross coordinated movements; irregular movements; difficulties with awareness, timing, and sequencing)
➤ Communication, affect, cognition, language, and learning style
   • Delayed expressive language and relies on gestures for communication
   • Mom reports that Jason learns by watching his brother and she would prefer home program on video in addition to being written

Tests and Measures

SPECIFIC TESTS AND MEASURES

Based on the findings of the History and System Review you determine which specific tests and measures you will use. The history and system review will identity clinical indicators for pathology/pathophysiology, impairments, functional limitations; disability; risk factors; and health, wellness, and prevention needs that will assist you in ruling in or ruling out specific tests and measures.

You can use the *Guide* to assist in identifying tests and measures categories, as well as specific tests and measures. Part 3 on the *Guide* CD will allow you to search either in the test categories or in the pattern. You will be able to find and review specific tools as well as link to specific articles to help you determine which tools you will use for Jason. Based on Jason's findings you select tests and measures from the following categories.

Tests and measures for this pattern include those that characterize or quantify the following:

➤ Anthropometrics characteristics (body dimensions): Jason is noted to have a slightly smaller right upper extremity (only noticeable in the upper arm as compared to the left). He is of average height and weight for his age

➤ Arousal, attention, and cognition (developmental inventory): Testing indicates that Jason's cognition falls within the average range. He has delayed expressive language using gestures to make needs known. During testing it was noted that tactile stimulation generally increased activity level.

➤ Assistive and adaptive devices (observation of during testing): Determined no assistive or adaptive devices needed

➤ Environmental, home, and work (job/school/play) barriers (observation and interview): Home: note six steps between levels, ceramic tile floor in kitchen, upper level open to main level with a metal railing. Wood chips under swing set and wood timbers around sand box. Community park has asphalt walking paths with irregular surfaces in grass. Mom reports Jason needs to be closely supervised as he falls frequently

➤ Gait, locomotion, and balance (ADL scale, observation): Results of the Pediatric Evaluation of Disability Inventory (PEDI) indicate that Jason has difficulty with transfers in and out of a tub, indoor locomotion in the areas of changing direction and carrying objects, outdoor locomotion on rough and uneven surfaces, and ascending and descending stairs in an upright position.

➤ Integumentary integrity (observation, interview): Normal

➤ Motor function (motor control and motor learning) (ADL scale, observation): On the PEDI, Jason was able to initiate movement, but had difficulty modulating and stopping movement especially with his right side. Difficulty with timing and sequencing of movement was noted when using his right arm and hand for self care activities. Understands two-step commands but has difficulty completing motor component of task

➤ Muscle performance (Functional muscle test): Weakness is evident in the right upper extremity, particularly in the triceps and supinators of the forearm

➤ Neuromotor development and sensory integration (developmental inventory): Gross motor skills range between 12 to 15 months. Just beginning to attempt running

➤ Orthotic, protective, and supportive devices (observation): Determined orthotic device not beneficial

➤ Pain (interview): None reported

➤ Posture (observation): Demonstrates asymmetrical posture in standing with excessive anterior tilt of the pelvis and excessive retraction of right shoulder. Tends to posture right arm in flexion at elbow, wrist, hand, and fingers with forearm in pronation

➤ Range of motion (functional tests and observation): Within normal limits for passive movement but demonstrates limitations in active movements on the right for reaching, grasping, extending hip, and rotating and flexing trunk. Limitations with active movement interfere with activities requiring two hands or use of right hand

➤ Reflex integrity (reflex tests): Hyperactive stretch reflexes are present to tendon tap at the ankle (plantar flexors), knee (quadriceps), and elbow (biceps) on the right. Normal stretch reflexes are evident on the left side of the body

> Self-care and home management (ADL scales, observation, interview): Results of the PEDI indicate difficulty with use of utensils, washing hands together, dressing, toileting. Jason drools occasionally, especially when concentrating on an activity. He is a "messy" eater, often losing food out of his mouth. He does not seem to notice when food escapes from his mouth

> Sensory integrity (observation): During administration of the PEDI, limited use and apparent lack of awareness of right arm for self-care activities were noted. Tactile defensive behaviors occasionally observed

> Ventilation and respiration/gas exchange (observation): Breathiness is noted during speech and consonants are limited in quantity and quality. He often gasps for breath after drinking

> Work (job/school/play), community, and leisure integration or reintegration (ADL scales, observation, interview): Jason enjoys age-appropriate play activities and demonstrates typical behaviors for a 24-month-old child when his brother or other children are present. Results of the PEDI, Social Function Domain, indicate difficulty with expressive communication, ability to report self-information (name), and safety within community. Parent reports difficulty with mobility in community park and backyard play areas

Evaluation (Clinical Judgment)

You now organize the data from the examination to determine which impairments are impacting Jason's functional abilities. You determine if the family's expectations for therapy are realistic, establish a diagnosis and a prognosis, and develop a plan of care.

Jason has impairments of motor function, weakness, and poor sensory appreciation on the right side. His gross motor skills are delayed, as is his expressive language. He relies on gestures for communication. He is a messy eater. Jason is starting to assist in dressing and has some interest in toilet training. He is walking, however, he has difficulty changing directions and stopping movement. He frequently falls.

Diagnosis

Based on the evaluation, you determine that deficits in motor function and sensory integrity are the primary impairments impacting Jason's functional abilities. The impairment of muscle performance appears to be secondary to impairments in motor function and sensory integrity. The impairment of communication appears related to the impairments in motor function and sensory integrity and you determine you need to refer Jason for an examination by a speech pathologist.

The data collected helped determine the primary dysfunction that will drive the interventions. Jason was placed in Practice Pattern 5C: Impaired Motor Function and Sensory Integrity Associated With Nonprogressive Disorders of the Central Nervous System—Congenital Origin or Acquired in Infancy or Childhood.

Prognosis (Including Plan of Care)

Using Pattern 5C, you review the prognosis statement, expected range of visits, and factors that may modify frequency of visits and duration of care. Then you develop a prognosis for Jason that addresses his and his family's expectations with an agreed upon frequency and duration of services. As part of the plan of care, you determine the anticipated goals and expected outcomes with Jason's family.

Over the course of 12 months, Jason will demonstrate optimal motor function and sensory integrity, and the highest level of function in the home and community within the context of his impairments, functional limitations, and disability. Specific prognosis statements for this episode of care would be linked to the functional outcomes proposed in the following chapters. Jason will receive private physical therapy for 3 months, once weekly with family education for his home program. After that, physical therapy will decrease to one time every 2 weeks.

The family has agreed to the program and the informed consent was signed. Jason will be discharged when the anticipated goals and expected outcomes have been met.

Interventions (for Clinical Consideration)

Using the anticipated goals and expected outcomes you developed as part of the plan of care, you review the interventions to determine which interventions will be appropriate. We have provided an example only for the two required interventions of coordination, communication, and documentation and patient/client-related instruction. You will need to select procedural interventions to complete his plan of care.

COORDINATION, COMMUNICATION, AND DOCUMENTATION

➤ Interventions: Coordination and communication with school providers; referral to speech pathologist

➤ Anticipated goals and expected outcomes: Family members will demonstrate enhanced decision-making skills regarding Jason's health and use of community resources

PATIENT/CLIENT-RELATED INSTRUCTION

➤ Interventions: Jason and family will receive instruction and education in a home program and updates. They will receive information on when it is appropriate to seek additional services

➤ Anticipated goals and expected outcomes: Jason's parents will have increased understanding of goals and outcomes and demonstrate his home program independently

PROCEDURAL INTERVENTIONS

You will need to select additional interventions from the nine procedural interventions described in Chapter 3 of the *Guide* to complete Jason's plan of care. Use the information presented in the pattern under the categories of "Interventions" and "Anticipated Goals and Expected Outcomes" and the information in Chapter 3 to assist in determining appropriate interventions and anticipated goals and expected outcomes for Jason. The following are examples of the most appropriate interventions for Jason:

➤ Therapeutic exercise

➤ Self-care and home management

➤ Functional training in work (job/school/play), community, and leisure integration or reintegration

➤ Manual therapy techniques

➤ Prescription, application, and as appropriate, fabrication of devices and equipment

➤ Electrotherapeutic modalities

Re-Examination

Global Outcomes for Patients (End of Episode of Care)

The global outcomes of physical therapy services are measured by impact of the interventions in the following areas:

➤ Pathology/pathophysiology (disease, disorder, or condition)
➤ Impairments
➤ Functional outcomes
➤ Disabilities
➤ Risk reduction/prevention
➤ Health, wellness, and fitness
➤ Societal resources
➤ Patient/client satisfaction

Criteria for Termination of Physical Therapy Services

➤ Discharge: Ending physical therapy services for this episode of care when anticipated goals and expected outcomes have been achieved
➤ Discontinuation: Ending physical therapy for this episode of care when the family declines intervention, Jason is unable to make progress toward outcomes, or it is determined that Jason will no longer benefit from physical therapy

Case Study #2: Jill

➤ Practice pattern 5C: Impaired Motor Function and Sensory Integrity Associated With Nonprogressive Disorders of the Central Nervous System—Congenital Origin or Acquired in Infancy or Childhood
➤ Medical diagnosis: Cerebral palsy, spastic quadriparesis, microcephaly, mental retardation, seizure disorder
➤ Age: 7 years

This case is an example of how to use the *Guide* to transition from an episode of care to an episode of prevention.

Examination

History

➤ General demographics: Jill is a 7-year-old white female
➤ Social history
  • Family/caregivers: Mother, father, aide at school
  • Social activities: Swimming class, horse back riding, enjoys watching videos and TV
➤ Employment/work (job/school/play): Jill is in school in a special education classroom, mainstreamed with other children part of the day, She has a classroom aide. She receives occupational, speech, and physical therapy

➤ Growth and development: Jill was born full-term following a normal pregnancy. Her Apgar scores were 5 at 1 minute and 8 at 5 minutes. Jill had seizures during the neonatal period and had an abnormal electroencephalogram (EEG). She was on mechanical ventilation for several days and initially had feeding difficulties. She was discharged from the NICU on antiseizure medication. At the time of discharge, she was drinking well from a bottle. At her 4-month follow-up visit with her pediatrician, decreased head growth was noted. She had a normal eye exam and brain stem auditory evoked response. Jill has continued to have occasional seizures despite being on antiseizure medication. She had orthopedic surgery (heel cord and adductor releases) at 5 years of age

➤ Living environment: Lives in a ranch style home. There are steps to enter home. Family is considering a ramp

➤ General health (report gathered from patient, family, or caregiver): Occasional seizures
  • Perception: She is generally healthy
  • Physical function: She is dependent on ADL and IADL
  • Role: Daughter, granddaughter, classmate

➤ Social function: Participating in a community-sponsored adaptive swimming class and therapeutic horseback riding (hippotherapy)

➤ Social/health habits (past and current): Not applicable

➤ Family history: Noncontributory

➤ Medical surgical history: Jill had orthopedic surgery (heel cord and adductor releases) at 5 years of age

➤ Current conditions/chief complaint: Parents are concerned about Jill's ability to access their home. Parents would like to know about appropriate modifications, adaptations, or equipment to assist in managing Jill as she grows

➤ Functional status and activity level: Jill is not ambulatory and is unable to maintain her balance in any position. She has a manual wheelchair with custom seating system. She is totally dependent on caregivers for self-care with the exception of assisting with arms through sleeves for dressing and weight-bearing for standing pivot transfers. She participates in a community-sponsored adaptive swimming class and therapeutic horseback riding (hippotherapy)

➤ Medications: Antiseizure medications

Systems Review

➤ Cardiovascular
  • Blood pressure: 78/128
  • Edema: None noted
  • Heart rate: 102 bpm
  • Respiratory rate: 25 bpm

➤ Integumentary
  • Presence of scar formation: Old scar on left arm—not necessary to assess
  • Skin color: Good
  • Skin integrity: Mild irritation on ischial tuberosities

➤ Musculoskeletal
  • Gross range of motion: Limited reach
  • Gross strength: Generalized weakness

- Gross symmetry: Asymmetrical
- Height: Fifth percentile
- Weight: Fifth percentile

➤ Neuromuscular: Gross motor skills at 3-month level

➤ Communication, affect, cognition, language, and learning style: Jill is able to make needs known through variations in vocalized patterns to familiar listeners

Tests and Measures

Based on the information presented in Chapter 4's Case Studies (in this text), you identified the impairments; functional limitations; disability; risk factors; and health, wellness, and fitness needs. Chapter 2 of the *Guide* (Tests and Measures), provides examples of pathology/pathophysiology; impairments; functional limitations; disability; risk factors; and health, wellness, and fitness needs for each test category. This information will help you in selecting the appropriate tests and measures as well as identifying impairments, functional limitations, and disability. Risk factors and health, wellness, and fitness needs also will be determined.

Selected Test Categories and Clinical Indications for Use

➤ Arousal, attention, and cognition (developmental inventory)
- Pathology/pathophysiology: Neuromuscular (cerebral palsy, seizures)
- Impairments: Arousal, cognition, distractibility, communication, motor function
- Functional limitations: Self-care, work, community/leisure (dependent in all areas)
- Disability: Self-care, work, community/leisure (unable to participate without assistance, vulnerable)
- Risk factors: Slow rate of learning, attending, seizures, inability to understand and interpret environment, inability to communicate, vulnerability
- Health, wellness, and fitness: Lack of awareness of need for fitness, inactivity, lack of education of caregivers on importance of health, wellness, and fitness

➤ Assistive and adaptive devices (observation, reports)
- Pathology/pathophysiology: Neuromuscular (cerebral palsy, seizures) musculoskeletal (secondary to neuromuscular pathology)
- Impairments: Motor function (positioning), posture, range of motion, joint integrity and mobility, integumentary, gait, locomotion and balance, muscle performance, sensory integrity, ventilation, and respiration
- Functional limitations: Self-care, work, community/leisure (dependent on devices to provide positioning)
- Disability: Self-care, work, community/leisure (dependent on devices to provide positioning for participation in activities)
- Risk factors: Inactivity, contractures, skin breakdown, osteopenia, digestive function, bowel and bladder function
- Health, wellness, and fitness: Inactivity, use of devices to address health, wellness, and fitness needs

➤ Environmental, home, and work (job/school/play) barriers
- Pathology/pathophysiology: Neuromuscular (cerebral palsy, seizures)
- Impairments: Locomotion (wheelchair, assisted standing pivot transfers), caregiver's ergonomics, and body mechanics (Mom reports back injury from lifting)

- Functional limitations: Self-care, play, community/leisure (needs to use wheelchair for mobility, devices for positioning)
- Disability: Self-care, play, community/leisure (dependent on caregivers, unable to control her environment)
- Risk factors: Decreased accessibility to home, work, community/leisure, evacuation plan
- Health, wellness, and fitness: Caregiver's health, wellness, and fitness

➤ Ergonomics and body mechanics: Examination of caregiver
  - Pathology/pathophysiology: None known
  - Impairments: Muscle performance, body mechanics
  - Functional limitations: Self-care (lifting, bathing, dressing, toileting), play, and community (accessing environments)
  - Disability: Inability to care for daughter
  - Risk factors: Repetitive stress, back injury of caregiver
  - Health, wellness, and fitness: Decreased understanding of importance of body mechanics and strength when lifting
  - Gait, locomotion, and balance (ADL scale, observation)

➤ Integumentary integrity (observations, risk assessment scale)
  - Pathology/pathophysiology: Neuromuscular (cerebral palsy, seizures)
  - Impairments: Locomotion (inactivity), integumentary (redness on tuberosities), questionable circulation
  - Functional limitations: Self-care, play, community/leisure (inactivity and inability to communicate discomfort)
  - Disability: Self-care, play, community/leisure (tolerance for sitting)
  - Risk factors: Skin breakdown, inactivity
  - Health, wellness, and fitness: Caregivers need understanding of the importance of positioning and devices to maintain skin

➤ Motor function (motor control and motor learning) (observations, ADL scale)
  - Pathology/pathophysiology: Neuromuscular (cerebral palsy, seizures)
  - Impairments: Motor function (limited voluntary movement, poor head, ocular motor, and oral motor control), locomotion (inactivity), range of motion, muscle performance, balance, posture
  - Functional limitations: Self-care, work, community/leisure (dependent on others)
  - Disability: Self-care, work, community/leisure (dependent on others for participation in actions, tasks and activities to fulfill required roles)
  - Risk factors: Inactivity, safety, vulnerability
  - Health, wellness, and fitness: Inactivity, understanding of the importance of devices to provide stability for movement

➤ Orthotic, protective, and supportive devices (observation, log reports)
  - Pathology/pathophysiology: Neuromuscular (cerebral palsy)
  - Impairments: Range of motion, motor function
  - Functional limitations: Self-care, work, community/leisure (need for standing and assistive standing pivot transfers)
  - Disability: Self-care, work, community/leisure (Ankle-foot orthotics needed to allow standing to complete role)
  - Risk factors: Contractures, loss of standing ability (digestive, bowel, and bladder function; osteopenia), skin breakdown

- Health, wellness, and fitness: Inactivity, use of devices to address health, wellness, and fitness needs

➤ Range of motion (observation, goniometry, contracture test)

- Pathology/pathophysiology: Neuromuscular (cerebral palsy), musculoskeletal (secondary to cerebral palsy)
- Impairments: Range of motion, joint integrity and mobility, integumentary, posture, muscle performance, motor control
- Functional limitations: Self-care, work, community/leisure (dependent on others for movement)
- Disability: Self-care, work, community/leisure (dependent on others to participate in actions, tasks, and activities to fulfill required roles)
- Risk factors: Contractures, skin breakdown, postural deviations, respiratory function
- Health, wellness, and fitness: Importance of maintaining joint motion and muscle length for adequate positioning as Jill ages

Evaluation

Using the information from the examination, what clustering of impairments, functional limitations, disability, risk factors, health, wellness and fitness were identified?

In Jill's case the following clusters were identified:

➤ Pathology/pathophysiology: Cerebral palsy, mental retardation, seizures

➤ Impairments: Motor function, range of motion, locomotion, cognition, caregiver body mechanics

➤ Functional limitations: Mobility, accessing environments, and dependency on others in the areas of self-care, work, and community/leisure

➤ Disability: Dependence on others to meet role of daughter, student, friend, child (barriers in home, evacuation plan)

➤ Risk factors: Inactivity, contractures, limited access to environment, skin breakdown

➤ Health, wellness, and fitness: Health and wellness of caregivers to assist Jill and prevent injury to caregivers, need understanding of the importance of positioning and devices to maintain range of motion, skin integrity, joint integrity and mobility, muscle length, and stable position to allow interaction with environment

Diagnosis

Based on your evaluation, the impairment that will drive intervention for Jill is motor function. The most appropriate practice pattern is 5C: Impaired Motor Function and Sensory Integrity Associated With Nonprogressive Disorders of the Central Nervous System—Congenital Origin or Acquired in Infancy or Childhood.

Prognosis (Including Plan of Care)

You also use the evaluation to determine the prognosis for Jill. The prognosis for 5C states that "Jill will demonstrate optimal motor function and sensory integrity and the highest level of functioning in home, school, play, and community and leisure environments, within the context of the impairments, functional limitations, and disabilities."

For Jill, the phrase "within the context of the impairments, functional limitations, and disabilities" has significance as she has a medical diagnosis that you know is a lifelong condition with impairments that will directly impact her ability to learn and move. Based on her age (7 years old), cognitive level (severe retardation), rate of change (motor skills still at 3 month level), motor control (limited voluntary movement, poor head, ocular motor and oral motor control), and functional skills (dependence), you determine that her needs are for appropriate devices to provide positioning for her to access and interact with her environment. You also determine that her home environment requires modifications and adaptations and that her caregivers should be trained to safely manage and assist Jill throughout her day.

Based on this prognosis you determine that Jill will benefit from an episode of care with the expected frequency to be two times per month the first month, then one time per month for the following 2 months. The anticipated goals and expected outcomes for this episode of care are to assess the home environment for modifications, equipment, and evacuation plan and to educate the caregivers in appropriate body mechanics, lifting, transfers, and use of devices. A home program also will be developed to address Jill's risk factors and health, wellness and fitness needs. Caregivers will demonstrate understanding and strategies used to implement her program.

Following achievement of anticipated goals and expected outcomes, it is anticipated that Jill will be discharged from her episode of care and placed in an episode of prevention. During the episode of prevention, Jill will be monitored quarterly through phone contacts or visits for the next six months. Parents also may contact the physical therapist as needed. Purpose of this episode of prevention is to update home program and evacuation plan, monitor orthotics and equipment, problem solve with caregivers, and advise family on community resources. If no new issues or medical interventions occur, Jill will be discharged from physical therapy.

Case Study #3: Taylor

➤ Practice pattern 5C: Impaired Motor Function and Sensory Integrity Associated With Nonprogressive Disorders of the Central Nervous System—Congenital Origin or Acquired in Infancy or Childhood

➤ Medical diagnosis: Myelomeningocele, repaired L1-2

➤ Age: 4 years

This case is an example of using the *Guide* for reclassification of the practice pattern. It also demonstrates how you can use two practice patterns at the same time.

Taylor has been in an episode of care, classified into practice pattern 5C, because his primary impairments that were driving the intervention were motor function and sensory integrity. Taylor was reexamined to determine if his primary impairments have changed and if reclassification into another practice pattern is necessary.

Reexamination

Summary of History and System Review from Initial Examination

➤ General demographics: 4-year-old male; he attends a preschool program three mornings a week

➤ Employment/work (job/school/play): Attends preschool program three mornings a week

➤ Living environment: Lives with parents' in ranch style house

➤ General health: Parents report generally good health

➤ Role: Son, classmate

MEDICAL/SURGICAL

At birth, a large myelomeningocele was noted and was closed surgically. A ventricular-peritoneal shunt was surgically inserted on day 5. Taylor had increased apnea and was on a respirator. He had questionable seizures, but his EEG was normal. He had a suspected Arnold Chiari malformation that was treated by surgical release of the posterior fossa. He had equinovarus deformities and underwent serial casting beginning at 2 weeks of age. He subsequently had surgery to correct bilaterally dislocated hips.

REEXAMINATION CURRENT CONDITION/CHIEF COMPLAINT

Taylor was seen by his physician who requested an evaluation of Taylor's equipment needs as he will be entering kindergarten this fall. He has a skin breakdown on the sacrum that needs dressing changes three times a week.

REEXAMINATION TESTS AND MEASURES

➤ Arousal, attention, and cognition (developmental inventory): Taylor has visual perceptual problems, which has made cognitive testing difficult. His performance suggests that his cognitive skills are in the average range. He has good attention skills and is usually cooperative and motivated in the classroom

➤ Assistive and adaptive devices (observations, ADL scales, IADL scales): Taylor currently uses an anterior walker and a freestanding orthosis (parapodium). He self-propels in a manual wheelchair. Has available loaner, manual wheelchair

➤ Gait, locomotion balance (ADL scales observations, mobility skills, functional assessments): External support is necessary for standing. Taylor ambulates with a swing-to gait using a parapodium and a walker, but is ready for long leg braces and crutches. Balance reactions are slow in sitting and standing. He has good protective reactions in sitting, but not in standing

➤ Motor function (motor control and motor learning) (observation, motor impairment tests, physical performance tests.): Taylor has loss of motor function in his lower extremities. He has good head control in all positions and normal upper extremity coordination

➤ Muscle performance (functional muscle tests, observation, palpation): Generalized weakness is noted in upper extremities and trunk, especially in abdominal muscles. Taylor tends to hold his breath when using his upper extremities for weight-bearing or strenuous tasks. He has inadequate abdominal strength to support sustained exhalation. He has poor active trunk extension. Overall endurance for physical activity is decreased compared to peers

➤ Neuromotor development and sensory integration (observation, motor function tests): Taylor rolls with poor leg dissociation. He can get in and out of sitting and into all fours independently. He attempts to pull to kneeling. In sitting and all fours he "hangs on his ligaments" rather than using muscle activity. He has normal grasp, manipulation, and release. He has visual acuity problems and wears glasses. He has particular difficulty with figure-ground discrimination and bending his head to look at the floor disturbs his balance. He has an average sentence length of three to four words and sounds produced are within normal limits. He is being evaluated for speech and language services

➤ Posture (observation): In all fours, Taylor demonstrates a lordotic posture and "hangs" on his shoulder girdle. In sitting, he slumps rather than using muscle activity to sit upright. Caregivers have noticed his posture when sitting has declined. He has a breakdown on the sacrum

➤ Range of motion (contracture tests, observations, goniometry): Range of motion is within functional limits. Taylor has slightly tight hip flexors and hip adductors

➤ Self-care and home management (observations, barrier identification, physical performance tests ADL, IADL scales): Taylor can put on and take off a T-shirt. He needs assistance for lower body dressing. Oral motor skills are normal and there are no feeding problems. He needs assistance with other self-cares such as toileting

➤ Sensory integrity (sensory tests): Taylor demonstrates loss of cutaneous and proprioceptive sensation below T12

➤ Work (job/school/play), community, and leisure integration (observation, interviews): Taylor is a sociable child who is interested in age-appropriate play and leisure activities. He is most interested in peer interaction in his home and in his classroom as he cannot keep up with peers outside or on the playground. He is enrolled in a Saturday karate class in the community

Evaluation

Based on the re-examination you determine that Taylor's primary impairments are no longer motor function and sensory integrity, but rather impaired muscle performance and integumentary. You review the practice patterns and determine that Taylor should be classified into practice pattern 4C: Impaired Muscle Performance and Practice Pattern 7C: Impaired Integumentary Integrity Associated With Partial-Thickness Skin Involvement and Scar Formation.

When determining the appropriate pattern it is important to review the first page of the pattern (Patient/Client Diagnostic Classification) reviewing the inclusion, exclusion, and note sections. You will see by reviewing this page for pattern 4C that it includes conditions of chronic neuromuscular dysfunction and musculoskeletal dysfunction. You also will note that this pattern can be used with any patient/client regardless of his or her pathology or condition as long as muscle performance is the primary impairment.

Taylor also is placed in pattern 7C to address the interventions for his skin breakdown. Placement in two patterns is appropriate when the interventions for the impairments cannot be address in only one pattern.

Diagnosis

The primary impairments that impact Taylor's functional abilities now fall into the pattern of 4C: Impaired Performance and 7C Impaired Integumentary Integrity Associated With Partial Thickness Skin Involvement.

Prognosis

When using two patterns it is important to know that you do not add the expected range of number of visits per episode of care of the two patterns, but rather use the factors column to adjust the range of number of visits for each pattern. In Taylor's situation, his prognosis statements would appear as follows:

"In 3 months, Taylor will demonstrate muscle performance and the highest level of functioning in the home, leisure and community within the context of his impairments functional limitations, and disabilities. In 4 weeks, Taylor will demonstrate optimal integumentary integrity and the highest level of function in home, school, and play." For this episode of care, the prognosis is that Taylor's area of skin breakdown will be healed and his family and school staff instructed in a program to maintain good skin integrity. Taylor also will demonstrate adequate upper extremity strength to reposition himself frequently in his chair throughout the day to prevent future skin breakdown.

Case Study #4: Ashley

➤ Practice pattern 5B: Impaired Neuromotor Development
➤ Medical diagnosis: Down syndrome
➤ Age: 15 months

This case is an example of using the *Guide* to select procedural interventions based on the examination, evaluation, diagnosis, and prognosis.

Examination

HISTORY

➤ General demographics: Ashley is a 15-month-old female
➤ Social history: Ashley lives with her mother and father who are the primary care givers
➤ Employment/work (job/school/play): Ashley enjoys observing other children, but does not interact with them
➤ Growth and development: Ashley was discharged from the hospital at 6 weeks of age. She was diagnosed with Down syndrome shortly after birth
➤ Living environment: She lives in a two-level home with her bedroom on the second level
➤ General health status (self report, family report, caregivers report)
  • Role: Daughter, grandchild
  • Social function: Ashley attends a mother–infant early intervention program twice weekly
➤ Medical/surgical history: Ashley was a full-term infant born to a 26-year-old primipara mother who had experienced an uncomplicated pregnancy. Ashley was diagnosed with Down syndrome shortly after birth. She had esophageal atresia and primary repair was not possible. A gastrostomy was present for the first 6 months of age. She had a ventricular-septal defect that was surgically repaired at eight months. Ashley has a history of chronic otitis media with mild conductive hearing loss. PE tubes were placed at 12 months
➤ Current conditions/chief complaint: Currently she is receiving consultative physical therapy, occupational therapy, and speech therapy services twice a week when she and her mother attend an early intervention program
➤ Functional status and activity level: Ashley has variety of movement patterns but is slow and postural reactions are delayed. She has poor oral-motor skills and does not assist in dressing. She observes other children but does not interact
➤ Medications: None

System Review

The systems review may include:

➤ Anatomical and physiological status
  • Cardiovascular: heart rate—WNL; respiratory rate—WNL
➤ Integumentary
  • Presence of scar formation: Scar present on chest from heart surgery, NA to assess
  • Skin color: Normal
  • Skin integrity: Normal
➤ Musculoskeletal
  • Gross range of motion: Hypermobility is noted in both proximal and distal extremities
➤ Neuromuscular
  • Gross coordinated movements: Ashley has good head control in all positions. She rolls independently, transitions in and out of sitting, and in and out of a hands and knees position. She also pulls to stand at furniture
➤ Communication, affect, cognition, language, and learning style
  • Beginning verbal communication, parent requests written home program with diagrams

Tests and Measures

➤ Anthropometrics characteristics (scales, observation): Ashley's height and weight are within the normal range for children her age with Down syndrome. Facial features are characteristic of children with Down syndrome
➤ Arousal, attention, and cognition (developmental inventory): Formal IQ testing has not been completed on Ashley, although she has mild retardation associated with her medical diagnosis. She is a passive child, needing encouragement and stimulation to attend to motor and cognitive tasks. She has several words that she uses singly rather than in combination (eg, "more," "mama," "dada")
➤ Gait, locomotion, and balance (ADL scale, observations): Ashley pulls to stand but is not yet attempting to cruise at furniture. She will walk with maximal assistance with two hands held. She has slow and usually ineffective protective and equilibrium reactions in sitting, all fours, and standing
➤ Joint integrity and mobility: Within normal range to passive movement
➤ Motor function (motor control and motor learning) (ADL scale, observations): Although Ashley appears to have a typical variety of movement patterns, her movements are very slow and postural reactions are delayed. Ashley needs multiple repetitions of cognitive and motor tasks for skill achievement and retention
➤ Muscle performance (ADL scales, observation): Ashley has poor muscle definition throughout her body, particularly noticeable in the shoulders and hips. She tends to lock her elbows into extension and externally rotate her arms when making movements transitions. She has poor stability in weight-bearing positions (eg, all-fours, kneeling)
➤ Neuromotor development and sensory integration (developmental inventories, motor assessment, observations): Ashley has good head control in all positions. She rolls independently. She transitions in and out of sitting and in and out of a hands

and knees position. She also pulls to kneeling and pulls to stand at furniture. She tends to use straight-line movements without using trunk rotation. She does not appear hypersensitive to tactile input. She generally is apprehensive about movement activities. She grasps objects but cannot release them with control. She cannot pick up pellet-sized objects

➤ Range of motion (observation): Hypermobility is noted in both proximal and distal extremities. She tends to keep her shoulders elevated with shortened capital extensors muscles

➤ Reflex integrity (reflex tests): Decreased tendon reflexes (hypotonia) are present throughout upper and lower extremities. Low muscle tone also is noted throughout the trunk

➤ Self-care and ADL (physical performance tests): Ashley has poor oral-motor skills. She uses a suckling pattern in feeding. Her tongue is thick in contour and protrudes from her mouth. She drinks from a cup only at snack time. Solids are inconsistently presented. She tends to lose food from her mouth. She does not assist in any other self-cares

➤ Sensory integrity: Vision is normal. Mild hearing loss has been noted. Ashley tends to avoid movement-based activities

➤ Respiration and ventilation: Ashley has decreased respiratory-phonotory functioning. She is a mouth breather and occasionally drools

➤ Work (job/school/play), community, and leisure integration or reintegration (disability inventory, observations): Ashley observes other children but does not interact with them. She tends to fling objects or toys to dispose of them. Play is seldom goal directed

Evaluation

Based on the examination you determine the following: Ashley has poor muscle definition throughout her body, with poor stability in weight-bearing positions. She has hypermobility in both proximal and distal extremities, and has low muscle tone. She is able to pull to standing at furniture but does not cruise. She has slow protective and equilibrium reactions in sitting, all fours and standing. She grasps objects but cannot release them with control. She is a mouth breather and occasionally drools. She has a mild hearing loss.

Diagnosis

The data collected help determine the primary dysfunction that will drive the interventions, which is her impaired neuromotor development. You place Ashley in practice pattern 5B: Impaired Neuromotor Development.

Prognosis

Ashley will demonstrate optimal neuromotor development and the highest level of functioning in the home and community, within the context of her impairments, functional limitations, and disabilities. Ashley's prognosis for independent ambulation at home and in community environments is good, as children with Down syndrome typically become ambulatory. The family declined home-based services but agreed to consultative services from occupational, physical, and speech therapy when Ashley and her mother attend early intervention program provided two times per week. Ashley will be discharged when anticipated goals and expected outcomes have been met.

Interventions (for Clinical Consideration)

COORDINATION, COMMUNICATION, AND DOCUMENTATION

➤ Interventions: Coordination and communication with occupational therapy, speech therapy, and early intervention program (teachers, classroom aides)

➤ Anticipated goals and expected outcomes: Available resources are maximally utilized. Care is coordinated with family and any other caregivers

PATIENT/CLIENT-RELATED INSTRUCTION

➤ Interventions: The family will receive instruction, education, and training in a home program and updates. They will receive information on when it is appropriate to seek additional services

➤ Anticipated goals and expected outcomes: Ashley's parents will have awareness of and use community resources. Parents and caregivers will have increased awareness of the impact of Ashley's diagnosis

PROCEDURAL INTERVENTIONS

To assist Ashley in achieving her anticipated goals and expected outcomes you select therapeutic exercise as one of her procedural interventions. When selecting a procedural intervention, you should review the information provided Chapter 3 of the *Guide* (Interventions), under the specific procedural intervention. Each procedural intervention provides examples of clinical indications for the intervention in the categories of pathology/pathophysiology, impairments, functional limitations, disability, risk reduction, and health, wellness, and fitness needs.

Each procedural intervention also lists categories of specific interventions and examples of anticipated goals and outcomes that impact pathology/pathophysiology, impairments, functional limitations, disability, risk reduction and health, wellness, and fitness as well as societal resources and patient/client satisfaction. You can use this section to assist you in determining appropriate goals and outcomes.

For Ashley you select Therapeutic Exercise, as it addresses her needs for neuromotor development training, gait and locomotion training, and strength training.

Case Study #5: John

➤ Practice pattern 5B: Impaired Neuromotor Development

➤ Medical diagnosis: Attention deficit hyperactivity disorder, developmental coordination disorder

➤ Age: 5 years

This case is an example of using the *Guide* for re-examination and termination from an episode of care.

Reexamination

Summary of History and System Review from Initial Examination

➤ General demographics: John is a 5-year-old male

➤ Employment/work (job/school/play): He attends half-day kindergarten, 5 days per week

➤ General health: Stated prior health was excellent

➤ Role: Son, grandson

➤ Medical/surgical: John was a premature infant who spent a short time in the NICU before being discharged to home. He was noted to have slightly delayed motor milestones (sat at 9 months of age; walked at 18 months.) He has always been considered to be very active child. He is easily frustrated with motor tasks and temper tantrums are frequent. He is noted to be "clumsy" and is unable to perform gross and fine motor tasks as well as peers (eg, cannot ride a bike without training wheels: has poor handwriting/ printing). He was evaluated by a developmental pediatrician and neuropsychologist and received dual diagnoses of ADHD and DCD

Re-Examination: Current Condition/Chief Complaint

John has improved in his functional status in the areas of self-care, and has learned to ride a bike without training wheels. He has not been cooperating in physical therapy and the parents would like to discontinue physical therapy and occupational therapy and continue with a home program. They are interested in information on community resources.

Re-Examination: Tests and Measures

➤ Arousal, attention, and cognition (observations; safety checklist): John's attention span has improved since he began taking medication. He still has difficulty with selective attention and often has to be redirected to task. Formal IQ testing on the Stanford-Binet suggests above average intelligence. John has an expressive language delay, often omitting consonants in words and words in sentences

➤ Gait, locomotion, and balance (ADL scales, observation, functional assessment): John walks independently, but occasionally walks on his toes. He can walk with a heel-toe gait when reminded. He tends to walk too quickly with poor balance, often bumping into environmental objects or other people. He cannot walk a 4-inch balance beam without falling off and only can maintain his balance on one foot for 1 to 2 seconds

➤ Motor function (motor control and motor learning) (observation, coordination screens, movement assessment scales): John is consistently characterized as being "clumsy." He has difficulty varying the speed of movement and coordinating upper and lower extremities, such as required when performing jumping jacks. He has motor planning problems and has difficulty learning new motor tasks. He requires increased practice to master each motor skill. Skills do not generalize easily

➤ Muscle performance (timed activity tests, ADL and IADL scales): Upper extremities strength is decreased for his age. For example, he has difficulty supporting his weight on his arms to "wheelbarrow." Endurance for age-appropriate activities, such as soccer, is decreased compared to his peers

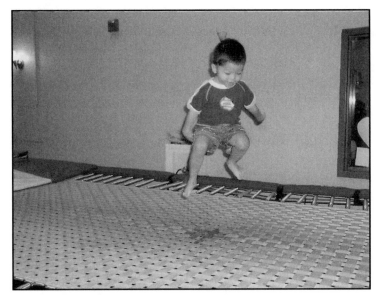

Figure 5-3. Child jumping on trampoline during circus gymnastics program.

➤ Neuromotor development and sensory integration (activity index, motor function tests, neuromotor assessment): John ambulates independently. He can run, although he does so in a poorly coordinated pattern. He cannot skip, but gallops instead. He has difficulty with ball skills (eg, catching, throwing, dribbling) and eye-hand coordination. He uses a modified lateral pinch for coloring and printing. He occasionally demonstrates signs of tactile defensiveness

➤ Posture (observation): John tends to walk with stiff legs and a decreased arm swing. He leans forward as he walks

➤ Range of motion: Range of motion is within normal limits

➤ Self-care and home management (ADL and IADL scales, interviews, observation): John has difficulty using utensils during meals and prefers finger foods. He is independent in dressing, but has difficulty with buttons, snaps, and zippers. He prefers velcro closures, t-shirts, and sweatpants. He is independent in toileting, but needs to be monitored to do an adequate job bathing and tooth brushing

Evaluation

John has been receiving physical and occupational therapy each two times a month from a private agency. He attends a half-day kindergarten program but does not qualify for special education. He has made progress in therapy especially in self care and gross motor skills, however he is refusing to cooperate with therapy and he has not met all his current anticipated goals and expected outcomes. Parents report that John enjoys and fully participates in a community based circus program where he works on coordination and motor skills as part of the routines (Figures 5-3 through 5-6). Parents report that staff members working with John are willing to incorporate ideas from therapists into his circus program activities.

Figure 5-4. Child swinging on trapeze and landing on foam incline during circus gymnastics program.

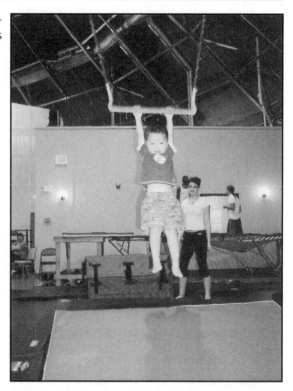

Figure 5-5. Child swinging on trapeze and landing on foam incline during circus gymnastics program.

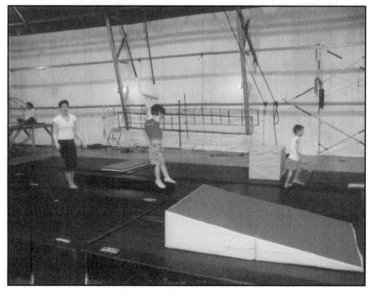

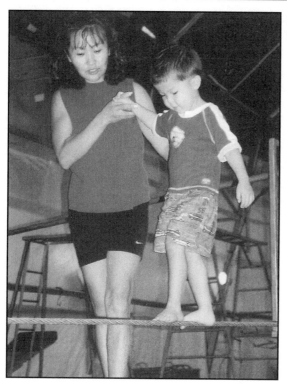

Figure 5-6. Assisted walking on a high wire during circus gymnastics program.

Diagnosis

The primary impairments that impact John's functional status continue to be consistent with Pattern 5B: Impaired Neuromotor Development.

Prognosis

Should John be discharged or discontinued? Discharge is the process of ending physical therapy services that have been provided during a single episode of care. It occurs when the anticipated goals and expected outcomes have been achieved. Discontinuation is the process of ending physical therapy services that have been provided during a single episode of care when the patient/caregiver, parents or legal guardian decline to continue intervention. When physical therapy services are terminated prior to achievement of anticipated goals and expected outcomes, the patient/client's status and the rationale are documented.

Based on John's lack of cooperation during therapy, parent's request to end therapy, and John's involvement in a community-based children's circus program, you determine that John will be discontinued from this episode of care following consultation with community-based circus staff and establishment of home program. Parents are in agreement with this plan. John will seen two times per month for 2 months at his community circus site, to consult with community-based staff and set up a home program and updates.

References

1. American Physical Therapy Association. Guide to physical therapist practice. 2nd ed. *Phys Ther*. 2001;81:9-744.

2. American Physical Therapy Association. Guide to physical therapist practice. Vol I: a description of patient management. *Phys Ther*. 1995;75:707-764.

3. American Physical Therapy Association. Guide to physical therapist practice. *Phys Ther*. 1997;77:1163-1650.

4. American Physical Therapy Association. Guide to physical therapist practice. Revisions. *Phys Ther*. 1999;81:623-629.

5. American Physical Therapy Association. Guide to physical therapist practice. Revisions. *Phys Ther*. 1999;81:1078-1081.

6. Bernhardt-Bainbridge D. What's new: guide to physical therapist practice. 2nd ed. *PTmagazine*. 2001;9:34-37.

7. Nagi S. Some conceptual issues in disability and rehabilitation. In: Sussman M, ed. *Sociology and Rehabilitation*. Washington, DC: American Sociological Association; 1965:100-113.

8. World Health Organization. *International Classification of Impairments, Disabilities, and Handicaps*. Geneva, Switzerland: Author; 1980.

9. National Advisory Board on Medical Rehabilitation Research. *Draft V: Report and Plan for Medical Rehabilitation Research*. Bethesda, Md: National Institutes of Health; 1992.

10. Nagi S. *Disability and Rehabilitation*. Columbus, Ohio: Ohio State University Press; 1969.

11. Nagi S. Disability concepts revisited: implications for prevention. In: *Disability in America: Toward a National Agenda for Prevention*. Washington, DC: Institute of Medicine, National Academy Press; 1991.

12. World Health Organization. *International Classification of Functioning, Disability, and Health* (ICIDH-2). Geneva, Switzerland: Author; 2000.

13. *Disability in America: Toward a National Agenda for Prevention*. Washington, DC: Institute of Medicine, National Academy Press; 1991.

14. Brandt EN Jr, Pope AM, eds. *Enabling America: Assessing the Role of Rehabilitation Science and Engineering*. Washington, DC: American Sociological Association; 1965:100-113.

15. Guccione AA. Physical therapy diagnosis and the relationship between impairments and function. *Phys Ther*. 1991;71:499-504.

16. Jette AM. Using health-related quality of life measures in physical therapy outcomes research. *Phys Ther*. 1993;73:528-537.

17. Jette AM. Physical disablement concepts for physical therapy research and practice. *Phys Ther*. 1994;74:380-386.

18. Guccione AA. Arthritis and the process of disablement. *Phys Ther*. 1994;74:408-414.

19. Rimmer JH. Health promotion for people with disabilities: the emerging paradigm shift from disability prevention to prevention of secondary conditions. *Phys Ther*. 1999;79:495-502.

20. Gill-Body KM, Beninato M, Krebs DE. Relationship among balance impairments, functional performance, and disability in people with peripheral vestibular hypofunction. *Phys Ther*. 2000;80:748-758.

21. Bartlett DJ, Palisano RJ. A multivariate model of determinants of motor change for children with cerebral palsy. *Phys Ther*. 2000;80:598-614.

22. Palisano RJ, Hanna SE, Rosenbaum PL, et al. Validation of a model of gross motor function for children with cerebral palsy. *Phys Ther*. 2000;80:974-985.

23. Ketelaar M, Vermeer A, Hart H, et al. Effects of a functional therapy program on motor abilities of children with cerebral palsy. *Phys Ther*. 2001;81:1534-1545.

24. Shumway-Cook A, Patala AE, Stewart A, et al. Environmental demands associated with community mobility in older adults with and without mobility. *Phys Ther*. 2002;82:670-681.

25. Fragala MA, O'Neil ME, Russo KJ, et al. Impairment, disability, and satisfaction outcomes after lower-extremity botulinum toxin A injections for children with cerebral palsy. *Pediatr Phys Ther*. 2002;14:132-144.

26. Steiner WA, Ryser L, Huber E, et al. Use of the ICF model as a clinical problem-solving tool in physical therapy and rehabilitation medicine. *Phys Ther*. 2002;82:1098-1107.

27. Kott KM, Held SL. Effects of orthoses on upright functional skills of children and adolescents with cerebral palsy. *Pediatr Phys Ther*. 2002;14:199-207.

28. Kim CM, Eng JJ. The relationship of lower-extremity muscle torque to locomotor performance people with stroke. *Phys Ther*. 2003;83:49-57.

29. Jones MA, McEwen IR, Hansen L. Use of power mobility for a young child with spinal muscular atrophy. *Phys Ther*. 2003;83:253-262.

30. Tokcan G, Haley SM, Gill-Body KM, et al. Item-specific functional recovery in children and youth with acquired brain injury. *Pediatr Phys Ther*. 2003;15:16-22.

31. Giallonardo L. Guide in action: patient with total hip replacement. *PT*. 2000;8:76-86.

CHAPTER 6

PHYSICAL THERAPY IN THE NEONATAL INTENSIVE CARE UNIT

Meredith Hinds Harris, EdD, PT
Rebecca Welch, MSPT, PCS

The neonatal intensive care unit (NICU) is certainly a window into the next high tech century (Figure 6-1). It is advanced technology in the highest degree. The medical dictionary defines the NICU as "a hospital unit containing a variety of sophisticated mechanical devices and special equipment for the management and care of premature and seriously ill newborns. The unit is staffed by a team of nurses and neonatologists who are highly trained in the pathophysiology of the newborn."[1] When entering the NICU we initially are aware of the brightness, the constant noise level, and the scurrying around of a variety of intense looking people.[2,3] On closer examination we are attracted to babies attached to an incredible number of monitors, electrodes, machines, and tubes. A different language is spoken here: terms like "spells," "ABG," "TCM," "CPAP," and "BPD" are often heard in addition to the medical terminology with which the physical therapist is more familiar.[4-6]

Ideally, care of a fragile infant in the NICU is orchestrated by a team working in concert to provide the best appropriate care for the infant and the family. Personnel in the NICU include the neonatologist (a pediatrician who has special training in how to deal with the preterm or critically ill full-term newborn) and the perinatologist (an obstetrician who specializes in high-risk pregnancies). The neonatologist directs the overall care of the infant. Nurses in the NICU have special training and/or education in supervised practice and in-service experience. Some units have nurses with specialty training and expertise, called neonatal nurse clinicians or practitioners. Their roles differ from unit to unit. In most units they provide primary care. In some units, they provide transport services to bring critically ill babies from distant places to the center. Many units also have a variety of medical residents from several different specialties, such as pediatrics, obstetrics, and family practice. Other people who help care for an infant in NICU are: the physician assistant who helps oversee the infant's progress, the respiratory therapist who oversees the breathing needs of infants who require oxygen or who are on ventilators, the social worker who helps families deal with the stress of having a sick infant and with discharge planning, and the physical, occupational, and speech therapists who evaluate the infant's developmental progress and develop individualized plans of intervention in the unit and after discharge. In some units, dietitians who oversee the nutritional care of the infant are becoming integral members of the team.[7]

Figure 6-1. Typical NICU.

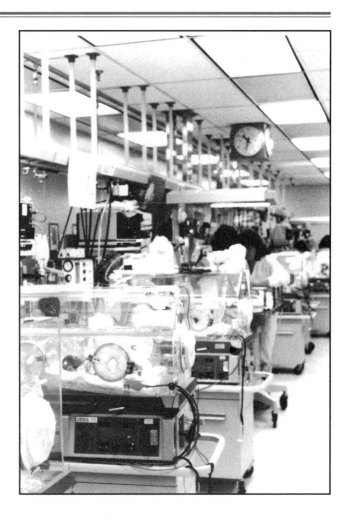

Indications for NICU

When we think of the babies admitted to the NICU the typical image is that of very tiny, preterm infants. This may be due to the publicity in the popular press regarding these babies. Another reason the small baby comes to mind is because the length of hospital stay is long and the cost enormous. Technological advances are making it possible for many babies born 3 months early and weighing less than 2 pounds to survive. Terminology associated with prematurity defines premature infants as those born before 37 weeks gestation and low birth weight (LBW) weighing between 1501 and 2500 g, very low birth weight (VLBW) 1001 to 1500 g, and extremely low birth weight (ELBW) below 1000 g. Infants who are small for gestational age (SGA) or medically fragile also may be seen in the NICU. These babies are at risk for potential damage to many organ systems. Possible problems include retinopathy of prematurity (ROP), affecting the visual system; intracranial hemorrhage (ICH), affecting the central nervous system (CNS); necrotizing enterocolitis (NEC), affecting the gastrointestinal system; respiratory distress syndrome (RDS), bronchopulmonary dysplasia (BPD), apnea, and bradycardia, affecting the cardiac and pulmonary systems; sepsis; and meningitis.[8] Long-term hospitalization often disrupts normal parent-child relationships. The need for continual medical intervention, often including the use of heart and respiratory rate monitors after discharge, makes it difficult for the parents of these children to believe that their babies are "normal."

Although the long-term prognosis for many of these infants is good, the cost both financially and emotionally is high and may result in irreparable damage to the structure of the family. In some cases, mothers of preterm infants may be young, have little financial or emotional support, and have received little if any prenatal care.[9] In some centers, particularly in urban or economically depressed settings, infants may be admitted to the NICU because of maternal drug and/or multiple substance abuse. Each type of substance carries with it a unique and not necessarily well-understood risk that compounds the issues of prematurity. With maternal substance abuse and sporadic or absent prenatal care, there is increased risk of prematurity, intrauterine growth retardation, gastro-urinary malformations, LBW, infections, cardiac and limb malformations, and risk to infection from human immunodeficiency virus (HIV). Infants affected by substance abuse also may have to cope with narcotic abstinence syndrome (NAS) characterized by neurobehavioral sequelae.[10,11] When there are the added issues of perinatal drug abuse, HIV infection, and economically depressed family situation, the premature or medically fragile newborn infants and their health care providers face problems about long-term outcome which is still undetermined.[12]

The best predictor of long-term outcome for preterm infants is not birth weight or medical complications, but the socioeconomic status of the family.[13,14] While smaller and earlier babies are surviving, it is important to note that in many units half of the admissions are for babies weighing 2500 g (approximately 5.5 pounds) or more. This weight is usually the target weight for discharge for LBW infants. However, many of these heavier babies are at significant risk for developmental disabilities, and therapists should concentrate time and effort on these infants, as well as the small preterm infants.

Examples of babies other than preterm infants who may be admitted to the NICU are those with neonatal sepsis or infection. Infants who are full term or preterm have few capabilities to combat infection. Infants may contract infections in utero, while passing through the birth canal, or after birth. Certain types of infections that may be virtually harmless to adults are potentially fatal to infants. Although there have been great advances in antibiotic therapy, infant infections often become systemic via the blood system and eventually may result in meningitis because of immaturity in the blood/brain barrier.[15] Even with advanced technology, infants may die as a result of "neonatal sepsis syndrome." Surviving infants may be neurologically impaired and certainly should be closely monitored by the physical therapist in the NICU and other members of the team. Infants at risk for HIV infection because of maternal HIV infection are at increased risk for frequent periodic opportunistic infections and sexually transmitted diseases. The potential for transmission of HIV infection from an infected woman to her child can be substantially reduced with pharmacological intervention during pregnancy. Women who are infected with HIV and who receive prenatal care have the opportunity to receive antiretroviral medication that can prevent the transmission of HIV infection to the infant. There are indications that the earlier prophylactic intervention is begun, the better the chance of preventing transmission. The long-term effects of prenatal antiretroviral medications appear to have low risk, but longitudinal developmental study is needed.[16] Infants who are in this high-risk category should be assessed carefully and closely monitored over time for potential neurological impairment or developmental delay.[17-20]

At first glance, the fat, rosy-cheeked infants of diabetic mothers (IDM) look healthy, and we assume that they are very healthy children. However, these babies are generally large for gestational age (LGA) and are at risk for congenital anomalies and difficulty with glucose metabolism. Unless they are managed medically immediately, hypoglycemic seizures may result. Another typical finding in IDM is feeding difficulties. The infants often are initially lethargic, and feeding patterns may be even less mature than gestational age would indicate.[21] Keeping gestational age in mind, the therapist can be of great assistance to both the nursing staff and the parents by offering techniques to increase alertness, as well as suggestions for positioning and oral motor facilitation.[22]

The differentiation between preterm, appropriate for gestational age (AGA), and small for dates or SGA, and intrauterine growth retarded (IUGR) babies is important. Causes of poor intrauterine growth include: maternal smoking, drugs, or alcohol; intrauterine infections; and placental insufficiency. Since brain growth is so critical prior to birth and during the first year of life, anything that compromises this growth may decrease both the number and size of neurons. Little or no evidence has been documented for regeneration of neurons following this critical period. In studies where SGA children were followed on a long-term basis, two outcomes were documented. The children generally did not catch up with their growth parameters and remained smaller when compared to same-age peers and other family members. Additionally, they often had difficulty in school, particularly with attending skills, even if they were intellectually normal.[23,24] If possible, the etiology of growth retardation should be ascertained, because certain types of intrauterine infections are particularly devastating to the CNS. TORCH infections (see Glossary) may result in significant microcephaly and in some cases visual or auditory defects.

Children with perinatal asphyxia have received inadequate oxygen prior to, during, or shortly after birth. Apgar scores[25] or blood pH may give an indication of the severity of oxygen deprivation, but some babies appear normal on follow-up even when early indicators seem predictive of significant impairment. Other infants sustain severe brain damage with minimal indication of asphyxia. Full-term babies seem to be at a greater risk for brain damage due to asphyxia. This may be because their CNS systems are relatively more mature, just as an adult has less capacity to demonstrate neural plasticity than a child. It also may be related to the relative oxygen needs of a full-term nervous system as compared to an immature nervous system. Certain drugs, such as cocaine, when ingested during pregnancy put the infant at risk for hypoxia, decreased cardiac output, uterine arterial vasoconstriction, impaired oxygen transport, intracranial hemorrhages, or infarct. Clinical symptoms may or may not be present immediately nor detectable early.[26] The severity of the neurological insult may be evaluated partially by the presence or absence of secondary complications, including seizures, the need for ventilator support, and kidney damage. All of these factors are indicators of significant neurological damage. If none of these indicators is present, but the child demonstrates feeding difficulties, long-term problems are still a possibility.[27] The use of appropriate neuromotor and/or neurobehavioral tests may yield helpful diagnostic and prognostic information.

A variety of syndromes and congenital anomalies are observed in infants in the NICU. Included in this category are chromosomal abnormalities, such as Down syndrome (trisomy 21), other lethal trisomies (13 and 18), birth defects (including myelomeningocele and cleft palate), congenital cardiac and limb defects secondary to maternal drug use, and problems related to lack of intrauterine space (eg, arthrogryposis and club foot). Medical diagnoses such as these indicate the necessity for therapeutic intervention in the NICU, parent counseling regarding long-term implications, and a variety of therapy services following discharge. Infants with specific medical diagnoses and early identified developmental disability are probably the easiest to identify regarding the need for services. However, some of these infants never are admitted to the NICU. Others remain in the unit for a very short period of time. Because of the need for a variety of other specialty consultations, referral to physical therapy may be overlooked. Depending on the setting, it may be appropriate for the acute hospital staff to provide long-term intervention for these babies and families. However, in most cases referral to local community agencies as out-patients or for comprehensive family-centered care through community early intervention programs usually better meets the needs of the infant and family. Children referred to social service agencies for foster care need to be carefully tracked to ensure that their health, therapeutic services, and developmental progress are carefully monitored and that they are not lost to follow-up during periods of family disruption or placement process.

The Role of the Physical Therapist in the NICU

Physical therapists are successful in identifying new frontiers to provide effective and cost-efficient physical therapy. Any physical therapist involved in pediatric therapy probably has considered that if only he or she had begun treatment earlier with a specific child, the results of intervention would be improved. Logically, then, we look to the NICU as the earliest type of "hands-on" treatment.

The role of the physical therapist in the NICU is similar to that in other settings. Effective care is based on using foundation knowledge in basic and clinical sciences and critical thinking and problem solving to address the needs of the fragile newborn and the family. This culmination of skills and knowledge and specialty training in the equipment, environment, and particular diagnoses and problems of these infants leads to: examination, evaluation, establishment of a physical therapy diagnosis, prognosis, plan of care, intervention strategies, and outcome measurements.

The NICU is a very complex and specialized world. Close coordination and communication with team members and with the family must occur for the best outcome in the management of fragile infants, Examination, evaluation, and establishment of a physical therapy diagnosis and prognosis are all part of the process that helps the physical therapist determine the most appropriate intervention(s) to achieve the most beneficial outcomes desired by the team.[28] Examination is best done through observation, conversation, and coordination with other team members to minimize excessive handling and overstimulation. Evaluation requires appropriate developmental tools designed for use with fragile and preterm infants. Diagnosis in physical therapy initially is guided by the medical diagnosis, but the physical therapist identifies motor, sensory, and developmental dysfunction. Prognosis is the determination of the predicted optimal level of improvement in function and the amount of time needed to reach that level. Prognosis also may include a prediction of levels of improvement that may be reached at various intervals during the course of therapy. In the infant in the NICU, establishing a prognosis is extremely difficult and can change rapidly depending on the fragility of the infant. Intervention requires coordination, communication, documentation, and instruction of other staff members and family members.

Physical therapy intervention encourages developmental progression of the infant and promotes understanding and acceptance of the family when intervention is needed after discharge. Through appropriate education and instruction, the family is encouraged to heal after the stress of the NICU period and promote growth and development in the infant. Physical therapy along with team intervention can provide the support, knowledge, and skills to take the child and family to the next and subsequent levels of care toward problem resolution.

When there has been adequate prenatal care, evaluation of the mother-infant system has already occurred. Information from obstetrics provides clues to interferences or stressors during the prenatal, perinatal, and immediate post-natal periods. The therapist uses this information as part of the history to determine the most appropriate approach to the examination of and subsequent intervention for the infant.

Figure 6-2. Typical extension of the preterm with supine positioning. Note lack of subcutaneous fat.

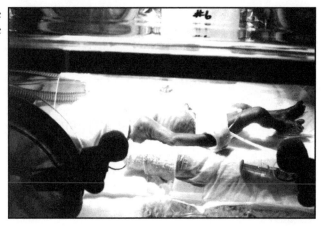

Fetal ultrasound films may have been used to assess movement to detect abnormalities. How we might intervene if abnormalities are noted must be carefully planned. Enthusiastic, energetic physical therapists may descend on the unsuspecting neonatal unit certain that they will be able to right the wrongs of years of delayed referrals, and that they will be able to improve the developmental outcome of any baby with whom they interact. The staff of most neonatal units are very protective of the needs of the babies and are, perhaps justifiably, suspicious of new personnel and new techniques. It is important to display competence and to provide evidence to support the type of intervention selected in order to gain the acceptance as an important member of the NICU team.

Understanding fetal development is a prerequisite for beginning intervention programs in the NICU. The last trimester of fetal development should be studied intensely to provide a framework for appropriate motor, sensory, and functional activities. Previous experience with full-term or older infants with movement abnormalities or impairments may be modified.[29] For example, the full-term child is generally flexed, while the more preterm the baby is, the more relative extension is noted[30] (Figure 6-2). Although non-nutritive sucking may begin as early as 17 weeks postconception, nutritive sucking and therefore bottle- or breastfeeding rarely is accomplished prior to 34 weeks. It would be as foolish to try bottlefeeding with a baby of 30 weeks gestation as it would be to begin self-feeding with a 2-month-old typically developing child.

Sick and preterm babies have difficulty maintaining homeostasis (ie, temperature, blood pressure, heart, and respiratory control). Their sleep cycles are brief and often disturbed.[31,32] Organization of sensory stimuli and state control often is disrupted or impaired in infants exposed to drugs or alcohol in utero. Overvigorous or mistimed activities that the therapist thinks may provide positive input to these fragile babies may be potentially life-threatening. The terminology "infant stimulation" is probably one of the most inappropriate concepts in treating any child, and particularly those in the NICU. These babies are already overstimulated both visually and auditorily. The tactile, vestibular, and proprioceptive input they are receiving is not comparable to the intrauterine environment, nor is it similar to what a full-term baby would receive in the first few days of life.[33]

Therapists can have an impact on the neonatal environment by helping parents and staff members understand the sensory and motor needs of the babies and to help provide as normalized sensory motor experiences within the infant's capabilities to cope with intervention and still maintain appropriate growth and medical stabilization.[34-36] Generally speaking, it is contraindicated to evaluate or treat a baby just after a feeding or stressful medical procedure. It is appropriate to gather information contributing to evaluation by observing the infant at various times of the day and by talking with physicians, nurses, and other team members involved in care. This early examination time is a good time to meet with parents and, when appropriate, gain information from them about their concerns and perceptions of care after discharge from NICU.

Because a baby's optimal time for intervention might occur when the therapist is not available, it is essential to train parents, nursing staff, and other caregiving staff in intervention strategies. Some therapists think that they alone are capable of providing these services. However, the most successful treatment strategies are those that are integrated into the total lifestyle of the baby and carried out throughout the waking hours. In-service education, as well as role modeling of useful techniques, will enhance normalization of the baby's sensory motor and behavioral environment.

Physical therapy in the NICU is a relatively new entity and continues to evolve with technology and evidence of intervention outcomes. There have been many studies showing both positive and negative outcomes related to short-term intervention techniques.[37-41] There have been very few studies on whether early NICU intervention techniques have long-term positive outcomes for children and families.[42-44] The guiding therapeutic principle should be to "do no harm." Benefits that result should be carefully documented and whenever possible measured through appropriate outcome tools. Information must be shared with other team members to ensure a comprehensive approach to care. Long-term effects are difficult to assess, because the older the child, the more difficult it is to differentiate whether the outcome is related to the primary insult, the intervention, the genetic complement, or the environment.

Evaluation

Changing practices in NICU are becoming more "infant and family friendly." Cluster care is a strategy used by the team to minimize handling and stress to an infant.[45] Members of the NICU team determine a plan of care that allows team members to gather information or provide intervention in the most supportive, least disruptive manner. [46] In addition, intervention in the NICU is increasingly involving parents in very early infant care.[47] The evaluation of the newborn begins long before being admitted to the NICU. Although the physical therapist is not directly involved in the earliest evaluations, it is important to become familiar with the terminology and to understand what has been done previously to enhance quality of life. Early in the pregnancy, the obstetrician monitors weight gain and fundal height of the mother. Ultrasound examination also may be done to evaluate fetal growth. Ultrasound is capable of evaluating the status of the heart and kidneys and can determine whether intrauterine hydrocephalus is present. Amniocentesis may be done to determine whether the fetus has certain genetic abnormalities such as Down syndrome and is used late in the pregnancy to determine lung maturity. Mothers are taught to monitor fetal movements and to inform their physicians of any change in these patterns.

Once labor begins, both external heart rate monitors and internal probes can be used to determine if the baby is well oxygenated. Immediately after birth, at 1 and 5 minutes of age, Apgar scores are obtained. The following five measures are assessed: heart rate, respiratory effort, muscle tone, reflex irritability, and color. Each item is scored 0, 1, or 2, with the best possible score being 2 and the lowest score being 0. The Apgar is an evaluation of neonatal well-being and is not meant to determine long-term neurological outcome. Rather, it is an indication for the delivery room personnel to act immediately, if the score is low, to resuscitate the infant.[48,49] On the other hand, low 5-minute Apgar scores may be indicative of long-term neurological sequelae, and these infants should be monitored carefully.

Another early evaluation is the gestational age assessment originally described by Dubowitz[30] (Figure 6-3). This assessment includes two broad categories: external signs (edema, skin texture, skin color, lanugo, plantar creases, nipple formation, breast size, ear form and firmness, and genitals) and neurological signs related to muscle tone, positioning, and response to handling. Physical therapists may be involved in the neurological part of this assessment, and it may be useful later as a determiner of neurological maturation of muscle tone.

A number of authors have described evaluations for newborn and preterm infants[50-54] (Figure 6-4). These evaluations stress assessment of positioning at rest, excursion of passive motion, and reflexes and are therefore quite passive in nature. Although there are differences in these evaluations, there also are similarities. Both Amiel-Tison[51] and Korner[53] considered gestational age in the development of their exams. The Prechtl examination[55] is designed for the full-term newborn, but it must be noted that a preterm infant at term is not precisely like a baby born at term because of differences in the environment. It is possible for a baby to have significant neurological abnormalities, including structural deficits (hydrocephalus, porencephaly, or intracranial hemorrhage), and still look "normal" on these initial evaluations. For this reason, we must consider carefully the medical history, including prenatal risk factors, and perform serial evaluations over a period of time to predict accurately long-term outcomes.

Prechtl[55] incorporated states of alertness of the newborn in the total assessment of neurological status. He noted that even the reflex character of the baby varied depending on whether he was in deep or light sleep, awake, drowsy, alert, or crying. Korner,[53] in an attempt to standardize her evaluation, noted state for each item.

Brazelton[52] refined the concept of state of alertness in his Newborn Behavioral Assessment Scale (NBAS). Although neurological reflex items are included, this is not the focus of the NBAS. Care is taken to assess the baby at his or her optimal time in the wake-sleep cycle. In addition, a variety of sensory modalities are presented to the sleeping infant to assess his or her initial responses, as well as his or her ability to accommodate sensory input. The NBAS is the only newborn assessment that recognizes individual differences and responses to environmental input. This assessment has been continually revised.

We need to consider the state of the infant in any type of evaluation. Although it may be possible to wake an infant to perform an evaluation, a more optimal picture of the infant's abilities will be obtained by waiting until the baby arouses naturally. In studies where babies were not awakened either for medical care or for other invasive procedures, medical personnel did not need to wait more than 10 minutes to perform a procedure. Babies also gained weight faster and were discharged from the hospital sooner when they were not wakened unnecessarily. From a financial perspective, anything that can be done to shorten hospital stay will be regarded as a positive intervention.

Individual variability occurs in infants with no two babies being exactly alike, even identical twins. The baby's state of alertness, the time of day, the general activity in the NICU, other procedures that have preceded the examination, medical concerns such as infection or anemia, and the gestational age of the infant need to be considered. In addition, the cultural background of the infant should be considered.[56] The *Guide to Physical Therapist Practice* provides a systematic approach to evaluation and is adapted for use in the NICU.

The examination has three components: the *patient/client history*, *systems review*, and *tests and measures*.

(Front)

CLINICAL ESTIMATION OF GESTATIONAL AGE

AN APPROXIMATION BASED ON PUBLISHED DATA

EXAMINATION FIRST HOURS

PHYSICAL FINDINGS		WEEKS GESTATION (20–48)
VERNIX		APPEARS · COVERS BODY, THICK LAYER · ON BACK, SCALP, IN CREASES · SCANT, IN CREASES · NO VERNIX
BREAST TISSUE AND AREOLA		AREOLA & NIPPLE BARELY VISIBLE NO PALPABLE BREAST TISSUE · AREOLA RAISED · 1–2 MM NODULE · 3–5 MM · 5–6 MM · 7–10 MM · >12 MM
EAR	FORM	FLAT, SHAPELESS · BEGINNING INCURVING SUPERIOR · INCURVING UPPER 2/3 PINNAE · WELL-DEFINED INCURVING TO LOBE
	CARTILAGE	PINNA SOFT, STAYS FOLDED · CARTILAGE SCANT RETURNS SLOWLY FROM FOLDING · THIN CARTILAGE SPRINGS BACK FROM FOLDING · PINNA FIRM, REMAINS ERECT FROM HEAD
SOLE CREASES		SMOOTH SOLES T CREASES · 1–2 ANTERIOR CREASES · 2–3 ANTERIOR CREASES · CREASES ANTERIOR 2/3 SOLE · CREASES INVOLVING HEEL · DEEPER CREASES OVER ENTIRE SOLE
SKIN	THICKNESS & APPEARANCE	THIN, TRANSLUCENT SKIN, PLETHORIC, VENULES OVER ABDOMEN EDEMA · SMOOTH THICKER NO EDEMA · PINK · FEW VESSELS · SOME DESQUAMATION PALE PINK · THICK, PALE, DESQUAMATION OVER ENTIRE BODY
	NAIL PLATES	APPEAR · NAILS TO FINGER TIPS · NAILS EXTEND WELL BEYOND FINGER TIPS
LANUGO		APPEARS ON HEAD · EYE BROWS & LASHES · FINE, WOOLLY, BUNCHES OUT FROM HEAD · SILKY, SINGLE STRANDS LAYS FLAT · RECEDING HAIRLINE OR LOSS OF BABY HAIR SHORT, FINE UNDERNEATH
		APPEARS · COVERS ENTIRE BODY · VANISHES FROM FACE · PRESENT ON SHOULDERS · NO LANUGO
GENITALIA	TESTES	TESTES PALPABLE IN INGUINAL CANAL · IN UPPER SCROTUM · IN LOWER SCROTUM
	SCROTUM	FEW RUGAE · RUGAE, ANTERIOR PORTION · RUGAE COVER · PENDULOUS
	LABIA & CLITORIS	PROMINENT CLITORIS LABIA MAJORA SMALL WIDELY SEPARATED · LABIA MAJORA LARGER NEARLY COVERED CLITORIS · LABIA MINORA & CLITORIS COVERED
SKULL FIRMNESS		BONES ARE SOFT · SOFT TO 1" FROM ANTERIOR FONTANELLE · SPONGY AT EDGES OF FONTANELLE CENTER FIRM · BONES HARD SUTURES EASILY DISPLACED · BONES HARD, CANNOT BE DISPLACED
POSTURE	RESTING	HYPOTONIC LATERAL DECUBITUS · HYPOTONIC · BEGINNING FLEXION THIGH · STRONGER HIP FLEXION · FROG-LIKE · FLEXION ALL LIMBS · HYPERTONIC · VERY HYPERTONIC
	RECOIL · LEG	NO RECOIL · PARTIAL RECOIL · PROMPT RECOIL
	ARM	NO RECOIL · PROMPT RECOIL MAY BE INHIBITED · PROMPT RECOIL AFTER 30° INHIBITION

(Back)

CLINICAL ESTIMATION OF GESTATIONAL AGE

AN APPROXIMATION BASED ON PUBLISHED DATA

CONFIRMATORY NEUROLOGIC EXAMINATION TO BE DONE AFTER 24 HOURS

PHYSICAL FINDINGS		WEEKS GESTATION (20–48)
TONE	HEEL TO EAR	NO RESISTANCE · SOME RESISTANCE · IMPOSSIBLE
	SCARF SIGN	NO RESISTANCE · ELBOW PASSES MIDLINE · ELBOW AT MIDLINE · ELBOW DOES NOT REACH MIDLINE
	NECK FLEXORS (HEAD LAG)	ABSENT · HEAD IN PLANE OF BODY · HOLDS HEAD
	NECK EXTENSORS	HEAD BEGINS TO RIGHT ITSELF FROM FLEXED POSITION · GOOD RIGHTING CANNOT HOLD IT · HOLDS HEAD FEW SECONDS · KEEPS HEAD IN LINE c TRUNK >40° · TURNS HEAD FROM SIDE TO SIDE
	BODY EXTENSORS	STRAIGHTENING OF LEGS · STRAIGHTENING OF TRUNK · STRAIGHTENING OF HEAD & TRUNK TOGETHER
	VERTICAL POSITIONS	WHEN HELD UNDER ARMS, BODY SLIPS THROUGH HANDS · ARMS HOLD BABY LEGS EXTENDED · LEGS FLEXED GOOD SUPPORT c ARMS
	HORIZONTAL POSITIONS	HYPOTONIC ARMS & LEGS STRAIGHT · ARMS AND LEGS FLEXED · HEAD & BACK EVEN FLEXED EXTREMITIES · HEAD ABOVE BACK
FLEXION ANGLES	POPLITEAL	NO RESISTANCE · 150° · 110° · 100° · 90° · 80°
	ANKLE	45° · 20° · 0 · A PRE-TERM WHO HAS REACHED 40 WEEKS STILL HAS A 40° ANGLE
	WRIST (SQUARE WINDOW)	90° · 60° · 45° · 30° · 0
REFLEXES	SUCKING	WEAK NOT SYNCHRONIZED c SWALLOWING · STRONGER SYNCHRONIZED · GOOD · GOOD HAND TO MOUTH · PERFECT
	ROOTING	LONG LATENCY PERIOD SLOW, IMPERFECT · HAND TO MOUTH · BRISK, COMPLETE, DURABLE · COMPLETE
	GRASP	FINGER GRASP IS GOOD STRENGTH IS POOR · STRONGER · CAN LIFT BABY OFF BED INVOLVES ARMS · HANDS OPEN
	MORO	BARELY APPARENT · WEAK NOT ELICITED EVERY TIME · STRONGER · COMPLETE c ARM EXTENSION OPEN FINGERS, CRY · ARM ADDUCTION ADDED · BEGINS TO LOSE MORO
	CROSSED EXTENSION	FLEXION & EXTENSION IN A RANDOM, PURPOSELESS PATTERN · EXTENSION BUT NO ADDUCTION · STILL INCOMPLETE · EXTENSION ADDUCTION FANNING OF TOES · COMPLETE
	AUTOMATIC WALK	MINIMAL · BEGINS TIPTOEING GOOD SUPPORT ON SOLE · FAST TIPTOEING · HEEL TOE PROGRESSION WHOLE SOLE OF FOOT · A PRE-TERM WHO HAS REACHED 40 WEEKS WALKS ON TOES · BEGINS TO LOSE AUTOMATIC WALK

Figure 6-3. Dubowitz's gestational age assessment (reprinted with permission).

Figure 6-4. Neonatal evaluation form.

Neonatal Evaluation Form*

Name: _____   Testing Date: _____
D.O.B.: _____ Gestational Age: _____ Day of Life: _____
Birth Weight: _____ Present Weight: _____
Type of Birth: _____
Apgar: _____ 1 min. _____ 5 min. _____ Diagnosis: _____
Parental History: Perinatal History: Neonatal History:

Predominant State:		Primary Walking:	
Posture:	N/Ext/Fl/other	response	N/absent
scissors	no/yes	scissors	no/plantigrade/
lateral preference	no/R/L		tiptoe
strong ATNR	no/R/L	symmetry	equal/↓R L/ab R L
Motor Activity:		Placing:	
amount	N/↑/↓	response	N/poor
symmetry	equal /R ⊃L/L⊃ R	symmetry	equal/R↓/L↓
focal twitching	no/R/L	Eyes:	
jittery/clonic	no/R/L	visual focus	yes/no
tremulous	no/yes	visual tracking-smooth/jerky/___ °	
Oral Motor:		doll eye/nystagmus	
head shape	symmetrical/R/L		yes/↓R L
rooting	N/↓R L/ab R L		
sucking	N/↓/ab/Asym/uncoord	Auditory:	
palate	N/nar/high/cleft	response (loud)	yes/no/startle
gag	N/↑/↓	symmetry (soft)	N/↓R L/ab R L
respiration	N/reverse/shal/	Moro:	
	labored/stridor	threshold	N/low/high
Pull to Sit:	N/sl.↓/sev.↓/↑tone	symmetry	equal/↓R L/ab R L
Palmar Grasp:		Cry:	
response	N/↑/↓	amount	N/↑/↓/ab
symmetry	equal/R /L	high pitch	no/yes
cortical thumb	occassional/oblig.	monotonous	no/yes
Hip Abduc. Resist.:	N/↑R L/↓R L	Primitive Crawl:	N/↓/absent
Planter Grasp:	N/↓R L/↑R L	Tactile:	
Toe Signs:	↑R L/↓R L	touch	N/hypo/hyper
Ventral Suspension:	N/floppy/↑	pain	N/hypo/hyper
Gallant:	equal/↓R L/ab R L	Tone:	
upright suspension:	N/slips/flops/R↓/L↓	amount	N/↑/↓
		symmetry	equal/↑R L/↓R L
		distribution	generalized/
			UE > LE/LE > UE
		State Change:	N/irrit./depr.

Feeding Problems:

Summary:

HISTORY

The history is a systematic gathering of data from both the past and the present related to why the infant is referred to the physical therapist for services. The data that are obtained (generally through physician, nurse, or parent interview; through review of the infant record; or from other sources) include demographic information; social history; prenatal, birth, or family history; growth and development; general health status; medical/surgical history; medications; and other clinical tests.

SYSTEMS REVIEW

After organizing the available history information, the physical therapist begins the "hands-on" component of the examination. The systems review is a brief or limited examination of the anatomical and physiological status of the cardiovascular/pulmonary, integumentary, musculoskeletal, and neuromuscular systems.

The systems review includes the following:

➤ For the cardiovascular/pulmonary system, the assessment of heart rate, respiratory rate, blood pressure, and edema

➤ For the integumentary system, the assessment of pliability (texture), presence of bruising or mottling, skin color, and skin integrity

➤ For the musculoskeletal system, the assessment of gross symmetry, gross range of motion, gross strength, length, and weight

➤ For the neuromuscular system, a general assessment of gross coordinated movement and developmental motor function

The systems review also assists the physical therapist in identifying possible problems that require consultation with or referral to another team member. As the examination progresses, the physical therapist may identify additional problems that were not uncovered by the history and systems review and may conclude that other specific tests and measures or portions of other specific tests and measures are required to obtain sufficient data to perform an evaluation, establish a diagnosis and a prognosis, and select interventions. The examination, therefore, must be dictated by the health of the infant and the therapist's ability to handle the child.

TESTS AND MEASURES

Tests and measures are the means of gathering data about the infant. From the comprehensive identification and questioning processes of the history and systems review, the physical therapist determines the infant's needs and generates diagnostic hypotheses that may be further investigated by selecting specific tests and measures. These tests and measures are used to rule in or rule out causes of impairment and functional limitations; to establish a diagnosis, prognosis, and plan of care; and to select interventions. The tests and measures that are performed as part of an initial examination should be only those that are necessary to: 1) confirm or reject a hypothesis about the factors that contribute to making the current level of the infant's function less than optimal, and 2) support the physical therapist's clinical judgments about appropriate interventions, anticipated goals, and expected outcomes.

The physical therapist may decide to use one, more than one, or portions of several specific tests and measures as part of the examination, based on the purpose of the examination, the complexity of the condition, and the directions taken in the clinical decision-making process.

Specific tests and measurements with good reported validity and reliability designed by and/or used by physical therapists in the NICU include: the Assessment of Preterm Infant Behavior (APIB),[57] the NBAS,[58] the Alberta Infant Motor Scales (AIMS),[59] the Test of Infant Motor Performance (TIMP),[60] Movement Assessment of Infants (MAI),[61] the Bayley Scales of Infant Development, Second Edition (BSID),[62] and the Peabody Developmental Motor Scales, Second Edition (PDMS-2).[63]

Before applying any standardized test to an infant in the NICU, the therapist must be aware of the appropriateness of the test for the infant under consideration. Most tests require special skill or training in the test administration. In addition, when applied to the special environment of the NICU, particular care must be used to exercise appropriate judgment in test selection and have considerable experience with a large number and variety of infants in order to correctly administer the test and interpret the test findings appropriately.

Therapeutic Techniques

Before beginning a therapeutic program in the NICU, therapists must be knowledgeable of neuromuscular and neurobehavioral development in full-term, preterm, and medically fragile infants. Therapists should be well-experienced in applying facilitation techniques and aware of expected outcomes when applied to the immature neonate.[24,60-62] A good understanding of the general principles of facilitation and inhibition is vital in establishing credibility with other professionals working with these babies. Any handling technique can be inhibitory or facilitatory depending on how it is administered. Slow, rhythmic movement tends to be calming, while rapid, irregular movement is alerting. Changing the position of the infant, even when using the same sensory input, may result in a different response. Unless the physical therapist understands the neuromuscular implications of handling and positioning, it is not possible to explain to other medical personnel why certain techniques are useful. Two basic principles must be adhered to when dealing with the fragile population in the NICU: **when in doubt, do nothing** and **do no harm.**

Many articles describe specific techniques of rocking, stroking, swaddling, positioning, talking, and providing certain types of tactile and visual input and report improved scores on infant motor behavior and intelligence scales.[64] Other studies demonstrate little or no change in outcome. These widely divergent results may be due to the fact that many of these intervention strategies do not address the total baby in the context of the environment, but instead attempt to manipulate isolated variables. The physical therapist must consider all the sensory and motor avenues available to the neonate: visual, auditory, tactile, olfactory, gustatory, kinesthetic, proprioceptive, and vestibular.[65] When observing motor responses to sensory input, changes in heart and respiratory rates, sweating, and color change should be considered. Als[50] described various avoidance techniques observed in preterm infants in response to overstimulation. These included sneezing, coughing, eye closing, and, in extreme circumstances, apnea, bradycardia, vomiting, and defecating. This is not to imply that whenever we observe these responses the infant is being overstimulated, but to consider sensory overload when we are not observing the desired motor output. When treating adults or older children, if the desired response is not elicited, the therapist may increase sensory input. This strategy may be potentially harmful with the neonate.

When developing an intervention plan it is helpful to compare the environments of the fetus, the NICU, and the home. The intrauterine environment is one of constant tactile input, decreased visual input, constant noise (maternal heart beat, digestion), and both active movement generated by the baby and passive movement generated by the mother. The NICU has constant bright lights, loud mechanical noises, and provides little movement for the infant. The home environment might include dim lights, children and animal noises, cooking smells, music, and varying amounts of movement. Parents and NICU staff can be encouraged to make the NICU environment either more like the intrauterine or the home environment by placing a light cloth cover over the top of the isolette to decrease the glare of bright lights and closing isolette doors carefully to decrease loud noises. Tactile input to the infant's body with the whole hand, rather than with the fingertips to the extremities, will help to calm the child. Mirrors, pictures of faces, and toys with faces may be placed inside the isolette when parents cannot be present (Figure 6-5). Care must be taken to prevent potential exposure to infection, so it is best to discuss the intervention with the NICU team to ensure infant safety. Water beds or hammock positioning can be used to encourage active movement and for increased vestibular input.[64] The preterm infant has little body fat and therefore has difficulty retaining body heat. Also, the temperature control mechanism is not fully mature. Care must be taken to avoid chilling that will increase caloric needs and energy requirements in these babies. Babies who have been in the NICU may not be able to adjust to the relative dark and quiet of home when discharged. If this is the case, the parents should be encouraged to use a nightlight and a radio until the baby is able to tolerate the decreased sensory input.

Theories of child development continually change. At one time it was believed that infants were without skills or preferences at birth. We now know that infants are born with certain preferences and capabilities. In the visual area, they prefer the human face. Even when the elements of a face are rearranged in a visual presentation, they are not as interesting to the baby as a face (Figure 6-6). In the area of color, the preference is for red and yellow, probably because these colors can be diffused through the mother's abdomen, and can be seen before birth. Sharp contrasts in color and lines, such as stripes or checker-

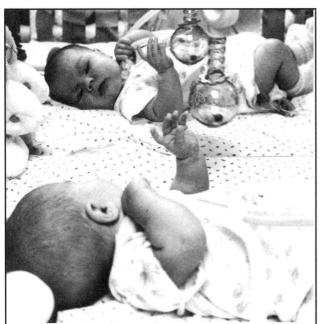

Figure 6-5. Use of a mirror in the crib.

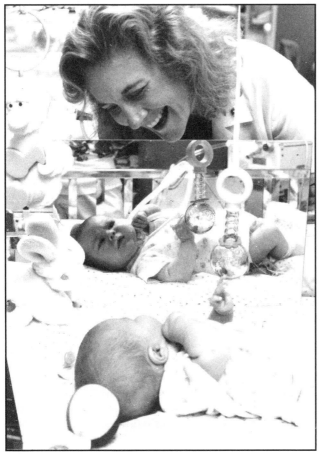

Figure 6-6. Infants prefer faces to objects.

Figure 6-7. Use of sidelying to enhance hands together and hand-to-mouth behavior.

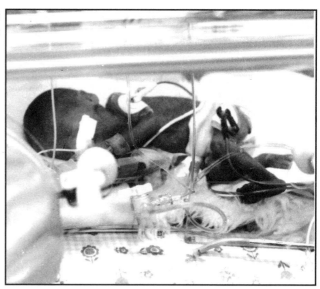

board patterns also are attractive. In the auditory area, babies prefer voices to other sounds and the female voice to the male.[66] Researchers now are trying to determine what types of music are most appealing to the newborn. Neonates prefer sweet to salty and bitter tastes.[67] Certain speeds of rocking are preferred, probably those most similar to the human heart rate. We now appreciate that the newborn comes into the world with certain specific sensory and motor systems for interacting with the environment. Less research has been done regarding the sensory capabilities of the preterm infant because of his fragile medical status. When providing an enriching environment, the therapist must be aware of infant signals being careful not to produce sensory overload. Research alerts us to specific caution on sensory stimulation for infants exposed to drugs as these infants may be hyperirritable and disorganized by visual, auditory, tactile, and vestibular input unless it is carefully modulated and monitored.

Before administering any intervention techniques, the therapist should observe the infant at rest and observe responses when nursing care or other procedures are done. Is the baby able to maintain his heart and respiratory rate? Does the infant startle whenever touched? Are movements smooth or jerky? Is the infant usually positioned on the back or facing only one direction? When are the eyes open? These and other questions should be asked before beginning to handle the baby. Do not begin physical therapy immediately following feeding. The baby will not be able to respond optimally, and the nursing staff will not welcome your services if the baby vomits. The battle to assist the infant toward gaining weight and growing must be attended to by all who interact with the infant.

Whenever possible, encourage sidelying positioning which allows the baby to bring his hands together and toward his mouth for self-calming (Figure 6-7). Sidelying promotes a balance between flexion and extension. Generally, skin-to-skin contact is a positive experience for infants, and bringing the hands together or to the mouth will provide more normal sensory input than putting a pacifier or your finger in the infant's mouth. Skin-to-skin contact can be both calming and alerting. When the baby is no longer on a respirator or is medically stable, visual responses can be enhanced by positioning him upright. As mentioned previously, use of the whole hand rather than the fingertips is preferable and less irritating to the baby. Physiological flexion develops in the last trimester, partially in

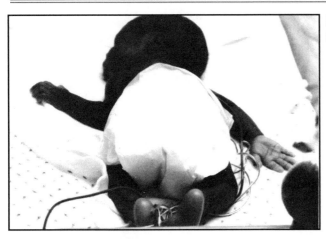

Figure 6-8. Use of a prone position to facilitate flexion.

response to decreased space and partially as an active process in neurological development.[68] Infants who are born before they have a chance to develop physiological flexion or who demonstrate extensor over-activity and are then placed supine for long periods of time may have difficulty developing flexor patterns because the supine position facilitates extension and because it is difficult for these babies to flex against gravity.[69] To help the infant develop normal movement patterns, prone positioning should be attempted if it is not medically contradicted (Figure 6-8). Sidelying with tactile input on the anterior surface of the infant's body also will facilitate flexion. Another method useful in encouraging flexor responses is the use of non-nutritive sucking. Swaddling can be used to provide tactile input and to encourage flexion.

The physical therapist often is asked to evaluate a baby because of difficulty with feeding. Therefore, being well-versed on normal oral motor reflexes, as well as potential pathological patterns that may occur, is important. Although non-nutritive sucking may begin as early as 17 to 18 weeks postconception, nutritive sucking (the skills necessary for successful feeding) do not emerge until approximately 34 weeks gestation, or 6 weeks before full-term delivery. The sucking response can be strengthened by encouraging non-nutritive sucking prior to the time that bottlefeeding is initiated.[70] In addition to waiting to begin feeding until the infant is gestationally ready, it is important to evaluate the strength and rhythm of sucking. Does the infant use coordinated "stripping" or back and forth movements of his tongue, seal the lips adequately to prevent loss of fluid around the nipple, and remember to breathe when feeding?

Before feeding an infant, assess muscle tone and state of alertness. A floppy, sleeping baby or an agitated, screaming baby is not in an optimal state for successful feeding. Facilitatory or inhibitory input, such as fast or slow rocking, can be used to prepare the baby and also to facilitate sucking. Mechanical problems might contribute to feeding difficulties. Certainly, cleft lip or palate presents unique problems and special nipples and bottles have been devised for these babies. Many babies with cleft palates also have small jaws which contribute to further difficulties because of airway obstruction by the tongue. Occasionally the airway obstruction becomes life-threatening and surgical intervention becomes necessary to correct this problem.

The preterm infant who has required mechanical ventilation for a prolonged period of time often has a very high palate because of distortion from the endotracheal tube. If this baby is weak, bringing the tongue up to the palate in order to begin sucking may be difficult. Gentle pressure with the nipple either up against the palate or down on the tongue may assist this infant to initiate feeding.

Figure 6-9. Positioning to encourage sucking.

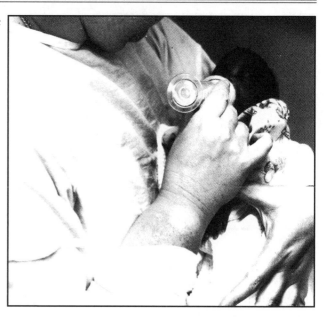

Generally, the principles for feeding any child or adult with feeding difficulties apply to the neonate as well. Avoid neck extension as it opens the airway and can result in aspiration. Jaw control might be necessary for the infant having difficulty with lip closure. Slight traction to elongate the neck may facilitate swallowing. Swaddling or other positioning to encourage flexion will facilitate sucking, which is a flexion activity (Figure 6-9). Rocking can be used to encourage sucking. In a preterm infant who has difficulty remaining awake for an entire feeding, it might be useful to unwrap the baby, hold him slightly away from your body, and use short bursts of periodic moderately fast rocking to increase alertness.

Babies should be watched carefully during the process of feeding (Figure 6-10). It is not uncommon for them to have periods of apnea or bradycardia during feeding.

Subtle changes in color, particularly perioral cyanosis, or just a pale appearance should be noted. There are many causes of these "spells" during feeding, including neurological immaturity and inability to coordinate sucking, swallowing, and breathing. Another cause of feeding bradycardia might be vagal hypersensitivity which may result when feeding tubes are passed down the throat. It is important to inform the medical staff if abnormal feeding patterns persist, because they may be indicative of more complex medical problems such as anemia or generalized infection. Necrotizing enterocolitis is closely associated with prematurity and gastrointestinal feeding so it is important to identify potential contributing feeding issues in intervention with neonates.[71]

There are many different kinds of feeding nipples used in the NICU. Our first inclination is to use the softest nipple with very small babies. Experience has shown that this may not always be the best strategy. Encouraging a stronger sucking pattern with a harder nipple may encourage a more mature pattern to develop and enhance muscle strength in the neck and oral motor areas. The formula may flow rapidly through the softer nipple, making it more difficult for the baby to handle a larger amount of fluid in his mouth, causing choking. Each infant should be evaluated carefully as to the type of nipple which will optimally suit his stage of development and his unique feeding problems.

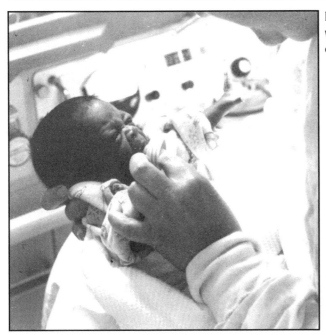

Figure 6-10. Evaluation of sucking, which produced a gag reflex and bradycardia.

Why is it important for the physical therapist to look at feeding problems? The most obvious reason is to address the whole child. Babies in the NICU generally feed every 4 hours. If it takes an hour or more to feed a baby each time, this is comparable to a full-time job for the parent. Difficulty with feeding may interfere with parent-child interaction and may diminish the mother's feelings of self-esteem if she feels that she is unable to successfully nourish her child. In addition to these issues, babies with unexplained feeding difficulties not related to immaturity are at risk for additional neurological abnormalities. Because so much of the newborn neurological examination is not predictive of long-term outcome, feeding is a very important factor in assessing neuromotor functioning. Infants with significant feeding difficulties, even when they do not develop major motor handicaps, are at risk for speech and language abnormalities because the same muscles necessary for successful feeding are used in speech production.[72]

Physical therapists in the NICU should view themselves as teachers and role models for both the staff and the parents. It is imperative to establish in-service education programs for parents and nursing staff and to provide orientation for resident physicians, which includes both practical examples of intervention strategies, as well as the theoretical basis for treatment. In addition, role modeling with proper positioning and handling techniques is essential. If in-service and orientation programs are successful, there will be an increase in referrals as staff members come to recognize the value of, and become comfortable in, requesting physical therapy consultation.

Parents often ask what kinds of toys to purchase for their infants. Care must be taken to not introduce potential sources of infection or safety hazards into the infant environment. As in all other intervention, members of the NICU team should be aware of the intervention plan to create the most effective growth and nourishing environment. Sometimes toys might be counterproductive to the infant environment. When parents and NICU staff understand the general sensory capabilities and the medical stability of the child, they can do a better job of selecting appropriate toys. There is nothing magical about any particular toy that will make babies happier or smarter. Although some toys may help to alert a certain baby, the best thing to use is the human touch, voice, and face. Toys are useful when there are not any caretakers to interact with the baby, but they do not take the place of people. The most expensive toys are not necessarily better than cheaper toys that are well made, safe, and provide interesting sensory experiences. Again, the caution—**when in doubt do nothing**—especially when it comes to toys brought into an NICU environment that might interfere with medical care.

It is not always possible to identify children with neuromuscular abnormalities in the NICU. For this reason, a systematic method of providing periodic follow-up for those children who are at high risk for long-term disabilities should be established. In reviewing criteria for follow-up in numerous NICUs,[73,74] it becomes apparent that similar categories are used. It is not necessary to follow every infant who briefly has been admitted to the NICU. Typical follow-up criteria include:

➤ LBW (this can mean anything from below 2000 to below 1250 g)

➤ Perinatal asphyxia, often determined by Apgar scores

➤ Infants requiring mechanical ventilation (the length of time on a respirator varies)

➤ Intrauterine growth retardation

➤ Neurological abnormality (seizures, abnormal muscle tone, intracranial hemorrhage, congenital or acquired hydrocephalus)

➤ Documented sepsis or meningitis

➤ Congenital anomalies, birth defects, and chromosome abnormalities

➤ Vision and hearing defects

➤ NAS or narcotic withdrawal

➤ Gastrointestinal abnormalities or prolonged feeding difficulties which may lead to failure to thrive

➤ High-risk indicators of potential HIV infection

These criteria generally encompass 40% to 50% of those children admitted to the NICU. Most clinics adjust for prematurity, using the child's due date as an estimation of birth date. There is some variation in how long clinics use this adjustment. If a child is not showing "catch up" by 2 years of age, long-term delays are suspected. Preterm infants, if they are appropriate for gestational age, are not destined to be small. Their ultimate growth is more determined by their genetic complement rather than the size at birth. Growth patterns of preterm infants are different from full-term babies. Often they show very rapid catch up growth with the head growing fastest. The weight catches up next, and finally, height. It is important to reassure parents that this rapid head growth is normal for their child. If the child is properly nourished, growth often reaches the normal growth parameters within the first year of life.

Most major neurological handicaps can be identified within the first year of life with careful attention to quality of movement, as well as to quantity of motor development.[75] Long-term language and cognitive development generally take longer to determine.

Approximately 5% of live births are transferred to tertiary centers for medical management. Of those infants who require such services, approximately 15% have major developmental abnormalities.[76] Although smaller babies are surviving, there have not been significant changes in the percentage of children with developmental disabilities. Therapists working in schools, hospitals, and other clinics mistakenly believe that few infants in NICU settings develop normally. It is difficult to accurately assess whether NICU graduates are at greater risk for problems such as dyslexia and other learning disabilities. Because environmental factors become more significant with increasing age, it is difficult to assess how much of the problem is related to prematurity and how much to other factors.[77] Therefore, it is important that comprehensive neonatal care includes follow-up after NICU and referral to community-based early intervention programs to address the whole family's need for skills and knowledge and assistance in family-centered care.[78,79]

The NICU is an exciting place for the physical therapist to work. Medical professionals and families work as a team to optimize the outcome of high-risk infants. The information presented in this chapter is only a brief introduction for the therapist interested in working in this setting. Previous pediatric experience as well as supervised clinical practice in the NICU is strongly recommended. It is important that any therapist interested in NICU care become familiar with the eight competencies and areas of knowledge base for physical therapy service in the NICU described by Scull and Deitz.[80] Attainment of these competencies in prevention of stress, physical examination, intervention design and modification, intervention implementation, consultation and coordination, research, education, and administration can help the physical therapist develop the expertise to become an integral member of the NICU team.

Case Study #1: Jason

➤ Practice pattern 5C: Impaired Motor Function and Sensory Integrity Associated With Nonprogressive Disorders of the Central Nervous System—Congenital Origin or Acquired in Infancy or Childhood

➤ Medical diagnosis: Cerebral palsy, right hemiparesis

➤ Age: 24 months

History

Jason was the first born of nonidentical twins delivered by Cesarean birth 8 weeks prematurely. His Apgar scores were 7 at 1 minute and 9 at 5 minutes. His birth weight, head circumference, and length were appropriate for gestational age. He did not require any mechanical ventilation at birth. A cranial ultrasound at 3 days of age showed a left-sided germinal matrix hemorrhage with normal sized ventricles. A follow-up ultrasound 1 week later, however, revealed complete reabsorption of the clot and normal ventricular size bilaterally. A Brazelton NBAS initially was performed when Jason was 3 weeks old (35 weeks postconceptional age). At that time, Jason demonstrated few self-calming strategies, such as non-nutritive sucking or hand-to-mouth activities, and his tendon reflexes generally were brisk. Jason's disorganized movement did not support his attempts at self-calming, such as hand to mouth and hand to face. He also had difficulty with positioning while in the NICU due to these diffuse disorganized movements that were extensor dominant. He maintained his head tilted to the right, which placed him at risk for neck muscle tightness. Trunk incurvation was diminished slightly on the right. There was significant ankle clonus bilaterally and he was jittery. He was on caffeine citrate, which was being used to control apnea and bradycardia spells that occurred, particularly during feeding. This medication has been noted to result in some generalized jitteriness and increased muscle tone in infants. Jason's visual focusing was minimal due to his apparent overstimulation in the NICU environment.

Jason was re-evaluated by the physical therapist at 7 weeks of age (39 weeks postconception). At that time, the asymmetry was no longer apparent, but he continued to be difficult to calm and was jittery. Jason and his twin were discharged at 40 days of age on caffeine citrate. Jason did not receive physical therapy services in the NICU, nor were any recommended at discharge, even though there were early, subtle, transient findings of asymmetry and jitteriness. The use of theophylline or caffeine citrate to control apnea and bradycardia spells can result in jitteriness, as well as increased muscle tone, thereby making it difficult to accurately assess the neurological status of these babies. The majority of children who present with a history like Jason's develop normally. However, there have not been comprehensive long-term studies done to evaluate the outcome of therapeutic doses of caffeine.

The twins were seen in follow-up clinic at 4 months of age (2 months corrected gestational age). Jason had decreased strength in his flexor muscles and tended to overuse his extensor muscles, but this was felt to be due to his " prematurity." He continued to be irritable and preferred to hold his head to the right, but his examination was otherwise "normal."

The next visit was scheduled at Jason's 6-month-adjusted chronological age (8 months true chronological age). At this time his mother remarked that Jason was "left handed." She also noted that Jason did not kick his right leg as frequently as his left. His mother remarked that Jason was more difficult to hold than his twin and that he didn't seem to mold to her body as easily. Jason's neurological evaluation was markedly asymmetrical, with a persistent asymmetrical tonic neck reflex to the right, fisting of the right hand with the thumb flexed in the palm, and 5 to 7 beats of ankle clonus on the right. The BSID was administered by the physical therapist at this visit but Jason was age appropriate when adjusted for prematurity.

The abnormal neurological findings were discussed with his parents, and a more complete neurological examination was recommended. Jason was referred for physical therapy intervention in their local community. Neurological abnormalities in children like Jason may not become obvious before 6 to 9 months of age. In some areas of the country, it is becoming more difficult to locate therapy services for "at-risk" infants without documented diagnostic criteria. For this reason, it is important for NICU follow-up clinics to monitory closely such infants and refer them for services as soon as abnormalities become apparent.

Case Study #2: Jill

➤ Practice pattern 5C: Impaired Motor Function and Sensory Integrity Associated With Nonprogressive Disorders of the Central Nervous System—Congenital Origin or Acquired in Infancy or Childhood

➤ Medical diagnosis: Cerebral palsy, spastic quadriparesis, microcephaly, mental retardation, seizure disorder

➤ Age: 7 years

History

Jill was the product of a full-term, uncomplicated pregnancy. She was the first child for her 30-year-old mother. The delivery was very rapid and Apgar scores were 5 at 1 minute and 8 at 5 minutes. There were no initial problems and Jill was placed in the normal newborn nursery. The nurses in the nursery noted some unusual eye movements and occasional stiffening of Jill's extremities when she was 4 hours old and called the staff from the neonatal intensive care nursery. Jill was immediately transferred to the NICU and given a loading dose of phenobarbital. Her seizures continued, and several other anticonvulsant

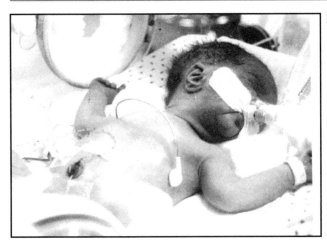

Figure 6-11. Jill on respirator.

medications were added, following an examination by the pediatric neurologist. The increase in medication resulted in respiratory depression, and Jill was placed on a respirator at 12 hours of age (Figure 6-11). The EEG was markedly abnormal at this time. Over the next several days, the seizures gradually subsided, medications were decreased, and Jill was weaned from the respirator. However, Jill had overall decreased responsivity to her environment. Her alertness was poor as well as her orientation to stimuli. She exhibited a general startle response that included whole body extension when stimulated.

Initial physical therapy evaluation at 5 days of age, using the Brazelton NBAS and Dubowitz Scales, revealed a sleepy child with generalized hypotonicity, absent suck, and diminished gag response. Over the next week, the feeding pattern improved and Jill was sent home bottlefeeding. Feeding techniques recommended by the physical therapist to the parents and nursing staff included rapid rocking prior to and during feeding for vestibular input, perioral stroking, positioning in midline with slight neck flexion, using a pacifier between feeding to strengthen the suck, and positioning upright as possible to improve alertness.

The physical therapist met with the parents, the pediatric neurologist, and the neonatalogist to discuss long-term prognosis and program planning. A brain stem auditory evoked (BAER) test was administered because of neonatal seizures, and the response time was slightly delayed. An eye exam was recommended at 2 months of age because Jill required assisted ventilation.

Prior to discharge, the parents were instructed in positioning and handling techniques. Jill initially presented as a child with low muscle tone, but with potential for increased tone with time, which mandated close monitoring of her home program. The parents were given a handout discussing the use of toys to enhance visual and auditory skills. Jill's stay in the NICU was short, but she will need long-term programming. It is extremely important for the physical therapists working in the NICU to maintain good communication with community agencies providing therapy services. Because of her history of prolonged seizures and early feeding problems, Jill was referred for home-based physical therapy services when she was discharged from the hospital.

When seen initially in follow-up clinic at 4 months of age, Jill was a very irritable child, with generalized increased muscle tone. The parents reported that Jill was difficult to hold because of her strong extensor pattern. Her extensor tone with a possible tongue thrust also made sucking on a bottle or on her pacifier frustrating for Jill and her parents. Jill also tended to keep her hands fisted with poor hands to face and hands to midline movements. Overall, she had decreased active movement in her head, trunk, and extremities. Visually, Jill's orientation and ability to focus was poor. At this visit, a decrease in her head growth was noted because of the significant neonatal insult. The eye exam and a repeat of the BAER were normal. The need for continued therapy services as well as future educational needs were discussed, and the parents were referred to the local agency for family support services.

Case Study #3: Taylor

➤ Practice pattern 5C: Impaired Motor Function and Sensory Integrity Associated With Nonprogressive Disorders of the Central Nervous System—Congenital Origin or Acquired in Infancy or Childhood
➤ Medical diagnosis: Myelomeningocele, repaired L1-2
➤ Age: 4 years

History

Taylor was a child born at full term who was delivered by cesarean section because of fetal distress and breech presentation. A large lumbar myelomeningocele was noted immediately at birth and he was transferred to the NICU. The neurosurgeon, after examining the infant, explained to the parents the long-term implications of myelomeningocele, including paralysis, potential mental retardation, hydrocephalus, bowel and bladder dysfunction, and the need for long-term care and many surgical procedures. They were given the option of an immediate operation, and they chose to have primary closure of the myelomeningocele.

Taylor was examined by the physical therapist prior to the surgery. It was noted that he had 90 degrees hip flexion contractures, and knee flexion was limited to 60 degrees. He also had severe equinovarus deformities of both feet. There was no response to sensory input of touch, pressure, or pin prick on either lower extremity.

Following primary closure of the myelomeningocele, the physical therapist met with the parents to discuss the long-term rehabilitation goals for Taylor, including the good potential for assisted ambulation. The parents were instructed in range of motion techniques and advised regarding skin precautions because of the sensory loss. Emphasis was placed on developing good head and trunk control, upper extremity skills, maintaining lower extremity mobility, and cognitive skills. They were given a list of books on normal development that were available in the hospital parent library. They were encouraged to be aware of the positive aspects of Taylor's development and not concentrate solely on his disability. Referral was made, with their permission, to the local spina bifida association, which has an excellent parent-to-parent support network. Referral also was made to state services for child with disabilities, to assist with some of the financial burden associated with having a child with a long-term disability requiring continuing medical and surgical intervention, as well as orthotic and transport equipment.

Three days following primary closure of the myelomeningocele, a bulging fontanelle was noted. Cranial ultrasound revealed enlarged ventricles, and a ventricular-peritoneal shunting was performed on day 5. Taylor continued to have severe apnea spells and was placed on a respirator. The neurosurgeon recommended an EEG to rule out seizures, and fortunately the EEG essentially was normal. An Arnold-Chiari malformation was suspected as causing compression of the brain stem and the resultant apnea spells. At 2 weeks of age, a surgical decompression of the posterior fossa was performed. The apnea

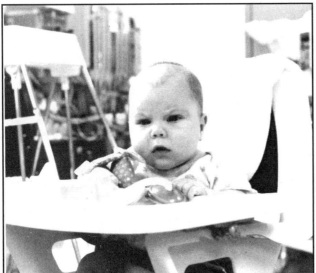

Figure 6-12. Four-month-old child in NICU experiences normal upright positioning.

improved and the respirator was discontinued, but Taylor continued to have apnea several times a day requiring stimulation to resume breathing.

Because of the medical concerns, little attention was paid to rehabilitation services. However, the foot deformities were being treated with serial casting by the orthopedic surgeon. During this time the physical therapist performed passive range of motion to the lower extremities of the child and instructed both parents and the nursing staff on range of motion and prone positioning to reduce hip flexion contractures. On the Infant Neurobehavioral Assessment Battery (INFANIB), Taylor had an overall score that was in the abnormal range due to his hypotonic lower extremities. Suggestions for toys were given to the family to encourage them to look at Taylor's need for normal sensory input in the relatively normal hospital environment.

The apnea spells continued and Taylor remained in the NICU for 4 months. Every attempt was made to provide a variety of sensory motor experiences appropriate for his age that would not compromise his medical status (Figure 6-12). Additionally, infant massage was taught to the parents and the nurses to increase tactile input to Taylor. A specialized water mattress was used with Taylor to provide vestibular input that may have been lacking because of decreased movement in utero as well as in the external environment. Discharge plans were eventually made, with a cardiorespiratory monitor for home use. The need for continuing range of motion activities and observing Taylor's skin integrity was reviewed with the parents. He was referred to a physical therapist for home services once a week and to the myelomeningocele clinic at the local children's orthopedic hospital outpatient department. Because so many community services were available to this family, Taylor was not scheduled to return to the NICU follow-up clinic.

Case Study #4: Ashley

➤ Practice pattern 5B: Impaired Neuromotor Development
➤ Medical diagnosis: Down syndrome
➤ Age: 15 months

Figure 6-13. Facilitating hand-to-mouth.

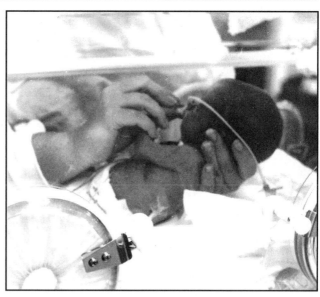

History

Ashley was the first child born to a 26-year-old woman. The pregnancy was uncomplicated, and Ashley was born at full-term. Characteristics of Down syndrome were noted in the baby at the time of delivery. She was transferred to the NICU because of a heart murmur. Cardiac echogram revealed a rather large ventricular septal defect. On further examination, an esophageal atresia was noted. Primary repair of the esophageal atresia was not possible, and a gastrostomy was performed. No oral feedings were permitted. However, Ashley had a fair suck on a NUK pacifier (Gerber, Parsippany, NJ), and this was encouraged.

Activities suggested to Ashley's parents included positioning in various ways: upright with as little support as necessary to enhance head and trunk control, prone to encourage head control and upper extremity weight bearing, and sidelying to encourage hands together and hand-to-mouth activities (Figure 6-13). There is no contraindication to prone positioning in a child with a gastrostomy. After the first week postoperatively, these children can be positioned safely in prone. Most children do not require any special devices for prone positioning, but for those that do, a small cut-out in a foam rubber block or wedge to accommodate the tube is sufficient. The earlier these children are placed in prone positioning, the easier it is for them, their parents, and the nursing staff. Other suggestions given to Ashley's parents included wrist rattlers and bells on her hands and feet to encourage movement, water toys to encourage movement against the resistance of water, holding her while in a rocking chair, use of a baby swing for vestibular input, and olfactory input with pleasant odors (cinnamon, cherry) during non-nutritive sucking.

Ashley was discharged from the hospital at 6 weeks of age. Because of concerns regarding medical complications, the family refused to become involved with an early intervention program. They were unwilling to follow a program of activities suggested to enhance motor development. They had many toys for Ashley, but these were used generally to provide visual and auditory stimulation and not movement.

At 6 months of age, the esophageal atresia was repaired. At 8 months of age, the heart defect was surgically corrected. At 10 months of age, the family consented to become involved with an early intervention program. When Ashley finally was evaluated by the physical therapist, she was 10 months of age and very hypotonic even for a child with Down syndrome. She was prop-sitting momentarily, had moderate head lag when pulled to sit, and would bear minimal weight on her legs. Ashley had many ear infections and finally received pressure equalizing tubes at 12 months of age. She has a mild conductive hearing loss.

In children like Ashley, with complex medical problems, the family may not be willing or able to participate even in non-stressful therapeutic activities. All of their energy is concentrated on the child's acute medical needs. Experience has shown that such families will eventually recognize the need for physical therapy services, as the child's delay becomes more apparent and the child grows larger as well as more difficult to handle. It is important to continue to reinforce the need for physical therapy services for the child. Often the best way to do this is for the primary physician or a specialist (cardiologist) to suggest programming to the family, because they will continue to see these children on a regular basis. The physical therapist in the NICU as well as those in the community constantly must work to keep physicians informed regarding the need for developmental physical therapy services and their availability.

Case Study #5: John

➤ Practice pattern 5B: Impaired Neuromotor Development
➤ Medical diagnosis: Attention deficit hyperactivity disorder, developmental coordination disorder
➤ Age: 5 years

History

John was born at 36 weeks gestational age to a 34-year-old mother. His Apgar scores were 8 at 1 minute and 10 at 5 minutes. He spent a short time in the NICU before being discharged to home but with no major medical problems noted at the time of birth or after birth. Many children who are later diagnosed with DCD have a history of prematurity but no abnormal neurological signs as infants. He was not referred for early intervention services at the time of discharge from the NICU.

Glossary

A and B SPELLS:
> Apnea-absence of respiration for 20 seconds;
> Bradycardia-heart rate less than 90 per minute, accompanied by cyanosis.

AGA: Appropriately grown for gestational age.

ANOXIA: Absence of oxygen.

ASPHYXIA: A condition in which there is a deficiency of oxygen and an increase in carbon dioxide in the blood and tissues. Perinatal asphyxia is lack of oxygen just prior to, during, or shortly after birth.

ASPIRATION: Breathing a foreign substance such as meconium, formula, or stomach contents into the lungs; may cause aspiration pneumonia.

ATELECTASIS: Collapse of the air sacks in the lungs.

BETAMETHASONE: A steroid given to a mother before a threatened preterm birth to help the baby's lungs mature.

BILIRUBIN: A yellowish substance produced when red blood cells break down; may cause jaundice, and in large amounts, kernicterus, with resultant basal ganglia damage and possible athetoid type cerebral palsy.

BLOOD GAS: A sample of blood which measures how much oxygen, carbon dioxide, and acid it contains; ABG—arterial blood gas; VBC—venous blood gas.

BRAIN STEM AUDITORY EVOKED RESPONSE TEST (BAER): A method for early detection of hearing loss in neonates in which brain wave response to a variety of sound levels is assessed.

BRONCHOPULMONARY DYSPLASIA (BPD): Iatrogenic condition, characterized by changes and alterations of the normal development of the air passages of the lungs and lung tissues generally following prolonged treatment with a respirator.

CHALASIA: Relaxation or immaturity of the sphincter between the esophagus and the stomach resulting in vomiting; also may be referred to as gastroesophageal reflux (GER).

CONTINUOUS POSITIVE AIRWAY PRESSURE (CPAP): The constant flow of air being blown into the lungs by a respirator.

DISSEMINATED INTRAVASCULAR COAGULATION (DIC): A condition in which the platelets and other clotting factors of the blood are consumed because of infection, hypoxia, acidosis, or other diseases or injuries; this results in excessive bleeding and often requires transfusions.

DUCTUS ARTERIOSUS: A fetal blood vessel extending from the pulmonary artery to the aorta; PDA—patent ductus arteriosus; a condition in which this vessel fails to close after birth which results in poor oxygenation and generally requires either medical or surgical intervention for closure.

ECLAMPSIA: Toxemia of pregnancy accompanied by high blood pressure, albuminuria, oliguria, tonic and clonic convulsions, and coma; may occur before, during, or after childbirth.

ENDOTRACHEAL INTUBATION: Passage of a small plastic tube through the trachea, past the vocal cords, and into the bronchial tree for assisted ventilation.

ERYTHROBLASTOSIS FETALIS: Blood type incompatibility between the mother and baby, causing maternal antibodies to attack neonatal blood cells, and causing severe anemia and jaundice in the newborn.

GAVAGE FEEDING: Feedings given through a tube passed through the nose or mouth and into the stomach in babies who are too immature to bottlefeed, or who are otherwise unable to feed orally.

HUMAN IMMUNODEFICIENCY VIRUS (HIV) INFECTION: Systemic fatal infection which severely compromises the immune system and causes neurological and developmental deficits; presents a widely variant clinical picture

HYALINE MEMBRANE DISEASE (HMD): Respiratory disease that affects preterm babies; it is caused by a lack of surfactant, a substance that prevents collapse of the alveoli.

HYPERALIMENTATION: Intervenous administration of glucose, protein, minerals, and vitamins; used when oral feedings cannot be initiated; this is also called total parenteral nutrition (TPN).

INDOMETHACIN: A drug used to close the patent ductus arteriosus.

INFANT OF A DIABETIC MOTHER (IDM): These babies are often LGA (large for gestational age) and are at high risk for both prenatal and postnatal complications.

LOADING DOSE: Sufficient amount of medication to obtain a therapeutic blood level.

LS RATIO: A ratio between two factors in surfactant (lecithin and sphingomyelin) in the amniotic fluid; this ratio is used as an indicator of lung maturity in the fetus.

MATERNAL SUBSTANCE ABUSE: Use of potentially teratogenic substances during pregnancy which may have adverse effect on the fetus; includes drugs such as heroin, cocaine, alcohol, and cigarettes.

MECONIUM: A greenish-black tarry material present in the fetal intestine before birth, and usually passed in the first few days after birth; this may be passed in utero if the baby is in distress before birth; aspiration of meconium results in asphyxia and severe respiratory complications.

NECROTIZING ENTEROCOLITIS (NEC): A condition in which there is diffuse or patchy necrosis of the mucosa or submucosa of the small or large bowel, probably due to ischemia and prematurity.

NEONATAL ABSTINENCE SYNDROME: Neurobehavioral sequelae identified in infants prenatally exposed to narcotic drugs.

NEONATE: A baby less than 4 weeks of age.

NON-NUTRITIVE SUCKING: Sucking on finger or pacifier, purpose is not for oral intake.

OCCIPITAL FRONTAL CIRCUMFERENCE (OFC): Head size measurement.

OLIGOHYDRAMNIOS: A greatly reduced amount of amniotic fluid.

$PaCO_2$: Partial pressure of carbon dioxide in arterial blood.

PaO_2: Partial pressure of oxygen in arterial blood.

PAVULON: A drug which acts on the myoneural junction and produces temporary paralysis; often used to prevent a baby from "fighting" the respirator.

PERIODIC BREATHING: Breathing interrupted by pauses of 10 or more seconds; common in preterm babies.

PERSISTENT FETAL CIRCULATION (PFC): A condition in which the blood continues to flow through the ductus arteriosus and bypass the lungs; this usually occurs in term and post-term infants following hypoxia.

PLACENTA ABRUPTIO: Premature separation of the placenta from the uterus with resultant bleeding and neonatal asphyxia.

PLACENTA PREVIA: A condition in which the placenta is abnormally positioned over the cervix, thereby preventing a normal vaginal delivery.

PNEUMOGRAM: Monitoring a baby's heart rate and respiratory patterns for several hours to detect any abnormalities either during waking or sleeping.

POLYCYTHEMIA: Abnormally high number of red blood cells, causing "sluggish" circulation; this is also called hyperviscosity.

POLYHYDRAMNIOS: Excessive amount of amniotic fluid.

POSITIVE END EXPIRATORY PRESSURE (PEEP): A constant amount of pressure exerted by the respirator to keep the lungs expanded.

PREMATURE RUPTURE OF MEMBRANES (PROM): The breaking of the membrane surrounding the fetus before the beginning of labor; this results in an increased possibility of infection.

RESPIRATORY DISTRESS SYNDROME (RDS): Terminology used interchangeably with hyaline membrane disease.

RETINOPATHY OF PREMATURITY (ROP): A condition of the eyes related to prematurity, oxygen concentration, and possibly other factors, affecting the blood vessels of the eyes that can result in blindness; previously called retrolental fibroplasia (RLF).

SEPSIS: Generalized infection characterized by proliferation of bacteria in the bloodstream, due to the fact the newborn has little capacity to localize or encapsulate infections.

SEPTAL DEFECTS: Congenital defects in the heart muscle; VSD—ventricular septal defect is an opening between the right and left ventricles; ASD—atrial septal defect is between the right and left atria; these defects generally require surgical repair.

SEXUALLY TRANSMITTED DISEASES: Infection passed prenatally or perinatally to the infant whose mother is infected; examples include syphilis, herpes, gonorrhea.

SMALL FOR GESTATIONAL AGE (SGA): Newborn whose growth parameters (weight, length, and head circumference) are less than the fifth percentile for gestational age; also called intrauterine growth retardation (IUGR).

SURFACTANT: A substance manufactured by the lungs to prevent alveolar collapse.

THEOPHYLLINE: A stimulant drug used in the treatment of apnea; caffeine citrate is also used for this purpose.

TOCOLYTIC DRUGS: Drugs used to stop premature labor (eg, ritodrine).

TORCH TITERS: A blood test to determine the presence of certain viral agents including toxoplasmosis, rubella, cytomegalovirus (CMV), and herpes.

TRANSCUTANEOUS MONITOR (TCM): A device to monitor oxygen concentration in the blood by means of a skin electrode.

TRANSIENT TACHYPNEA NEONATORUM (TTN): Rapid respiratory rate generally seen in term infants born by cesarean or with precipitous deliveries, related to poorly absorbed lung fluid; also called wet lung.

VERNIX: White, fatty substance that protects the fetus skin in utero.

References

1. Anderson KN. *Mosby's Medical, Nursing, and Allied Health Dictionary*. 5th ed. St. Louis, Mo: Mosby-Year Book; 1998.
2. Lawson K, Daum C, Turkewitz G. Environmental characteristics of a neonatal intensive care unit. *Child Dev.* 1977; 48:1633-1639.
3. Bell PL. Adolescent mothers' preconceptions of the neonatal intensive care unit environment. *Journal of Perinatal and Neonatal Nursing.* 1997;11:77-85.
4. Harrison H. *The Premature Baby Book.* New York, NY: St. Martin's Press; 1983.
5. Klaus MH, Fanaroff AA. *Care of the High Risk Neonate.* Philadelphia, Pa: WB Saunders Company; 1973.
6. Korones SB. *High Risk Newborn Infants.* 2nd ed. St. Louis, Mo: CV Mosby; 1976.
7. Thompson M, Price P, Stahle D. Nutrition services in neonatal intensive care: a national survey. *J American Dietetic Association.* 1994;94:440-442.

8. Philip AGS. *Neonate Sepsis and Meningitis*. Boston, Mass: GK Hall; 1985.

9. Johnson SH. *High Risk Parenting: Nursing Assessment and Strategies for the Family at Risk*. Philadelphia, Pa: JB Lippincott; 1979.

10. Frank DA, Augustyn M, Stuart DG. Review: prenatal exposure to cocaine does not independently affect physical growth, cognition, or language skills. *Evid Based Ment Health*. 2001;4:121.

11. Neuspiel DR, Hamel SC. Cocaine and infant behavior. *Developmental and Behavioral Pediatrics*. 1991;12:55-64.

12. Bryson YJ. *Perinatal Acquired Immunodeficiency Disease. Report of the 100th Ross Conference in Pediatric Research*. Columbus, Ohio: Ross Laboratories; 1991.

13. Lewis M, Wilson CD. Infant development in lower class American families. *Hum Dev*. 1972; 15:112-127.

14. Newberger CM. The cognitive structure of parenthood: designing a descriptive measure. *New Directions for Child Dev*. 1980;7:45-67.

15. Philip AGS. *Neonate Sepsis and Meningitis*. Boston, Mass: GK Hall Company; 1985.

16. Connor E, McSherry G, Yogev R. Antiviral treatment of pediatric HIV infection. In: Yogev, Connor, eds. *HIV Infection in Infants and Children*. St. Louis, Mo: Mosby-Year Book; 1992:505-532.

17. Belman AL. AIDS and pediatric neurology. *Neurologic Clinics*. 1990;8:571-603.

18. Grosz J, Hopkins K. Family circumstances affecting caregivers and brothers and sisters. In: Crocker AC, Cohen HJ, Kastner TA, eds. *HIV Infection and Developmental Disabilities*. Baltimore, Md: Paul H. Brookes; 1992:43-52.

19. Cohen HJ, Diamond GW. Developmental assessment of children with HIV infection. In: Crocker AC, Cohen HJ, Kastner TA, eds. *HIV Infection and Developmental Disabilities*. Baltimore, Md: Paul H. Brookes; 1992:53-62.

20. Harris MH. Habilitative and rehabilitative needs of children with HIV infection. In: Crocker AC, Cohen HJ, Kastner TA, eds. *HIV Infection and Developmental Disabilities*. Baltimore, Md: Paul H. Brookes; 1992:85-94.

21. Cowett RM, Schwartz R. The infant of the diabetic mother. *Pediatr Clin North Am*. 1982: 29:1213-1231.

22. Morris SE. *The Normal Acquisition of Oral Feeding Skills: Implications for Assessment and Treatment*. New York, NY: Therapeutic Media Inc; 1982.

23. Babson S, Kongos, J. Preschool intelligence of undersized term infants. *Am J Dis Child*. 1969; 117:553-169.

24. Fitzhardinge PM, Steven EM. Small for date infants: neurological and intellectual sequelae. *Pediatr*. 1972;50:50.

25. Apgar V, Beck J. *Is My Baby All Right*. New York, NY: Trident Press; 1973.

26. Zuckerman B, Frank DA, Hingson R, et al. Effects of maternal marijuana and cocaine use on fetal growth. *N Engl J Med*. 1989;320:762-768.

27. Gluck L. *Intrauterine Asphyxia and the Developing Fetal Brain*. Chicago, Ill: Year Book Medical; 1977.

28. American Physical Therapy Association. *Guide to Physical Therapist Practice*. Alexandria, Va: Author; 1998.

29. Moore KL. *The Developing Human*. 2nd ed. Philadelphia, Pa: WB Saunders; 1977.

30. Dubowitz LM, Dubowitz V. Clinical assessment of gestational age in the newborn infant. *J Pediatr*. 1970:77;1-10.

31. Barnard KE. The effect of stimulation on the sleep behavior of the premature infant. *Commun News Res*. 1973:6;12-40.

32. Dreyfus-Brisac C. Organization of sleep in prematures: implications for caregiving. In: Lewis M, Rosenblum LA, eds. *The Effect of the Infant on Its Caregivers*. New York, NY: John Wiley; 1974.

33. Ludington-Hoe S. *Parents Guide to Infant Stimulation*. Los Angeles, Calif: Infant Stimulation Education; 1983.

34. Blackburn S. Fostering behavioral development of high risk infants. *J Obstr Gyn Nurs.* 1983;12(Suppl):76-86.

35. Long JG, Lucey JR, Philip AG. Noise and hypoxia in the ICU. *Pediatr.* 1981;65:143-145.

36. Martin RJ, et al. Effect of supine and prone position on arterial oxygen tension in the preterm infant. *Pediatr.* 1979;63:528.

37. Korner AF, Kraemer HC, Haffner ME, Cosper LM. Effects of waterbed floatation on premature infants: a pilot study. *Pediatr.* 1975;56:361-367.

38. Korner AF, Schneider P, Forrest T. Effects of vestibular proprioceptive stimulation on the neurobehavioral development of preterm infants: a pilot study. *Neuropediatr.* 1983;14:170-175.

39. Orgill AA, Astbury J, Bajuk B, Yu VY. Early development of infants 1000 grams or less at birth. *Arch Dis Child.* 1982; 57:823-827.

40. Scarr-Salapatek S, Williams ML. The effects of early stimulation on low birth weight infants. *Child Dev.* 1973; 44:94-101.

41. VandenBerg K. Revising the traditional model: an individualized approach to developmental interventions in the intensive care nursery neonatal network. *Journal of Neonatal Nursing.* 1985;3.

42. Clark D, Ensher G, LeFever J. From newborn nursery to public school: comprehensive services for high risk infants. Presented at: Contemporary Issues in High Risk Infant Follow-Up; October, 1982; Madison, Wisc.

43. Kitchen WH, Ryan MM, Richards A, et al. A longitudinal study of very low birth weight infants: an overview of performance at 8 years of age. *Dev Med and Child Neurol.* 1980;22:172-198.

44. Weiner G. The relationship of birth weight and length of gestation to intellectual development at ages 8-10. *J Pediatr.* 1970;76:694.

45. Buehler D, Als H, Duffy FH, McAnulty GB, Liederman J. Effectiveness of individualized developmental care for low-risk preterm infants: behavioral and electrophysiologic evidence. *Pediatrics.* 1995;96:923-933.

46. McGrath J. Developmentally supportive caregiving and technology in the NICU. *Journal of Perinatal and Neonatal Nursing.* 2000;14:78-90.

47. Als H, Lawhon G, Duffy FH, et al. Individualized developmental care for the VLB preterm infant: medical and neurofunctional effects. *JAMA.* 1994;272:853-864.

48. Daksha P, Zdzislaw HP, Merwyn RN, Robert S. Effect of a statewide neonatal resuscitation training program on APGAR scores among high-risk neonates in Illinois. *Pediatrics.* 2001;107:648-656.

49. Casey BM, McIntire DD, Leveno KJ. The continuing value of the APGAR score for the assessment of newborn infants. *N Engl J Med.* 2001;344:519-520.

50. Als H, Lester BM, Brazelton TB. Dynamics of the behavioral organization of the premature infant: a theoretical perspective. In: Field T, ed. *Infants Born at Risk.* New York, NY: Spectrum; 1979.

51. Amiel-Tison C, Grenier A. *Neurological Evaluation of the Newborn and the Infant.* New York, NY: Mason Publications; 1983.

52. Brazelton TB. Neonatal behavioral assessment scale. *Clinics in Developmental Medicine.* 1973; 50.

53. Korner AF, Thom A, Forrest T. Neurobehavioral maturity assessment for preterm infants (NB-MAP). Presented at: Sensori-Motor Integration seminar; July 1985; San Diego, Calif.

54. O'Doherty N. Neurological examination of the newborn. In: Drillion CM, Drummond MB, eds. *Neurodevelopmental Problems in Early Childhood.* Oxford, England: Blackwell Scientific; 1977.

55. Prechtl H, Beintema D. The neurological examination of the full term newborn infant. *Clinics in Developmental Medicine.* 1964;12.

56. Freedman DG. Ethnic differences in babies. *Hum Nature*. 1979;Jan.

57. Als H, Lester BM, Tronick EC, Brazelton TB. Towards a research instrument for the assessment of preterm infants' behavior (APIB). In: Fitzgerald HE, Lester BM, Yogman MW, eds. *Theory and Research in Behavioral Pediatrics*. Vol 1. New York, NY: Plenum; 1982:85-132.

58. Brazelton TB. Neonatal behavioral assessment scale. 2nd ed. *Clinics in Developmental Medicine*. 1984;88.

59. Piper MC, Pinnell LE, Darrah K, Byrne PJ, Watt MJ. Construction and validation of the Alberta Infant Motor Scales (AIMS). *Can J Pub Health*. 1992;83:46-50.

60. Campbell SK, Kolobe THA, Osten ET, et al. Development of the test of infant motor performance. *Phys Med Rehabil Clin North Am*. 1993;4:541-550.

61. Chandler LS, Andrew MS, Swanson MW. *Movement Assessment of Infants: A Manual*. Rolling Bay, Wash: Child Development and Mental Retardation Center; 1980.

62. Bayley N. *Bayley Scales of Infant Development*. 2nd ed. San Antonio, Tex: The Psychological Corporation; 1993.

63. Folio R, Fewell R. *Peabody Developmental Motor Scales*. 2nd ed. Austin, Tex: Pro-Ed Publishing; 2000.

64. Keller A, Arbel N, Merlob P, Davison S. Neurobehavioral and autonomic effects of hammock positioning in infants with very low birthweight. *Pediatric Physical Therapy*. 2003;1:3-7.

65. Mueller CR. Multidisciplinary research of multimodal stimulation of infants born premature: an integrated review of the literature. *Matern Child Nursing J*. 1999:24:18-31.

66. Bower TGR. *A Primer of Infant Development*. San Francisco, Calif: WH Freeman and Co; 1977.

67. McCall R. *Infants: The New Knowledge*. Cambridge, Mass: Harvard University Press; 1979.

68. Nilsson L. *A Child is Born*. New York, NY: Dell Publishing; 1966.

69. Georgieff MK. Abnormal shoulder girdle muscle tone in infants born premature during their first 18 months of life. *Pediatrics*. 1986;77:664-669.

70. Measil CP, Anderson GC. Non-nutritive sucking during tube feedings: effect upon clinical course in premature infants. *J Obst Gynec Neonatal Nurs*. 1979;8:265-272.

71. Kamitsuka MD, Horton MK, Williams M. The incidence of necrotizing entercolitis after introducing standardized feeding schedules for infants between 1250 and 2500 grams and less than 35 weeks gestation. *Pediatrics*. 2000;105:379-392.

72. Illingworth R. Sucking and swallowing difficulties in infancy: diagnostic problems of dysphagia. *Arch Dis Child*. 1969;44:238.

73. Wisconsin Association for Perinatal Care. *Contemporary Issues in High Risk Infant Follow-up*. Madison, Wisc: Author; 1985.

74. Division of Neonatal/Perinatal Medicine and the Office of Continuing Education-School of Medicine, University of California, San Diego. *Tomorrow: A Follow-Up On Perinatal Care*. San Diego, Calif; 1980.

75. Prechtl HFR, Einspieler C, Cioni G, Bos A, Ferrari F, Sontheimer D. An early marker for neurological deficits after perinatal brain lesions. *Lancet*. 1997;339:1361-1364.

76. Cohen SE, Sigman M, Parmelee AH, Beckwith L. Perinatal risk and developmental outcome in preterm infants. *Seminars in Perinatology*. 1982;6:334-339.

77. Hunt JV, Tooley WH, Harvin D. Learning disabilities in children with birthweights 1500 grams or less. *Seminars in Perinatology*. 1982;6:280-287.

78. Grunwald P. Family-centered care in the NICU: from vision to reality. *Exceptional Parent*. 1997; 27:58-59.

79. McNab T, Blackman JA. Medical complications of the critically ill newborn: a review for early intervention professionals. *Topics in Early Childhood Special Education*. 1998;18:197-198.

80. Scull S, Deitz J. Competencies for the physical therapist in the NICU. *Ped Physical Therapy*. 1989;1:11-14.

Suggested Reading

Banus BS. *The Developmental Therapist*. New York, NY: Charles Slack Publishing; 1971.

Bly L. *The Components of Normal Movement During the First Year of Life and Abnormal Development*. Chicago, Ill: Neuro Dev Treatment Assoc; 1983.

Bobath B. The very early treatment of cerebral palsy. *Develop Med Child Neurol*. 1967;9:171-190.

Brown CC. Infants at risk: assessment and intervention: an update for health care professional and parents. *Pediatric Round Table Series*. No. 5. Calverton, NY: Johnson and Johnson Pediatrics; 1981.

Connor FP, Williamson GG, Siepp JM. *Program Guide for Infants with Neuromotor and Other Developmental Disabilities*. New York, NY: Teachers' College Press; 1978.

Crocker AC, Cohen HJ, Kastner A. *HIV Infection and Developmental Disabilities*. Baltimore, Md: Paul H. Brookes Publishing; 1991.

Dickson JM. A model for physical therapy in the neonatal intensive care nursery. *Phys Ther*. 1981; 61:45-48.

Drillien CM, Drummond MB, eds. *Neurodevelopmental Problems in Early Childhood: Assessment and Management*. Oxford, England: Blackwell Scientific Publications; 1977.

Egan DF, Illingworth RS, MacKeith RC. Developmental screening: 0-5 years. *Clinics in Developmental Medicine*. 1969;30.

Erickson M. *Assessment and Management of Developmental Changes in Children*. St. Louis, Mo: CV Mosby; 1976.

Espenschade AS, Eckert HM. *Motor Development*. Columbus, Ohio: Charles E. Merrill Publishing; 1967.

Finnie NR. *Handling the Young Cerebral Palsy Child at Home*. 2nd ed. New York, NY: E.P. Dutton; 1975.

Gabel S, Erickson MT. *Child Development and Developmental Disabilities*. Boston, Mass: Little Brown; 1980.

Holle B. *Motor Development in Children*. New York, NY: JB Lippincott; 1977.

Holt K, ed. Movement and child development. *Clinics in Developmental Medicine*. 1975;55.

Illingworth RS. *The Development of the Infant and Young Child: Normal and Abnormal*. 4th ed. Edinburgh: ES Livingstone; 1971.

Illingworth RS. *The Normal Child: Some Problems of the Early Years and Their Treatment*. Edinburgh: Churchill Livingstone; 1983.

Kaback MM. *Genetic Issues in Pediatric and Obstetric Practice*. Chicago, Ill: Yearbook Medical Publications; 1981.

Klaus MH, Kennell JH. *Parent-Infant Bonding*. St. Louis, Mo: CV Mosby; 1983.

Lewis M, Taft LT. *Developmental Disabilities: Theory Assessment and Intervention*. New York, NY: SP Medical and Scientific Books; 1982.

Lowrey GH. *Growth and Development of Children*. Chicago, Ill: Medical Publishers; 1978.

Paine RS, Oppe TE. *Neurological Examination of Children*. London: Wm Heineman Medical Books; 1966.

Papile L, Burstein J, Burstein R, Koffler H. Incidence and evaluation of subependymal and intra-ventricular hemorrhage: a study of infants with birth weightless than 1500 grams. *J Pediatr*. 1978;92:529.

Ramey CT, Trohanis PL. *Finding and Educating High Risk Handicapped Infants*. Baltimore, Md: University Park Press; 1982.

Van Blankenstein M, Welberger UR, LeHaas JA. *The Development of the Infant*. London, England: Wm Heineman Medical Books; 1978.

Volpe JJ. Perinatal hypoxic ischemic brain injury. *Pediatr Clin North Am*. 1976;23:383.

Wilhelm JJ. The neurologically suspect neonate. In: Campbell SK, ed. *Pediatric Neurologic Physical Therapy*. New York, NY: Churchill Livingstone; 1984.

Wright JM. Fetal alcohol syndrome: the social work connection. *Health and Soc Work*. 1981;6:5-10.

CHAPTER 7

Sensory Considerations in Therapeutic Interventions

David D. Chapman, PhD, PT
Rebecca E. Porter, PhD, PT

Studies suggest that learned movements can be performed in the absence of sensory input.[1,2] Sensory input and feedback are essential, however, during learning or relearning motor skills. Many children with developmental disabilities face the challenge of learning and performing movements with diminished or discrepant sensory information. The multitude of neuroanatomical pathways communicating afferent information to the motor control centers of the central nervous system (CNS) supports the critical nature of sensory input. Therefore, therapists rely on theoretical models such as dynamic systems theory that enable us to examine and evaluate multiple factors including sensory processes, that influence how children learn to move.

The sensory systems provide a primary media through which therapists can influence the motor behavior of a child with a developmental disability. Our touch, voice, and way of moving a child provide the CNS with a multitude of sensory data to be received, processed, and acted on. The effectiveness of our handling techniques depends, in part, on our orchestration of the sensory information reaching the child's CNS. Our intervention techniques are based on the manipulation of sensory input through one or more sensory systems.

The information in this chapter addresses the broad general category of developmental disabilities. An assumption has been made that the movement problems of children are of central origin and that mechanics of processing and responding to sensory information are affected. We present these problems from a dynamic systems perspective to illustrate how contemporary theory, when coupled with basic knowledge of anatomy and neuroanatomy, can be used to guide therapeutic interventions. It is our premise, that although different treatment approaches may be needed for children with a peripheral nerve lesion or lower motor neuron dysfunction, the theoretical basis for treatment would remain consistent. We begin with a brief overview of dynamic systems theory.

Dynamic Systems Theory

Principles and concepts from dynamic systems theory can be used to guide our interventions as we assist children with developmental disabilities to learn to move more effectively.[3] Proponents of this approach suggest that new motor skills emerge through the process of *self-organization* rather than by prescribed or hard-wired neural templates.[4] This means the movements children produce are the result of the "real-time" interactions between their multiple intrinsic subsystems such as the quality of sensory information, perceptions of the task, and fat-to-muscle ratio in the legs, as well as extrinsic factors such as handling techniques and available assistive device(s).[3,5]

Figure 7-1. Specially designed infant seat for infants with lumbar or sacral spina bifida.

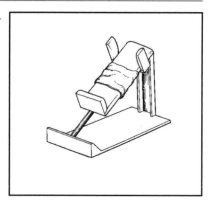

Additional principles and concepts from dynamic systems theory used to guide treatment sessions include *control parameters, rate-limiters,* and *attractors.* A control parameter is a component or factor that helps the child move differently in more functional and effective ways. For example, when infants with lumbar or sacral spina bifida are placed in a specially designed infant seat, they flex and extend their legs at their hips and knees (eg, kick) significantly more often than when they are seated in a conventional infant seat. (Figure 7-1).[3,6] Kicking is an important behavior because babies who kick their legs more often begin to walk earlier in life than infants who kick less frequently.[7] This example shows that the environmental context, an extrinsic factor, may be a control parameter that is used to facilitate specific movement patterns.

Additionally, as this example illustrates, the context for movement also may function as a *rate-limiter.* A rate-limiter is an element that limits the ability of the child to demonstrate a given movement. In this case, the conventional infant seat inhibited the ability of the infant with limited or absent sensory information to kick with flexion and extension at the hips and knees. As a result, this environmental context can be viewed as a rate-limiter for leg and knee kicks—one that may contribute to the delays these infants experience in learning to kick and then learning to walk.[6]

Control parameters and rate-limiters are not always located in the treatment environment or movement context. Instead, they may be found within the child. For instance, Ulrich, Ulrich, and colleagues found that when infants with Down syndrome periodically were held over a pediatric-sized treadmill over several months of time they produced more alternating steps when they showed an increased rate of weight gain and a decrease in their thigh and calf skin-fold measures.[5] These researchers suggested a relationship existed between these two variables. They stated that an increase in lower extremity strength was sufficient enough to enable the infants to produce more alternating steps on the treadmill when their rate of weight gain was less and/or their thigh and calf skin-fold measures were larger.

Attractors are the final concepts from dynamic systems theory that we will present as a construct to help us design effective treatment strategies. Within a dynamic systems approach, attractors are thought of as stable behavioral patterns or, in this case, movement patterns.[8-10] Attractors are perceived to be preferred, but not obligatory, movement patterns that result from the cooperation of the child's intrinsic subsystems within a given environment.[9,11] Within a particular context at a given point in development (time) the child will "settle into" preferred and perhaps limited range of movement patterns.[9] This means that certain behaviors are more likely to occur than others given the demands of the task, the status of the child and multiple subsystems, and the movement context.[10,12]

For example, young typically developing infants between the ages of 7 and 11 months when held over a pediatric-sized treadmill seem to prefer producing alternating steps vs other types of stepping patterns, such as single or parallel steps.[5,11,13,14]

An attractor represents a stable movement pattern for a child at a given point in time within a specified context. Over time and with intervention, we should expect the stability of a specific attractor to change. This loss of stability can be viewed as an increase in variability.[9] Therapists can measure this by monitoring the variability (eg, standard deviation) for that movement pattern. For example, the relative consistency or variability of a child's step length with each lower extremity may provide insight into how "stable" the child's gait pattern has become in a given context (eg, on a smooth level indoor surface with a reverse walker). We then can evaluate the child's progress by comparing the consistency of the step length on a level surface without the reverse walker to the consistency of the step length when walking on a similar surface with the reverse walker.

The loss of a stable attractor should not be interpreted as an inherently negative event in the therapeutic process. Clearly, children with developmental disabilities need to develop stable movement patterns in order to function effectively. However, children with developmental disabilities also need to develop adaptability in their movement patterns if they are going to successfully confront changes in environments and the expectations that come with different contexts. Thus, we advocate that an increase in variability simply be viewed as a sign or indicator that children are trying out new ways of moving or trying to develop new ways of coping with change within their internal systems or within a given environment. It becomes our responsibility as therapists to work to uncover what has changed (discover the control parameter) that will facilitate children developing new more functional, yet stable, ways of moving within a given environment.

Motor control theory principles and concepts from the dynamic systems perspective enable us see how important sensory information is to children with developmental disabilities as they seek to move more effectively and efficiently. Conceptual models of motor learning also highlight the significant function that sensory information plays in the production of functional movement patterns. For example, sensory feedback, in Adam's closed-loop theory of motor learning, is necessary for the ongoing production of skilled movement.[15] Schmidt, in his schema theory, suggested that the sensory consequences of a movement—how it felt, looked, and sounded—play an important part in learning to move in an effective manner.[16] More recently, Newell in his attempts to interface perception with action in an ecological theory of motor learning emphasized the significant role that perception of sensory information plays as the mover seeks to find (learn) optimal movement strategies given selected task and environmental constraints.[17]

None of these theories alone can explain the complex task confronting children with developmental disabilities who seek to move effectively and efficiently. Each theory, however, reinforces how dependent children with developmental disabilities are on the quality and quantity of sensory information available to them as they learn to generate well-controlled coordinated movements. With these ideas in mind, let us shift our attention to sensory information and the role it plays in the development of stable functional movement patterns.

Sensory Information

Within the normal process of motor learning, the ability to use sensory information appropriately is a critical component—an important subsystem—that impacts how children learn to perform coordinated movements. Edelman suggested in his *theory of neuronal groups selection* (TNGS) that when movements in a given category (eg, kicks) repeatedly are performed, the information generated from the efferent activations that result from these movements and the afferent sensory consequences are continuously and temporally correlated within and between local neuronal groups.[18,19] Thus, when movement patterns are repeated over time this ongoing multimodal flow of information strengthens the neural connections between localized groups of neurons within the motor cortex. Connections among related groups of neurons in other areas of the CNS, such as the visual and somatosensory areas, also are strengthened. This implies that movement patterns that are repeated frequently generate stronger neural connections that provide the basis for stable movement patterns.

Experimental support for Edelman's theory was provided by Ulrich et al[7] who found that infants with and without Down syndrome who kicked more often walked significantly earlier in life than similar infants who kicked less often. These results suggest that the infants strengthened the neural connections within the CNS that supported the stable action pattern of walking when they repeatedly produced a pattern of movement that was similar to the walking pattern (ie, kicked their legs). As a result, they were able to walk earlier in life than babies who kicked their legs less often.

Therapists who create a therapeutic environment through their touch, voice, equipment, and home programs in which the child can perform certain movement patterns such as alternating steps, consistently from session to session and between sessions will help strengthen the neural connections that support alternating steps. This will lead to the development of a stable attractor for alternating steps. In other words, the child will be more likely to produce alternating steps in the future given similar sensory input to the system. Alternatively, the therapist who disregards the need for consistent sensory information being available to the child and the CNS will, in effect, interfere with the child developing the stronger neural connections that support stable movement patterns. This will force the child into a situation where he is required to learn or "relearn" how to produce a given pattern of movement.

During movement, the CNS must differentiate between movement-related and non-movement-related information. As we consider the processing of sensory information, keep in mind that the CNS is analyzing sensory input available prior to the movement as well as the data generated as the result of the movement (feedback). Figure 7-2 diagrams the categorization of sensory information. As discussed in Chapter 3, intrinsic and extrinsic feedback in the form of both knowledge of results and knowledge of performance are critical variables in motor learning.

Peripheral feedback helps to strengthen neural connections and provides the CNS with information about the results of movement. Was the movement of the arm successful in positioning the hand to grasp the cup? Was the speed of movement of the protective extension reaction sufficient to stop the displacement of the child's center of gravity? The child gains knowledge of the results of his movements from internal and external sources. Internal sources of feedback include information from the sensory receptors, such as the muscle spindles and golgi tendon organs (which contribute to our "feel" of the movement), and the vestibular receptors (which contribute to our sense of position in space). External sources of information include visual and auditory input. Depending on the characteristics of the visual and auditory input, the information may be used as intrinsic feedback in which the information is compared to a learned reference of correctness which provides an error-detection mechanism or as extrinsic feedback which supplements or augments the intrinsic feedback.[2] Both internal and external feedback help strengthen the neural connections that support stable movement patterns.[18,19]

The therapist can act to augment intrinsic or extrinsic feedback or both. If the therapist provides a guiding resistance to the movement pattern, intrinsic proprioceptive informa-

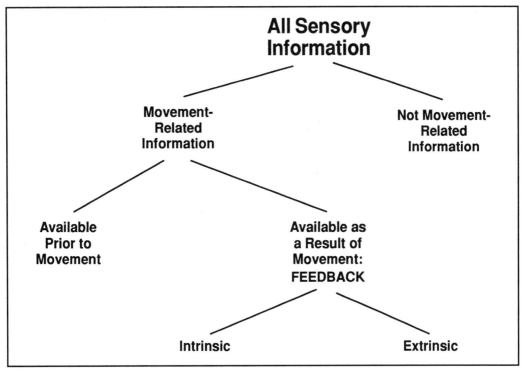

Figure 7-2. Utilization of sensory information in the process of motor control (adapted from Schmidt RA. *Motor Control and Learning.* 2nd ed. Champaign, Ill: Human Kinetics Publishers; 1988).

tion is increased. Extrinsic feedback can be increased by the therapist providing verbal commentary on the quality of the movement task—"Good hold!" (knowledge of performance) or commentary on the outcome of the movement—"Good step!" (knowledge of results).

While peripheral feedback plays a role in learning movement, once movements are learned, central monitoring of the movement increases in importance. As you first learn a motor pattern such as playing a piano, multiple sources of peripheral feedback inform you of the results of your finger movements. You attend to the feel of the movement, the sound produced by the movements, or the scowl of your teacher as you hit the wrong key. Once the movement is learned, the movements flow into each other without the need for delayed internal or external verifications of correctness of one movement before the next movement is made. Therapeutic handling techniques are designed to lead to this progression of motor learning and control.

Before developing balance within a posture, the child must have the sensory experience of being in the posture. Proprioceptive, vestibular, tactile, and visual information received by the CNS are unique to each particular posture. No amount of practice of head control in prone on elbows can provide an equivalent sensory picture of the responses necessary for head control in sitting or standing (see discussion of Transfer of Learning in Chapter 3). As the therapist handles the child within and moving between postures, the handling techniques should not interfere with the experience of being in the posture. The therapist's role is to assist the child in producing an appropriate movement response. Incorrect sensory feedback due to overcontrol or undercontrol of the child by the therapist will act as a rate-limiter and weaken the supporting neural connections. This will result in altered or inappropriate postural alignment and movement. In either case, the therapist must correct or compensate for the problem to assist the child in learning to produce the most efficient and effective movements possible.

Multiple mechanisms are available within the normally functioning CNS to protect higher centers from bombardment of sensory information. Some receptors, particularly the exteroceptors, demonstrate adaptation to a maintained stimulus. Awareness of a bandage on your finger fades quickly after it is placed on the skin, as the cutaneous receptors adapt to the continuous stimulation. With other receptors, it is crucially important that adaptation does not occur. Imagine the difficulties we would have moving if the vestibular macula did not inform us continuously of our position in relation to gravity.

With the magnitude of divergence of sensory information, a system of inhibition is necessary for the cortex to receive a clear representation of sensory input. The systems of feed-forward, feedback, and local inhibition ensure that a clear sensory message ascends through the long ascending pathways and synaptic connections to the cerebral cortex and other motor control centers. If these inhibitory mechanisms are not functioning appropriately, the cortex may receive a confused sensory picture, resulting in an inappropriate movement.

Sensory pathways not only have ascending but also descending connections with the higher centers of the CNS. The descending connections allow the higher centers to support or shut down ascending information from receptors. The CNS can attend selectively to or enhance a particular set of sensory information while ignoring or suppressing another set. This ability of the CNS allows the student to concentrate on the teacher's instructions despite the noise of other children in the hallway. Deficits with the complex mechanism of selectively attending to particular avenues of sensory information present major problems for a child attempting to learn in an unstructured school environment.

Characteristics of Sensory Systems

No sensory system should be classified as inherently facilitory (control parameters) or inhibitory (rate-limiters). Each system has the potential for increasing or decreasing the level of activity of the CNS as well as strengthening or weakening the neural connections that support stable movement patterns, depending on the manner in which the sensory stimulus is delivered. Rood formulated general guidelines that assist in predicting the types of motor response that will be elicited based on the characteristics of the delivery of the sensory input.[20] A quick brief stimulus results in a burst of motor activity. One can predict that a light stroke to the arm of a child may elicit a phasic burst to withdraw from the stimulus. Rapid, repetitive stimulation results in a more maintained response. Repetitive tapping or mechanical vibration of a muscle are techniques that have been used to induce a sustained contraction of the muscle.

Slow, rhythmical, repetitive stimuli decrease the level of responsiveness of the individual. Parents instinctively rock fussy infants to calm them. Monotone, droning instructors have deactivated the minds of students for centuries. A maintained stimulus, such as gravity, should elicit a maintained response. The influence of gravity should elicit continuously the automatic responses necessary to maintain a posture. When considering the response to a maintained stimulus, we must evaluate the potential adaptation of the receptor to the stimulus. A maintained cutaneous input should result in accommodation of the receptors and therefore a decreased rate of firing of these sensory pathways.

The therapist should consider additional influences on a child's response to sensory input. The set point of the autonomic nervous system (ANS) is a potential rate-limiter. For example, a child who is tense and sympathetically dominated may respond to a friendly pat with a startle and withdrawal. Variations in the sympathetic or parasympathetic set point of the child result in variations in the response to a particular handling technique. The technique which was a control parameter and effective yesterday may be a rate-limiter today and produce less optimal responses because the child's ANS is activating sympathetic responses.

Past experiences also influence the interpretation of sensory data. A particular cologne or aftershave may elicit parasympathetic responses if associated by the child with the scent of a loving parent. The same scent could elicit sympathetic responses if it were associated with the scent of an abusive parent.

The therapist must evaluate the number of sensory channels being stimulated by a particular handling technique. Depending on the functional and maturational level of the CNS, the child may not be able to respond appropriately to techniques or environments that provide multimodal stimulation. The child may be able to attend to controlling the position of his head when he is sitting with the therapist controlling the position of his pelvis, only if there are no other distractions such as the therapist talking. Gradually, and in a controlled manner, the therapist should introduce additional sources of input so that the child can function within a more typical environment. Responsibility to control the amount and type of sensory input requires the therapist constantly to analyze the stimuli the child is receiving to avoid inappropriate stimulation.

Our motor responses are specific to the environmental context of the moment. It is input from sensory systems that provides the CNS with the internal and external information necessary to assess the constraints under which the movement is to be performed. Gentile's Taxonomy of Motor Tasks provides therapists with a system for analyzing the complexity of different movement tasks.[21] Inherent in understanding the complexity of the movement is an analysis of the spatial and temporal attributes of the environment and the body's movement. From the perspective of the child's nervous system, the larger the quantity and diversity of sensory information that must be received and processed, the more difficult the process becomes—a rate-limiting process for the child who needs to move more efficiently and effectively. Walking and chewing gum at the same time is a more complex task than either performed independently. The addition of an object to carry or manipulate further complicates the task. As treatment progression is planned for a particular child, one must remember to consider the potential rate-limiting aspect of the amount of sensory information that must be analyzed in order to produce the appropriate movement pattern under a given set of environmental constraints.

Selection of Sensory Input

Each intervention technique should be selected to facilitate or act as a control parameter for the child in producing an adaptive response. A response is considered to be adaptive if it indicates a higher level of function than the previous behavior of the child. Farber defined an adaptive response to sensory stimuli as a "behavior of a more advanced, organized, flexible, or productive nature than that which occurred before stimulation."[20] We attempt to assist the child to produce higher level, more appropriate, and more functional movement. This is the measurement tool we can use to determine if we selected correctly the appropriate intervention techniques. How consistently the child produces a more functional movement provides us with an indicator of how stable that attractor or movement pattern has become.

The concept of using sensory input to provide guidance as a teaching technique to assist the individual in learning to perform a specific movement pattern was introduced in Chapter 3. Remember that the strongest effect of guidance is to alter the performance of the movement pattern during a specific trial. When the child is unable to execute a movement pattern which is effective and efficient, the physical therapist is responsible for selecting the control parameter (ie, treatment technique) that will enable the child to make a better response. Guidance in the form of therapist-enhanced sensory input is reduced as the child takes more responsibility for producing an adaptive response and movement independently.

The process of selecting an appropriate technique can seem overwhelming to the inexperienced clinician. The following general guidelines may assist in the process of selecting sensory techniques to be used in a particular program.

➤ The therapist should select sensory stimuli that are more naturally occurring in preference to those that are artificial. An electric vibrator may elicit the contraction of a muscle, but is not the type of stimulus to which the child will respond in a typical movement situation. Preferentially, the activation of muscles can be achieved by weight bearing, vestibular input, or cutaneous facilitation. These are the types of sensory information that the child will be required to respond to outside of the therapeutic setting and that can be administered by a parent or other caregiver

➤ Interventions should be developmentally appropriate for the child. Appropriateness must be considered in terms of physical, mental, and social development. Working on locomotion in all fours may be perceived as demeaning by a teenager with a developmental delay. Although quadruped may be therapeutically appropriate for the movement problems, the therapist must either convince the teenager to accept the rationale or select another posture

➤ The type of sensory stimulation should be appropriate to the activity. The postural neck muscles respond to vestibular input and to proprioceptive information such as approximation through the cervical spine. Rapid, quick stretch is not a stimulus to which these muscles routinely are subjected. Intervention techniques based on approximation or vestibular input would be more appropriate to activate these muscles than a quick stretch

➤ The quality of the adaptive response frequently is enhanced if the child can respond to sensory cues other than cortically processed verbal commands. In our daily activities, many postural movements are made in response to intrinsic sensory cues. We hold our heads erect in response to vestibular, proprioceptive, and visual information, not in response to being told to pick up our heads and tuck our chins. Therapy should attempt to elicit automatic postural adjustments in response to the demands of the situation or the desire to accomplish the task. The more automatic movement becomes (a function of strengthened neural connections), the more likely it will be incorporated in the child's repertoire of movements outside the therapeutic setting (a stronger or more stable attractor)

➤ The therapist should use the least amount of control or sensory input necessary to elicit an adaptive response. Throughout the intervention process, the therapist must remember that a primary goal is to remove the intervention. The therapist must assess constantly if components of the intervention strategy can be withdrawn. If the child is working on head control in sitting with the therapist controlling the position of the pelvis in all planes, the therapist could challenge the child by gradually relinquishing control in movements requiring flexion. As this control is beginning to be mastered by the child, control of extension gradually is relinquished by the therapist. As long as the therapist retains total control, the child will not have the opportunity to actively strengthen the neural connections that support the appropriate movements and as a result will be less likely to learn the appropriate movements in response to incoming sensory messages

Examination and Evaluation

In examining the status of sensory systems in children with developmental disabilities, the therapist basically is evaluating the perception of sensation. We are looking for indications that the information is being received and processed, thus producing appropriate motor responses or providing correct feedback for internally produced movement. This intent is different from the purpose of sensory testing in children with peripheral nerve or spinal cord lesions. In these cases, the therapist is more concerned with the presence of sensation rather than the interpretation of sensory information.

The goal of the examination is to determine which sensory systems are functionally intact. The therapist then can design intervention strategies based on these systems. For example, if the child does not respond to vestibular input or responds inappropriately, techniques that use other sensory systems should be the primary focus in the initial interventions.

Guard against overtesting of the sensory systems. A complete neurological sensory examination can be time consuming, fatiguing, and tedious for the child. Before beginning a comprehensive evaluation, try to target specific sensory systems on which your examination and evaluation should focus. If the physician's neurological examination is available, review the results to identify areas that should be explored further. Interviews of parents, teachers, or other caregivers may provide indications of sensory dysfunction. Does the child seem to attend to visual or auditory input consistently? Does the child explore or attempt to explore tactilely objects with his mouth or with both hands equally? Does the child withdraw from touch which could indicate tactile defensiveness? How does the child react to being moved through space? Does the child appear to enjoy movement or is the child fearful? How accurate is the child in reaching for objects? Answers to questions such as these will provide the therapist with insight to the functioning of the various sensory systems. Additionally, the use of standardized sensory profiles such as the Infant/Toddler Sensory Profile or the Sensory Profile allows the therapists to determine the child's responses in a "natural environment" and to compare the child's responses with peers (see Chapter 2).

Therapists can gather similar information by examining the child's movements. Does the child orient appropriately to gravity? Does the child seem to perceive correctly the relation of his body parts? Can the child accurately place the extremities for support or for reaching? From this process, the therapist should be able to target specific sensory systems for further evaluation. For information on the specifics of a detailed neurological examination, refer to the Suggested Reading at the end of the chapter. Examples of examining and evaluating each sensory system within a therapeutic framework will be discussed in combination with intervention strategies.

The sensory examination and evaluation should not only establish the level of integrity of a particular sensory system, but also must attempt to determine the child's sensory preferences. A child might enjoy vestibular input while being less comfortable with cutaneous/proprioceptive input. The therapist must investigate if this indicates a like/dislike or represents a dysfunction within a system. Although the determination may be difficult to make, the therapist should attend to behavioral cues. For example, consistent increases in activity level and aversion responses to tactile input may indicate tactile defensiveness.

Examination and evaluation of function of the sensory systems should encompass more than examining each system in isolation. The child may attend preferentially to a particular input or to input on one half of the body when presented with multiple inputs. In the presence of auditory distractors (a potential rate-limiter), the child may be unable to process visual input. The child with hemiplegia may be able to attend to cutaneous input on the involved side only if it is presented in isolation. If the child is touched on both sides simultaneously, only the touch on the uninvolved side (cortical inattention or bilateral extinction) may be reported. Preferential attending to certain sensory modalities may account for the difficulties a child has in making the transition from a controlled therapeutic environment to a more typical environment with its multitude of simultaneous, competing information.

Postural control or balance requires the integration of sensory input to construct an awareness of the location of the body's center of gravity in relation to the base of support as well as the ability to perform an appropriate musculoskeletal response. Visual, vestibular, and somatosensory information are combined into the perception of one's orientation in relationship to gravity, the support surface, and surrounding objects.[22] Deficits in any of these systems will affect balance control, particularly in situations when the remaining alternative sensory inputs are not available or are in conflict. A child with reduced vestibular function may increase the reliance on visual references to maintain postural control. For this child, the performance of balance tasks will be increasingly difficult as the level of illumination is decreased or the eyes are closed. The therapist must monitor the child's responses throughout the assessment process for indications of difficulties with intersensory integration in relationship to postural control (see Chapter 8).

Intertwining Examination and Intervention Strategies

In this section, we present examples of treatment techniques based on input via the major sensory systems. Methods of examining and evaluating the child's response to the sensory input will be discussed. Examination, evaluation, and intervention are integrated in this section since therapists frequently conduct these processes simultaneously. The therapist may use the child's responses during intervention to evaluate the function of one or more sensory systems.

Cutaneous Input

Receptors located in the skin are responsible for touch and temperature information. Therapists can stimulate touch receptors to either inhibit or facilitate motor activity. Static, maintained contact of a surface with the child's skin should result in adaptation of touch receptors and inhibition of the muscles underlying the skin.[23] Therapists use this technique by resting their hands on the skin overlying spastic muscles to inhibit the muscles. Care must be taken to maintain constant, even pressure on the child's skin. Changing pressures could result in an increase in the activity of the underlying muscle. This concept is used in the construction of splints.[21] The static surface should be in contact with the surface overlying the spastic muscle. Straps are placed preferentially over the antagonists to the spastic muscles. The therapist assesses the success of the use of inhibitory, maintained touch by the response of the child. Has the muscle relaxed? If the child is able to make more functional movements then the inhibitory, maintained touch has functioned as a control parameter enabling the child to move more effectively.

When the therapist attempts to facilitate the response of a muscle, manual contacts should be placed over the muscle belly. A changing, nonstatic pressure is used. Cutaneous receptors make spinal cord level synaptic connections with gamma motoneurons.[24]

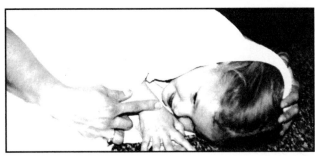

Figure 7-3. Child positioned in sidelying with sheet blanket for neutral warmth to decrease overall level of activity. Note therapist's control of the hand position of the child and use of approximation to control head position (photo courtesy of William D. Porter).

Cutaneous input may enhance the sensitivity of the muscle spindle and, therefore, positively influence the response of the muscle. Just as with inhibitory touch, the effectiveness of the technique is assessed by evaluating changes in the child's response.

Temperature receptors increase their rate of firing as the skin temperature changes. The concept of neutral warmth can be used when the therapist attempts to decrease the overall level of the child's activity or stiffness in a limb. The therapist attempts to create an environment in which neither the temperature nor cutaneous receptors are being stimulated to fire above the base firing rate. This environment is created by wrapping the child or the body part in lightweight toweling or a sheet blanket (Figure 7-3). The neutral environment is maintained until the desired response occurs. If the child is wrapped for too long, the increase in skin temperature may result in an increase in activity rather than a decrease. This is analogous to the restlessness created when you become too warm while sleeping and attempt to kick off the covers.

Therapists should attend to the temperature of the room in which they are working with a child. In the optimal setting, the temperature would be adjusted to meet the needs of each child. A child with limited body fat or high activity level would be treated in a warmer room. In selecting the appropriate room temperature, the therapist should consider the baseline skin temperature of the child. The baseline skin temperature will vary with the child's health and the temperature of the child's previous environment. Remember that the temperature receptors are reporting deviations from baseline. It is important, therefore, to consider whether the child has been in a warm, muggy environment or a windy, cold environment prior to therapy. This may affect the baseline of muscle activity and the type of temperature input the therapist chooses to use.

When considering the effects of temperature changes on the child, remember to consider your hand temperature. Therapist-child rapport can quickly be disturbed by a cold hand placed on a warm abdomen.

In general, sensory inputs that evoke a withdrawal response or that are interpreted by the child as noxious or painful are functioning as rate-limiters and will be counterproductive to the goal of learning to make adaptive movements. A child with a developmental disability may demonstrate an aversive response to light touch which may be described as tactile defensiveness. The therapist can help the child prepare for the therapy session by allowing him to desensitize the skin by vigorous rubbing with various textures and media. The child may tolerate the process better if he is allowed to control the input. When the therapist uses cutaneous input to guide the child through a movement pattern, a firm touch should be employed.

Figure 7-4. Use of a scooter to facilitate postural extension. The child can control the amount of vestibular stimulation being provided (photo courtesy of William D. Porter).

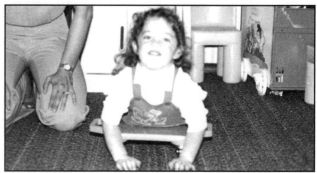

Vestibular Input

Vestibular input can either arouse or depress the level of activity of postural extensors and the level of alertness of the child, depending on the characteristics of the stimuli. Slow, rhythmical, repetitive rocking, rolling, or swinging typically relaxes and calms the child. Parents combine the concepts of neutral warmth and repetitive vestibular input by wrapping a fussy baby in a blanket and slowly rocking the child to sleep. Rapid, non-rhythmical stimulation with stops, starts, and changes in direction of movement is arousing and increases postural tone. Encouraging a child to move prone on a scooter board requires the use of postural extensors, while allowing vestibular input to reinforce the activity of the postural muscles (Figure 7-4).

Inversion is a technique used by therapists to stimulate the vestibular receptors to elicit a response similar to the Landau response or pivot prone posture. Infants who have had limited exposure to being placed in prone (as may occur when parents avoid any time in prone as a misinterpretation of the "Back to Sleep" campaign) may require additional stimulation to develop the postural extensors to work against gravity. According to McGraw, the child progresses through four developmental stages in response to inversion.[25] Initially, the infant responds to inversion with increased flexion and emotional arousal. The next stage is the extension response, which is the response sought when inversion is used as a therapeutic intervention. Crying is seldom heard during this phase. Later, inversion of the infant results in attempts to appropriately right the head to the horizon. Crying is frequent since these attempts are not successful. In the final stage, the child seems to recognize the futility of reversing the inverted position and hangs relaxed. Therapists should be aware of these developmental stages. If a child responds to inversion with a flexion response rather than the expected extension response, inversion may not be a developmentally appropriate technique. The therapist may need to use other forms of sensory stimulation to activate extension and introduce inversion later.

Some therapists have used the postrotatory nystagmus test developed by Ayres as an indicator of the integrity of the vestibular system.[26] The duration of nystagmus is measured following 10 rotations of the child in a 20-second period. The head of the child must remain flexed at 30 degrees during the duration of the rotation. Other sensory stimuli, particularly visual, should be controlled during the rotations since they may influence the results. This test indicates the integrity of the vestibulo-ocular connections, but does not necessarily provide information concerning the multiple diverse connections between the vestibular system and other parts of the CNS.

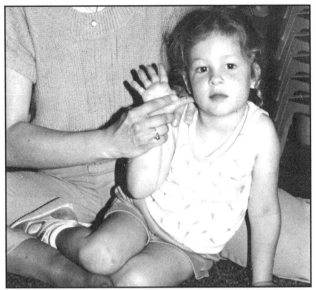

Figures 7-5. The therapist applies a quick stretch to the triceps brachii (photos courtesy of William D. Porter).

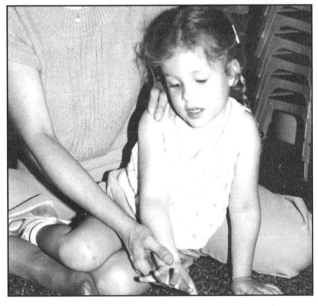

Figures 7-6. The therapist applies resistance to extension to augment the contraction of the triceps brachii (photos courtesy of William D. Porter).

Proprioceptive Input

Proprioceptive or, more generally, somatosensory input is provided by almost every handling technique used by therapists. Many techniques have used the concept of reciprocal innervation to affect spasticity. The antagonist of the spastic muscle is activated (a potential control parameter) to achieve inhibition of the spastic muscle (a likely rate-limiter). A therapist might use a quick stretch to the triceps brachii (Figures 7-5 through 7-7). The quick stretch elongates the equatorial region of the muscle spindle, increasing the discharge rate of the Ia fiber. The Ia fiber monosynaptically connects with an alpha motoneuron innervating a motor unit in the triceps resulting in a contraction of those

Figure 7-7. This demonstrates the target posture with the activated triceps being used in a support response (photo courtesy of William D. Porter).

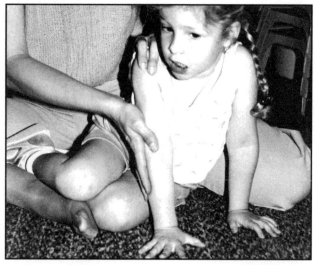

fibers. Resistance helps maintain the contraction response of the muscle, so that the phasic burst following the quick stretch becomes a maintained or tonic response. Activation of the triceps reciprocally should inhibit the spastic biceps. If the therapeutic goal is to facilitate a particular muscle, a quick stretch followed by resistance can be used to attempt to activate the hyporesponsive muscle.

A mechanical vibrator with the appropriate characteristics will produce a muscle contraction. The vibrator should have an amplitude of 1.0 to 2.0 mm[27] with a frequency of 100 to 125 Hz (cycles per second).[23] The vibration increases the discharge rate of the Ia fiber from the muscle spindle resulting in a contraction of the muscle being vibrated. Although the technique may be effective in producing a contraction, it is difficult to use a vibrator within the context of producing functional, adaptive behaviors. Since vibration is not a stimulus that evokes movement responses in a normal framework of movement patterns, it should be reserved for occasions when other techniques are not effective.

Joint receptors appear to influence the type of contraction produced by the muscles crossing the joint. Approximation, or compression of the joint space, seems to elicit a holding contraction, particularly in the joint alignment typical for weight bearing (see Figure 5-7). Traction or separation of the joint spaces assists with movement. As the therapist assists the child with movement between postures, traction can be added to an extremity to facilitate the transition. Once the child has assumed a posture, traction can be added through the extremities in weight bearing positions or through the vertebral column to reinforce the holding contraction necessary to maintain the position.

The therapist may alter the child's proprioceptive input (and to some extent, other system input) by using guidance assistance/resistance to facilitate movement. The purpose of the guidance assistance/resistance is to enable the child to experience movement within the environmental context in which the response should occur. This technique is employed when the child has been unable to use trial-and-error learning to refine a movement pattern.

Tests for proprioception frequently are not appropriate for the child with developmental disabilities. The young child or a child with marked limitations cannot reproduce the postures with one extremity that a therapist has created with the opposite extremity. This represents deficits in position sense which is a common rate-limiter in children with developmental disabilities. The child may not understand or be able to communicate when the therapist moves a toe or finger up or down (kinesthesis or movement sense). In these cases, the therapist must evaluate how the child moves and uses the extremities to gain an understanding of the child's ability to act on proprioceptive information. A child may allow an extremity to lag behind when moving between postures or fail to appropriately position the extremity when assuming a resting position despite having the ability to move the extremity. In this case, the therapist would suspect that the child lacks proprioceptive input or is unable to process the input in order to know the location of the extremity. The therapist's observational skills will be the primary tool to evaluate proprioception in the majority of children with developmental disabilities.

Visual Input

As discussed previously, visual information is one of the critical elements for maintaining postural control, particularly in individuals with vestibular system deficits. Assessment of static and dynamic balance tasks with and without vision will provide clues to the child's reliance on visual input.

Woollacott reported that young infants commit more errors in their responses to perturbations when visual information also is being processed.[28] Apparently infants learn to use the visual input in conjunction with other sensory information over time as motor control is mastered in various postures.

When children have difficulty in maintaining appropriate vertical alignment in sitting or standing, some therapists use positioning in front of a mirror to provide visual cues on the alignment. This tactic encourages the substitution of visual information for attention to internal cues (somatosensory and vestibular input) indicating appropriate alignment. Attention to internal cues is necessary to remain aligned when the mirror is removed. The reversal of movements that occurs when viewing actions in a mirror may function as a rate-limiter and cause some children initially to hesitate in moving, resulting in errors in moving toward a target. Therapists should consider the effects of substituting visual information for proprioceptive/vestibular cues when deciding to use mirrors in teaching maintenance of vertical alignment postures or movements within those postures with various children.

Auditory Input

If a child has difficulty processing multiple sensory inputs selectively, extraneous sounds from the environment often are districting. With this child, the therapist should select a treatment environment that eliminates extraneous auditory inputs. As the child masters a particular task, background noises should be added. The goal should be eventually to progress the child to performing the task within a non-isolated environment.

The therapist's voice is an important therapeutic tool. Tone, volume, rate, and rhythm of speech must be modulated to meet the needs of the child. A child who is easily upset would respond best to a soothing, slow-paced, repetitive speech pattern. The child who is lethargic may need more authoritative, brisk verbal cues. Therapists should not confuse the need to be authoritative with being loud. Therapists can apply general rules of sensory input discussed previously to the therapeutic use of their voices.

Summary

The most effective therapists engage in constant analysis of the child's response to their handling and the environment. This analysis includes consideration of all the sensory input the child is receiving. The therapist should note the conditions under which appropriate and inappropriate responses are made. Evaluation of these observations can help the therapist identify control parameters and rate-limiters which will lead to the construction of more effective intervention programs. Suggested readings to explore these topics further are included at the end of this chapter.

As examination, evaluation, and treatment intervention are discussed in other chapters of this text, consider the type and quality of sensory input that underlies the technique. For example, in Chapter 8, the types of sensory stimuli that elicit postural reactions are presented. If the child cannot appropriately process one type (or types) of sensory input, the response may not be demonstrated or the response may be degraded. This represents a very different problem from the child who cannot demonstrate the appropriate response due to muscle weakness. Just as the CNS must integrate input from multiple sensory systems, the reader is encouraged to integrate the information from this chapter with the concepts throughout this text.

Conclusion

Therapists working with children with developmental disabilities use manipulation of sensory input as a primary means of improving movement abilities. Some handling techniques obviously are designed to alter sensory input (inversion, quick stretch); other techniques evoke more subtle changes in postural alignment altering the proprioceptive inflow and changing the motor response. While this chapter has surveyed sensory considerations in handling children from a dynamic systems perspective, information from other chapters can be included within the scope of this topic. The challenge offered to us by children is to observe skillfully, analyze objectively, and manipulate creatively their movements, the tasks, and the environment until the highest and most functional level of independence is achieved.

Case Study #1: Jason

➤ Practice pattern 5C: Impaired Motor Function and Sensory Integrity Associated With Nonprogressive Disorders of the Central Nervous System—Congenital Origin or Acquired in Infancy or Childhood
➤ Medical diagnosis: Cerebral palsy, right hemiparesis
➤ Age: 24 months

Examination

In observing Jason's play, the therapist notes that Jason does not spontaneously use his right upper extremity to assist in manipulating objects. This observation plus others made during the initial intervention session leads the therapist to conclude that Jason is demonstrating sensory neglect of the involved extremities, particularly the right upper extremity. Jason will turn his head to look at an object that touches him on the right. However, if the therapist touches both the right and left sides simultaneously, Jason seems to notice only the contact on the left. This observation reinforces the therapist's conclusion that Jason demonstrates sensory neglect. Jason's mother reports that he does not like to snuggle on her lap. He cries or fidgets when she tries to kiss his neck. Jason grimaces, fusses, or pulls away when the therapist lightly touches him on the right side. The therapist concludes that Jason is tactilely defensive on the right side. When objects are placed in Jason's right hand, he grasps them tightly and cannot control release.

Jason is able to stand independently from the middle of the floor by assuming a bear stance (support on hands and feet) and rising. The therapist notes that when Jason stands, he has a slight anterior tilt of his pelvis with pelvic retraction on the right. His standing posture improves when the therapist controls the position of the pelvis and approximates through the right lower extremity to reinforce weight bearing through the heel. The therapist observes that contact of the ball of the foot with the floor results in a plantar grasp response. During gait, Jason demonstrates a short stride length on the right due to backward rotation of the right pelvis with genu recurvatum and a valgus foot position during stance. Jason's mom reports that he frequently falls, has difficulty keeping up with his peers, and usually falls when he tries to run. The results of testing for righting and equilibrium reactions suggest that the vestibular system information is being interpreted appropriately; however, motor control dysfunction interferes with a complete response on the right side.

FUNCTIONAL LIMITATIONS

Jason does not use his right arm and hand effectively for self-care tasks or for manipulation of toys during play. He does not protect himself well when falling backwards or to the right side in sitting or in standing and frequently bumps his head. He demonstrates poor coordination during gross motor tasks. He falls frequently when walking and cannot run and keep up with peers. Jason is a "messy" eater, frequently losing food out of his mouth. He has difficulty eating food with texture and often spits it out or chokes on it.

IMPAIRMENTS

Jason demonstrates poor sensory awareness on the right side of his body. He has poor motor control of the right upper extremity and slow protective reactions. He demonstrates poor lip closure, difficulty in moving his tongue laterally, and an immature chewing pattern. He does not seem to notice when food is escaping from his mouth. Jason's balance in standing is poor and he relies on his left side to control initiation and propulsion during gait.

GOALS

Treatment goals are for Jason to:

1. Increase sensory awareness of right side of body, especially the right upper extremity and right side of mouth
2. Increase speed and effectiveness of upper extremity protective reactions
3. Improve lip closure and tongue control
4. Improve balance reactions, especially in standing
5. Improve coordination during gross motor tasks, such as running
6. Improve coordination during fine motor tasks, such as manipulation of toys

FUNCTIONAL OUTCOMES

Following 3 months of intervention, Jason will:

1. Use both hands to take off socks
2. Use both hands to catch and throw a 12-inch ball
3. Fall less than three times/day
4. Use his arms to catch himself when he falls

5. Eat soft meats without losing food out of his mouth

6. Run 10 to 20 feet and keep up with peers

Intervention

To assess the progress being made toward meeting the general treatment goals, the therapist establishes several measurable functional objectives for Jason. Jason's ability to perform the tasks will be evaluated at the conclusion of each intervention session and at the initiation of the subsequent session in order to determine both changes in performance and motor learning. Following treatment, Jason will:

1. In sitting, lift an 8-inch diameter ball 5 inches from the table top using both upper extremities (with the therapist assisting the right extremity). Jason must be seated in an appropriate chair to permit his feet to rest on the floor. The table height should be adjusted to provide a comfortable working surface. The therapist can use approximation through the right lower leg to reinforce a flat position of the foot

2. In sitting, with his right hand placed on an 8-inch diameter ball placed 12 inches in front of him, roll the ball from side to side five times without losing contact with the ball

3. Tolerate contact of the handler (his therapist or one of his parents) on his right upper extremity for 1 minute without signs of emotional distress

4. In spontaneous play, attempt to use the right upper extremity in an appropriate manner five times during a 3-minute observation period

5. In standing at a table, maintain a neutral foot flat position of the right lower extremity for 1 minute while playing with a toy

6. In standing, will use two hands (with therapist assistance for the right arm/hand) to throw a 6-inch in diameter lightweight playground ball at a target that is 8 to 10 feet away while stepping forward with his right foot. (*Note:* The therapist will need to emphasize heel contact through visual or auditory cues)

7. Practice walking on different types of surfaces (eg, level, single-thickness tumbling mat, double-thickness tumbling mat, up/down a 10-foot ramp) using different types of stepping patterns such as long steps, marching, or running with minimal hand-held assistance

To progress Jason toward meeting these objectives, the therapist could include the following activities as part of the intervention program. The session should begin with Jason, one of his parents, or the therapist rubbing different textures or materials over the left and right sides of Jason's body. The contact with Jason's skin should be steady and continuous. Materials with rougher textures such as toweling or cotton sheet blankets should be used initially (Figure 7-8). The handlers also should use their hands to rub Jason's skin so that Jason is comfortable with the touching that will follow during the session. The therapist can assist Jason in rubbing body lotion over his extremities as a reward for tolerating the contact (Figure 7-9).

Appropriately seated at the table, the therapist should position Jason's right arm so that he is weight bearing through the elbow with his hand flat on the table. Jason is allowed to play in this position for a few minutes. Then he is encouraged to participate in activities such as water play or finger painting with his right arm. These activities are designed to increase his awareness of his right arm and to decrease tactile defensiveness.

Following inhibition of inappropriate upper extremity posturing as discussed in Chapter 12, Jason should engage in two-handed activities with an 8-inch diameter ball.

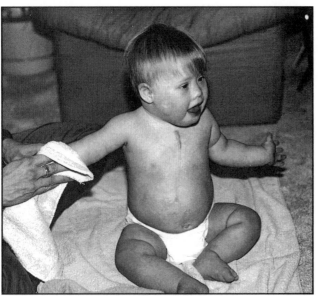

Figure 7-8. Use of toweling to increase the child's tolerance for the therapist's manual contacts with the extremity during the treatment session (photo courtesy of William D. Porter).

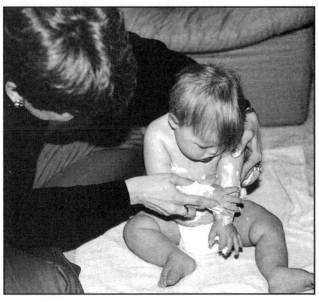

Figure 7-9. Participation of the child in activities such as spreading foam over the trunk and extremities may increase the child's tolerance for these types of interventions (photo courtesy of William D. Porter).

With the therapist controlling the position of the right extremity and the weight of the ball, Jason should push the ball away from his chest and pull it back. After several repetitions, Jason should be guided to lift the ball from the support surface and return it (Figures 7-10 through 7-12). The therapist should attempt to reduce the amount of external control required to keep Jason's right hand in contact with the ball. The therapist also should assist Jason in pronation and supination movements (Figure 7-13). This activity will require more control by the therapist since this is a developmentally advanced activity. It is included to work toward appropriate range of motion and to promote inhibition of inappropriate movements.

Figures 7-10. Ball activities to promote inhibition of inappropriate overflow in the right upper extremity and to promote two-handed activities.

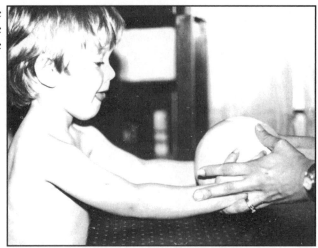

Figures 7-11. Ball activities to promote inhibition of inappropriate overflow in the right upper extremity and to promote two-handed activities.

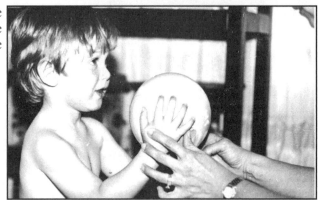

Figures 7-12. Ball activities to promote inhibition of inappropriate overflow in the right upper extremity and to promote two-handed activities.

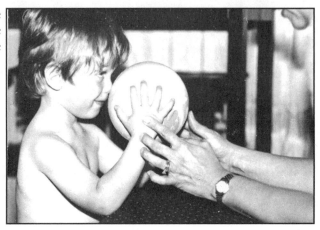

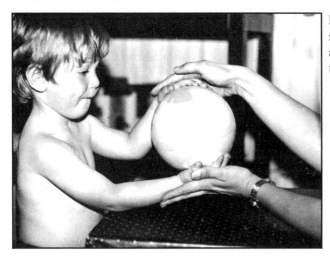

Figure 7-13. Use of ball to promote supination range of motion of right forearm and inhibition of inappropriate posturing.

Chapter 11 addresses developing ambulation skills. The weight-bearing activities presented in the treatment sequence are effective activities in inhibiting the influence of the plantar grasp reflex. When an appropriate weight-bearing posture is achieved, approximation through the pelvis reinforces maintenance of the position. Throwing the ball at a target is included to promote forward rotation of the right side of his pelvis along with a more normal heel contact with his right foot while giving Jason experience with a gross motor skill that he can perform with his peers. Practicing walking in a variety of ways on multiple surfaces is designed to increase his movement repertoire as well as improve his dynamic balance and motor control.

Case Study #2: Jill

➤ Practice pattern 5C: Impaired Motor Function and Sensory Integrity Associated With Nonprogressive Disorders of the Central Nervous System—Congenital Origin or Acquired in Infancy or Childhood

➤ Medical diagnosis: Cerebral palsy, spastic quadraparesis, microcephaly, mental retardation, seizure disorder

➤ Age: 7 years

Examination

Jill's parents report that she does not like to be moved between positions. Her therapist notes that movement through space results in signs of autonomic distress, such as increased respiration and heart rate, increased perspiration, crying, and increased stiffness. Righting reactions are not present beyond her ability to maintain her head in neutral when she is held vertical; however, the assessment of her ability to respond to vestibular input is complicated by the pattern of muscle tightness. She typically postures with her head extended and her mouth open with her lips and tongue retracted. Any touch to the lips or skin overlying the oral musculature results in increased lip retraction and increased head extension.

FUNCTIONAL LIMITATIONS

Jill is nonambulatory and is unable to maintain her balance in any position. She demonstrates poor head control in all positions, except when held vertically when she can maintain a neutral head position. She is unable to maintain her balance in any position. Jill requires physical support to sit and cannot roll over. She presents with no independent floor mobility. Her protective and equilibrium responses to movement are absent. It is difficult for Jill to voluntarily grasp and release objects. Jill has difficulty eating and drinking. Her ocular control is poor.

IMPAIRMENTS

Jill has limited cognitive ability and demonstrates poor selective attention. Her motor control is diminished secondary to generalized muscle weakness, especially for trunk, head, and neck control. She presents with a kyphotic posture in the upper back with a mild scoliosis and an indented sternum. Jill responds to movement through space with autonomic distress and shows hypersensitivity in the oral area.

GOALS

Treatment goals are for Jill to:

1. Increase her ability to attend to visual and auditory stimuli
2. Improve her strength and motor control, especially of her head, neck, and trunk muscles
3. Improve her ability to tolerate movement through space with little to no autonomic distress
4. Decrease her sensitivity to stimulation in the oral area

FUNCTIONAL OUTCOMES

Following 3 months of intervention, Jill will:

1. Hold her head erect for 5 minutes when positioned in her vertical stander to watch a classroom activity or video
2. Tolerate being lifted out of her wheelchair and carried during movement transitions without signs of distress
3. When positioned in her adapted wheelchair, maintain lip closure for 1 minute with no more than one assist from the handler during feeding
4. When positioned in her adapted wheelchair, maintain jaw closure for 1 minute with no more than one assist from her handler during feeding
5. When positioned in her adapted wheelchair, appropriately close lips and jaw on the rim of a drinking glass with no assistance from the handler other than to position and hold the glass

Intervention

Jill's intervention program must include a systematic introduction of activities to stimulate the vestibular system to increase her tolerance for movement. Positioned securely in supine in a hammock, she can be rocked gently in an antero-posterior direction. The initial excursion of the swing would be small. The amplitude and frequency of swings gradually will increase as Jill's tolerance increases. Given the autonomic signs of distress Jill displayed during the examination, the therapist takes baseline measurements of pulse,

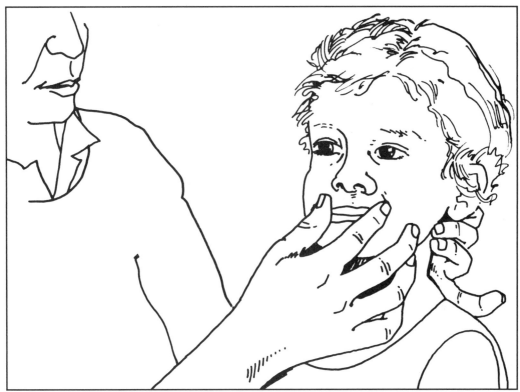

Figure 7-14. Quick stretch to orbicularis oris to facilitate lip closure.

respiration rate, or blood pressure to determine Jill's response to intervention. Other vestibular activities would include antero-posterior rocking with Jill positioned in her wheelchair or positioned sidelying in a wagon. It is important that Jill experience movement in a variety of positions. It is equally important that Jill feel secure while she is being moved.

As Jill's tolerance for antero-posterior movement increases, movements in other directions would be added. Movements to be introduced would include medio-lateral, cephalo-caudal, non-repetitive rotation about the body axis (as in rolling prone to supine to prone), diagonal, and finally rotatory movements. Tolerance of each new movement would be carefully assessed.

As Jill's control of her head and trunk position improve (Chapter 9), problems with control of the oral musculature can be addressed. Maintained jaw closure will be difficult to achieve as long as Jill continues to posture with her head and neck extended. The skin overlying the oral musculature can be desensitized by the therapist's use of maintained manual contact around the mouth. This should assist in decreasing withdrawal responses. The therapist must be sure to approach Jill's face carefully so that a visual startle or withdrawal is not elicited.

Jaw and lip closure can be facilitated by a quick stretch (Figure 7-14) or fingertip vibration of the appropriate musculature. The therapist should desensitize the skin prior to application of these techniques. Functional activities such as drinking from a straw will assist Jill in consolidating her gains (Figure 7-15). The therapist can use finger pressure to the orbicularis oris to facilitate lip closure or can construct a mouthpiece as suggested by Farber to provide a similar response.[20]

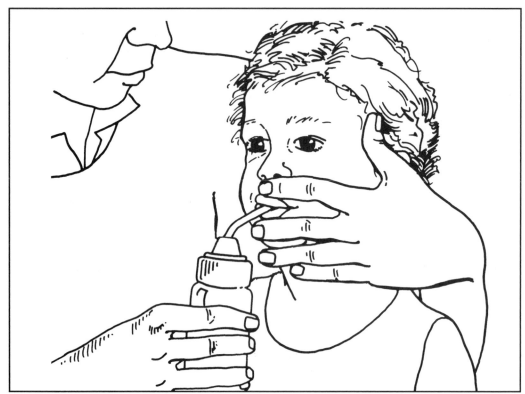

Figure 7-15. Therapist facilitation of jaw and lip closure to assist Jill in drinking through a straw.

The therapist should attend to the stimulation of intra-oral muscles as well as extra-oral musculature. Oral hygiene swabs can be used to stroke the gums, to stretch the insides of the cheeks, or to resist tongue motions (Figure 7-16). The therapist must select an instrument that will not harm the child in case a bite reflex is triggered.

Jill's progress in control of her mouth and tongue will be linked with her progress in developing head and trunk control. Activities in these two areas will reinforce her attempts at oral motor control.

Case Study #3: Taylor

➤ Practice pattern 5C: Impaired Motor Function and Sensory Integrity Associated With Nonprogressive Disorders of the Central Nervous System—Congenital Origin or Acquired in Infancy or Childhood

➤ Medical diagnosis: Myelomeningocele, repaired L1-2

➤ Age: 4 years

Examination

The examination of Taylor related to his sensory problems reveals a loss of cutaneous and proprioceptive sensation below the level of T-12. The lack of proprioceptive information from hips, knees, ankles, and feet present difficulties in Taylor's attempts to maintain a challenged sitting posture, static all-fours position, or standing posture in an orthosis.

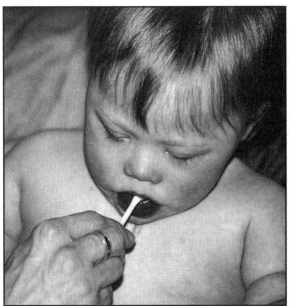

Figure 17-16. Introduction of an oral hygiene swab for stimulation of intraoral muscles. Note that the child's head is positioned in flexion to counter the tendency to withdraw from the stimulus (photo courtesy of William D. Porter).

Taylor's visual acuity problems necessitate the wearing of eyeglasses at all times. Taylor has figure-ground discrimination difficulties and has difficulty locating small objects on a visually distracting background. In standing, when he bends his head to look at the floor through his glasses, his balance is disturbed. This presents difficulty in correct placement of his crutches among objects on the floor.

The therapist must extrapolate information from the overall examination to suggest the origin of the balance deficit when Taylor looks down in standing. Since somatosensory information from the lower extremities is lacking, Taylor has an increased reliance on vestibular and visual information for balance. Normal head righting and protective extension reactions in sitting suggest that vestibular responses are within normal limits. The therapist concludes that visual perceptual problems are the primary contributors to balance problems in standing with head movement. Taylor must learn to produce the appropriate compensatory movements when his center of gravity is displaced by motion of the head.

Functional Limitations

Taylor requires external support to stand and ambulates with a swing-to gait using a parapodium and a walker, but is ready for long leg braces and crutches. Although he attempts to pull to kneeling, Taylor demonstrates poor sitting and standing balance. Taylor requires assistance for lower body dressing. Taylor has difficulty placing his crutches in the correct location on the floor.

Impairments

Taylor demonstrates loss of cutaneous and proprioceptive sensation below T-12. Taylor has visual acuity and perceptual problems, especially figure-ground discrimination, with slow balance reactions in sitting and standing. He experiences frequent skin breakdowns and has a loss of motor function in his lower extremities. Taylor shows generalized muscle weakness and a lack of endurance in his upper extremities and trunk, particularly his abdominal muscles.

GOALS

Treatment goals are for Taylor to:

1. Improve his visual perceptual skills, especially figure-ground discrimination

2. Improve his balance reactions in sitting and standing

3. Decrease the frequency of his skin breakdowns

4. Improve the strength and endurance of his upper extremity and trunk muscles, especially his abdominals

FUNCTIONAL OUTCOMES

Following 3 months of intervention, Taylor will:

1. Correctly don his shoes and socks eliminating potential pressure areas every time

2. Maintain correct body alignment in his new orthosis while reciprocally lifting his crutches 10 times in 30 seconds

3. Maintain standing balance in his new orthosis for 15 seconds with his eyes closed (with crutches)

4. Maintain standing balance in his new orthosis for 1 minute while moving his head up, down, right, and left (with crutches)

5. In standing, identify numbers placed on shapes on the floor with 80% accuracy. (This outcome assumes that Taylor can visually identify numbers and shapes on a plain background)

Intervention

Included in Taylor's intervention program would be education of Taylor and his parents on techniques of providing good skin care. The parents and Taylor will learn to monitor the condition of the skin with each change of his shoes or orthosis. The therapist should evaluate the consistency of the parents' visual inspection of Taylor's legs at each preschool session they attend. If the behavior is established at school, it should generalize to other situations. The objective would be stated as follows: Taylor's parents will visually inspect his lower extremities for indications of skin irritation or pressure following every removal of shoes and socks, or orthosis.

Activities addressing balance and figure ground training should be conducted both in the freestanding orthosis and his new orthosis (long leg braces with a pelvic band). Taylor eventually can learn to maintain his balance while hitting a ball with one crutch. A variety of floor backgrounds can be used, progressing from plain to visually distracting patterns. Initially, he should be stationary with the ball position being varied for different trials (Figure 7-17).

As Taylor increases his balance and skill, the ball can be rolled to him so that he can bat it with his crutch. Objects of varying heights can be placed around Taylor with the goal of touching the top of each object with his crutch without knocking over the object (Figure 7-18). These types of activities also address problems discussed in Chapter 9 such as lack of trunk rotation.

Taylor may benefit from activities such as a wheelchair obstacle course. Manipulation of his chair will increase upper extremity and trunk strength and endurance. Successful completion of the course requires good visual perceptual skills and motor planning. This activity can be a fun reward for successful completion of more difficult tasks during the therapy session.

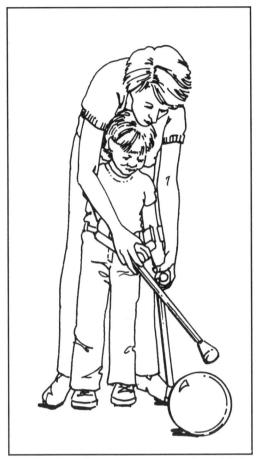

Figure 7-17. Balance activities in standing while hitting a stationary ball with one crutch.

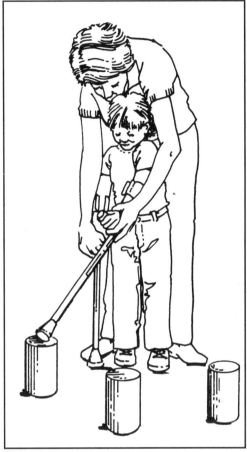

Figure 7-18. Trunk rotation in standing promoted by touching objects placed in a semicircle around Taylor.

Case Study #4: Ashley

➤ Practice pattern 5B: Impaired Neuromotor Development
➤ Medical diagnosis: Down syndrome
➤ Age: 15 months

Examination

Ashley demonstrates a lack of stability in all positions as well as generalized hypotonia (Figure 7-19). During her examination, she was noted to respond to rapid, irregular vestibular input with more appropriate postural tone and stability. Proprioceptive and cutaneous input also improved her ability to maintain postures.

Ashley was noted to be generally apprehensive about movement. Discussion with the parents indicates that Ashley's ongoing series of medical problems have resulted in her being treated by the family as a "fragile" child. Ashley has not had the opportunity to experience motion as a part of typical games parents play with infants. The therapist must

Figure 7-19. Ashley's posture in moving from prone to sitting indicates the exaggerated flexibility present in the hips due to her generalized hypotonia.

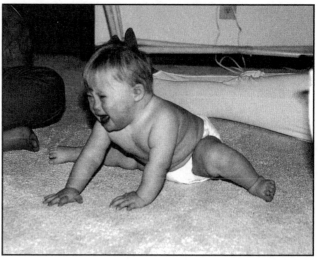

not only introduce Ashley to the fun of movement activities, but also reassure her parents that the activities are appropriate for her.

FUNCTIONAL LIMITATIONS

In general, Ashley avoids movement, demonstrates slow movements, and has delays in postural reactions. She relies on a wide base of support with lumbar lordosis, knee hyperextension, and foot pronation when she stands. Ashley is not attempting to cruise at furniture at this time. She has difficulty performing grasp and release tasks and shows limited oral motor skills.

IMPAIRMENTS

Ashley presents with hypermobile joints, low muscle tone (hypotonia), a mild hearing loss, and mental challenges associated with her medical diagnosis.

GOALS

Treatment goals are for Ashley to:
1. Increase her stability in all positions, especially at the shoulder and hip joints
2. Increase strength and endurance in all positions, particularly in sitting and standing
3. Reduce her and her parents' apprehension regarding movement experiences

FUNCTIONAL OUTCOMES

Following 3 months of intervention, Ashley will:
1. Maintain an appropriate alignment in a quadruped position during play for 30 seconds with no more than one cue from the handler
2. Maintain appropriate alignment in standing with upper extremities on a support for 1 minute with the handler providing no more than two cues
3. Move from standing to sitting to all-fours position with no indications of apprehension
4. Tolerate therapist-assisted movements between various developmentally appropriate postures with no indications of apprehension

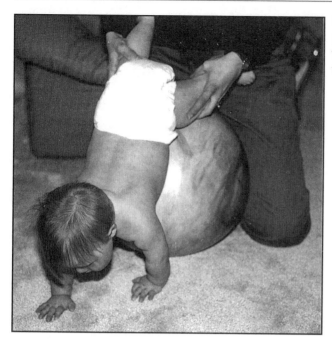

Figure 7-20. Inversion over a ball to promote shoulder girdle stability with weight-bearing through upper extremities.

Intervention

Activities in the intervention program are designed to increase postural stability. Ashley can be inverted on a ball leading to weight-bearing support through her arms (Figure 7-20). Sitting on the ball, she can be bounced. This provides vestibular stimulation and approximation through the vertebral column (Figure 7-21). Ashley should be encouraged to rock in the all-fours position while the therapist approximates through the head or pelvis in the long axis of the vertebral column (Figure 7-22). The therapist may approximate through the long axis of the upper extremities or the femurs to reinforce postural holding contractions through the extremities. Following the inversion activity on the ball, Ashley could be moved into a standing position. Approximation through the pelvis with the force vector through the correct alignment of the lower extremities should improve Ashley's standing posture. Ashley should be involved in upper extremity play activities as the therapist reinforces correct standing alignment (Figures 7-23 through 7-25). This should assist Ashley in integrating the control she is learning in situations outside of therapy.

Following inversion or other vestibular facilitory techniques, the therapist should assist Ashley in moving between developmental positions. The therapist is assisting Ashley in using the increased postural control developed during the intervention session.

Figure 7-21. Bouncing on ball with therapist assisting in maintaining appropriate postural alignment.

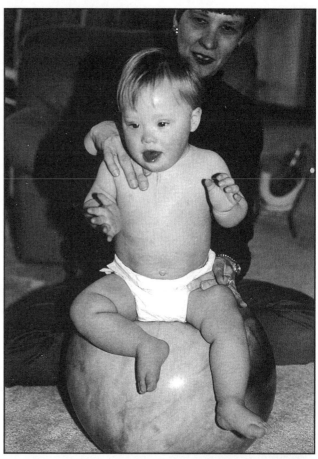

Figure 7-22. Rocking in all fours with therapist approximating through the long axis of the vertebral column to reinforce postural alignment.

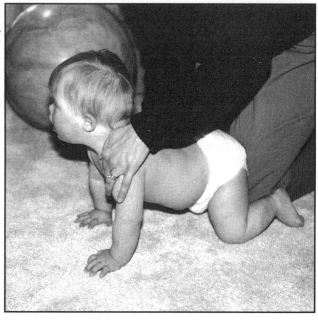

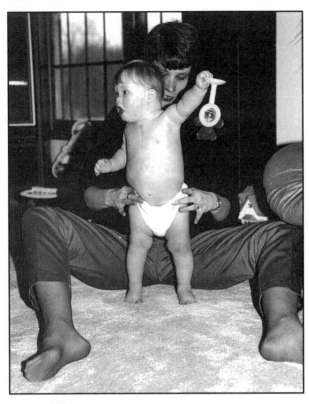

Figure 7-23. Practice of standing balance while involved in upper extremity play activities.

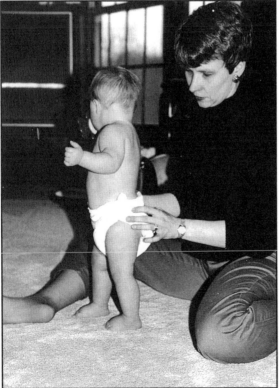

Figure 7-24. Practice of standing balance while involved in upper extremity play activities.

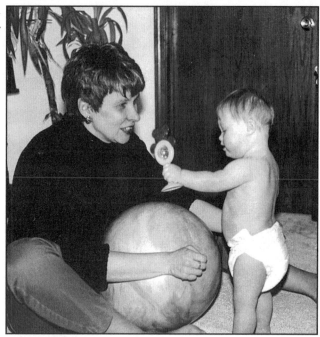

Figure 7-25. Practice of standing balance while involved in upper extremity play activities.

Case Study #5: John

➤ Practice pattern 5B: Impaired Neuromotor Development
➤ Medical diagnosis: Attention deficit hyperactivity disorder, developmental coordination disorder
➤ Age: 5 years

Examination

In observing John's play and after conferring with John's parents it became apparent that John changes activities very quickly for someone his age—usually after just 1 to 2 minutes. His parents indicate that his short attention span also is a concern at school as is his reluctance to participate in any structured gross motor activities. John tends to move by walking or jogging. When provided with a demonstration, John was able to gallop but had difficulty with single leg balance as well as hopping and skipping. John attempted to catch an 8-inch lightweight ball, but after two tries he simply moved to another area of the gym and began to play with small toy animals.

John's parents report that he does not yet ride a bike independently and does not seem to like to play on playground equipment at their neighborhood park. During this examination, John completed an obstacle course by playing Simon Says with the therapist in which he completed each obstacle separately rather than linking each task into a complete series of movement challenges. The series of tasks revealed that John has normal range of motion in all of his extremities, but has difficulty in supporting his body weight with just his upper extremities.

FUNCTIONAL LIMITATIONS

In general, John tends to avoid physical activity and is described as "clumsy" and is unable to perform gross and fine motor tasks as well as his peers, such as skipping, throwing and catching a ball, using utensils during his meals, and manipulating buttons, snaps, and zippers. He also has difficulty with maintaining balance when standing still, walking on a 4-inch balance beam, and climbing over and under barriers.

IMPAIRMENTS

John has difficulty with selective attention and demonstrates an expressive language delay. His motor planning ability is poor and he has difficulty generalizing motor skills from one situation to another. John has decreased upper extremity strength and lower than normal cardiovascular endurance. Testing indicates that tactile discrimination, kinesthesia, and stereognosis are all lower than average for John.

GOALS

Treatment goals are for John to:

1. Improve his motor planning ability
2. Increase the fluidity of his movement sequences
3. Use his motor skills in multiple settings
4. Increase his upper body strength
5. Increase his cardiovascular endurance

FUNCTIONAL OUTCOMES

Following 3 months of intervention, John will:

1. Use both hands to throw and catch a 10-inch ball
2. Participate in directed physical activities in the physical therapy gym, in physical education at school, and in the neighborhood playground
3. Use both hands to hit a stationary ball with a lightweight bat or racquet
4. Participate in physical activity for 15 to 20 minutes without undue fatigue
5. Move in a variety of ways (eg, skipping, galloping, hopping, running) in the treatment gym as well as at school and in the neighborhood playground

Intervention

Initially, John should be treated in a well-controlled 1:1 setting with limited interruptions and distractions. The equipment used with John from session to session should remain consistent in the early phases of therapy. Over time and with experience, the therapist will need to gradually introduce different pieces of equipment (eg, different sized and colored balls) as well as people into the treatment sessions.

Timing of activities and sequencing of activities will be crucial to John's success. The therapist will need to be sensitive to John's "rhythms" during early treatment sessions. This will necessitate having equipment ready and the treatment area well-controlled so that the therapist can transition between activities according to John's needs/schedule rather than some external or fixed factor (eg, time or someone else needing a piece of equipment). This will maximize John's ability to have success when moving which will facilitate his attention to the movement task as well as his motivation to keep moving, both of which will be critical to helping him learn that it is fun to move in different ways and in different environments. As John's skills develop and his ability to complete movement tasks successfully are established, the therapist should move to more of an "on demand" approach so that John develops the ability to attend to and comply with requests that come from outside of his internal schedule/rhythms. This can be accomplished by having John help develop a schedule of events for his treatment sessions by offering John structured choices from a preselected array of activities.

As John progresses with his skill development and his ability to attend to the task the therapist will need to introduce "controlled" distractors such as a sibling or friend who participates in therapy with John or moving to a treatment area that has windows or a door that John must learn to ignore. Moving to a more open treatment setting will be the next step in advancing John's development. Communication and coordination with the physical therapist in John's school district is essential. At this point, John will begin to transition to school services and community activities designed to build on his progress and to continue to expand his motor planning skills.

During the final phase of this episode of care, John should be expected to participate in various physical activities for increasingly longer periods of time. The therapist should set expectations that are similar to what other 5-year-old children can meet successfully. For example, 10 to 15 minutes of active gross motor movement is not uncommon for most 5-year-olds. This expectation may need to be developed in the more controlled therapeutic setting initially before being applied in more open environments, such as the school or a public playground.

References

1. Polit A, Bizzi E. Characteristics of motor programs underlying arm movements in monkey. *J Neurophys*. 1979;42:183-194.

2. Schmidt RA. *Motor Control and Learning*. 2nd ed. Champaign, Ill: Human Kinetics Publishers; 1988.

3. Chapman D. Context effects on spontaneous leg movements of infants with spina bifida. *Ped Phys Ther*. 2002;14:62-73.

4. Kamm K, Thelen E, Jensen JL. A dynamical systems approach to motor development. *Phys Ther*. 1990;70:763-775.

5. Ulrich BD, Ulrich DA, Collier DH. Developmental shifts in the ability of infants with Down syndrome to produce treadmill steps. *Phys Ther*. 1995;75:14-23.

6. Chapman D. The ability of young infants with spina bifida to generate complex patterned leg movements. *Ped Phys Ther*. In review.

7. Ulrich BD, Ulrich DA. Spontaneous leg movements in infants with Down syndrome and nondisabled infants. *Child Dev*. 1995;66:1844-1855.

8. Abraham RH, Shaw CD. *Dynamics—The Geometry of Behavior. Part 1: Periodic Behavior*. Santa Cruz, Calif: Aerial Press; 1982.

9. Thelen E. Self-organization in developmental processes: can systems approaches work? In: Gunnar G, Thelen E, eds. *Systems in Development: The Minnesota Symposia in Child Psychology*. Hillsdale, NJ: Erlbaum; 1989:77-117.

10. Ulrich BD, Ulrich DA. Dynamic systems approach to understanding motor delay in infants with Down syndrome. In: Savelsbergh GJP, ed. *The Development of Coordination in Infancy*. Holland: Elsevier Science; 1993:445-459.

11. Thelen E, Ulrich BD. Hidden skills: a dynamic systems analysis of treadmill stepping during the first year. *Monographs of the Society for Research in Child Development, Serial No. 223*. 1991; 56(1).

12. Thelen E, Smith L. *A Dynamic Systems Approach to the Development of Cognition and Action*. Cambridge, Mass: The MIT Press; 1994.

13. Thelen E. Treadmill elicited stepping in seven-month-old infants. *Child Dev.* 1986;57:1498-1506.

14. Chapman D, Angulo-Kinzler R. Mechanisms for the Initiation of Infant Treadmill Steps. Paper presented at: North American Society for the Psychology of Sport and Physical Activity; 1995; Clearwater, Fla.

15. Adams JA. A closed-loop theory of motor learning. *J Motor Behav.* 1971;3:111-150.

16. Schmidt RA. A schema theory of discrete motor skill learning. *Psychol Rev.* 1975;82:225-260.

17. Newell KM. Motor skill acquisition. *Annu Rev Psychol.* 1991;42:213-237.

18. Edelman GM. *Neural Darwinism: The Theory of Neuronal Group Selection.* New York, NY: Basic Books; 1987.

19. Edelman GM. *The Remembered Present.* New York, NY: Basic Books; 1989.

20. Farber SD. *Neurorehabilitation—A Multisensory Approach.* Philadelphia, Pa: WB Saunders; 1982.

21. Gentile AM. Skill acquisition: action, movement, and neuromotor processes. In: Carr JH, Shepherd R, Gordon J, Gentile AM, Held JM, eds. *Movement Science Foundations for Physical Therapy in Rehabilitation.* Rockville, Md: Aspen Publishers; 1987:155-177.

22. Nasher LM. Sensory, neuromuscular, and biomechanical contributions to human balance. In: Duncan PW, ed. *Balance: Proceedings of the APTA Forum.* Alexandria, Va: American Physical Therapy Association; 1990:5-12.

23. Umphred DA. Classification of treatment techniques based on primary input systems. In: Umphred D, ed. *Neurological Rehabilitations.* 3rd ed. St. Louis, Mo: CV Mosby; 1995:118-178.

24. Noback CR, Strominger NL, Demarest RJ. *The Human Nervous System.* Malvern, Pa: Lea & Febiger; 1991:160.

25. McGraw MN. Neuromuscular mechanism of the infant. *Am J Dis Child.* 1940;60:1031-1042.

26. Ayres AJ. *Southern California Postrotatory Nystagmus Test.* Los Angeles, Calif: Western Psychological Services; 1975.

27. Hagbarth KE, Eklund G. The muscle vibrator—a useful tool in neurological therapeutic work. In: Payton O, Hirt S, Newton R, eds. *Therapeutic Exercise.* Philadelphia, Pa: FA Davis; 1978:138.

28. Woollacott MH. Postural control and development. In: Whiting HTA, Wade MG, eds. *Themes in Motor Development.* Boston, Mass: Martinus Nijhoff; 1986.

Suggested Reading

Campbell SK, ed. *Clinical Decision Making in Pediatric Neurological Physical Therapy.* New York, NY: Churchill Livingstone; 1999.

Campbell SK, Vanderlinden D, Palisano R, eds. *Physical Therapy for Children.* 2nd ed. Philadelphia, Pa: WB Saunders; 2000.

Carr JH, Shepherd R, Gordon J, Gentile AM, Held JM, eds. *Movement Science Foundations for Physical Therapy in Rehabilitation.* Rockville, Md: Aspen Publishers; 1987.

Montgomery PC, Connolly BH, eds. *Clinical Applications for Motor Control.* Thorofare, NJ: SLACK Incorporated; 2003.

Schmidt RM, Lee TD. *Motor Control and Learning: A Behavioral Emphasis.* 3rd ed. Champaign, Ill: Human Kinetics Publishers; 1999.

Umphred D, ed. *Neurological Rehabilitation.* 3rd ed. St. Louis, Mo: CV Mosby; 1995.

CHAPTER 8

DEVELOPING POSTURAL CONTROL

Patricia C. Montgomery, PhD, PT, FAPTA
Susan K. Effgen, PhD, PT

Introduction

For a child to have functional mobility, whether by rolling, crawling, or walking, a variety of active movements and postural adjustments must be made. Postural adjustments are necessary if a child is to move freely and efficiently and adjust rapidly to the demands of the environment. As the child matures, he displays a number of distinct movements, some anticipatory and some reactive, which orient his head and body in space, protect him when he falls, and assist him in attaining and maintaining his balance. These postural and extremity movements fall under the broad description of *postural control*. The term postural control often is used interchangeably with the terms *balance* or *stability*. One definition proposed for balance is "the ability to maintain the position of the body within stability limits (ie, the center of mass within the base of support)."[1] Balance also has been described as the ability to maintain an appropriate relationship between the body segments and the body and environment to complete a task.[2] Stability and orientation are two distinct goals of the postural control system.[2-4] Seeger stated that "some tasks, needing a particular orientation, are accomplished at the expense of stability. Examples are looking at a high corner shelf while standing on a ladder and extending sideways and riding a bicycle around a tight corner thereby leaning into the curve. In both instances, the person would have orientation against gravity, but would be vulnerable to instability... therefore, most tasks have postural control as a requirement, but the demands of stability and orientation change with each task."[3]

Multiple intrinsic systems (eg, musculoskeletal, cognitive, neuromuscular) as well as environmental context play a role in the development of postural control. The underlying mechanisms and the development of postural control in children continue to be areas of interest for research. Physical therapists must evaluate empirical evidence as it is obtained and be prepared to modify the theoretical framework regarding postural control as well as the examination tools and intervention strategies used with children.

Reflex Hierarchical Approach to Postural Control

Until the early 1990s, the reflex hierarchical model was the most prevalent model used in physical therapy practice to explain the development of postural control. The reflex hierarchical model was an integral component of traditional neurophysiological theories and treatment strategies proposed by clinicians including Berta Bobath[5] (Neurodevelopmental Theory [NDT]), Margaret Rood,[6] Sidney Brunnstrom,[7] and Margaret Knott and Dorothy Voss[8] (proprioceptive neuromuscular facilitation [PNF]).

These individuals were experienced physical therapists who found certain techniques to be helpful in treatment of their patients with pathology of the central nervous system (CNS). As these therapists were disseminating information regarding their approaches in the 1950s and 1960s, they attempted to apply scientific rationale to intervention techniques.[9] To develop a theoretical framework they had to refer to basic brain research that was done in the 1930's to 1950s.[10] Compared to the sophisticated research techniques being employed today, this brain research would be considered quite crude. Most of the studies were done with animal models and consisted of ablating or stimulating areas of the brain and observing resulting effects. In addition, much of the work on sensory receptors was directed at the isolated muscle spindle. As a result, the stretch reflex was extensively studied along with postures that occurred in decerebrate animals. The focus then, was on "reflexes" and "attitudinal" postures as the basis of movement and the development of postural control.

Reflexes were described as being hierarchical, with spinal cord reflexes being the most primitive, then brain stem reflexes, followed by midbrain righting reactions, and finally higher level cortical or equilibrium reactions.[11] The development of postural control was proposed to be dependent on hierarchical, developmental processes. For example, the infant was described as demonstrating primitive reflexes that became "integrated" with maturation. Eventually, when higher-level reflexes "emerged," the infant became able to control his posture.

Systems Approach to Postural Control

The II STEP Conference,[12] in 1991, sponsored by the Foundation for Physical Therapy and the Neurology Section and Section on Pediatrics of the American Physical Therapy Association (APTA) was an initial attempt to present evolving systems approaches and applications to patient treatment in physical therapy. Contemporary systems theories are based on research that has demonstrated that the brain does not function as a discrete control model, but in a more complex manner through multiple loops involving many areas (eg, distributed control model).[13,14]

Information related to systems theories has resulted in many premises proposed in the reflex hierarchical model being modified or discarded. For example, in traditional models, development was proposed to proceed in a proximal to distal fashion.[15] Depending on the developmental process studied, this progression varies. Studies on the development of automatic postural responses in standing have demonstrated a distal (ankle) to proximal sequencing in typically developing children.[16,17] This is in contrast to the response of children with cerebral palsy (eg, older, nonwalkers). The children with cerebral palsy demonstrated immature muscle activation patterns, some of which were proximal to distal and were considered atypical or inefficient.[16]

Postural Responses to Perturbations

A child's responses to being tilted while on an unstable surface often are used clinically to assess postural control. Forssberg and Hirschfeld[18] studied postural responses to perturbation during sitting on a moveable platform in adults and formulated a functional model of organization. One level of organization is involved in basic direction-specific response patterns (ie, forward sway of the body results in activation of dorsal muscles; backward sway of the body results in activation of ventral muscles). The second level of organization is "fine tuning" of the basic response patterns on the basis of multisensory afferent input (eg, somatosensory, visual, vestibular). Hadders-Algra et al[19] studied the ontogeny of postural adjustments during sitting in typically developing infants. Because infants who were unable to sit independently (5 to 6 months of age) already showed direction-specific muscle activation when balance was perturbed in sitting (during a brief period of sitting without support), an innate model of origin for the motor response patterns was suggested by the authors. Presumably, the children had not "practiced" sitting for the skill to be dependent on experience alone.

Postural responses in sitting following platform movement were assessed in 21 typically developing children ages 1½ to 4½ years of age.[20] Comparable data also were obtained for 11 infants seen three times between the ages of 5 to 10 months. There was a transient period between the ages of 9 to 10 months to 2½ to 3 years during which perturbations in sitting resulted in high activity in the direction-specific agonist muscles as well as the antagonist muscles. With maturation, agonist activity became more variable and antagonist activity disappeared.

Hadders-Algra and coworkers[21] tested postural responses in sitting on a moveable platform in three groups of children (ages 1½ to 4½ years). One group consisted of 13 preterm infants who had lesions of the periventricular white matter (PWM) of the brain that occurred in the neonatal period. The second group consisted of 13 preterm infants with normal neonatal brain scans, and the third group consisted of 13 healthy children born at term. The children whose history included PWM lesions demonstrated a limited repertoire of response variation to platform movement. Preterm birth was related to a decreased ability to modulate postural responses (eg, higher sensitivity to platform velocity and difficulty modulating electromyogram [EMG] amplitude with respect to the initial sitting position). The authors proposed two hypotheses to account for the differences in postural adjustments between preterm children (without PWM lesions) and age-matched children born at term. One hypothesis was that the neural circuitries producing direction-specific responses are not developed in the preterm infants. The second hypothesis was that sensory pathways may not be sufficiently integrated to elicit activity in the necessary synergies. They noted that variation in development of postural control is important to selection of the most appropriate response pattern.

Brogren and coworkers[22] studied postural adjustments during sitting in either an erect or crouched (eg, forward flexed) position on a movable platform of 10 children (3 to 7½ years of age) with mild-to-severe spastic diplegia and 10 age-matched children without disabilities. Children with severe spastic diplegia exhibited responses that suggested a basic deficit in postural control as well as marked dysfunction in the precise tuning of postural adjustments to task-specific conditions.

In another study using EMGs, muscle responses were recorded from eight children with spastic diplegia (2 to 10 years of age) recovering from balance threats in standing of varying magnitude and velocities.[23] In two control groups of typically developing children (one matched by chronological age and one matched by developmental level), response magnitudes increased as larger and faster perturbations occurred, whereas, in the group of children with cerebral palsy, response magnitudes did not increase. Because there was no difference in muscle onset latency or antagonist co-contraction between the two groups, the authors concluded that the primary constraint on balance recovery in the children with spastic diplegia was insufficient levels of contraction of agonist postural muscles.

Postural Adjustments During Active Movement

Scientists also are studying the development of postural movements or "adjustments" that accompany active movements. Van der Fits and Hadders-Algra[24] discussed reaching movements in adults that are accompanied by complex postural adjustments controlled by spatial, temporal, and quantitative parameters. They studied the development of postural adjustments during reaching over time in infants 3 to 18 months of age when placed in supine and sitting positions. The data suggested that, by 4 months of age, reaching patterns were accompanied by complex postural adjustments with features similar to adults. There was a transient period of less extensive postural activity at 6 to 8 months, the age at which mobility skills such as rolling, sitting up, and crawling develop. In a similar study, Van der Fits et al[25] described two transition periods. The first was at 6 months of age (as previously noted) when postural muscles were infrequently activated during reaching. At 8 months postural activity reappeared and infants were able to adapt postural adjustments to task-specific constraints, such as arm movement velocity or initial sitting position. The second transition occurred at 12 to 15 months. Consistent "anticipatory" postural activity was not present before 15 months, but became consistent after that age, particularly in the neck muscles. Refer to Chapter 12 for more information on the development of reaching.

Anticipatory Postural Movements

Researchers, therefore, are not only examining postural "responses" and postural "adjustments," but also are attempting to define "anticipatory" movements that are essential in feed-forward motor control. For example, the development of anticipatory postural adjustments was studied in children from 4 to 8 years of age in a task that required maintaining the stabilization of forearm position despite imposed or voluntary unloading of the forearm.[26] A clear developmental sequence was noted. First the selection of an efficient EMG pattern underlying forearm stabilization occurred, followed by mastery of timing adjustments. Grasso and coworkers[27] studied the emergence of anticipatory head orienting strategies during goal-directed locomotion in children. Eight children ranging from 3½ to 8 years of age walked along a 90-degree right corner trajectory to reach a goal, both in light and in darkness. The results demonstrated that predictive head orienting movements occurred, even in the youngest children. The authors suggested that feed-forward control of goal-directed locomotion appears very early in the development of gait.

In a study of 64 children (8 to 10 years of age), the performance of 32 children with developmental coordination disorder (DCD) was compared to the performance of 32 typically developing children during a rapid, voluntary, goal-directed arm movement.[28] Children with DCD demonstrated altered activity in postural muscles including early activation of shoulder muscles and postural trunk muscles with anterior trunk muscles demonstrating delayed activation. In children with DCD, anticipatory function was not present in three of the four anterior trunk muscles studied. The authors hypothesized that altered postural muscle activity may contribute to poor proximal stability and poor upper extremity control for goal-directed movement in children with DCD.

Postural Strategies

Scientists have begun to study the development in children of "postural strategies" that have been described in healthy adult subjects.[29,30] One example is an "ankle strategy" (swaying around the ankles with knees and hips extended) that is typically used when perturbations are small and the support surface is firm. In contrast, a "hip strategy" controls the center of mass (COM) by large rapid motions at the hip joints with anti-phase rotations of the ankles. A hip strategy typically is used when larger, faster perturbations are present or when the support surface is compliant or small, such as standing on a foam cushion or a balance beam. With larger perturbations that displace the COM outside the base of support (BOS), a series of steps or hops ("stepping strategy") is used to bring the BOS back into alignment under the COM. Roncesvalles and Woollacott[31] studied the ability to use a step for balance recovery in 25 children between 9 and 19 months of age. New walkers (up to 2 weeks walking experience) used a step infrequently and ineffectively when balance was threatened. Intermediate walkers (1 to 3 months walking experience) showed an increasing tendency to step and a significant improvement in execution as compared to new walkers. Advanced walkers (greater than 3 months walking experience) did not fall during backward support surface translations and were able to maintain balance with their feet in place or by using a step response. The authors concluded that there was a significant developmental transition in the emergence of compensatory stepping with 3 to 6 months of experience being required for an effective step response to develop.

Sensory Processing

Physical therapists are aware of the ongoing contribution of sensory processing to postural control. This is not in the reflex framework of "stimulus-response," where sensory input is considered to evoke reflex movement, but rather in the framework of the role of sensory input in developing and maintaining postural control. The CNS coordinates information from multiple sensory systems in order to produce different motor commands in different sensory environments.[32] Sensorimotor integration consists, therefore, of flexible, dynamic ongoing processes.

Nudo, Friel, and Delia,[33] in a study of ischemic lesions in the hand representation of the primary motor cortex in squirrel monkeys, suggested that the primary motor cortex plays a significant role in somatosensory processing during the execution of motor tasks. They stated that "motor" deficits, previously considered purely motor, may, at least partially, be due to a sensory deficit or "sensory-motor disconnection."

There are developmental changes and maturational processes that occur in sensory systems as well as in motor systems. Sundermier and Woollacott[34] demonstrated that visual cues contribute to or help modulate automatic postural responses of typically developing children who are in the developmental transition to independent walking. Adults rely primarily on somatosensory information for balance control in standing and visual inputs do not appear to contribute significantly (in automatic postural muscle responses of 90 to 100 msecs latency).[29,30] Children at this stage of development, therefore, are much more influenced by visual inputs than adults.

Sensory organization can be evaluated by using a visual enclosure and moveable platform that allows computerized measurements of postural stability and the strategies used to maintain balance. Testing usually is completed in six conditions: 1) eyes open, 2) eyes closed, 3) sway referenced visual surround, 4) sway referenced support surface, 5) eyes closed and sway referenced support surface, and 6) sway referenced support surface and visual surround referenced. Rine, Rubish, and Feeney[35] used this protocol to compare the performance of 23 typically developing children (3½ to 7 years of age) and 11 adults. Results indicated that children demonstrated adult-like use of somatosensory information between 4 to 6 years of age. Measures of vestibular and visual effectiveness in postural control, however, were not similar to adults by 7½ years of age, indicating that sensory integrative mechanisms were still maturing.

Hatzitake and coworkers[36] examined the relationship between specific perceptual and motor skills and static and dynamic balance performance in fifty 11- to 13-year-old typically developing children. Correlation analysis suggested that balancing (one-legged tasks) under static conditions was associated with the ability to perceive and process visual information (suggesting the use of feedback-based control). Under dynamic balancing conditions, however, ability to respond to destabilizing hip abductions-adductions was associated with motor response speed (suggesting use of a descending, feed-forward control strategy). The authors concluded that 11- to 13-year-old children have the ability to select varying balance strategies depending on task constraints.

Nashner et al[37] found that when children with cerebral palsy were asked to balance under changing sensory contexts (eg, eyes closed or with visual or ankle joint cues minimized), they lost their balance more than typically developing children. Children, as well as adults, must have accurate information regarding their position in space as well as the position of their body parts and be able to process this information efficiently for optimal motor control. Because perception is preparatory to movement, sensory functions are an integral part of the examination of children with deficits in motor control. Sensory systems, examination, and intervention strategies are discussed in Chapter 7.

Cognition

Cognitive functions also impact postural control.[38] Cognitive processes involved in attention, memory functions, organization, and sequencing compete with neural processes underlying balance. Deficits in cognitive processes have been identified as increasing the risk of falling and impeding progress in the elderly, as well as in patients with Parkinson's disease, multiple sclerosis, and Alzheimer's disease.[3] Huang and Stemmons[39] reviewed the literature related to dual-task methodology in adults and children, particularly in the areas of gait and postural stability. They suggested that information about how concurrent cognitive tasks influence motor performance in children would help physical therapists design more effective interventions.

Musculoskeletal Considerations

Range of motion must be adequate to allow postural control to occur. Shoulder flexion, extension, and abduction, as well as elbow, wrist, and finger extension, are necessary for upper extremity protective movements. Hip flexion and extension, knee extension, and ankle dorsi- and plantarflexion are needed for appropriate hip or ankle strategies in standing. The child must have sufficient muscle strength to resist the forces of gravity and environmental perturbations.

Woollacott and coworkers[16,17] asked normal children to stand in a crouched posture. This posture caused muscle response patterns to resemble those of children with cerebral palsy. The authors suggested that differences in balance control in children with cerebral palsy are due to both CNS deficits and biomechanical changes in postural alignment. The question is whether biomechanical changes alter motor control strategies or whether deficits in motor control require different postures. For example, Brogren et al[22] found that in children with spastic diplegia a crouched (eg, forward flexed) sitting position during perturbations on a movable platform did not induce postural deficiency but seemed to provide a solution to the sensorimotor problem of instability. The childrens' deficient adaptational capacity to platform perturbations was much more pronounced in an erect posture when compared to a crouched posture. Therefore, the crouched posture may be a functional adaptation that provides improved stability in sitting.

Practice or Experience

The reflex hierarchical model inferred that postural control developed automatically through reflex integration (eg, appearance and disappearance of primitive reflexes and appearance of higher level righting and equilibrium reactions). Some early developmental theorists, such as McGraw,[40] considered the maturation of the CNS to be the single driving force for developmental change. In other words, function emerges from structure. Research has shown that structure also can emerge from function.

Researchers have demonstrated that certain experiences are capable of inducing massive changes in the structure and function of visual, somatic, and motor cortex of otherwise normally reared kittens.[41] These plasticity triggering experiences have been shown to "induce adaptive changes in dendritic trees, dendritic bundles, functional properties of single cells in visual and somatosensory cortex, and even in the shape of the cortical representation of the body surface and motor map."[41] The changes that occur appear to be permanent and result in modifications of the animal's behavior. The brain responds to experience with adaptive changes in its structure, a structure that is initially determined by genetic factors.

Plautz et al[42] demonstrated that repetitive motor behavior during motor learning (not repetitive motor activity alone) produced changes in representational organization of the motor cortex in adult squirrel monkeys. Research with animal models also has shown that learning dependent synaptogenesis can occur within physiologically defined regions of the motor cortex.[43] Rats trained on a skilled reaching task exhibited expansion of wrist and digit movement representations within the motor cortex. Paralleling the physiological changes, trained animals also had more synapses per neuron than control animals within a specific neuronal layer representing the caudal forelimb.

Using functional magnetic resonance imaging, Schaechter and coworkers[44] assessed motor cortical reorganization in four human subjects post-stroke treated with constraint-induced movement therapy (CIMT). Data suggested that motor improvements were associated with a shift in laterality of motor cortical activation toward the undamaged hemisphere. In a similar study, transcranial magnetic stimulation was used to map the motor cortex and positron emission tomography was used to measure changes in motor-related activation.[45] CIMT was provided to patients who were 1 year or more following stroke. Results indicated that, compared to a control group of patients post-stroke who did not receive CIMT, the motor map size increased in the motor cortex of the affected hemisphere.

Byl[46] reviewed brain research that demonstrated that changes in structure and function of the CNS can occur throughout the life span through engaging in highly attended, repetitive, rewarded behaviors. Children also have demonstrated that practice or experience plays a role in developing "automatic" postural responses. Hadders-Algra et al[47] recorded postural responses during sitting on a moveable platform in 20 healthy infants at 5 to 6, 7 to 8, and 9 to 10 months of age. After the first session, parents of nine infants had their child practice sitting daily. During subsequent sessions, it appeared that training (ie, practicing sitting) facilitated response selection during platform perturbations in both forward and backward directions. The authors suggested that this demonstrated a training effect on the first level of the central pattern generator model of control (ie, direction-specific movement patterns) as well as response modulation. Sveistrup and Woollacott[48] studied 15 infants (ages 36 to 48 weeks) who were able to pull themselves into standing, but who were not able to walk independently. The infants were tested using a postural task that required them to stand and balance, with support, following a forward or backward movement of the support surface. One-half of the infants were given intense platform perturbation training on days between test sessions. EMGs of six leg and trunk muscles were recorded during test sessions. The infants who received training demonstrated significant increases in the probability of activating functionally appropriate muscles and in the number of functionally appropriate postural muscles activated in a single trial as compared to the nontrained infants. The authors suggested that during development, selective parameters of the automatic postural response are affected by experience with the postural task. Roncesvalles, Woollacott, and Jensen[49] studied developmental changes in the kinematics and kinetics underlying balance control in 61 children (ages 9 months to 10 years). The children experienced support-surface translations (platform perturbations) of varying size and speed. Children with greater locomotor experience were able to withstand larger threats to their balance without collapsing or stepping. The authors concluded that with increased experience and changing muscle torque regulatory abilities, balance skills became more robust.

Role of "Reflexes"

Now that the hierarchical reflex model has been discarded as the framework for the development of postural control, does that mean children no longer demonstrate a Moro response, primitive stepping, or an asymmetrical tonic neck "reflex"? No, of course not. Early motor behavior has not changed, but how we conceptualize what that motor behavior represents has changed.

Primitive Spinal Cord Reflexes

Consider the "primitive spinal cord reflexes" described in the reflex model. Included in this category are "flexor withdrawal," "positive supporting," "placing," and "stepping."[50] Research over the past 10 years has demonstrated the presence of central pattern generators (CPGs).[51,52] CPGs consist of neurons and interneurons in the spinal cord and brain stem that can spontaneously generate a motor pattern or movement without sensory or higher brain center input. The CPG for stepping has been demonstrated to be located in the spinal cord by many studies of animals. A similar CPG has been proposed to be present in the spinal cord of the human infant. This hypothesis is based on studies of fetal and early infant stepping,[53,54] as well as the ability of children with anencephaly to produce stepping movements.[55] Lamb and Yang[56] examined the idea that the same CPG for locomotion can control different directions of walking in humans. They studied 52 infants (ages 2 to 11 months) who were supported to walk on a treadmill at a variety of speeds. Forward stepping as well as sideways and backward stepping were attempted. The relationships between stance and swing phase durations and cycle duration were the same regardless of the direction of stepping or speed of the treadmill. The authors suggested that the results support the idea that the same locomotor CPG controls different directions of stepping in human infants.

One hypothesis, then, is that many of the movements historically described as "spinal reflexes" are present in a CPG located in the spinal cord and can be elicited through sensory input or used actively by the child for early kicking, supported stepping, and later for independent ambulation. CPGs for stepping, however, are not sufficient to generate a mature gait pattern. Supraspinal influences are necessary for transformation to a normal, mature gait pattern (eg, transition from digitigrade to plantigrade, development of upright balance).[51]

Some of our long-held assumptions regarding primitive reflexes are not supported by empirical studies. For example, one notion has been that precursors to early motor behaviors, such as placing and stepping reflexes, are determinants of fetal presentation at the end of pregnancy. Bartlett et al[57] demonstrated that this is not the case and proposed that spontaneously generated active whole body movements of the fetus may be more significant influences on fetal orientation at the time of birth.

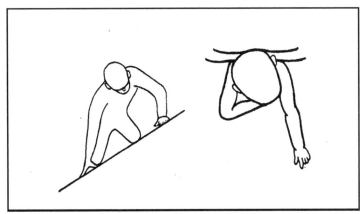

Figure 8-1. The asymmetric tonic neck reflexes (to the right in a child) are the antagonistic partners of the labyrinthine tilting reflexes (to the left). When the head is turned with the nose toward the left, the neck reflex induces extension of the left arm and the right arm flexes. Rapid lateral tilt with the nose to the left, however, causes extension of the right with flexion of the left arm. Labyrinthine tilting reflexes prevent falling during rapid tilt; neck reflexes prevent falling due to labyrinthine reflexes when only the head is moved (reprinted with permission from Kornhuber HH. The vestibular system and the general motor system. In: Kornhuber HH, ed. *Handbook of Sensory Physiology.* Heidelburg, Germany: Springer-Verlag; 1974).

Tonic Neck and Labyrinthine Reflexes

Another example of how we conceptualize what "reflex" patterns represent is how we view tonic neck reflexes and labyrinthine righting reflexes. A close examination of the effects on the extremities of the tonic neck reflexes and the labyrinthine righting reflexes demonstrates that these two postural mechanisms represent exactly opposite changes in postural tone or movement patterns (Figure 8-1).[58] In the classic studies of Magnus and DeKleijn,[59] side-down tilting of decerebrate cats resulted in a decrease in extensor tone of the limbs toward which the chin pointed. In the decerebrate cats without labyrinths, rotation of the head with the body upright resulted in an increase in extensor tone of the limbs toward which the chin rotated. The common description of the asymmetrical tonic neck reflex (ATNR) as producing increased extensor tone on the face side and increased flexor tone on the skull side is not technically correct. A more precise definition would be that increased extensor tone or extensor movement pattern is produced on the face side, and less extensor tone is elicited on the skull side, with resulting flexion.

In phylogenetically early animals that did not have a neck (eg, fish), the vestibular apparatus was sufficient for determining body position. In animals that developed the ability to move the head on the body, vestibular input was no longer sufficient to monitor body position. For example, in Figure 8-2, if the CNS only has information from the labyrinthine receptors, it cannot tell whether the head has moved on the body or the body has moved in space, as the vestibular input is the same. In Condition A, neck receptors inform the CNS that the head has moved on the body (not the body through space). In Condition B, the neck receptors inform the CNS that the head has not moved on the body (therefore, the body must have moved through space). In a normal situation, changes in somatosensory information related to weight shift (or the absence of weight shift) as well as visual information also provide information to the CNS regarding movement of the body, head, and extremities.

Although the role of the ATNR in eye-hand coordination has face validity, the relationship between movements associated with labyrinthine and neck inputs suggests a role in postural control. In 1974, Kornhuber[58] stated that Magnus, who initially described the neck "reflexes," failed to appreciate the functional relationship with labyrinthine

Figure 8-2. If the body is tilted (B) or the head moved on the trunk (A) in the same plane of motion with identical excursion and rate of movement, the labryrinths receive the same stimulus. Information from neck receptors provide the CNS with information to determine whether the body has moved in space or if the head has moved on the body. Body proprioception, signaling the presence or absence of weight-shift, and visual input also contribute to the orientation process (reprinted with permission from

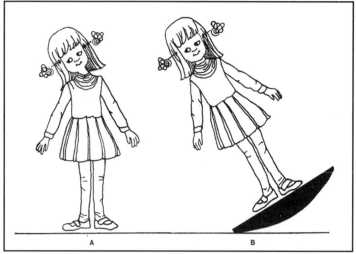

the Haworth Press, Inc. Birmingham, NY. From Montgomery PC. Vestibular processing in children. *Phys Occup Ther Pediatr.* 1985;2/3:33-55).

responses and his erroneous interpretation of the neck reflexes as "static" or "attitudinal" persists.

Anderson and coworkers[60] studied quadruped animal models and stated that movement at low frequencies, as a static position is approached, resulted in predominance of motor output to limb extensors from the neck reflexes, whereas for movement at faster frequencies, labyrinthine reflexes predominated. By monitoring H-reflexes of the lower extremities, Aiello et al[61] studied the interaction of tonic labyrinth and neck reflexes in three healthy adult human subjects to both lateral tilting of the body and neck rotations. Their data indicated that in man, as in animals, labyrinth and neck reflexes are organized reciprocally and contribute equally to postural stabilization.

The human infant learns to differentiate various combinations of head movement on the body in relation to movement of the body in space as he creeps on hands and knees (ie, quadruped). If the infant creeps onto an unstable surface and tips to the left side, increased weight bearing must occur on the down side of the tilt and less weight bearing must occur on the up side of the tilt to prevent a fall. If the infant were to continue to bear weight symmetrically when tipping, he would fall off the unstable surface. If the infant is creeping on a stable surface and turns his head to look to his right, he must bear weight equally on both arms (and not produce asymmetrical weight bearing as on the moveable surface). If the degree of tilt in the first example (unstable surface) results in the same labyrinthine information as active head turning to the right on a stable surface, the infant has to use somatosensory information from the neck receptors (as well as somatosensory information from the extremities and visual input) to determine whether he has moved through space or the head has moved on the body or both.

Locomotion and reaching have been regarded as separate motor tasks. Georgopoulos and Grillner[62] suggested, however, that they may be closely connected both from an evolutionary and neurophysiological perspective. Reaching appears to have evolved from the neural systems responsible for precise positioning of the limb during locomotion (eg, in quadrupeds). These authors suggested that the underlying neural mechanism is organized in the spinal cord. It could be hypothesized that the ATNR represents a CPG or neural circuitry in the spinal cord used during balance and postural control, limb placement, and reaching in animals as well as in humans (in hands and knees positions as well as in upright). Neuromodulatory control pathways from higher brain centers, however, are necessary to enable spinal cord and brain stem circuits to generate meaningful motor patterns.[63]

Reflexes and Medical Diagnosis

Physical therapists who work in neonatal intensive care nurseries or who are responsible for the examination of young infants need to have a working knowledge of early motor responses to sensory stimulation. Reactions to sensory stimulation that, for example, elicit a palmar grasp, rooting reflex, sucking reflex, walking reflex ("stepping"), or Moro and startle responses are used in the neurological assessment of preterm and full-term newborn infants[50,64] and to determine gestational age.[65]

If Moro and startle responses are absent in the neonatal period, it is considered a sign of disordered cerebral function. The persistence (after 6 months of age) of a response that normally "wanes" by 4 months of age (such as palmar grasp) is considered a sign of neurodevelopmental abnormality. Zafeiriou, Tsikoulas, and Kremenopoulos[66] prospectively examined eight primitive reflexes in 204 high-risk infants, of whom 58 developed cerebral palsy, 22 had developmental retardation, and 124 were normal at follow-up examination at 2 years of age. A change in the retention time of the reflexes studied was associated with each category of neurological abnormality on follow-up. Asymmetry in motor responses also can be of diagnostic value.[67] For example, asymmetry in a Moro response may result from a brachial plexus injury or a hemiparesis.

In summary, persistence of early motor patterns is suggestive of pathology to the motor control areas and functions of the CNS. If neuromodulary influences from higher brain centers do not occur during development, motor synergies will not be used efficiently for meaningful movement and early appearing movements will not be modified. If children with cerebral palsy, for example, do not begin to develop typical movement strategies and postural control by 12 to 18 months of age, and early motor patterns persist, it is highly predictive of nonambulation.[68-70]

Development of Postural Control (Nature vs Nurture)

The conceptualization of CPGs varies from "hard-wired" neuronal circuitry to "soft-wired" patterns of movement. Friesen and Cang stated: "experiments of the neuronal basis of animal movements… have demonstrated that central oscillators—termed central pattern generators [CPGs]—are at the core of all rhythmic movements."[71] Another view of CPGs is that the human CNS solves the problem of multiple motor possibilities for postural control through functional organization of basic direction-specific synergies that can be adapted to specific biomechanical constraints.[18,19,72] These direction-specific synergies are variable. For example, studies by Hadders-Algra and coworkers[19,72] of the postural responses of children during sitting on a moveable platform demonstrated more variability in flexor muscle responses to forward translations (backward sway) than in extensor muscle responses to backward translations (forward sway). The authors hypothesized that flexor muscles might be more affected by supraspinal mechanisms as compared to antigravity muscles that might be more dependent on spinal mechanisms, such as stretch reflexes. Other authors also have suggested that flexor control is more dynamic than extensor control.[73]

One model for the development of postural control is Edelman's "neural group selection theory."[74] In this theory, the fundamental step in development of postural control is the generation of genetically predetermined neuronal groups that are not precisely "wired." The second step in development is "tuning" of the innate circuits that are subject to experientially driven selection and mediated by synaptic modifications of the neuronal group response.

Thelen and coworkers[75,76] proposed an alternative view, mainly that self-organization occurs as a result of "learning by doing." They rejected the application of the term CPGs to infant muscle patterns and reviewed evidence that peripheral input can modulate movement patterns at birth. They also cited the high variability and number of possible combinations of movements that infants demonstrate. The dynamic systems approach views postural control as emerging from the interaction of the system's components within a particular task and environmental context.

The debate on the nature vs nurture contributions to motor development is an old one and has not been resolved.[77] Dynamic systems theorists recognize "the fact that infants are born with a species-typical neuronal anatomy, and that this anatomy forms the basis for further epigenetic changes."[76] Theorists adhering to the importance of genetically predetermined repertoires of direction-specific responses acknowledge that "experience plays an obvious role and probably helps to find the best connections among the myriad options provided by genetic information."[47]

Dynamic systems theory suggests that motor development is driven mainly by practice. This has obvious implications for pediatric intervention as physical therapists contribute to decisions regarding what motor behaviors are to be practiced and how children will practice (eg, direct intervention, home programs, community-based activities). On the other hand, it is unclear how amenable the child who has damage to genetic motor programs and CNS structures will be to motor interventions, and, in the presence of pathology, what neural mechanisms are available for achieving postural control. Our knowledge will continue to expand as researchers document ontogenetic changes that occur in the development of postural control, the variables that contribute to this process, the neuroplastic features of the brain, and the effects of various interventions.

Examination and Evaluation Principles

As therapists, we are concerned with at least three aspects of postural control. These are the "responses" that occur to maintain balance following a perturbation (eg, being bumped in a crowd); the postural "adjustments" that occur during active movement; and the "anticipatory" muscle activity that occurs in feed-forward planning of movement. These three functional components of postural control are not, however, proposed to be exclusive and, of course, are interrelated. They are intended to serve as a temporary framework for physical therapy examination, evaluation, and intervention as our understanding of the mechanisms contributing to postural control evolves.

Examination of Righting, Protective, and Equilibrium Reactions

Postural reactions are divided traditionally into three groups: *righting, protective,* and *equilibrium or balancing* reactions. They are not, however, separate distinct entities because they are interdependent and represent interactive subsystems.

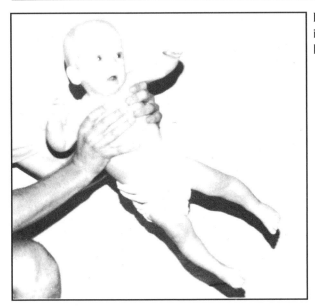

Figure 8-3. Vertical neck righting reaction in infant when suspended upright and tilted laterally.

RIGHTING REACTIONS

Righting reactions orient the head in space so that the eyes and mouth are in a horizontal plane or the body parts are restored to a normal alignment following rotation to any position in space. Righting reactions have been classified according to the receptor stimulated, the proposed regulating area of the brain, or the response given. Righting reactions depend on a number of different stimuli, including visual, vestibular, and somatosensory.

Vertical Righting Reactions

Vertical righting reactions refer to the ability to orient the head to vertical in a number of different positions. If a child is held upright and tilted 30 to 45 degrees in a lateral, anterior, or posterior direction (Figure 8-3), alignment of the head to vertical with the mouth horizontal is the expected response. Maintaining the head in alignment with the body is a partial response. The child should be able to right his head by 2.5 to 6 months of age.[11,78-80] If visual input is eliminated by blindfolding the child, the head still should right to vertical (in response to vestibular and somatosensory input). This response also has been called labyrinthine righting.[11]

Vertical righting reactions in prone occur when the child extends his head. These are present by 1½ to 4 months of age (Figure 8-4).[78,79,81,82] Lifting the head to 45 degrees is considered a partial response. Capital hyperextension frequently is observed in the child with CNS dysfunction. By 3 to 10 months of age, the child should be able to extend his entire trunk and pelvis when suspended in prone so an upward concavity is observed.[79,81] This posture is referred to as the Landau reaction; however, Milani-Comparetti and Gidoni[79] termed the response "body in sagittal plane." The ability to achieve antigravity extension and to display a response to prone suspension is an excellent example of the complex interaction among multiple systems. By 6 months of age, an infant has the cognitive ability to cooperate (or not cooperate) in movement. If the infant is unhappy or tired, he may choose not to extend the body when suspended in prone. An overweight infant may not be able to produce enough muscle force to volitionally lift his body against gravity. In a comprehensive study of 51 low-risk infants, Touwen[81] found that the Landau response was highly inconsistent and a definite developmental sequence could not be established.

Figure 8-4. Head righting reaction in prone position.

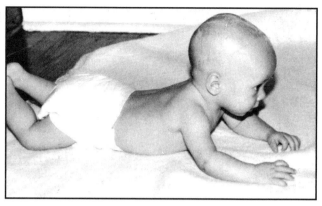

Figure 8-5. Head righting reaction seen in the supine position.

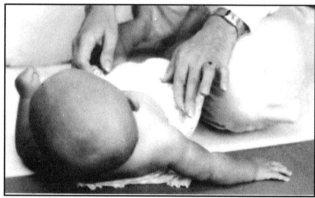

In supine, the child should be able to lift his head from the supporting surface by 5 months of age (Figure 8-5).[79] This is not a frequent spontaneous activity and gently pulling the child up to sitting and observing for chin tuck may be necessary for testing. Haley[78] reported that, when testing in this manner, a complete chin tuck throughout the entire movement did not occur in a sample of infants without disabilities until 8 to 10 months of age.

Head righting also should be present in sidelying and other positions. If the child can sit or stand with proper head positions, it can be assumed the righting reactions have developed and they do not have to be tested.

Rotational Righting Reactions

The rotational righting reactions[83] or body righting reactions[84] have many different, confusing, and contradictory names. It is best to describe the stimulus and response to avoid misleading terminology. The rotational righting reactions restore the body parts to normal alignment following rotation of some body segment. In the neonate, when the head is turned or the leg is flexed and adducted, the infant rotates like a log (nonsegmentally). This nonsegmental roll can be seen as late as 6 to 12 months of age,[11,85] after which it is considered an immature response. A mature response occurs when the head is turned or the leg is flexed and adducted and the child rolls showing distinct rotation between the pelvis and shoulder girdle with head and trunk rotation around the central body axis. Somatosensory input results from asymmetrical body contact, joint proprioception, and muscles stretch, and, as the head turns, vestibular and visual inputs also occur.

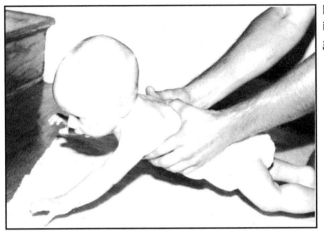

Figure 8-6. Protective reaction when infant is moved forward towards the ground.

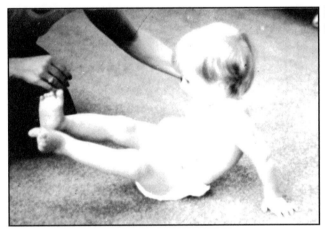

Figure 8-7. Backward protective reaction noted in sitting.

PROTECTIVE REACTIONS

Protective reactions, also called parachute[79] or propping reactions,[86] consist of extension movements of the extremities generally in the same direction of a displacing force that shifts the body's COM past the limits of stability. They can be facilitated by vestibular input caused by movement in space, somatosensory input to the weight bearing skin surfaces or changes in joint angles, and visual or auditory input from the impending displacing force.

Protective reactions can be elicited in many different positions. If the child's body is thrust downward, feet first from the upright vertical position, leg extension and abduction are expected by 4 months of age.[79] If adduction and internal rotation occur, a pathological condition might be suspected. When a child is moved forward toward the ground head first, arm extension and abduction should be observed by 6 to 7 months of age (Figure 8-6).

In sitting, a child can be pushed gently in all directions to facilitate protective reactions of the arms. Protective reactions in sitting are related to experience and are context dependent. It has been suggested that they develop laterally or sideways by ages 6 to 11 months, then forwards, and finally backwards by 9 to 12 months of age (Figure 8-7).[78,79,81] A study by Touwen[81] indicated that lateral protective reactions improved along with a parallel increase in sitting duration.

The amount, speed, and point of application of force, as well as the child's anticipation will affect the protective reaction observed. For example, less force is needed at the shoulder than at the pelvis to shift the COM. If the child anticipates the stimulus, he may prepare his body and an equilibrium reaction might occur instead of a protective reaction. If the speed of the force is too rapid, and there is not enough time for a protective response, a fall will occur. If the speed of the force is too slow, an equilibrium reaction may occur. Facilitating a protective reaction in a child who has already developed equilibrium reactions is difficult. The child usually will employ equilibrium movements initially and only display a protective reaction when pushed past the limits of stability.

EQUILIBRIUM REACTIONS AND BALANCE

Numerous terms have been used to describe the ability of an individual to maintain an upright posture and there has been a distinction between shifts of posture on a stable or unstable BOS. The terms postural fixation or balance have been used to describe reactions on a stable base, where the body moves over the support surface.[82] Equilibrium reactions,[78] tilting reactions,[79] and balance[87] have been used to describe movements on an unstable base of support (eg, tilt board, ball, foam rubber surface, or moving platform) where the supporting surface moves under the body.

Clinical observations consist of noting counter-movements of the head, neck, trunk, or extremities to displacement of the body's COM. The movement generally is in a direction opposite the opposing force, unlike protective reactions that are in the same direction as the force. When pushed or tilted laterally, the response can include a spinal concavity on the side pushed or elevated. Rotation of the upper trunk and head toward midline and counter-rotation of the lower trunk may occur.[83] Extension and abduction of the extremities on the elevated side or side being pushed may occur to help bring the body alignment back to center. Abduction and extension of the extremities on the depressed side or in the direction of a push also might occur in preparation for a protective reaction if the limits of stability are surpassed. When pushed or tilted forward so the anterior support surface is lowered, extension of the legs and trunk occurs. When pushed or tilted in a posterior direction, hip and trunk flexion occur. The amount of flexion or extension will depend on numerous factors, such as the position of the child, the amount of sensory input, and the ability of the child to respond. Reactions also can be tested in diagonal planes and should result in rotational responses. Balance reactions are tested by pushing the child gently while the child is supported on a stable base of support or with the child on an unstable base of support, such as a ball, bolster, moving platform, or adult's lap. Speed of tilt and length of time allowed for a response are important variables that determine the movement patterns observed.

Generally, balance reactions develop on a stable base of support before an unstable base of support in that position. Equilibrium reactions usually occur first in prone (5 to 9 months) (Figure 8-8), then supine (7 to 11 months), sitting (7 to 8 months), quadruped (8 to 12 months), and standing (12 to 21 months).[78,79] Haley[78] suggested that equilibrium reactions in sitting might occur before those in prone and supine. The age of achievement of these reactions is related to the achievement of motor skills in that position and interaction with the environment. Therefore, variability can be expected.

Examination of Postural Adjustments and Anticipatory Movements

Clinical examination of self-initiated components of postural control in children is in its infancy. Most physical therapists do not use EMG or computer-controlled platforms in their examination of pediatric patients. We currently rely on our clinical observation skills

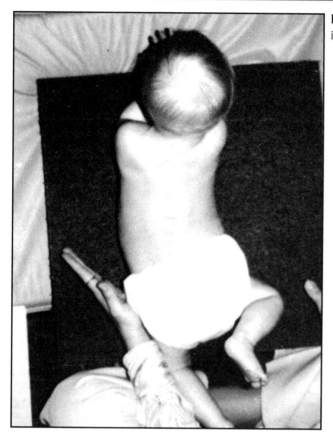

Figure 8-8. Equilibrium reactions seen in prone position.

as we watch children move or attempt to move in various environments to accomplish specific gross and fine motor tasks.

Where do we start? One determinant will be the age and expected motor competency of the child. What we observe and expect in a 3-month-old infant certainly will be different than what we observe and expect in a 3-year-old child. A traditional approach to evaluation of postural control in children has been to examine "static" and "dynamic" balance abilities. Static balance refers to maintaining balance in a specific posture, such as sitting or standing. Maintaining balance while actively moving is categorized as dynamic balance. Westcott et al[88] reviewed current pediatric assessment tools for testing postural control and related areas (eg, sensory processing, biomechanical factors) and stated that few measurements have acceptable documentation of reliability and validity. These authors suggested that one approach to evaluation is to closely examine the child's performance on the sections related to postural control on standardized tests that do have good reliability and validity (see Chapter 2). These test items will help determine the skill level of the child and whether the skill level falls below the expected competency of the child at a specific age. Even if a child is able to accomplish expected motor skills, however, the child still may have problems with postural control. This is especially applicable to children with mild motor delays or DCD who accomplish age-appropriate motor skills, but who are considered "clumsy."

An observational examination of postural control is accomplished by observing the child as he spontaneously moves through his environment, whether this is by rolling, crawling, scooting on his bottom, or walking. Physical therapists usually include an observational analysis in their overall examination of children. In regard to postural control specific observations should be made. Are the child's movements smooth and controlled? Is he steady or unsteady? Can he navigate obstacles in his path? Can the child make transitions in and out of positions with control or does he "fall" into positions assisted by gravity? Can the child maintain his balance in various positions including sitting, all fours, kneeling, and standing? Does the child use active muscle contractions to maintain postures or positions or does he "hang on his ligaments?"

The types of postural strategies used by the child (eg, ankle, hip, or stepping) should be determined. The more strategies the child has available, the more flexibility he has when selecting the most efficient strategy required by various environmental contexts. Some children will rely primarily on one strategy to maintain balance. For example, a child may not be able to "stand still," but can maintain his balance by continually "stepping" or bringing the BOS under his COM. The child who wears static ankle ankle-foot orthoses (AFOs) will be prevented from using an ankle strategy and will have to rely on a hip or stepping strategy to maintain upright balance.

Observing "anticipatory" components of postural control is particularly difficult. Is the child able to lift his arm in sitting, kneeling, or standing without falling or leaning forward? If the child consistently falls forward, he may not be "anticipating" the load of his arm in front of him and is not pre-setting back extensor muscles in anticipation of a load. Can the child stand in place and swing a bat without losing his balance? Does the child demonstrate clumsiness or loss of balance when lifting objects off a table or from the floor?

There may be a cognitive component to postural difficulties. For example, if the child does not accurately judge the anticipated weight of the object to be lifted, he cannot efficiently preset his back extensor muscles in anticipation of counteracting a specific load. Can the child maintain balance when asked to talk or when distracted (eg, cognitive interference)? Can the child imitate unfamiliar positions and maintain his balance (eg, motor planning)?

The therapist should note any additional variables that might impact the child's postural control. For example, what is the health status of the child? Are the child's levels of arousal and attention appropriate for the task? Is the child on any type of medication (eg, antiseizure medication) that might affect arousal states or balance?

Observe the child during daily activities or interview the parents or other caregivers to determine functional anticipatory movements and control. For example, does the child judge the height of curbs and steps to successfully clear the obstacles with his foot without tripping? Can he step on to an escalator or a moving walkway and maintain his balance? In ambulatory children who are considered "clumsy," ask the parent or teacher to describe the specific situations or tasks in which the child is observed to have difficulty.

An observational analysis can be helpful in determining postural control during basic movements such as: rolling, batting at ball from a hands and knees position, putting pellets in a bottle, or completing a pencil and paper task in a sitting position.[89] For example, during rolling, does the child spontaneously lift his head off on the floor in all positions, or does the head touch or remain on the floor (Figure 8-9)? Does the child assume anti-gravity extension when prone and anti-gravity flexion when supine? In a fine motor task while sitting, does the child need to adjust his posture often or does he appear secure during the task? Does the child need to lean on the table to stabilize himself (Figure 8-10)? Are extraneous, nonessential movements obvious during the task? Does the child use the optimal upper extremity positions and control for the fine motor task?

Because it is difficult to simultaneously direct the child, observe, and record performance, videotaping may be used to provide a permanent record that can be replayed and

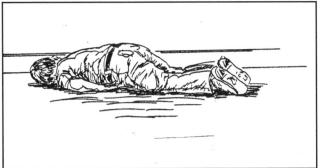

Figure 8-9. TASK: Rolling. SCORING: (Key: 1 =most atypical performance; 5=typical performance). *Head righting*: Score (1) head touches floor in prone. *Antigravity extension*: Score (1) flexed posture when prone (hips, knees, arms) (reprinted with permission from Richter EW, Montgomery PC. *Sensorimotor Performance Analysis.* Hugo, Minn: PDP Press; 1989:97-133).

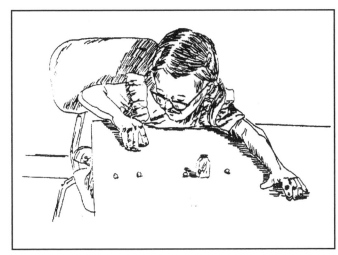

Figure 8-10. TASK: Pellets in bottle. SCORING: (Key: 1 =most atypical performance; 5=typical performance). *Trunk stability*: Score (1) leans on table. *Head position*: Scores (3) rotates; (3) flexed-eyes close to table. *Grasp adequate for age*: Score (5). *Changes hands at midline*: Score (1). *Inconsistent hand usage*: Score (1) (reprinted with permission from Richter EW, Montgomery PC. *Sensorimotor Performance Analysis.* Hugo, Minn: PDP Press; 1989:97-133).

objectively graded. An area of research that will be particularly helpful to physical therapists as we evaluate and treat children is to determine the correlation between clinical observations of postural control and quantitative analyses through the use of EMG recordings of muscle activity and sophisticated methods of measuring activity of the CNS. It is important to determine if our clinical observations and inferences regarding motor control are accurate and correct.

Intervention Considerations

Treatment of children with deficits in postural control and balance is very complex. Multiple systems are involved and each system may need to be addressed directly and then as part of an interaction of several systems to achieve functional outcomes.

Figure 8-11 outlines some of the areas to be considered in physical therapy intervention. These have been discussed previously in this chapter and include sensory processing, cognitive functions, musculoskeletal considerations, and practice and experience. In addition, other issues may become evident during the examination process. For example, the child may have generally poor health and be deconditioned. Deconditioning frequently is present in children with chronic health problems or after recovery from long illnesses or surgery. If necessary, a reconditioning program similar to that used for any deconditioned child should be implemented.

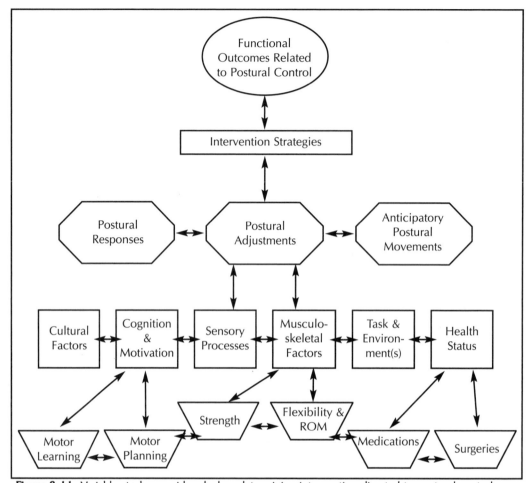

Figure 8-11. Variables to be considered when determining intervention directed to postural control.

The child's emotional and arousal state should be considered. An active alert state is best to participate in and benefit from intervention. The inability to perform a movement must be distinguished from refusal. Children who are "posturally insecure" and fearful may be hesitant to participate in movement-based activities, therefore, activities need to be presented in a non-threatening manner. Generally it is best to start intervention with activities where the child perceives he is "safe" and where he will have some success. Activities can be gradually increased in complexity relative to various requirements of postural control.

Principles of motor learning should be incorporated into sessions (see Chapter 3). The therapist needs to determine the target behavior, how frequently it will be practiced, and how frequently the child will be provided with knowledge of results. A systems approach suggests that the therapist needs to consider the environments and materials used during treatment. Practice of specific daily functional tasks needed by the child in his normal environments should be a primary consideration in treatment. Practice should occur in each of the environments with different materials and different individuals, so that generalization of the task can be achieved. Similarly, the percentage of time spent practicing postural responses to perturbations (such as being tilted on a therapy ball) should be

Table 8-1
Activities to Promote Various Postural Strategies

Ankle Strategy

➤ In standing, with hips and knees straight, raise both arms slowly up in front of body and hold 5 seconds, return arms to sides; extend both arms slowly behind body and hold 5 seconds, return arms to sides

➤ In standing, with hips and knees straight, "sway" like trees in a breeze (forward/ backward) or "dance/sway" to music

➤ Standing on tiltboard with hips and knees straight, sway forward and backward very slowly

Hip Strategy

➤ Balance on tiptoes

➤ Walk forward and backward on tiptoes—stop on verbal command and maintain balance

➤ Walk on narrow balance beam or 4-inch wide elastic band placed on floor (pretend you are walking a "tightrope" in the circus)—start and stop on verbal command without stepping off beam or band

Stepping Strategy

➤ March to music (forward, backward, sideways)

➤ Twirl to the left three times, then twirl to the right three times—vary speed

➤ Walk on uneven terrain outside (eg, grass, gravel, pea rock)

Hip and Stepping Strategies

➤ In standing on a tiltboard, tip board faster until hip or stepping strategy demonstrated

➤ Play "statue" or "freeze" (ie, child moves spontaneously then attempts to maintain his posture when the adult says "freeze")

➤ Bounce ball to child outside his base of support

small in comparison to the practice of postural adjustments and anticipatory postural control needed during active movement (such as lifting the arm to reach for a toy while seated on a bench or swinging a bat at a suspended ball). This reflects the relative amount of time during the day the child reacts to perturbations vs the amount of time active movement is attempted.

Specific activities can be used, for example, to facilitate different postural strategies (Table 8-1). Examples of general intervention strategies for improving various aspects of postural control and specific treatment techniques are provided in the following case studies.

Case Study #1: Jason

➤ Practice pattern 5C: Impaired Motor Function and Sensory Integrity Associated With Nonprogressive Disorders of the Central Nervous System—Congenital Origin or Acquired in Infancy or Childhood

➤ Medical diagnosis: Cerebral palsy, right hemiparesis
➤ Age: 24 months

Examination and Evaluation

POSTURAL RESPONSES TO PERTURBATION

➤ Righting reactions: Jason rights his head in all planes
➤ Protective reactions: In sitting, Jason has left anterior, lateral, and posterior protective reactions in response to tilt. The right arm initiates movement in response to tilt forward and sideward, but without full extension and weight bearing. The right arm does not respond effectively when Jason is tilted backward
➤ Equilibrium reactions: In sitting and standing when his balance is perturbed, left trunk musculature appears to respond appropriately, but trunk movement on the right is delayed or absent. Jason tends to use a protective stepping reaction. This response is not consistent and he often falls. He is more successful maintaining his balance during slow tilt

POSTURAL CONTROL DURING ACTIVE MOVEMENT

➤ Mobility skills: Jason rolls easily on the floor and pushes up on all fours. He can creep on all fours, but does not fully bear weight on the right arm. He can assume standing independently from the middle of the floor and walks independently. He attempts to runs, but is unsteady and falls frequently
➤ Transitions: Jason transitions independently from sitting on the floor to quadruped or kneeling positions. He can assume a bear-stance to move into standing. Some unsteadiness is noted in transitions, but Jason is generally successful and does not lose his balance
➤ Fine motor skills: Jason has more difficulty maintaining his balance in sitting when lifting or manipulating objects and in standing when lifting or carrying objects. When attempting to lift heavy objects, he does not appear able to anticipate the load he needs to counteract, and he tends to fall forward

FUNCTIONAL LIMITATIONS

Jason has difficulty bearing weight on and balancing on his right leg to shift his weight or to turn to his right. For example, when "dancing" to music he leans to the left and circles to his left, but does not circle to his right. He falls frequently during the day, especially when trying to walk rapidly or run. When he falls forward or to his left side he effectively uses his left arm to catch or protect himself. He does not use his right arm effectively to catch himself when falling toward his right side, often bumping his head against the wall or objects. He often assumes an asymmetrical posture when playing with toys, leaning and orienting toward his left side, and has difficulty playing with toys that require bilateral hand use.

IMPAIRMENTS

Jason demonstrates weakness and poor motor control of his right extremities, especially the right upper extremity. He appears to have a mild disregard for the right side of his body and the right side of space, tending to use the left side of his body for motor tasks and to orient objects to the left side of space. He demonstrates tightness in the muscles of the right upper extremity and in the right hip muscles and lateral trunk flexors. His balance reactions in sitting and standing are adequate to slow tilt or mild perturbations but are too slow to be effective during rapid tilt or perturbations. Postural adjustments also appear adequate during slow active movements, but are less efficient during rapid active movements or when lifting, carrying, or manipulating objects.

GOALS

Treatment goals are for Jason to:

1. Increase strength of right upper and lower extremities
2. Improve standing balance
3. Increase frequency of orienting to the right side of space
4. Increase range of motion of right extremities and trunk
5. Improve protective reactions of the right upper extremity

FUNCTIONAL OUTCOMES

Following 3 months of intervention, Jason will:

1. Be able to play leapfrog bearing weight on both extremities for several seconds
2. Walk up and down three to five steps, holding on to a railing, using a reciprocal pattern
3. Decrease the number of falls from 10 times to two to three times daily
4. Spontaneously position toys at midline or slightly to the right side of the body during play, two of five trials
5. Attempt to extend the right upper extremity when losing his balance or falling toward his right side three of five occurrences

Intervention

Strengthening activities (Goal #1) can include practicing "wheelbarrowing" with adult assist. Using both arms to push open doors or to push against resistance offered by an adult or object (eg, pushing over a bench, pushing a chair across the kitchen floor) may improve elbow extension, shoulder protraction, and general upper extremity strength. In quadruped Jason can be encouraged to bear weight equally on both extended arms. He can be encouraged to shift his weight onto the right arm and attempt to bat a suspended balloon or reach for a toy with the left arm.

Supporting the body by leaning with both arms on a bench or holding an adult's hands while trying to do one leg knee bends is an example of a lower extremity strengthening activity. Reciprocal stair climbing and descent with assistance for balance also will improve strength and weight shift onto the right leg (Goals #1 and #2). Using small Velcro weight cuffs (eg, 1 pound) around the wrists or ankles during "weight-lifting" games can be used to improve strength and increase proprioceptive input.

Walking and attempting to run on uneven terrain outside as well as slight inclines will improve upright balance control (Goal #2). Walking straddling a 4-inch wide elastic band laid flat on the floor or a 2" x 4" board placed on the ground will facilitate a weight shift to the right side (Goals #2 and #3). Placing paper footsteps on the carpet or making footsteps with chalk on the sidewalk can be used to try to get Jason to shift his weight to the right leg. Placing toys or the television at midline and eventually to the right side of his body will help Jason orient to that side of space (Goal #3).

To increase range of motion (Goal #4), passive mobility activities such as placing Jason in sidelying and gently rotating the pelvis and shoulders in opposite directions can be done. Since Jason has tight right hip and lateral trunk flexors, active right hip extension and lateral trunk flexion to the left should be encouraged. "Swimming" prone over a bolster or reaching for a suspended toy with the left arm while sidelying on the right can be tried.

Playing games in sitting (eg, "rocking boat" on sofa cushion) and standing (eg, "dancing" to music) that require increased weight shifts will provide practice with losing his balance and catching himself effectively (Goal #5). Activities specific to improving equilibrium on an unstable base might include prone on a scooter, use of a vestibular board, therapy ball, or seesaw. The therapist will have to structure activities to emphasize falling to the right to promote active participation of the right upper extremity.

Case Study #2: Jill

➤ Practice pattern 5C: Impaired Motor Function and Sensory Integrity Associated With Nonprogressive Disorders of the Central Nervous System—Congenital Origin or Acquired in Infancy or Childhood

➤ Medical diagnosis: Cerebral palsy, spastic quadriparesis, microcephaly, mental retardation, seizure disorder

➤ Age: 7 years

Examination and Evaluation

POSTURAL RESPONSES TO PERTURBATION

➤ Righting reactions: Jill can maintain her head in neutral when held vertical. However, she cannot right her head when tilted more than 30 degrees from upright. She raises her head momentarily in prone, but not in supine

➤ Protective reactions: Protective reactions of the extremities are not present in response to imposed movement in any position

➤ Equilibrium reactions: These reactions are not present in response to imposed movement in any position

POSTURAL CONTROL DURING ACTIVE MOVEMENT

➤ Mobility skills: Jill can shift her position when lying on the floor and rolls from supine to sidelying. She is unable to maintain her balance in any position (eg, sitting, all fours, kneeling, standing)

➤ Transitions: Jill does not make any independent transitions of movement between positions. She is able to assist in standing pivot transfers by momentarily bearing weight on her legs

➤ Fine motor skills: Jill attempts to grasp, but her hand often closes involuntarily prior to obtaining an object. She cannot manipulate objects with her fingers

FUNCTIONAL LIMITATIONS:

Jill has not developed functional balance or postural control in any position (eg, sitting, kneeling, all fours, standing). She has poor head control and needs maximal support in all positions, either through adult assistance or through the use of adaptive equipment (eg, wheelchair, stander).

IMPAIRMENTS

Jill has a severely compromised motor control system as a result of pathology involving her CNS, including a seizure disorder and microcephaly. She does not demonstrate balance or protective reactions to passive tilt or actively during attempts to move. She has generalized stiffness in her extremities and trunk with associated tightness, especially in the end excursions of joint range of motion. Jill has severe mental retardation that often limits her ability to understand and cooperate during motor activities. In addition, she often is lethargic and during those times active movement appears to be more difficult and fatiguing. The periods of decreased arousal may be associated with her antiseizure medications.

GOALS

Treatment goals are for Jill to:

1. Maintain current range of motion
2. Maintain ability to bear weight in standing
3. Achieve adequate trunk support for stability in sitting and standing through proper positioning and adaptive equipment
4. Improve head control in supported sitting and during caregiver handling

FUNCTIONAL OUTCOMES

Following 3 months of intervention, Jill will:

1. Maintain range of motion to be comfortable in her wheelchair and stander and while positioned prone on the floor
2. Maintain standing balance for 3 to 5 seconds to assist in standing pivot transfers
3. Maintain upright head control for 5 minutes in supported sitting during a classroom activity
4. Right and maintain her head in vertical when being lifted or carried as part of her daily care at home and school

Intervention

Jill has a school and home schedule of positioning that is designed to maintain her range of motion (Goal #1). This includes being in her prone stander and lying prone on the floor to maintain hip and knee extension. When in prone she is assisted in bringing her arms up over her head to maintain forward flexion and external rotation of her shoulders as well as elbow extension. During some classroom activities she long sits on the floor with support from a classroom aide (eg, leaning back against the adult). At home her family places her in her wheelchair for 15 minutes each evening with her legs in extension and propped on a footstool. Both activities assist in maintaining range of motion of the hamstrings and extension of the knee joint.

Part of Jill's daily routine at home and school is to assist in standing pivot transfers (Goal #2). She currently has a well-fitting seat insert for her wheelchair and a lap tray which positions her well for classroom activities (Goal #3).

Because Jill has some head control in an upright position, she is provided opportunities throughout the day to actively control her head position (Goal #4). For example, Jill is placed astride the adult's lap, and while proper support is given to the trunk, a vertical head position and active contraction of the cervical muscles are encouraged. Jill is most successful when working at the end of the range near sitting, where gravity offers the least resistance. Slowly moving in a small arc of motion in supported sitting encourages both concentric and eccentric muscle contractions. In supported sitting, either in a chair, rocking chair, or on an adult's lap, Jill is tilted from side to side and forward and back. The adult usually starts with 5 to 10 degrees of slow tilt, giving adequate time for a response. If no response occurs, Jill's head is positioned and a holding contraction required. Progression to larger degrees of tilt and more rapid movement can occur. It is helpful to make this activity more fun and meaningful by having her look out a window or in a mirror.

Case Study #3: Taylor

➤ Practice pattern 5C: Impaired Motor Function and Sensory Integrity Associated With Nonprogressive Disorders of the Central Nervous System—Congenital Origin or Acquired in Infancy or Childhood

➤ Medical diagnosis: Myelomeningocele, repaired L1-2

➤ Age: 4 years

Examination and Evaluation

POSTURAL RESPONSES TO PERTURBATIONS

➤ Righting reactions: Taylor rights his head in all directions when tilted in sitting and in a supported upright position (held by an adult)

➤ Protective reactions: All upper extremity protective reactions in sitting are present to passive tilt. Standing reactions are not testable

➤ Equilibrium reactions: In prone and supine, on a stable and unstable base of support, the upper trunk response to tilt is present. In sitting, the upper trunk response also is present, however, the quality of the response is poor. Taylor responds slowly to tilt and frequently has insufficient muscle strength or endurance to maintain an upright posture without reverting to a protective response. Equilibrium reactions were not tested in standing

POSTURAL CONTROL DURING ACTIVE MOVEMENT

➤ Mobility skills: Taylor can roll consecutively, sit with good balance, and attempts to pull to kneeling. He tends to "hang on his ligaments" rather than use active muscle contractions to maintain his posture. He uses his arms to pull and belly crawl or to "scoot " on his bottom

➤ Transitions: Taylor is able to get in and out of sitting and into an all-fours position independently. He is working on transitions from his wheelchair, such as on and off a classroom chair and on and off the toilet. In these transitions, he demonstrates trunk instability and frequent loss of balance

➤ Fine motor skills: Taylor has normal grasp, manipulation, and release. He has difficulty manipulating large or heavy objects due to difficulty in stabilizing his trunk

FUNCTIONAL LIMITATIONS

Taylor cannot walk independently, but uses an anterior walker and a parapodium. He also has begun practicing standing balance wearing a reciprocal gait orthosis (RGO) and using forearm crutches. He has good independent sitting balance. When reaching for objects outside his base of support, however, he tends to fall. If he falls to the side in sitting, he usually catches himself with his arms and returns to sitting. When he loses his balance in standing in his parapodium or with crutches he does not use his arms effectively to catch himself. His balance during transitions in and out of his wheelchair and on and off classroom chairs or toilet are precarious and he needs moderate assistance for safety.

IMPAIRMENTS

Taylor has loss of motor and sensory function in his lower extremities secondary to his myelomeningocele. He has poor active trunk extension and demonstrates generalized weakness in his arms and trunk. Balance reactions to passive tilt in sitting and supported standing are slow. Taylor has visual-perceptual problems, particularly figureground discrimination. In addition, when he bends his head to look at the floor his balance often is disturbed.

GOALS

Treatment goals are for Taylor to:

1. Increase strength in trunk and upper extremities
2. Increase independence in transfers
3. Improve balance in standing with walker
4. Improve balance in sitting.
5. Decrease sensitivity to head bending in standing
6. Increase endurance for ambulation with his walker
7. Improve protective reactions in standing

FUNCTIONAL OUTCOMES

Following 3 months of intervention, Taylor will:

1. Independently lift his body weight with his arms during transfers
2. Transfer in and out of his wheelchair to a classroom chair with minimal assist
3. Lean laterally to either side in his parapodium (with walker) and correct his balance without assistance
4. In sitting, reach laterally to the limits of his base of stability for an object without using a protective reaction
5. Use his walker and follow a visual pattern (trail) on the floor without becoming unsteady or losing his balance
6. Walk around the classroom area intermittently with his walker for 10 to 20 minutes without fatiguing
7. From standing, actively fall forward on a 3-inch mat and catch himself with his arms without hitting his head on the mat

Intervention

General upper extremity strengthening activities such as prone push-ups and wheelchair push-ups can be included in Taylor's program (Goal #1). Using small weights, pulleys, or elastic bands for upper extremity strengthening would add variety to his program. Active trunk extension in prone, upper trunk flexion in supine, and lateral flexion in sidelying should be incorporated for trunk strengthening. These anti-gravity movements will help increase muscular endurance in those muscles necessary for equilibrium movements. Once Taylor can perform these antigravity movements, resistance can be added and diagonal patterns encouraged.

Taylor should practice a variety of transfers at home and at school (Goal #2) to improve his efficiency and independence. Moderate assistance should be gradually lessened to minimal assistance, and, eventually, to standby assist for safety.

In standing with his parapodium, Taylor could practice reaching outside his base of support as far as possible for objects (Goal #3). Swaying in standing or "dancing" would also improve his balance. When in sitting, he should be encouraged to reach for toys placed on the floor and hung at ear level in an area around his body (Goal #4). When he reaches for a toy, resistance can be provided either by using elastic bands attached to the hanging toys or using heavy toys on the floor. Goals #3 and #4 also can be addressed by having Taylor respond to tilt on an unstable base of support, such as a ball. Tilting could be done in prone and supine to strengthen trunk muscles as well as in sitting. In addition to anterior, posterior, and lateral tilting, diagonal tilting should be provided.

Repetitive head bending in standing should be done to tolerance to try to habituate Taylor to the visual and vestibular inputs (Goal #5) that occur. Activities that require him to look down while walking, such as following a pattern on the floor, should help him accommodate to the sensory input. As part of his classroom routine, Taylor should be encouraged to use his walker for longer periods of time (Goal #6). In addition to using the walker in his classroom, moving to other areas in the school (eg, to the cafeteria or music room) should be gradually added to his routine. Taylor would benefit from specific activities to help him develop the ability to catch himself when he falls (Goal #7). Controlled (by an adult) falls from standing will give him experience with these movements and the upper extremity responses that he needs to produce for protection. Eventually, he should be able to rock, fall forward on his own, and catch himself.

Case Study #4: Ashley

➤ Practice pattern 5B: Impaired Neuromotor Development
➤ Medical diagnosis: Down syndrome
➤ Age: 15 months

Examination and Evaluation

POSTURAL RESPONSES TO PERTURBATION

➤ Righting reactions: All vertical and rotational reactions are present
➤ Protective reactions: In sitting, Ashley has anterior and lateral responses, but an inconsistent response to tilt in a posterior direction. All of her protective reactions are slow
➤ Equilibrium reactions: Equilibrium responses are present in prone and supine on a stable base of support. In sitting, anterior and posterior responses are present, but lateral equilibrium responses are delayed. Ashley was too fearful to permit testing in all fours or standing or on an unstable base of support

POSTURAL CONTROL DURING ACTIVE MOVEMENT

➤ Mobility skills: Ashley can roll, sit independently, creep on hands and knees, pull to kneeling, and pull to stand. She does not cruise at furniture and does not walk independently. In standing she has a wide base of support with lumbar lordosis, knee hyperextension, and foot pronation. She does not use active muscle contraction to maintain her posture, but "hangs on her ligaments"

➤ Transitions: Ashley transitions in and out of sitting and in and out of a hands and knees position. She uses straight plane movements without trunk rotation. She is unsteady, particularly when trying to move quickly

➤ Fine motor skills: Ashley grasps objects but does not have controlled release. She has difficulty manipulating small objects and will not attempt to lift or manipulate heavy objects

FUNCTIONAL LIMITATIONS

Ashley has achieved some basic motor skills such as sitting, creeping on hands and knees, and pulling to stand. However, she is unsteady in all positions and easily loses her balance when perturbed or when she moves quickly or becomes distracted. When she loses her balance she tries to correct her position using her head, trunk, and extremities. Her attempts to right herself often are too slow to be effective. Protective reactions of the arms and legs also are noted with loss of balance, but she tends to rigidly lock her extremities and becomes upset if she falls. She avoids interacting during gross motor activities with her peers, especially if they are moving quickly around her. When seated at a small table, Ashley tends to lean on the table with her arms. She has difficulty maintaining an erect trunk position for more than 1 to 2 minutes to free both hands to play with toys.

IMPAIRMENTS

Ashley has low muscle tone and joint hypermobility. She appears to have difficulty stabilizing her joints when in weight bearing positions. She tends to move slowly and is fearful about participating in movement activities. She has slow protective and balance reactions. Ashley is a passive child and is not physically active unless encouraged or assisted by an adult. She appears to have generalized weakness and poor endurance for gross motor activities. Ashley has a general developmental delay, including cognitive and language deficits, associated with her diagnosis of Down syndrome.

GOALS

Treatment goals are for Ashley to:

1. Increase strength of trunk and extremities
2. Improve balance in all positions (sitting, all fours, kneeling, standing)
3. Improve protective responses
4. Increase physical activity level
5. Decrease fear of movement and falling

FUNCTIONAL OUTCOMES

Following 3 months of intervention, Ashley will:

1. Maintain her balance in sitting when passively tipped or tilted 30 degrees to the left or right

2. Maintain her balance in all fours when slightly perturbed at the hip or shoulder

3. Be able to reach laterally for a toy while on all fours without loss of balance

4. Begin to cruise three to four steps to the left or right

5. Move around her parent-infant classroom (any method) to obtain a toy without prompting or assist from an adult

6. Respond positively to being swung in a playground swing or sliding down a small incline

Intervention

The therapist works with the classroom teacher and parent to determine what movement activities Ashley will tolerate. Examples may be repetitive tilting while sitting on an adult's lap, slowly progressing to using a therapy ball or bolster to encourage trunk activity and strengthening (eg, abdominal muscles, back extensors) (Goal #1). Playing tug of war with elastic bands and batting and kicking at a suspended balloon will help increase extremity strength.

Ashley's classroom has a small waterbed mattress in the play area. This is a safe environment to have Ashley work on her balance skills (Goal #2) by having her sit, creep on all fours, and attempt to kneel on the waterbed. If she falls she will not be injured and may begin to enjoy movement and learn to use her extremities and trunk more effectively for controlling her balance and using protective responses (Goals #2 and #3). Favorite toys or rewards could be used to motivate her to move independently (Goal #4). Games, such as "chasing" her on hands and knees, might motivate her to move more and faster.

The play area also has a small playground set which includes a swing and slide. Ashley should be assisted in swinging and sliding to her tolerance (Goal #5). Her family should be encouraged to assist Ashley in participating in movement-based activities at home, such as being held by an adult while the adult "dances," "sways," "bounces," and "turns in circles." A small rocking chair can be used to encourage Ashley to move herself in a controlled, non-threatening activity and can be used in both the home and school environments.

Case Study #5: John

➤ Practice pattern 5B: Impaired Neuromotor Development

➤ Medical diagnosis: Attention deficit hyperactivity disorder, developmental coordination disorder

➤ Age: 5 years

Examination and Evaluation

Postural Responses to Perturbation

➤ Righting reactions: John rights his head in all directions in all positions tested (ie, sitting on ball, tilting in hands and knees, kneeling, and standing on a vestibular board

➤ Protective reactions: John demonstrates protective reactions in all positions tested

➤ Equilibrium reactions: John demonstrates equilibrium reactions in all positions tested

Postural Control During Active Movement

➤ Mobility skills: John ambulates independently, but is described as being "clumsy." He has difficulty with age-appropriate motor skills, such as running, hopping, skipping, and riding a bicycle. John appears to have difficulty doing two things at once, such as participating in a motor activity while talking

➤ Transitions: John is independent in transitions of movement, although he demonstrates some slowness and incoordination with higher-level transition skills, such as moving on and off playground equipment

➤ Fine motor skills: John has difficulty with "tool use" (eg, pencils, knife, and fork). His is independent in dressing, but has difficulty with buttons, snaps, and zippers. When carrying large or heavy objects, he more frequently bumps into furniture or walls

Functional Limitations

John demonstrates poor motor coordination as compared to other children his chronological age. He has difficulty with motor skills such as bike riding (eg, still must use training wheels). He demonstrates incoordination and poor endurance for play activities such as jumping rope, skipping, ball games, and performing "jumping jacks." He avoids physical play and games with his peers. John is clumsy and often bumps into environmental objects or people.

Impairments

John easily becomes frustrated when trying to learn new motor skills. He has a poor attention span and is very distractible. He tends not to stick with a task long enough to perform enough repetitions to improve his performance. He also fatigues quickly when participating in gross motor activities. Upper extremity strength is decreased as compared to other children his age.

Goals

Treatment goals are for John to:

1. Increase overall strength
2. Increase endurance for motor activities
3. Improve balance and coordination during gross motor activities and walking
4. Improve eye-hand coordination in conjunction with balance activities

Functional Outcomes

Following 3 months of intervention, John will:

1. Be able to complete five prone push-ups
2. Ride his bike (with training wheels) for 5 miles during family bike trips
3. Perform three repetitions of jumping jacks, one of three attempts
4. Walk in a crowded environment (eg, mall, grocery store) without bumping into objects or people
5. Catch and throw a tennis ball from a kneeling or standing position, seven of 10 trials

Intervention

John's family will carry out a home program designed to improve his overall strength, endurance, and coordination. Family activities, such as bike riding, playing tag, and participating in school activities, such as soccer and T-ball, will encourage John's participation (Goals #1 and #2). The physical therapist also should suggest appropriate community activities for John. For example, the family could investigate having John participate in a "Karate for Kids" class to improve his strength, endurance, and motor control. In addition, John can accompany his father to the local health club and work with small weights as his father does strength training.

Cognitive strategies can be used to assist John in remembering to walk slower and pay attention to his environment (Goal #3). He can practice walking around the local playground on various terrains (eg, sand, gravel, grass) with environmental objects (eg, swings, slide, merry-go-round) to navigate. This activity can be increased in complexity by having John carry objects of various sizes and weights and by having him talk while walking. John's father can work with him on throwing and catching balls of different sizes and weights as John usually is motivated to do activities when his father participates (Goal #4). The physical therapist will monitor John's motor program and progress, adapting or adding activities as John improves his motor skills.

Communication and coordination of services should occur between school and private therapists. If John does not qualify for school physical therapy services, the private physical therapist should try to coordinate services with his physical education and classroom teachers.

References

1. McCollum G, Leen T. Form and exploration of mechanical stability limits in erect stance. *J Motor Beh*. 1989;21:225-238.

2. Horak FB. Assumptions underlying motor control for neurological rehabilitation. In: Lister M, ed. *Contemporary Management of Motor Control Problems. Proceedings of the II STEP Conference*. Alexandria, Va: Foundation for Physical Therapy; 1991:11-27.

3. Seeger MA. Balance deficits: examination, evaluation, and intervention. In: Montgomery PC, Connolly BH, eds. *Clinical Applications of Motor Control*. Thorofare, NJ: SLACK Incorporated; 2002:271-307.

4. Shumway-Cook A, Woollacott MH. *Motor Control: Theory and Practical Application*. 2nd ed. Philadelphia, Pa: Lippincott,Williams & Wilkins; 2001.

5. Semans S. The Bobath concept in treatment of neurological disorders. *Am J Phys Med*. 1967;46:732-788.

6. Stockmeyers SA. An interpretation of the approach of Rood to the treatment of neuromuscular dysfunction. *Am J Phys Med*. 1967;46:900-961.

7. Perry CE. Principles and techniques of the Brunnstrom approach to the treatment of hemiplegia. *Am J Phys Med*. 1967;46:789-815.

8. Voss DE. Proprioceptive neuromuscular facilitation. *Am J Phys Med*. 1967;46:838-899.

9. NUSTEP. *Northwestern University Special Therapeutic Exercise Project*. Baltimore, Md: The Waverly Press; 1967.

10. Payton OD, Hirt S, Newton RA. *Neurophysiologic Approaches to Therapeutic Exercise: An Anthology*. Philadelphia, Pa: FA Davis; 1977.

11. Fiorentino MR. *Reflex Testing Methods for Evaluating CNS Development*. Springfield, Ill: Charles C. Thomas; 1963.

12. Lister M. *Contemporary Management of Motor Control Problems: Proceedings of the II STEP Conference.* Alexandria, Va: Foundation for Physical Therapy; 1991.

13. Newton RA. Neural systems underlying motor control. In: Montgomery PC, Connolly, BH, eds. *Clinical Applications of Motor Control.* Thorofare, NJ: SLACK Incorporated; 2002:53-77.

14. Hikosaka O. Neural systems for control of voluntary action—a hypothesis. *Adv Biophys.* 1998;35:81-102.

15. Gesell A. The ontogenesis of infant behavior. In: Carmichael L, ed. *Manual of Child Psychology.* 2nd ed. New York, NY: John Wiley & Sons; 1954:335-373.

16. Woollacott MH, Burtner P. Neural and musculoskeletal contributions to the development of stance balance control in typical children and in children with cerebral palsy. *Acta Paediatr Suppl.* 1996;416:58-62.

17. Woollacott MH, Burtner P, Jensen J, et al. Development of postural responses during standing in healthy children and children with spastic diplegia. *Neurosci Biobehav Rev.* 1998;22:583-589.

18. Forssberg H, Hirschfeld H. Postural adjustments in sitting humans following external perturbations: muscle activity and kinematics. *Exp Brain Res.* 1994;97:515-527.

19. Hadders-Algra M, Brogren E, Forssberg H. Ontogeny of postural adjustments during sitting in infancy: variations, selection, and modulation. *J Physiol.* 1996;493:273-288.

20. Hadders-Algra M, Brogren E, Forssberg H. Postural adjustments during sitting at preschool age: presence of a transient toddling phase. *Dev Med Child Neurol.* 1998;40:436-447.

21. Hadders-Algra M, Brogren E, Katz-Salamon M, et al. Periventricular leukomalacia and preterm birth have different detrimental effects on postural adjustments. *Brain.* 1999;122:727-740.

22. Brogren E, Forssberg H, Hadders-Algra M. Influence of two different sitting positions on postural adjustments in children with spastic diplegia. *Dev Med Child Neurol.* 2001;43:534-546.

23. Roncesvalles MN, Woollocott MW, Burtner PA. Neural factors underlying reduced postural adaptability in children with cerebral palsy. *Neuroreport.* 2002;13:2407-2410.

24. Van der Fits IB, Hadders-Algra M. The development of postural response patterns during reaching in healthy infants. *Neurosci Biobehav Rev.* 1998;22:521-526.

25. Van der Fits IB, Otten E, Klip AW, et al. The development of postural adjustments during reaching in 6- to 18-month-old infants. Evidence for two transitions. *Exp Brain Res.* 1999;126:517-528.

26. Schmitz C, Martin N, Assaiante C. Building anticipatory postural adjustment during childhood: a kinematic and electromyographic analysis of unloading in children from 4 to 8 years of age. *Exp Brain Res.* 2002;142:354-364.

27. Grasso R, Assaiante C, Prevost P, et al. Development of anticipatory orienting strategies during locomotor tasks in children. *Neurosci Biobehav Rev.* 1998;22:533-539.

28. Johnston LM, Burns YR, Brauer SG, et al. Differences in postural control and movement performance during goal directed reaching in children with developmental coordination disorder. *Hum Mov Sci.* 2002;21:583-601.

29. Nashner L, McCollum G. The organization of human postural movements: a formal basis and experimental synthesis. *Behav Brain Sci.* 1985;8:135-172.

30. Horak F, Nashner L. Central programming of posture control: adaptation to altered support surface configurations. *J Neurophysiol.* 1986;55:1369-1381.

31. Roncesvalles MN, Woollacott MH. The development of compensatory stepping skills in children. *J Mot Behav.* 2000;32:100-111.

32. McCollum G, Shupert CL, Nashner LM. Organizing sensory information for postural control in altered sensory environments. *J Theor Biol.* 1996;180:257-270.

33. Nudo RJ, Friel KM, Delia SW. Role of sensory deficits in motor impairments after injury to primary motor cortex. *Neuropharmacology.* 2000;39:733-742.

34. Sundermier L, Woollacott MH. The influence of vision on the automatic postural muscle responses of newly standing and newly walking infants. *Exp Brain Res.* 1998;120:537-540.

35. Rine RM, Rubish K, Feeney C. Measurement of sensory system effectiveness and maturational changes in postural control in young children. *Pediatr Phys Ther.* 1998;10:16-22.

36. Hatzitake V, Zisi V, Kollias I, et al. Perceptual-motor contributions to static and dynamic balance control in children. *J Mot Behav.* 2002;34:161-170.

37. Nashner LM, Shumway-Cook A, Marin O. Stance posture control in select groups of children with cerebral palsy: deficits in sensory organization and muscular coordination. *Exp Brain Res.* 1983;49:393-409.

38. Shumway-Cook A, Woollacott M. Attentional demands and postural control: the effect of sensory context. *J Gerontol A Biol Sci Med Sci.* 2000;55:10-16.

39. Huang Hsiang-Ju, Stemmons V. Dual-task methodology: application in studies of cognitive and motor performance in adults and children. *Pediatr Phys Ther.* 2001;13:133-140.

40. McGraw MB. *The Neuromuscular Maturation of the Human Infant.* New York, NY: Hafner Press; 1945.

41. Spinelli DN. Plasticity triggering experiences: nature and the dual genesis of brain structure and function. In: Gunzenhauser N, ed. *Infant Stimulation: Pediatric Round Table: 13.* Skillman, NJ: Johnson & Johnson Baby Products; 1987.

42. Plautz EJ, Milliken GW, Nudo RJ. Effects of repetitive motor training on movement representations in adult squirrel monkeys: role of use versus learning. *Neurobiol Learn Mem.* 2000;74:27-55.

43. Kleim JA, Barbay S, Cooper NR, et al. Motor learning-dependent synaptogensis is localized to functionally reorganized motor cortex. *Neurobiol Learn Mem.* 2002;77:63-77.

44. Schaechter JD, Kraft E, Hilliard TS, et al. Motor recovery and cortical reorganization after constraint-induced movement therapy in stroke patients: a preliminary study. *Neurorehabil Neural Repair.* 2002;16:326-338.

45. Wittenberg GF, Chen R, Ishii K, et al. Constraint-induced therapy in stroke: magnetic-stimulation motor maps and cerebral activation. *Neurorehabil Neurol Repair.* 2003;17:48-57.

46. Byl NN. Neuroplasticity: applications to motor control. In: Montgomery PC, Connolly BH, eds. *Clinical Applications of Motor Control.* Thorofare, New Jersey: SLACK Incorporated; 2002: 79-106.

47. Hadders-Algra M, Brogren E, Forssberg H. Training affects the development of postural adjustments in sitting infants. *J Physiol.* 1996;15:289-298.

48. Sveistrup H, Woollacott MH. Practice modifies the developing automatic postural response. *Exp Brain Res.* 1997;114:33-43.

49. Roncesvalles MN, Woollacott MH, Jensen JL. Development of lower extremity kinetics for balance control in infants and young children. *J Mot Behav.* 2001;33:180-192.

50. Prechtl HFR. *The Neurological Examination of the Full-term Newborn Infant. Clinics in Developmental Medicine. No. 63.* 2nd ed. Philadelphia, Pa: JB Lippincott. 1977:39-56.

51. Leonard CT. Motor behavior and neural changes following perinatal and adult-onset brain damage: implications for therapeutic interventions. *Phys Ther.* 1994;741:753-767.

52. MacKay-Lyons M. Central pattern generation of locomotion: a review of the evidence. *Phys Ther.* 2002;82:69-81.

53. DeVries JIP, Visser GHA, Prechtl HFR. Fetal motility in the first half of pregnancy. In: Prechtl HFR, ed. *Continuity of Neural Functions from Prenatal to Postnatal Life.* Oxford, England: Spastics International Medical Publications; 1984:46-64.

54. Forssberg H. Ontogeny of human locomotor control, I: infant stepping, supported locomotion and transitions to independent locomotion. *Exp Brain Res.* 1985;57:480-493.

55. Andre-Thomas M, Autgaerden S. Locomotion from pre- to post-natal life. In: *Clinics in Developmental Medicine. No. 24.* London, England: Medical Books Ltd; 1966:1-88.

56. Lamb Y, Yang JF. Could different directions of infant stepping be controlled by the same loco-motor central pattern generator? *J Neurophysiol.* 2000;83:2814-2824.

57. Bartlett D, Piper M, Okun N et al. Primitive reflexes and the determination of fetal presentation at birth. *Early Hum Dev.* 1997;48:261-273.

58. Kornhuber HH. The vestibular system and the general motor system. In: Kornhuber HH, ed. *Handbook of Sensory Physiology. Vestibular System Part 2: Psychophysics, Applied Aspects, and General Interpretation. Vol VI/2.* New York, NY: Springer-Verlag; 1974:581-586

59. Magnus R (Abstracted by Signe Brunnstrom). Haltung. *Phys Ther Rev.* 1953;33:281-290. Reprinted in: Payton OD, Hirt S, Newton RA, eds. *Neurophysiologic Approaches to Therapeutic Exercise.* Philadelphia, Pa: FA Davis; 1977:64-66.

60. Anderson JH, Soechting JF, Terzuolo CA. Role of vestibular inputs in the organization of motor output to forelimb extensors. In: Granit R, Pompeiano O, eds. *Reflex Control of Posture and Movement. Progress in Brain Research.* New York, NY: Elsevier/North-Holland Biomedical Press; 1975;413-421.

61. Aiello I, Rosata G, Sau GF, et al. Interaction of tonic labyrinth and neck reflexes in man. *Ital J Neurol Sci.* 1992;13:195-201.

62. Georgopoulos AP, Grillner S. Visuomotor coordination in reaching and locomotion. *Science.* 1989;245:1209-1210.

63. Marder E, Bucher D. Central pattern generators and the control of rhythmic movements. *Curr Biol.* 2001;11:986-996.

64. Dubowitz L, Dubowitz V. *The Neurological Assessment of the Preterm and Full-Term Newborn Infant. Clinics in Developmental Medicine. No. 79.* Philadelphia, Pa: JB Lippincott; 1981:334-338.

65. Dubowitz LM, Dubowitz V. Clinical assessment of gestational age in the newborn infant. *J Pediatr.* 1970;77:1-10.

66. Zafeiriou DI, Tsikoulas IG, Kremenopoulos GM. Prospective follow-up of primitive reflex profiles in high-risk infants: clues to an early diagnosis of cerebral palsy. *Pediatr Neurolol.* 1995;13:148-152.

67. Egan DF, Illingworth RS, MacKeith RC. Developmental screening 0-5 Years. *Clinics in Developmental Medicine. No. 30.* London: William Heinemann Medical Books Ltd; Philadelphia, Pa: JB Lippincott; 1969:9–16.

68. Effgen SK. Integration of plantar grasp as an indicator of ambulation potential in developmentally disabled infants. *Phys Ther.* 1982;4:433-435.

69. Sala DA, Grant AD. Review article: prognosis for ambulation in cerebral palsy. *Dev Med Child Neurol.* 1995;37:1020-1026.

70. Montgomery PC. Predicting potential for ambulation in children with cerebral palsy. *Pediatr Phys Ther.* 1998;10:148-155.

71. Friesen WO, Cang J. Sensory and central mechanisms control intersegmental coordination. *Current Opinion in Neurobiology.* 2001;11:678-683.

72. Hadders-Algra M, Brogren E, Forssberg H. Development of postural control—differences between ventral and dorsal muscles? *Neurosci Biobehav Rev.* 1998;22:501-506.

73. Dietz V, Horstmann GA, Berger W. Interlimb coordination of leg-muscle activation during perturbation of stance in humans. *J Neurophys.* 1989;6:680-693.

74. Sporns Q, Edelman GM. Solving Bernstein's problem: a proposal for the development of coordinated movement by selection. *Child Dev.* 1993;64:960-981.

75. Thelen E, Cooke DW. Relationship between newborn stepping and later walking: a new interpretation. *Dev Med Child Neurol.* 1987;29:380-393.

76. Thelen E, Spencer JP. Postural control during reaching in young infants: a dynamic systems approach. *Neurosci Biobehav Rev.* 1998;22:507-514.

77. Hadders-Algra M, Brogren E, Forssberg H. Nature and nurture in the development of postural control in human infants. *Acta Paediatr Suppl.* 1997;422:48-53.

78. Haley SM. Sequential analysis of postural reactions in non-handicapped infants. *Phys Ther.* 1986;66:531-536.

79. Milani-Comparetti A, Gidoni EA. Routine developmental examination in normal and retarded children. *Dev Med Child Neurol.* 1967;9:631-638.

80. Bayley N. *Bayley Scales of Infant Development.* New York, NY: Psychological Corporation; 1969.

81. Touwen B. *Neurological Development in Infancy, Clinics in Developmental Medicine. No. 58.* Philadelphia, Pa: JB Lippincott; 1976.

82. Knobloch H. *Manual of Developmental Diagnosis.* New York, NY: Harper & Row; 1980.

83. Gilfoyle EM, Grady AP, Moore JC. *Children Adapt.* Thorofare, NJ: SLACK Incorporated; 1981:57-77.

84. Tower G. Selected developmental reflexes and reactions—a literature search. In: Hopkins HL, Smith HD, eds. *Willard and Spackman's Occupational Therapy.* 6th ed. Philadelphia, Pa: Lippincott; 1983:175-187.

85. Peiper A. *Cerebral Function in Infancy.* New York, NY: Consultants Bureau; 1963:156-210.

86. Saint-Anne D'Argassies S. Neurodevelopmental symptoms during the first year of life. *Dev Med Child Neurol.* 1972;14:235-246.

87. Barnes MR, Crutchfield CA, Heriza CB, et al. *Reflex and Vestibular Aspects of Motor Control, Motor Development and Motor Learning.* Atlanta, Ga: Stokesville Publishing; 1990;379,451.

88. Westcott SL, Lowes LP, Richardson PK. Evaluation of postural stability in children: current theories and assessment tools. *Phys Ther.* 1997;77:629-645.

89. Richter EW, Montgomery PC. *The Sensorimotor Performance Analysis.* Hugo, Minn: PDP Press; 1989.

Developing Head and Trunk Control

Janet Sternat, PT

Therapists have a long history of trying to foster development and improve movement abilities in children who have impairments, functional limitations, or issues that interfere with quality of life. The information in Chapter 8 addressed general issues and research related to postural control. The purpose of Chapter 9 is to focus specifically on the role of the head and trunk in motor development and control. Suggestions for qualitative evaluation strategies and interventions reflect various current clinical approaches. Empirical evidence needs to be gathered regarding the short- and long-term effects of these interventions.

Development of head and trunk control is important to the overall motoric development of the child. To look closely at the head and trunk is somewhat like putting a drop of water under a microscope. What appears at first to be a simple whole is in fact a dynamic system made up of many parts. Through movement, the skin, bones, muscles, and fascia all contribute to what appears to be the static function of maintaining postural alignment. This apparent mechanical alignment, as well as neurophysiological control systems, and basic synergistic patterns form the substrates of body-mind expression.[1-3]

From a reflex hierarchical model, spinal movements and their underlying reflexes are simple enough to delineate but are not sufficient to explain motor control.[1] Functional motion analysis is a more contemporary way to view movements of the head, neck, thorax, and related parts. The head and trunk should be able to extend, flex, laterally flex, and rotate in a variety of pro- and antigravity positions.[4] To accomplish these fundamental movements, the musculoskeletal and nervous systems are interdependent in a motor-sensory-motor relationship.[5,6] This relationship includes emotional and excitement levels (arousal) that affect motivation, intent, attention, and muscle tone.[7,8] Related nervous system structures, specifically the cerebellum, limbic system, reticular system, and proprioceptors, participate in preparing for and monitoring motor activity. [5,8-10]

As if the head and trunk are not complex enough, the development of "control" requires the additional perspective of intrauterine progression of fetal movement. The potential for competent movement is a composite of many factors including the practiced movement of the fetus in utero.[11] Fetal movement also is related to intrauterine development (as differentiated from post-natal development) of passive muscle tonus, which has been found to occur in a caudal to cephalic and distal to proximal direction.[9] Descriptions of fetal movement support a motor-sensory-motor basis.[11] Trunk and head movements occur initially, followed by isolated and differentiated movements of head, limbs, diaphragm, and then jaw. Limb and head movements have been reported to precede tactile exploration of the face, followed by sucking and swallowing. Spontaneous movements have been documented to occur even before reflexive movements (see Chapter 1).

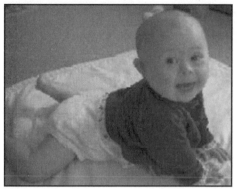

Figure 9-1. Ability to extend lumbar spine; extend elbows, open fingers, turn head and eyes within head, vocalize, orient to visual or auditory stimulation, support head above shoulders, move in and out of raised head position.

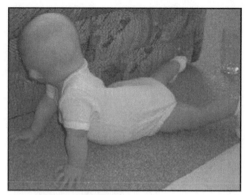

Figure 9-2. Ability to vary foot position, shift shoulders forward with head turning, shorten one side of the trunk and lengthen the other; flex or extend hips and knees (compare to Figure 9-1).

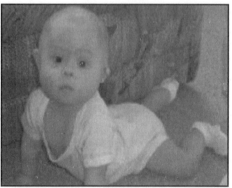

Figure 9-3. Ability to lift lower ribs off the floor, focus eyes, flex one leg while extending the other, extend one hip with flexing the other, shift the central axis to left or right of center—all without increasing effort or loss of smooth quality.

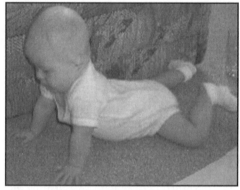

Figure 9-4. Ability to tuck chin to follow eye gaze downward.

The relationship of the neck to head and trunk movement, of the spine and ribs to respiration and posture, of the pelvis to posture and movement, and the interrelationships of muscles to postural tone, dynamic stability, and movement patterns must be considered in relation to motor control. By 6 months of age, a typically developing child exhibits the following movements that are related to organized movement of the head, neck, ribs, spine, and pelvis (Figures 9-1 through 9-9).[3]

Additionally, in order to organize the cervical, thoracic, and lumbar spine in relationship to the pelvis, the child must be able to[12-16]:

1. Use the eyes for gazing, tracking, focusing, orienting, leading movement, and early social interactions

2. Use the mouth for eating, breathing, vocalizing, mouthing, talking, kissing, tasting, and communicating

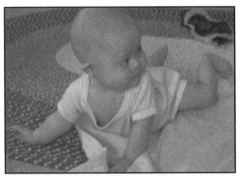

Figure 9-5. Ability to shift weight over diagonal axis and lift left side of pelvis off floor in preparation to move, ability to bend both elbows and keep head above shoulders.

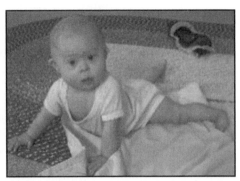

Figure 9-6. Ability to shorten one side of the neck and lengthen the other for gaze and listening.

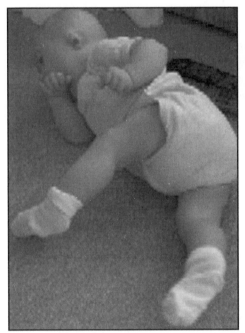

Figure 9-7. Ability to transition by rolling, vary foot position from plantar to dorsiflexion, use ground forces to assist the movement.

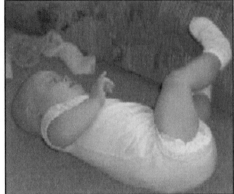

Figure 9-8. Ability to lengthen all spine components at once, flex hips, and extend knees.

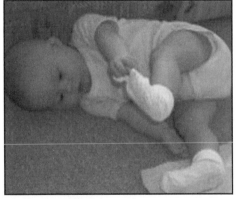

Figure 9-9. Ability to roll from back to side, tuck chin, lift head off support surface, perform hand function with eyes guiding.

3. Use the breathing mechanism for sustaining life, producing and changing sounds, coughing, and expressing emotion

4. Use movement for balance, mobility, orientation, play, and exploration

5. Use posture and alignment for play, socialization, activities of daily living (ADL), and learning

Additionally, physical and cognitive requirements that impact motor development of the head and trunk include[17-19]:

1. Freedom of the joints to move and to be held in place

2. Adequate balance of muscle strength and power across various joints

3. Variation of muscle tone from active to resting states in coordination and timing with various muscle groups in an action sequence

4. A desire or interest in something

5. The ability to respond appropriately to stimulation

These requirements encompass interrelationships of body parts and neuromechanisms. To function adequately, a child must be able to maintain a desired posture while freely using distal components of the body (ie, hands, feet, mouth, and eyes). A child must have thoracic and rib movements that are combined to promote stability and mobility at the same time as respiration is occurring and change as demands vary from resting to active states.[20,21] Changes in body position must occur with graded control between supported and upright positions.[22,23] The ability to move with grace, power, lightness or coordination, and speed variation depends on awareness, perception, balanced muscle strength, and tonus, as well as patterns of movement.[24-30]

Opposing muscles must be able to elongate, "letting go" through the full excursion of joint range while other muscle groups are contracting to provide a stable point from which movement can occur.[31,32] The active muscle groups must have sufficient contractile force to carry the body part in the desired direction. Antagonists must grade the elongation or decelerate the moving part to prevent loss of control.[31,33] Specific muscle groups related to trunk control include the capital flexors and extensors, spinal flexors and extensors, intercostals, and hip flexors and extensors. The latter two groups are mentioned as they pertain to function of the pelvis. As these muscles work to balance one another, they enable the head and trunk to respond with movements of lateral flexion and rotation.[8,27]

In treatment, two goals are primary. The first goal is to establish firm somatic proprioceptive responses that become the basis for sensory perception and interplay with movement.[2] The second goal is to develop the potential for muscle groups to be used in a functionally appropriate manner to respond as movement demands occur from internal states or environmental situations.[1,34,35] Functional movement should be possible with a sense of lightness and ease, as well as incorporating the element of reversibility.[6,36] This amount of control allows for the expression of postural reactions and the integration of innate motor programs with the execution of skilled, learned movements.[8,27,32,37]

Control of Movement

Seven basic principles that should be considered as they pertain to motor control include muscle elongation, mobilization, body biomechanics, tonus gradation, balanced muscle function, activation, and repetition.

In infant motor development, shortened muscles must elongate from physiologic flexion to achieve the full variety of postures associated with normal movement.[4] *Elongation* is the ability of a muscle to release its hold or tension and lengthen through the full excursion of joint movement. This need for muscle elongation as a preparation for movement continues throughout life.[27] Skin, ligaments, and subcutaneous tissue all have visco-elastic properties that may take over the function of postural holding. When low muscle tone, inadequate strength, or trauma result in an imbalance of muscle function, these structures may begin to restrict movement and cause pain.[27] Movement restricted by the unnatural holding of muscles, skin, fascia, or ligaments may require specialized preparation that includes techniques for soft tissue *mobilization*, myofascial release, and massage.[17,27]

Biomechanical influences of the body also may produce changes in muscle function and create the malalignment often associated with disorganized motor function.[2] If the spine is collapsed into flexion, realignment of the thoracic spine will have a direct effect on trunk flexors through elongation produced by lifting the thorax. Biomechanical influences may be produced passively during handling and positioning or actively during facilitation of specific muscle groups (eg, promotion of active upper back extension in prone or sitting).

The ability to produce normal variations (ie, tonus gradations) in postural tone is one of the desired outcomes of treatment. To achieve this requires an understanding of the events that produce and change body tone. Emotional states and thought patterns have an effect on body tone.[18] These conditions may vary from moment to moment with different levels of excitement, worry, fear, anger, depression, or within a sleep/wake cycle. Each condition produces a definite effect on the body that can be felt through the muscles and fascia.[18,19,27] External events or stimulation also may have an effect on body tone. Children may respond differently to direct input such as percussion, tapping, bouncing, or jumping. While some children may calm to increased proprioceptive input, others may become more active. Techniques such as slow rhythmic rocking, deep massage, myofascial release, muscle elongation, and soft rhythmic sound generally result in inhibition. However, children who do not feel like taking a nap or quieting may instead become quite irritable and tense. The physical environment and the feelings of others in the immediate environment have a direct effect on body tone and behavior. Events such as changes in barometric pressure, extreme temperatures, or even the attitude and/or expectations of the therapist may help to explain mood swings, comfort level, and body tension.[19,20] Muscles have a natural level of tension at rest that increases with active motion and reduces again when activity ceases. This often is not seen in children with lesions of the central nervous system (CNS), emotional arousal problems, or genetically predisposed extremes of muscle tone.

Normally, muscles function optimally and a feeling of lightness and ease of movement results.[27,36] The muscles used to control the head and trunk must work synergistically to achieve this ease in maintaining spinal alignment. Once this *balance of muscle function* is achieved, the expression of righting reactions, postural responses, and active head and trunk movements become possible in all planes of movement.[1,2,32]

A familiar phrase from an unknown source goes, "if you don't use it, you'll lose it." This pertains to most living cells and tissue including the nervous and musculoskeletal systems.[9] It pertains to initial fetal development and continuing growth. Muscles that are inactive and do not produce movement become atrophied and, through disuse, sensory awareness of that body part also may be diminished.[38] Movement can be initiated (ie, *activation*) from at least two levels of the brain.[8] On a consciously directed level, new skills can be learned in isolation and executed in component parts. The young child actively may practice parts of higher level skills. For example, reciprocal kicking observed in play uses many of the same muscles required for walking, although it is not the same task as walking. Although this kicking may be automatic and not always be directed through conscious effort, the child is conscious of and delights in the movement sensation. Early isolated attempts at movement may become incorporated into patterns of movement as postural control develops. After actively practicing weight shifting, the body may be more responsive to changes in position (ie, weight shift producing the need to realign posture). Automatic and semiautomatic responses are desired for adaptation to the environment and to provide the ability to act on the environment with efficient, fluid execution. Both types of actively produced responses, volitional and automatic, can be used in treatment. The first goal is to establish the ability to move. The second goal is to improve the efficiency of movement through practice in a functional context.

In the process of motor development the infant can be observed to produce specific movements thousands of times. This practice (ie, *repetition*) enhances communication between the sensory and motor systems of the body.[27] The more often a motion is produced, the easier it becomes to produce and eventually to incorporate with more complex patterns of movement.[10]

Examination and Evaluation

In order to determine intervention strategies for the head and trunk, a baseline of current function must be determined and examination procedures delineated. In order to look systematically at factors related to developmental levels and functional ability as well as factors interfering with movement of the head and trunk, the therapist may use a combination of examination tools (see Chapter 2) and methods. The methods that may be used during the examination and evaluation follow.

Method I: Observe-Effort, Strength, and Muscle Tone Changes With Various Positions and Activities

Posture should be observed when the child is in supine, prone on extended arms, side sitting, long sitting, and bench sitting. An examiner must note if:

➤ There are any asymmetries that should be investigated further or if invariant skeletal deformities exist

➤ The child is showing any undo effort, such breath holding, retracting or clenching the jaw, pressing out the tongue, or making unnecessary movements in the mouth, extremities, and shoulders when movement is attempted

➤ Fluctuations of muscle tone can be observed as changes of posture occur from supported (resting) to unsupported (active) positions

➤ The child's breathing patterns are congruent with movement and resting states

➤ The child's breathing pattern indicates comfort or distress

At rest, ease of passive movement should be evident. When the child is excited or stimulated, emotional tone can be expressed as increased muscle tension. During active movement of isolated body parts or of the total body through space, compensatory tone or stability patterns may be noted.[2,4]

When muscle tonus or motor control are insufficient to support posture, predictable compensations result.[4,9] These compensatory stability patterns may be observed or felt during active movement. For example, an increase in muscle tone or exaggerated extension posture might be apparent at the shoulders (elevation and retraction) and spine (cervical and lumbar hyperextension).[2,6,8] The use of a Valsalva maneuver or breath holding might be observed when the upper back extensors or trunk flexors are insufficient to maintain an erect spine.[8] Hip flexor "fixing" or holding might be a substitute for inadequate pelvic control. Fixing also may occur in the pectoral muscles to provide increased shoulder stability.[4] Such compensatory use of muscles generally interferes with efficient movement.[29] As the use of compensatory patterns continues, additional problems may result, such as shortening of the muscles used for "holding" and weakness of other muscles (due in part to hypotonia or to disuse). A distorted body image and maladaptive patterns of movement may occur instead of balanced responses for postural holding.[2,38,39]

Problems associated with poor head and trunk control are different in the infant as compared to the older child. Initial problems with sucking and respiration may be early indicators of trunk instability in the infant.[4,6,8,34] Secondary more obvious problems develop as the infant attempts to use the control that is available to gain mobility or an upright position. If problems with head and trunk control remain unresolved, they become easier to recognize because of the compounding effects of effort and repeated abnormal use of compensatory movement patterns.[4]

Method II: Handle and Feel for Mobility, Stability, and Flexibility

Mobility should be examined from two perspectives:

➤ First, actual flexibility of the joints and subcutaneous tissue must be palpated. Are joints hypermobile? Is full range of motion possible passively? In particular, the atlanto-occipital, lumbo-sacral, hip, and intervertebral joints must be able to move freely. When evaluating spinal rotation, the pelvis should be able to remain stationary while the upper trunk turns, and the shoulders should be able to remain stationary while the head turns on the neck. When all segments of the spine are able to move freely, the motions of flexion/extension and rotation combined with the straight planes of motion will have a segmental look. Differentiated movement then becomes possible and the thoracic skeleton has a chain-like relationship with itself and its related parts

➤ Second, active flexibility of the motor kinematic system must be checked. The examiner must determine whether joint excursion is blocked by shortened muscles, limited by weak agonists, or prevented by muscle holding. Examination should include requests for movement (eg, "look here," "roll over") as well as elicitation of movement during handling and function (eg, removal of clothing). Does the child turn and lift the head with ease and efficiency? Does the child demonstrate anticipatory shifts in the pelvis and postural changes in response to movement facilitation? Is the child breathing freely with all efforts?

Method III: Request or Elicit Motor Skills, Then Observe and Record Performance Using Various Normative or Checklist Tools (See Chapter 2)

Automatic reactions and skilled movements, such as catching or kicking a ball, are dependent on learned motor ability and intact neural mechanisms for efficient execution. Skilled observation is necessary to determine the level of congruency of head and trunk organization with any given task or function. The skills should be observed in relationship to a child's developmental level or functional expectations in a specific environment.

Method IV: Continue the Examination During Intervention

Additional information can be gathered by combining examination with intervention. Determining what will benefit a child who has a unique medical and genetic history is best derived from experience with the child responding to a variety of experiences with the examiner. In children with complex histories, emotional difficulties may obscure accurate findings. The examination must include consideration of attachment issues, nutritional priorities, sleep patterns, allergies, and other medical and health factors.[16,40-42]

Skilled observation is necessary to determine the quality of head and trunk control. Does the head right sufficiently during rolling? Are the eyes able to locate objects and monitor the hands without excessive head movement? Does movement occur from the pelvis to position the head and trunk in anticipation of reaching for a desired object or taking a drink from a cup? Is there observable disorganized motor function during attempts to balance?[2] Is there lack of automatic proprioceptive control during facilitated weight shifting?[2] Is there a variety of postures observed during play?[2]

Following examination using one or more methods, the therapist must draw conclusions related to goals and intervention strategies. The results of examination simply will delineate a list of needs related to essential requirements, essential movement abilities, or developmental issues. Not all findings will indicate a need for intervention. The provision of therapy must be determined by the effect of those needs on the child's functional capabilities and on the child's developmental and movement potential.

Intervention Strategies

In the same way that head and trunk control have been dissected and defined by the underlying biomechanics, kinesiology, and components of movement, treatment can be analyzed by looking at basic principles. If the basic principles are understood, treatment techniques can be selected from a variety of approaches and combined to achieve optimal results.

Three aspects of intervention are especially relevant in the organization of head and trunk control and motor learning. One aspect is to establish clear somatic proprioceptive responses that become the basis for sensory feedback and interplay with movement. Accurate somatosensory information is needed for optimal motor control and learning. This information is considered to be derived from the bottom up in brain function.[43] A second aspect is to consider perception as preparatory for movement. Visual input is most important for children when they are learning to move. This input drives the system from the top down and must connect with pathways from the bottom up. Auditory channels and kinesthetic channels are necessary to translate rhythm and to follow directions when language develops. These are part of the feed-forward or top-down loops. The third aspect to consider is the actual potential for muscle groups to be used in a function. There must be an optimal resting state or turgor and capabilities for strength related to task demands.[17,22,23,29] That is, the muscle must be able to respond as movement demands occur from internal states or environmental situations. This means the necessary range of motion must be available throughout hips, spine, and shoulder girdle. The musculoskeletal structures underlie and create the kinematic links to function.[17]

One approach to effective intervention is to discover and follow the child's developmental progress and movement sequences. Using the guidelines from Transdisciplinary Play-Based Assessment, an intervention program is easy to initiate.[15] This means a child can be viewed as the leader or the guide for intervention. The intervention activities are

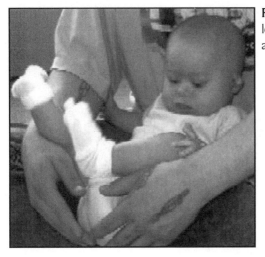

Figure 9-10. Gentle support and positioning to lengthen the spine. Note the gentle open hands of the adult, leaving the child to move freely.

selected after observing functional deficits suggested by the child's play, interactions, or breathing patterns. The therapist determines the following:

➤ What activities or handling techniques or equipment will enhance what a child is already doing?

➤ How can the total body be incorporated more fully into a task or movement pattern?

➤ What supports can be provided to allow for a child's successful interaction with the environment?

Something as simple as hand placement by the therapist on a child's body part can increase the awareness of that part by the CNS at conscious and subconscious levels. Touch seldom goes unnoticed by the brain. This contact can lead to a direct change in function of the part by reducing or enhancing muscular effort and by increasing perception. Contact, when there is a history of negative contact, may yield an avoidance or defensive response if the touch is interpreted by the child's nervous system as threatening. It becomes the therapist's responsibility to monitor a child's response to touch and at the same time monitor how the touching is presented from the therapist's own state of arousal, physical comfort, intention of outcome, and skill at establishing physical and emotional rapport. Time too often is a factor that plays a significant role in setting the emotional tone of the therapist. Rushed work often reduces sensitivity and complicates effective intervention. It is necessary, therefore, for the therapist to develop an intervention plan that matches comfortably with the time allotted for treatment.

Figures 9-10 through 9-23 are offered to demonstrate possibilities most likely to invite active movement of the child, while setting up some constraints to elicit specific motor responses. The figures show strategies that can be used to target and support development and improve functional abilities associated with the head, neck, ribs, thoracic/lumbar spine, and pelvis. The techniques selected and suggested in Figures 9-10 through 9-23 are used to optimize independent muscle activity for a given function. A child should be invited to use more or less muscle effort depending on the need to develop strength, coordination, or competence. These strategies generally fall into three categories: 1) techniques used to activate specific muscles or movement patterns, 2) techniques used to elicit typical movement responses, and 3) techniques used to enhance breathing.

In the least restrictive environment for therapy, simply motivating a child or assisting the child to move may be sufficient to improve function. The therapist also must be

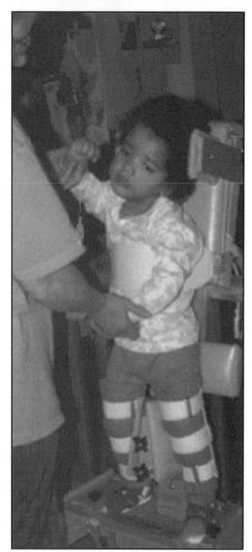

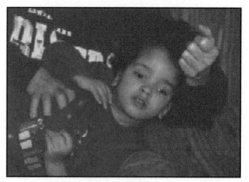

Figure 9-12. Active assistance to produce a natural head position in sidelying. Two points of contact introduce the movement pattern of shortening the lateral trunk flexors for stability and lifting the head for orienting. Note the forearm, not fingers, is used at the head. Note the hand on the ribs makes contact with the bones of the ribs for greater feedback.

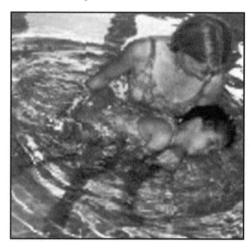

Figure 9-11. Maximum support of night splints, body jacket, and stander to afford active practice of head and eyes with help to move arms in play with music.

Figure 9-13. Using buoyancy to afford comfort in sidelying with practice of active head turning to move supine or prone.

accepting of any of the child's movement patterns (quantity as well as quality). This means supplying approval and support for what already is occurring and introducing change only after the therapist understands what is meaningful to the child. This means avoiding correcting a child by saying "Don't move that way!" and instead assisting a child to access the environment in easier and more meaningful ways. The therapist also might simply reflect verbally what is observed by describing in words understood by the child.

In a more structured setting more specific postural requirements can be promoted. For example, the therapist's hands can be used to apply sensory input to direct or support the musculoskeletal system and to perceive what changes are occurring in temperature, underlying muscle tension, or movement. The therapist's hands also can communicate to

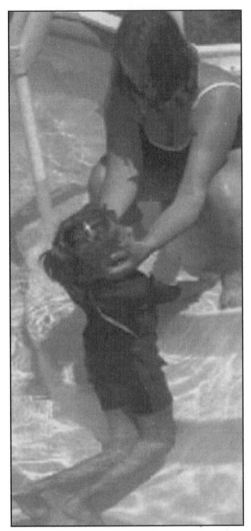

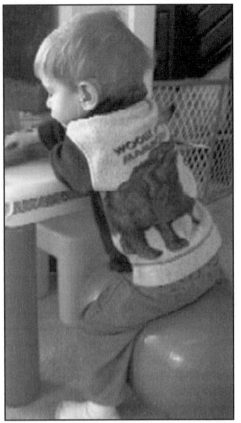

Figure 9-15. Using a peanut-shaped therapy ball to facilitate the practice of postural control during functional activity.

Figure 9-14. Steps are used to accommodate for lack of mobility in lower extremities while the child practices moving from kneel to tall kneel. Adult handling is minimal to help initiate and time the movement practice.

the child a sense of caring and confidence more directly than words can communicate. This use of the hands is referred to as "informative touch" and has been well-documented in the domains of bodywork and massage.

Additionally, the therapist can set up specific conditions by using equipment or suggesting imagery to restrain or require specific movements.

The ultimate measure of effectiveness of any intervention is observing the child playing with the sensation of movement, practicing isolated movements (eg, kicking or waving), or using movement patterns in a functional activity or skill (eg, rolling, climbing, creeping, or looking).

Breathing, pulmonary function, respiration, and phonation are related to aspects of trunk development and intervention. Abdominal muscle strength and freely moving

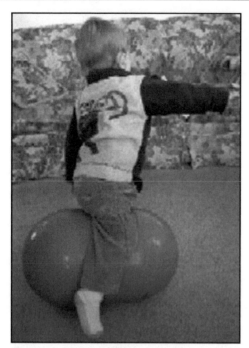

Figure 9-16. Using the same equipment to practice dynamic balance and weight shifting with bouncing.

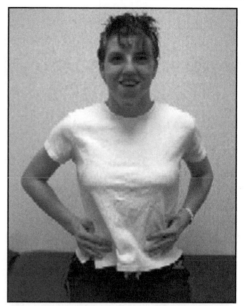

Figure 9-17. Inhalation with self-feedback at the base of the ribs. Alternative method could be to use therapist's hands for feedback and to vary the positions to include supine and standing. The inhalation can be accomplished with intention or during an activity such as singing or reading out loud.

intercostal muscles are two required factors for airway pressure to increase for secretion clearing and sustained phonation. One way of assisting breathing patterns is for the therapist to place his or her hands on the child's chest or shoulders. This hand placement can enhance particular phases of breathing or promote graded exhalation. Note that Figures 9-17 through 9-22 combine breathing strategies with movement pattern practice.

This brief section on breathing is to indicate its usefulness as a place to start treatment as well as its importance as a functional outcome. Breathing is essential in sustaining life, enriching development through the oxygenation of CNS cells, and communication. Changes in breathing can signal comfort or distress during intervention and care should be used at all times to monitor intervention, handling, and rapport.

Case Studies

Suggested intervention strategies and therapeutic activities for the case studies are based on the least restrictive approach to setting up opportunities for motor learning to improve the quality of movement coordination and to enhance functional capabilities. This protocol is suggested when selecting and combining treatment strategies:

➤ Determine the child's priorities through observation and conversation

➤ Know where the child is developmentally

➤ Know what the child's interest is in peer and family member interactions

➤ Know what interests the child in the areas of fine and gross motor play

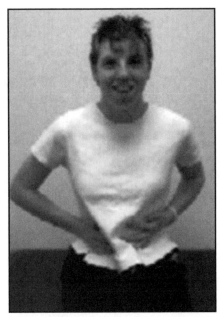

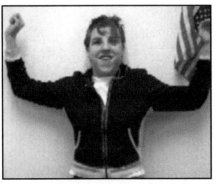

Figure 9-19. Sitting so as to lean against the wall for support and feedback, inhale with arms apart.

Figure 9-18. Exhalation slow and with sound production. Note hands stay in place to help push the ribs inward and hold them as the diaphragm becomes ready to again inhale. This is unhurried breathing practice to better engage the diaphragm without auxiliary muscles. An alternative method to that in Figure 9-17.

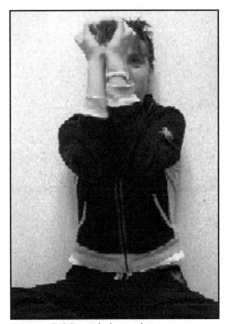

Figure 9-20. Exhale with arms coming together. Alternative position can be to use supine and standing (also against a wall). Exhalation is again held until the diaphragm automatically initiates inhalation.

➤ Know how the child receives information—from touching or being touched, looking, listening, or all three

➤ Know that the child always has an idea (image of achievement) and that this image may need to be addressed to improve coordination

➤ Know what the child desires for motivation and interest

➤ Know how to reflect what the child is doing either verbally or physically using one or two points of touch (Both forms of feedback are very powerful in the brain and essential for motor learning. This is one method for the child to learn if his image of achievement is the same [success] as his outcome)

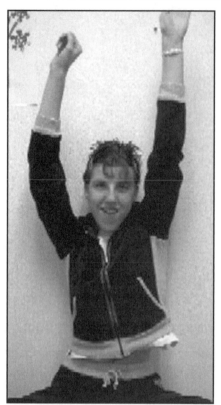

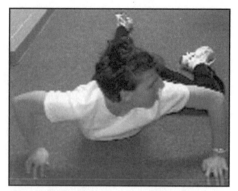

Figure 9-22. Playing with active movement in prone by doing the "alligator." The knee comes headward as the child looks over the same shoulder towards the knee. This is practice of extension with rotation and lateral flexion.

Figure 9-21. Using reciprocal reaching coordinated with breathing to practice lengthening the lateral flexors on the weight bearing side while shortening on the opposite side. Movement is practiced so as to become lighter and executed with more freedom speed. Vocalization is added once the movements are well-coordinated.

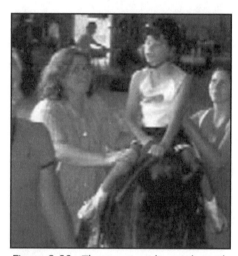

Figure 9-23. Therapeutic riding with tactile input to guide movement of thoracic spine in relationship to movements made by the horse. Side walkers ensure safety by maintaining leg position on either side of the rider. The horse is guided as needed by a lead when neck reining needs clarification.

➤ Know how to be creative and change your idea about what might be acceptable during a motor learning session

➤ Know how to develop a nurturing supportive relationship with the child by being positive about his capabilities and interests

➤ Consider opportunities for reciprocal or interdependent events (Initially a child can lead the session after being offered specific constraints of equipment or environment)

➤ Be ready to take the lead and begin to vary or focus the movement experiences by varying the orientation or complexity of the chosen activity or by providing informative touch (An observant adult can increase a child's opportunities and feedback for motor learning by adding visual, auditory, or breathing variation to freely selected movements)

➤ Use the floor as a constraint for movement play as a safe starting point for the child who is posturally insecure

➤ Facilitate physical and motor organization that will be most congruent with a child's desire for function or achievement

➤ Support and enhance a child's ideas so that the outcome will occur with greater degrees of independence and ease

➤ Work within constraints and parameters that will improve the child's awareness of the performance

➤ Practice slow movement and draw attention to specific aspects of the pattern to increase awareness and perception

➤ Teach one variation to already accomplished movements and patterns of movements

➤ Use simple basic materials such as balloons or beach balls on a string, the floor or a low table, foam balls, styrofoam rollers, peanut-shaped therapy balls, elastic bands, and therapy tubing

➤ Provide instruction in successful techniques to caregivers to ensure repetition and maximize motor learning

Case Study #1: Jason

➤ Practice pattern 5C: Impaired Motor Function and Sensory Integrity Associated With Nonprogressive Disorders of the Central Nervous System—Congenital Origin or Acquired in Infancy or Childhood

➤ Medical diagnosis: Cerebral palsy, right hemiparesis

➤ Age: 24 months

Examination and Evaluation

Examination reveals the following problems with head and trunk control. As Jason is observed walking, an asymmetrical posture is evident with a slight anterior tilt of the pelvis. The pelvis is retracted on the right. He has an observable asymmetry in the rib cage. When moved passively, the hip flexors are shortened on the right side as compared to the left. The lateral trunk flexors also are shortened on the right side. When tested on responses to passive tilt in sitting and standing and when watching Jason move independently, equilibrium reactions are inadequate due to poor quality of trunk control that results in poor ability to weight shift, especially to the right side. Head righting is adequate for protection, but asymmetry is apparent, associated with shoulder retraction on the right. When observing Jason play, it appears that capital flexion is poor in isolation and does not balance use of capital extensors during functional movement. Trunk rotation is limited to the left more than to the right.

FUNCTIONAL LIMITATIONS

In relation to head and trunk control when Jason is active, he tends to move stiffly, especially through the trunk. This contributes to his difficulties with upright balance. Jason is ambulatory, but falls frequently, especially when trying to move quickly or to run. Right shoulder and hip retraction interfere with balance and protective reactions during active movement, making Jason "unsteady" so that he has difficulty moving quickly and keeping up with his peers in play situations.

IMPAIRMENTS

Jason demonstrates asymmetry in muscle flexibility with muscles on the right side of his trunk and extremities less flexible than on the left. Weakness is evident in shortened muscle groups. Jason has difficulties with motor control of the right side of his body with slower reactions to loss of balance and decreased ability to use his right extremities and trunk during functional activities. He appears to have some sensory disregard for the right side of his body. Respiratory control appears to be poor as Jason is often "out of breath" and cannot sustain volume for singing simple songs.

GOALS

Treatment goals are for Jason to:

1. Increase mobility of the hips and spine
2. Increase ability to shift weight to the right side
3. Increase ability to activate cervical and abdominal muscles
4. Improve respiratory function
5. Improve body awareness of the right side of his body

FUNCTIONAL OUTCOMES

Following 3 months of intervention, Jason will:

1. Sit independently on a bench showing symmetrical position of the pelvis with weight on the right ischium equal to weight on the left ischium, 80% of the time
2. Rise from supine to sitting by rotating the trunk to the left, 25% of the time when observed during play
3. Climb on and off furniture using reciprocal movement in the lower extremities, 100% of the time
4. Move actively through full range of motion in all joints of the trunk, neck, and hips 80% of the time when required by a gross motor activity such as climbing and squatting
5. Demonstrate the ability to run 10 to 20 feet without falling more than three times per day
6. Demonstrate ability to change direction quickly when walking without falling, two of three attempts
7. Sustain the volume of vocal sounds for simple songs and noises

Intervention

To prepare Jason for movement activities, the following muscles require elongation:

right hip flexors and lateral trunk flexors, capital extensors, and scapular abductors. Passive movement of the thoracic spine must be possible for rotation to occur during active movement.

When muscle elongation is possible, active responses should be facilitated in the capital flexors and trunk flexors/extensors. Treatment positions should include supine activities such as reaching up and putting scarves on the feet or grabbing the feet and rocking to promote use of neck and trunk flexor muscles. Prone activities (on the floor, a therapy ball, or bolster) can be used to promote head and trunk extension through games such as "flying" or reaching for objects. Sitting activities (as on the therapist's lap or therapy ball) are helpful for facilitating trunk rotation to either side. Activities might include reaching to one side to obtain a puzzle piece and then reaching to the other side to place the piece in a puzzle.

Functional activities that might be incorporated into Jason's play routines include swinging, climbing, and jumping. Independent climbing and jumping can be encouraged by piling blankets and pillows in front of a couch. In a hammock, Jason could be positioned prone with a pillow to support the trunk. Jason could be encouraged to use extended arms to push himself forward and backward to facilitate head and trunk extension and bilateral extremity use.

Jason will be asked to imitate animal-like movements (eg, "walk and swing your trunk [arms] back and forth like an elephant"). Walking around increasingly difficult obstacle courses (first slowly, then more rapidly) will improve his ability to shift his weight and change his direction. Music in the background might be helpful to establish a rhythm for play and weight-shifting activities.

To address sensory issues, massage and tactile input will be used to increase muscle length and body awareness and to draw Jason's attention to his body (particularly to movement capabilities on his right side).

Use of toys that require "blowing," such as pinwheels and horns will be provided. Manual assistance applied to the rib cage can be used to facilitate the desired movement. Jason will be asked to imitate sounds and exaggerate his exhalation as the therapist gives percussion or vibration to his back, side, or chest.

Treatment sessions in a pool that stress bilateral activities and walking and running in the water might be incorporated into Jason's intervention. An unweighted walking device, such as a treadmill, also might be used to increase lower extremity weight shift and symmetry of the pelvis in an upright position.

Case Study #2: Jill

➤ Practice pattern 5C: Impaired Motor Function and Sensory Integrity Associated With Nonprogressive Disorders of the Central Nervous System—Congenital Origin or Acquired in Infancy or Childhood

➤ Medical diagnosis: Cerebral palsy, spastic quadriparesis, microcephaly, mental retardation, seizure disorder

➤ Age: 7 years

Examination and Evaluation

Assessment reveals the following problems with head and trunk control. Jill's upper spine is collapsed forward into a kyphotic posture with head and neck hyperextension. When moved passively, tightness and limitation of movement are exhibited in capital extensor, pectoral, shoulder girdle, hip flexor, and lumbar spine muscles. A deformity (an indented sternum) is noted in the chest. When moved passively, or when observed during attempts at active movement, Jill has limited control of her head and trunk in any position.

FUNCTIONAL LIMITATIONS

Jill has poor ability to lift her head in prone, to maintain it in upright, or to turn it in unsupported positions to visually explore her environment. She cannot roll over and has no method of independent mobility. Jill has limited ability to communicate with individuals in her environment.

IMPAIRMENTS

Jill has decreased range of motion and limited motor control in her head, trunk, and extremities. Jill has intellectual and attention deficits and a seizure disorder.

GOALS

Treatment goals are for Jill to:

1. Improve postural control of upper back extension, abdominal function, and freedom of the thorax for breathing and sound production
2. Increase flexibility in shoulder girdle and hips
3. Improve head control and symmetrical posture

FUNCTIONAL OUTCOMES

Following 3 months of intervention, Jill will:

1. Support and turn her head with equal ability to the right or left while sitting with assistance, to select a preferred activity, 50% of the time
2. Lift her head in prone on elbows position and maintain the position for 5 seconds to visually locate a toy placed in front of her
3. Produce a vowel sound for 2 to 3 seconds to communicate that she wants an adult's attention
4. Roll from prone to supine, one of five attempts

Intervention

To prepare muscles for activation and to achieve upright postures, elongation of the following muscles should be accomplished: cervical extensors, pectorals, lumbar extensors, hip flexors, and trunk flexors. Jill will require supported positions during manual facilitation and stretching of muscle groups. For example, with Jill's arms extended over her head to extend the upper back and the therapist or classroom aide supporting her in sitting, a bouncing movement can be produced to increase activation of muscles in the neck and trunk. This will be most effective if Jill can be sitting on a moveable surface, such as a sofa cushion, bolster, or ball. Positioning devices such as a sidelyer and prone stander can be incorporated into her daily routine to assist in maintaining muscle length.

Vibration, percussion, and tactile input to the ribs, sternum, and spine may be effective in producing relaxation and decreasing general stiffness. Jill should be encouraged to vocalize during these techniques. Having the classroom staff or therapist verbalize about Jill's body parts and movement during these activities will assist Jill to sense her own body.

Visual stimulation (looking in a mirror or at preferred toys or people) may assist in facilitating head movements while in various positions. Orientation to sound also could be used to encourage Jill to turn her head actively in different directions.

Aquatic therapy is very beneficial for Jill in promoting general relaxation. The buoyancy of the water allows her to control some movements of the head and trunk that she has difficulty performing against gravity. For example, suspending her in the pool with flotation devices allows her opportunities to experiment with head and trunk as well as extremity movements. This is an activity the family can participate in and will help maintain her range of motion.

Jill's therapeutic horseback riding program also is beneficial in maintain lower extremity joint and muscle range (eg, sitting on the horse) and desensitizing her to movement through space. Although she currently has maximum support when astride the horse, she has some opportunities during transfers and when riding to attempt to maintain her head and trunk erect.

Case Study #3: Taylor

➤ Practice pattern 5C: Impaired Motor Function and Sensory Integrity Associated With Nonprogressive Disorders of the Central Nervous Ssytem—Congenital Origin or Acquired in Infancy or Childhood

➤ Medical diagnosis: Myelomeningocele, repaired L1-2

➤ Age: 4 years

Examination and Evaluation

Evaluation reveals that Taylor is motivated to walk with braces and assistive devices. He is able to maintain and change positions as needed when he is on the floor using some compensatory strategies such as breath holding, hanging on ligaments, and using increased muscle tone. Taylor has a loss of muscle function below the level of T12 and will have to develop as much strength as he can in the muscle groups above this level. He will have to learn movement strategies unique to his sensory and motor capacity.

Functional Limitations

Taylor is slow when using his walking devices compared to his peer group and tires from the extra effort. Taylor moves about in his wheelchair with ease but fatigues quickly.

Impairments

Taylor has visual perceptual problems particularly with figure-ground discrimination. Bending his head to look at the floor disturbs his balance and this may interfere with his safety when ambulating with his walker. He has poor active trunk extension but has good head control in all positions and normal upper extremity coordination. Generalized weakness is present in his upper extremities and especially in his trunk muscles. Additionally, Taylor has slightly tight hip flexors and hip adductors. He demonstrates a loss of cutaneous and proprioceptive sensation below T-12 and has had frequent skin breakdowns in the sacral area and in his feet/ankles.

Goals

Treatment goals are for Taylor to:

1. Increase his strength in all active muscle groups, especially the trunk flexors and extensors as well as his shoulder girdle musculature
2. Increase his speed of ambulation
3. Decrease number of skin breakdowns in the sacral area and in his feet/ankles
4. Improve his endurance during play activities

FUNCTIONAL OUTCOMES

Following 3 months of intervention, Taylor will:
1. Actively participate in movement games and activities for 30 minutes daily without needing a rest
2. Be able to walk with his walker, wheel his wheelchair, and make movement transitions while producing coordinated sounds such as in singing, yelling, or counting for up to 30 seconds
3. Repeat specific required movements to strengthen abdominal muscles, back extensors, and gluteal muscles for up to 10 minutes a day while lying on the floor participating in group exercises with classmates

Intervention

Attempts can be made to make movement experiences fun and rewarding so that Taylor becomes self-motivated to build up his strength. Staging wheelchair races using ramps will increase upper body strength. Going on long "walks" where Taylor is allowed to set the pace will increase his curiosity and confidence with movement in general. Taylor should be included in more community movement recreational activities where he could participate using his walker. Ready-made audio- and videotapes that encourage floor activities should be used at least two times a week. Tapes such as *YogaKids* and *Monkey Moves* would be examples. An intensive program to address strength needs using push-ups, head lifts, bridging, resistive reaching, and commando crawling as challenges should be used along with a program with active breathing exercises. Once Taylor is in a school program, periodic intensive intervention should be used to keep up with changing strength needs as Taylor grows. Resistive materials such as theraband and rubber tubing could be used in combination with active arm and breathing exercises.

Case Study #4: Ashley

➤ Practice pattern 5B: Impaired Neuromotor Development
➤ Medical diagnosis: Down syndrome
➤ Age: 15 months

Examination and Evaluation

Examination reveals that Ashley has a history of fragile health and medical intervention. She now is healthy, but significantly delayed in her play and cognitive skills as well as in the area of motor ability.

FUNCTIONAL LIMITATIONS

Ashley likes to move on the floor on her terms. She is apprehensive when moved too quickly and is slow with her own movement abilities. Ashley likes to throw things more than she likes to interact with children or play with toys. Ashley is delayed in all motor development and lacks variety in what she does. She stands with poor alignment and is not cruising or walking. Ashley compensates for low muscle tone by "hanging on her ligaments." She needs many repetitions to incorporate a new movement pattern in her motor coordination and developmental skills. Ashley drinks from a cup that is held by her caregiver. She does not assist in self-cares.

IMPAIRMENTS

Ashley has low muscle tone in her trunk and extremities. She also demonstrates poor muscle definition throughout her body, particularly noticeable in the shoulders and hips. Hypermobility is noted in all upper and lower extremity proximal and distal joints. She has poor stability in weight-bearing positions such as all fours and kneeling. Ashley has slow and usually ineffective protective and equilibrium reactions in all positions. She has decreased respiratory-phonotory functioning and drools occasionally.

GOALS

Treatment goals are for Ashley to:

1. Tolerate moving more quickly in her environment
2. Demonstrate a greater variety of movement patterns
3. Improve stability of her upper and lower extremities as well as her trunk during weight bearing activities

FUNCTIONAL OUTCOMES

Following 3 months of intervention, Ashley will:

1. Seek movement in her environment by climbing over objects, into a ball pit, or onto the sofa during free play
2. Smile or produce sounds during riding or movement activities such as swinging in a swing, rocking in a chair, or propelling a small riding toy
3. Maintain a stable trunk during sitting while she plays with a toy using both hands

Intervention

Ashley's family should be shown how to use a variety of touching techniques such as infant massage, joint compression, hugging, vigorous rubbing, and squeezing of the limbs to provide her with more sensory input. Play activities should include the introduction of tactile materials and movement stimulation. Ashley should be encouraged to climb into a bin of dried beans, heavy plastic balls, or in a large cardboard box with pillows and blankets. She might like to be pushed around in the box or plastic bin while supported well with the pillows or blankets. Additionally, Ashley could be pulled around while lying on a blanket to increase her tolerance of movement while still feeling secure. She also could be jostled or swung as long as she feels safe and secure. Unweighted walking protocols to facilitate ambulation could be used as soon as the family is ready for intervention on a formal basis. Ashley's family should be provided with written information on outcomes and possibilities for children who have Down syndrome. Videotapes and other curriculum guides could offer information about specific movement development.

Case Study #5: John

➤ Practice pattern 5B: Impaired Neuromotor Development

➤ Medical diagnosis: Attention deficit hyperactivity disorder, developmental coordination disorder

➤ Age: 5 years

Examination and Evaluation

John has a good imagination and likes to be involved with visually stimulating activities, such as videogames. He does not have significant neuromotor deficits as seen in children with cerebral palsy and spina bifida. Control of head and trunk movements, therefore, is adequate for motor activities. The Sensory Integration and Praxis Tests were administered by a therapist in his school district and John had particular difficulty with tests that involved tactile and kinesthetic processing.

FUNCTIONAL LIMITATIONS

John avoids motor activities or tasks where he believes he is not skilled and does not participate in many age-appropriate motor activities with his peers. As a result, he does not practice motor skills and does not improve his coordination abilities. He has difficulty remembering the sequence of multi-task activities and is slow to learn new motor skills. He tends to be impulsive and demonstrates a low tolerance for frustration. He also has poor social skills when interacting with peers.

IMPAIRMENTS

John has generalized weakness in his upper body. He has attention deficits that interfere with his remembering instructions and following through with practice of motor skills. He has difficulty modulating his rate of movement with any consistency and, therefore, attempts to do most transitions of movement by running.

GOALS

Treatment goals are for John to:

1. Improve motor planning
2. Increase frequency and duration of participation in age-related motor activities with peers
3. Increase upper body and shoulder strength
4. Increase frequency of practice of self-selected motor activities

FUNCTIONAL OUTCOMES

Following 3 months of intervention, John will:

1. Be able to weight-bear on his arms to "camel" walk and "crab" walk as part of an imitative game
2. Participate in a video instruction exercise session for 10 to 15 minutes without fatiguing
3. Play on the playground with peers for 15 minutes without adult prompting
4. Access three of five available playground equipment structures (eg, slide, swing, merry-go-round) independently within a 15-minute observation period

Intervention

John may benefit from a structured exercise program or perceptual motor activities using videotapes from *YogaKids* or *Move Like the Animals*. These activities would be incorporated to improve his interest and feelings of competence in using his body. Sensory information embedded in motor activities using swings, ball baths, tunnels, and large motor or playground equipment would help improve his body awareness. Walking and running outside on uneven terrain will increase proprioceptive input and challenge his balance. Movements that occur in these activities will necessitate appropriate use of head and trunk control.

References

1. Cohen B. *The Alphabet of Movement: Primitive Reflexes, Righting Reactions, and Equilibrium Responses, Part 2.* Northhampton, Mass: Contact Quarterly; 1989:14.

2. Magrun WM. *Clinical Observation of Posture* [video]. Tucson, Ariz: Therapy Skill Builders; 1985.

3. Nadis S. The energy efficient brain. *Omni Magazine.* 1992:2.

4. Bly L. *The Components of Normal Movement During the First Year of Life and Abnormal Motor Development.* Chicago, Ill: NeuroDevelopmental Treatment Association; 1983.

5. DiJoseph L. *Motor Behavioral vs Motor Control: Holistic Approach to Movement.* Rockville, Md: American Occupational Therapy Association; 1984:7.

6. Dubowitz V. *The Floppy Infant.* 2nd ed. Lavenham, Suffolk, England: The Lavenham Press; 1980.

7. Brazelton TB. *Neonatal Behavioral Assessment.* Lavenham, Suffolk, England: Spastics International Medical Publications; 1973.

8. Casaer P. *Postural Behavior in Newborn Infants.* Lavenham, Suffolk, England: The Lavenham Press; 1979.

9. Gilles FH, Leviton A, Dooling EC. *The Developing Human Brain, Growth, Epidemiology, Neuropathology.* Boston, Mass: John Wright PSG; 1983.

10. Restak R. *The Brain.* New York, NY: Bantam Books; 1984.

11. Prechtl H. *Continuity of Neural Functions from Prenatal to Postnatal Life.* London, England: Spastics International Medical Publications; 1984.

12. Shonkoff JP, Phillips DA. *From Neurons to Neighborhoods. The Science of Early Childhood Development.* Washington, DC: National Academy; 2000.

13. Stokes B. *Amazing Babies. Essential Movements for Babies.* Santa Barbara, Calif: Malcom; 2002.

14. Bricker B, Wadell M. *AEPS Curriculum for Three to Six Years.* Baltimore, Md: Brookes Publishing; 1996.

15. Linder TW, Paul H. *Transdisciplinary Play-Based Assessment (TPBA).* Baltimore, Md: Brookes Publishing; 1993.

16. Brazelton TB. *Touchpoints—Your Child's Emotional and Behavioral Development.* Reading, Ma: Perseus; 1992.

17. Simons DG, Simons L, Travel JG. *Myofascial Pain and Dysfunction: The Trigger Point Manual, Vol. 1: The Upper Half of Body.* 2nd ed. Hagerstown, Md: Lippincott, Williams and Wilkins; 1999.

18. Banal J. *The Thorax.* Seattle, Wash: Eastland Press; 1991.

19. Brooks-Scott S. *Mobilization for the Neurologically Involved Child: Assessment and Application Strategies for Pediatric OTs and PTs.* Tucson, Ariz: Therapy Skill Builders; 1998.

20. Brazelton TB. *Neonatal Behavioral Assessment Scale.* 2nd ed. Hagerstown, Md: JB Lippincott; 1984.

21. Ginsburg C. Body-image, movement, and consciousness: examples from a somatic practice in the Feldenkrais method. *Journal of Consciousness Studies*. 1999;6:79-91.

22. Boehme R. *Developing Midrange Control and Function in Children with Fluctuating Muscle Tone*. Tucson, Ariz: Therapy Skill Builders; 1990.

23. Boehme R. *The Hypotonic Child*. Tucson, Ariz: Therapy Skill Builders; 1990.

24. Thorpe D. *The Effects of Aquatic Resistive Exercise on Strength, Balance, Energy Expenditure, Functional Mobility, and Perceived Competence in a Person With Cerebral Palsy*. San Antonio, Tex: American Physical Therapy Association Combined Sections Meeting; 2001.

25. Alon R. *Mindful Spontaneity Lessons in the Feldenkrais Method*. Berkeley, Calif: North Atlantic Books; 1996:71.

26. Feldenkrais M. *The Master Moves*. Capitola, Calif: Meta; 1984.

27. Feldenkrais M. *Awareness Through Movement*. New York, NY: Harper & Row; 1977.

28. Hanna T. *The Body of Life*. New York, NY: Alfred A. Knopf; 1983.

29. Kendall F, McCreary E. *Muscles Testing and Function*. 3rd ed. Baltimore, Md: Williams and Wilkins; 1983.

30. Dull HW. *Freeing the Body in Water*. Merrickville, Ontario: Worldwide Aquatic Bodywork Association; 1997.

31. Wells KF. *Kinesiology: The Scientific Basis of Human Motion*. 4th ed. Philadelphia, Pa: WB Saunders; 1978.

32. Campbell S. *Pediatric Neurologic Physical Therapy*. New York, NY: Churchill Livingstone; 1984.

33. Alter J. *Surviving Exercise*. Boston, Mass: Houghton Mifflin; 1983.

34. Massery M. *Respiratory Rehabilitation Secondary to Neurological Deficits: Understanding the Deficits. Chest Physical Therapy and Pulmonary Rehabilitation*. 2nd ed. Chicago, Ill: Year Book Medical Publishers; 1987.

35. Massery, M. Chest development as a component of normal motor development: implications for pediatric physical therapists. *Ped Phys Ther*. 1991;3:3-8.

36. Seifert M. Gerda Alexander's Eutony: its theory, its practice and its teaching. *Somatics Journal*. 1985;Spring-Summer:17-32.

37. Ayres AJ. *Sensory Integration and Learning Disorders*. Los Angeles, Calif: Western Psychological Services; 1983.

38. Upledger JE, Vredevoogd JD. *Craniosacral Therapy*. Seattle, Wash: Eastland Press; 1973.

39. Feldenkrais M. Bodily expressions. *Somatics*. 1988;Spring-Summer:15-24.

40. Lehane L. Neuropeptides, emotion and the bodymind. *Nexus New Times*. 2003;10:39-42.

41. Pert C. *Molecules of Emotion. The Science Behind Mind-Body Medicine*. New York, NY: Touchstone/Simon and Schuster; 1999.

42. Porges SW. *Orienting in a Defensive World: Mammalian Modifications of Our Evolutionary Heritage. A Polyvagal Theory*. College Park, Md: Department of Human Development, University of Maryland; 1995.

43. Ratey MD. *A User's Guide to the Brain*. New York, NY: Vintage Books; 1994.

10 RESPIRATORY AND ORAL-MOTOR FUNCTIONING

Rona Alexander, PhD, CCC-SP

Speech is a complex and highly sophisticated means by which information can be exchanged or communicated among individuals.[1] It requires the effective and efficient integration of a variety of features, including pitch, loudness, resonance, duration, vocal quality, articulation, rate, and rhythm. The integration of these features for proficient speech functioning has its foundation in the development of the motor control system. This motor control system is influenced by an extensive number of anatomical, physiological, kinesiological, neurological, neuromotor, sensory-motor, perceptual, acoustical, cognitive, and environmental factors.[2,3]

Speech cannot be viewed as a total reflection of a child's level of language functioning. As described by Bloom and Lahey,[4] language consists of an element of content or meaning (eg, semantics of a message). Content or meaning is represented by a linguistic form (eg, an expressive mode of communication used according to specific phonological, morphological, and syntactic rules). Language use or function is specific (eg, the purpose of a message and the context of the utterance). As children interact in their environment, they develop a base of language competence that is the interaction of language content, form, and use. Although speech is significant because of its general acceptance as our primary form of expressive language, it must not be equated with overall language competence. Speech should not be regarded as the only form in which knowledge can be communicated to others.

This chapter will present information specifically relevant to the evaluation and treatment of oral-motor, feeding/swallowing, and respiratory-phonatory function because of their intricate relationship to and effect on general movement development. However, this emphasis should not negate the importance of the evaluation and treatment of receptive and expressive language function by a qualified speech-language pathologist when developing programming for children with developmental disabilities.

Oral-Motor, Feeding/Swallowing, and Respiratory-Phonatory Function

To understand the significance of oral-motor, feeding/swallowing, and respiratory-phonatory function in pediatric evaluation and intervention, it is necessary to understand their role in typical development.[5] From birth, the typical, full-term infant uses the oral, pharyngeal, laryngeal, esophageal, and respiratory mechanisms for feeding, breathing, crying, sound production, and sensory exploration. Liquids presented by bottle or breast are ingested using a negative-pressure sucking pattern. This sucking pattern

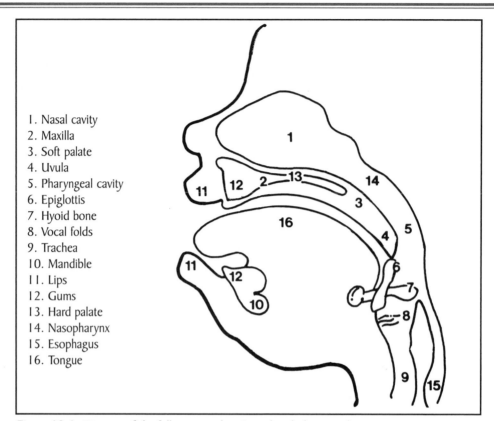

1. Nasal cavity
2. Maxilla
3. Soft palate
4. Uvula
5. Pharyngeal cavity
6. Epiglottis
7. Hyoid bone
8. Vocal folds
9. Trachea
10. Mandible
11. Lips
12. Gums
13. Hard palate
14. Nasopharynx
15. Esophagus
16. Tongue

Figure 10-1. Diagram of the full-term newborn's oral and pharyngeal areas.

is created by a combination of jaw, tongue, and cheek/lip movements. These movement patterns are related directly to the newborn's physiological flexion and small infra-oral space.[6] The newborn can breathe through the nose and suck simultaneously, since liquids are moved back over a cupped tongue and pass around the sides of the epiglottis directly into the esophagus. This process avoids the high-positioned laryngeal area which is protected by the hyoid bone, pharyngeal musculature, and the close approximation of the uvula and epiglottis (Figure 10-1).

Once the infant begins to turn and lift the head with neck extension against gravity, the influence of physiological flexion on the mouth is reduced, resulting in wider ranges of jaw and tongue activity. Suckling now becomes the active oral pattern of the infant and is composed of large up/down and forward/backward movements of the jaw and large, rhythmical, forward/backward movements of a thin, cupped tongue. Minimal muscle activity occurs in the cheeks and lips. Oral movements for sucking still will occur when the infant's head is held in a more stable flexed position by the feeder.

The newborn's respiratory function at rest is characterized by obligatory nasal breathing and an open pharyngeal airway. There is close approximation of the back of the tongue to the soft palate.[7] The rib cage is elevated within the trunk with the upper ribs at almost a 90-degree angle to the spine. The rib cage is limited in its skeletal mobility and active movements (Figure 10-2). On inhalation, abdominal or belly breathing occurs as the diaphragm contracts and lowers causing expansion of the abdominal wall and lower ribs. With effortful crying, movement, or stress, strong contraction of the diaphragm may pull the anterior ribs and sternum downward and posterior while expanding the abdominal

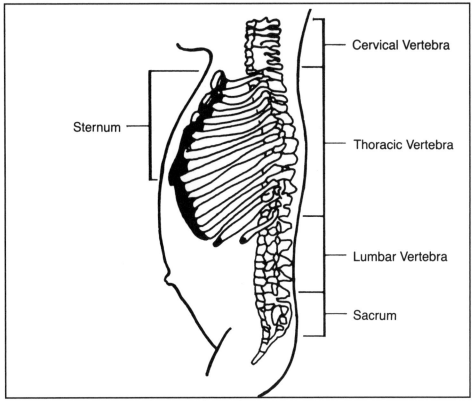

Figure 10-2. Diagram of the full-term infant's rib cage.

wall and pushing the lower ribs outward. This lower rib expansion often is referred to as rib flaring.

A direct relationship exists between sound production and body movement starting at birth. Sounds are produced spontaneously on expiration and crying is nasal in quality. Short duration and low intensity vegetative sounds are produced by the infant, especially during feeding.

The infant's development of more controlled movement against gravity throughout the first year of life establishes a basis on which more functional oral-motor, oral-pharyngeal, respiratory-phonatory, and sound production activity can be produced. Changes in oral-motor, oral-pharyngeal, and respiratory function also have a major influence on general movement development. This is apparent in the development of well-controlled head and neck flexion, which depends on the active use of the suprahyoid and infrahyoid muscles that have primary control of jaw, tongue, and hyoid movements.[8]

Developmental changes in the respiratory system have a profound effect on general movement, as well as on oral-motor, feeding/swallowing, and respiratory-phonatory function. As the child of 4 to 6 months of age begins to use the abdominal musculature in supine and is held passively upright against gravity in sitting, the ribs are drawn downward, creating an angle between the ribs and spine of less than 90 degrees. Stabilization of the rib cage by the abdominals in a more downward direction will modify the contour and alignment of the rib cage. The intercostals and levator costarum then are prepared for future active use in more adult abdominal/thoracic respiratory functioning. Abdominal activity will provide the musculature of the head, neck, shoulder girdle, mouth, and pharynx with a base of stability from which more integrated, controlled movements can be developed.

Oral-motor development is affected by a variety of factors, including growth, contour, and alignment changes; the introduction of new varieties of oral sensory stimulation (eg, puréed foods, solids, toys); the child's active coordinated movements against gravity; and changes in the respiratory mechanism. The 6-month-old infant reflects the interaction of these factors in the use of the cheeks, lips, and tongue in bottle- or breast-feeding for more active negative-pressure sucking. However, the wider range of movements that compose suckling continue to predominate in spoon feeding and cup drinking, facial expression, and sound production. Although solid food generally will be handled using sucking or suckling movements, some new movements of the tongue and jaw may appear as a munching pattern develops. Sound production will modify to include a greater variety of vowels and consonants with changes in duration, loudness, intonation, and vocal quality.

By 12 months of age, the child has developed more highly coordinated general movement abilities. These skills provide an integrated neuromotor and sensory-motor foundation from which more coordinated oral-motor, oral-pharyngeal, and respiratory-sound production activity can be produced and developed. Movements of the jaw, tongue, cheeks, and lips for sucking and fine coordination of these movements with breathing now are predominant in bottle drinking, breast feeding, and spoon feeding. Greater sucking activity is evident in cup drinking, although excessive jaw activity is compensated for by use of tongue protrusion under the cup or by biting on the cup rim for stability. The tongue exhibits lateral movements as it transfers and maintains food on the side-biting surfaces in coordination with cheek musculature activity during chewing. The jaw uses a variety of up and down, diagonal, and circular-diagonal movements as it breaks up the solid food in preparation for swallowing. More controlled abdominal/thoracic respiratory function and oral-pharyngeal function provide a foundation for long chains of sounds, with varying consonant-vowel combinations and occasional single word productions.

Impairments in Oral-Motor and Respiratory Coordination Function

As is true in typically developing infants, infants with neuromotor involvement begin to function using the oral-motor and respiratory mechanisms at birth. The type and severity of their neuropathology, however, may result in impairments of the neuromuscular, musculoskeletal, sensory, perceptual/cognitive, respiratory, cardiovascular, and gastrointestinal systems. Such impairments may result in the infant's attempt to obtain stability at the head, neck, mouth, and shoulder girdle through the use of abnormal head and neck hyperextension, tongue retraction (ie, the pulling back and holding of the tongue body in a more posterior position in the oral mechanism), and humeral extension with adduction and internal rotation. With the head and neck in a hyperextended position, the cheeks and lips will be drawn back into retraction and the jaw will depress or thrust open and retract. Compensatory shoulder elevation and oral movements such as: 1) lip pursing (ie, purse-string positioning of the lips and cheeks), 2) tongue thrusting (ie, strong forward pushing of a thickly bunched tongue), 3) tongue retraction with anterior tongue elevation against the hard palate, 4) jaw thrusting with protrusion, and 5) exaggerated jaw closure may develop as the infant attempts to function in feeding, sound production, and general movement activities

The infant may not be able to suck or suckle liquids efficiently from the bottle or breast due to cheek-lip and tongue retraction. He may be able only to swallow with strong head and neck hyperextension and tongue thrusting, which may result in choking, coughing, or gagging. Jaw thrusting and exaggerated jaw closure may occur due to jaw instability whenever the nipple or spoon is presented. The variety of oral movements that the child can use for vowel and consonant sounds will be limited to those that can be produced only when there is head and neck hyperextension, tongue retraction, jaw thrusting, and cheek-lip retraction.

Respiratory-phonatory coordination will be affected directly by atypical or inadequate development of the head, neck, shoulder girdle, and extrinsic tongue musculature. Problems that may develop include: prevention or restriction of active stability and mobility of the upper rib cage, active use of the abdominals in expiration, and active thoracic expansion for inhalation. Compensatory shoulder elevation and use of a shortened rectus abdominus for stability may result in severe retraction of the sternum and anterior ribs with excessive lateral flaring of the lower ribs on inhalation. This will negatively influence the quality, duration, pitch, rhythm, loudness, and rate of phonation and early sound production. Immobility or deformities of the rib cage, as well as immobility of the laryngeal area, will develop. This restricts adequate breath support for sound production and adequate coordination between respiration, laryngeal function, and oral-motor activity.

Although early oral-motor, oral-pharyngeal, and respiratory coordination function may appear adequate in some children with neuromotor involvement, there generally is an abnormal quality to their movements. This abnormal quality may interfere with the development of *refined* motor coordination required in activities such as chewing, cup drinking, and speech. When abnormal lumbar extension with hip flexion, abduction, and external rotation (frog-leg posture) is maintained for stability, the hip flexors remain in a shortened position. This posture places the pelvis in an anterior tilt and does not allow for active abdominal muscle activity. Therefore, a shallow belly breathing pattern will be used. Changes in the contour and alignment of the structures of the rib cage as well as activity of its musculature will be limited, giving the thoracic area a more barrel-shaped appearance. Longer, controlled exhalations for sound production and speech cannot be developed. If compensatory humeral extension with adduction is used to reinforce spinal extension in prone, sitting, or standing, additional compensations at the head, neck, and mouth may result, which interfere with development of coordinated oral-motor and oral-pharyngeal control.

When adequate thoracic and lumbar extension and abdominal muscle activity do not develop, some children attempt to stabilize the trunk using the hip adductors and hamstrings. This may result in abnormal hip extension and adduction. To shift the center of gravity forward in sitting and standing, compensatory humeral extension with adduction, abnormal upper trunk flexion, and compensatory head and neck hyperextension are used. Limitations in the expansion of the upper thoracic area and abnormal contraction of the rectus abdominus may occur. Rib cage mobility as well as rib cage and abdominal musculature activity for respiratory coordination with feeding, phonation, and sound production activities will be restricted.

Intervention Framework

Subsequent to the completion of a thorough clinical examination and evaluation of a child's oral-motor, feeding/swallowing, and respiratory coordination function, recommendations are made regarding the need for other evaluations; the appropriateness of the procedures presently being used for nutritional intake; the need for instrumental assessment of the swallowing process; and the need for future treatment programming. A comprehensive treatment plan will include delineation of goals and objectives for both direct patient treatment by the therapist and carryover activities such as mealtime feeding and tooth brushing.

During mealtime feeding, the primary goal always will focus on nutritional intake and its presentation in the safest manner possible for the child. The implementation of new strategies to modify a child's oral function or head and neck position during mealtime may lead to reduced nutritional intake. This will result in the caregiver's rejection of these new strategies. It is essential to further investigate the child's oral, pharyngeal, and general movement activities, their coordination with respiration, and other factors that may be influencing the child's activity as a component of the intervention plan prior to making changes in procedures being used in mealtime feeding. New strategies can be introduced during direct treatment and carried over into mealtime when the child's response does not negatively impact the primary mealtime feeding goal.

Direct patient treatment should improve function through active preparation and handling. Intervention strategies are based on knowledge of typical and atypical developmental processes. Treatment must reflect understanding of the relationship between general movement, oral-motor activity, oral-pharyngeal function, and respiratory coordination development. The importance of repetition for learning and the therapist's ability to analyze the specific movements required for task accomplishment also are essential components. Once specific objectives begin to be accomplished in direct treatment, they can be incorporated into carryover activities.

Clinical Examination and Evaluation

When evaluating a child's oral motor, feeding/swallowing, and respiratory-phonatory-sound production functioning, information should be obtained on the movements of the child's oral mechanism during feeding, sound production, and general movement. The quality and coordination of these oral movements and the effect of postural control, movement, and sensory stimulation on oral-motor and respiratory-phonatory-sound production function also should be assessed. In addition, the coordination of respiration with feeding, sound production, and general movement must be observed. The child's use of different modes of communication during movement, play, and feeding activities are important components of the examination process. This information is gathered through careful questioning of the parent or caregiver, observation of the child with the caregiver during various activities, and, when appropriate, direct testing by the evaluator.[9-12]

Analysis of the child's oral-motor and respiratory coordination function during feeding activities is a significant part of the evaluation process. Questions should be posed to the caregiver to obtain information on feeding and respiratory history as well as on mealtime length, nutritional intake, preferred food textures, feeding utensils, positioning used, and the child's feeding activity. Often the information gathered from caregivers helps the evaluator discover factors that may be influencing a child's function, especially in the areas of feeding and swallowing, which may not be evident during observation of a mealtime feeding activity.

Careful observation of the interactions of the caregiver and child, the procedures used, and the child's oral-motor and respiratory function during feeding is an essential component of the examination process. Special emphasis should be placed on describing the initial body alignment of the child for feeding and any changes that occur in alignment over time. How food and liquid are presented, the child's response to these presentations, the oral movements used during feeding, and the coordination of respiration with oral movements also are noted.

After observing the child and caregiver, direct testing may be appropriate to analyze movements already observed or to try to modify function through changes in handling, positioning, food textures, or food presentation. Handling to stimulate more active anti-gravity postural control and movement may be provided to evaluate the child's potential for changes in oral-motor, respiratory-phonatory, sound production, and general communication function. Direct testing by the evaluator should focus on obtaining maximum information through discussions with the parent or caregiver and observation of the caregiver and child during general movement, feeding, and communication activities.

If aspiration is suspected based on the child's history (eg, chronic respiratory illnesses; frequent coughing, choking, or gagging during feeding; consistent wet, gurgly vocalizations; and increased respiratory distress during feeding), and observations made during the clinical examination, an oral-pharyngeal motility study (ie, videoswallow study, modified barium swallow) or a fiberoptic endoscopic evaluation of swallowing (FEES) may be conducted.[13,14] These studies more directly evaluate if, when, and under what conditions aspiration may be occurring. The findings of these instrumental evaluations should be obtained prior to implementing changes in the child's mealtime feeding.[15]

A child's oral-motor activity, body position, and head/neck position during and after feeding may be influenced by gastrointestinal problems. Gastroesophageal reflex (GER) is the return flow of the stomach contents into the esophagus. GER may be suspected if the child has a history of excessive spitting up or vomiting during or after meals, increased irritability after specific amounts of nutritional intake, poor weight gain, fussiness in regard to changes in food types or textures, or aspiration pneumonia. The child's primary physician should be contacted if GER is suspected for discussion of the possibility of further testing or referral for examination by a pediatric gastroenterologist.[16] If GER exists, the child will be resistant to changes in food textures. This may limit the possibility of improving oral-motor function for feeding as well as the potential for increasing the child's nutritional intake for weight gain.

Treatment Programming

Treatment to improve oral-motor activity, oral-pharyngeal function, and respiratory-phonatory coordination must address goals and strategies that help the child develop the motor components required to more successfully use the oral, .pharyngeal, laryngeal, esophageal, and respiratory mechanisms for feeding/swallowing, crying, sound/speech production, and communication. Emphasis must be placed on developing functional activity of the cheeks, lips, tongue, and jaw as well as their coordination with respiration. Strategies for direct treatment services leading to progressive improvement in function may not be immediately incorporated into activities such as mealtime feeding if their use initially interferes with overall nutritional intake. Therefore, a well-coordinated program for improved function through both direct treatment and carryover activities should be designed.[17-24]

Underlying all treatment for improved oral, pharyngeal, and respiratory coordination is the developmental relationship between active movement in these areas and coordinated anti-gravity movement in general. Dynamic handling during direct treatment is necessary to facilitate more normal active movements of the head, neck, mouth, shoulder girdle, spine, rib cage, pelvis, and hips. Appropriate handling will lead to the development of active functional movements that can be repeated and generalized to a wide variety of activities.

Proper body alignment through positioning may provide a base of central stability for better oral-motor, oral-pharyngeal, and respiratory functioning during carryover activities such as mealtime feeding. However, this alignment will not provide a foundation for the generalized integration of these new movements to other activities (eg, general movements, sound/speech production). Both dynamic handling, which facilitates the integration of active anti-gravity movements, and proper body alignment through positioning play important roles in the child's overall treatment program.[25,26]

When aspiration and GER are not primary issues, there are strategies that may be implemented during mealtime feeding to support the primary goal of nutritional intake. These strategies often include the establishment of proper positions for feeding, the modification of food textures and feeding utensils being used, and the incorporation of other methods or procedures for food presentation. There is not one piece of equipment or way to adapt equipment that is successful in establishing good feeding positions for all children. However, proper positioning for better function at mealtime requires good body alignment. This includes neutral head flexion with neck elongation; symmetrical, stable shoulder girdle depression with scapulohumeral dissociation; and symmetrical trunk elongation. Good body alignment also includes neutral positioning of a stable, symmetrical pelvis; hip stability with neutral abduction and rotation; and stable, symmetrical positioning of the feet flat on a surface (Figure 10-3). Any deviation from this central base of good body alignment due to physical deformity or inappropriate equipment will restrict the positive effects of positioning on function during mealtime.

Although proper positioning will have a significant effect on mealtime feeding, the wide variety of sensory experiences that occur during mealtime may continue to make feeding difficult. Thickened textures of food and liquid, rather than thin or pureed food and liquid, may provide sensory-motor information and stimulate more active oral-motor functioning.[10,11] The selection of appropriate feeding utensils can be essential to the encouragement of greater functional activity of the cheeks, lips, tongue, and jaw during mealtime. The presentation of food and liquid by the feeder must be modified so that visual, auditory, and tactile input do not result in atypical postures. Atypical postures may reduce nutritional intake and restrict or limit oral activity and its coordination with respiration.

Strategies directed toward mealtime feeding are important but narrow in focus. Strategies for direct treatment are of primary significance to the modification of overall oral-motor, oral-pharyngeal, and respiratory coordination function. As function is modified through direct treatment, changes may be made in positioning and procedures used during mealtime.

Preparation through handling is necessary for developing the motor components required for coordinated oral-motor and respiratory-phonatory functioning. Handling is combined with specific activities to facilitate the development of neutral head flexion with neck elongation and stable shoulder girdle depression with scapulohumeral dissociation. Active rib cage mobility and stability with abdominal musculature activity are important. Additionally, handling should facilitate active lip closure, rounding, and spreading, as well as active jaw movements up/down, forward/backward, and in diagonal, and circular-rotary directions similar to those seen in the normal developmental process.

Special emphasis in treatment must be placed on handling to enhance respiratory coordination with oral function. Facilitation of active thoracic and lumbar spinal extension in supine, prone, and through transitional movements will help elongate shoulder girdle and abdominal musculature (see Chapter 9). This may lead to development of greater rib cage mobility and stability. As the child begins to sit and move in and out of sitting and stand-

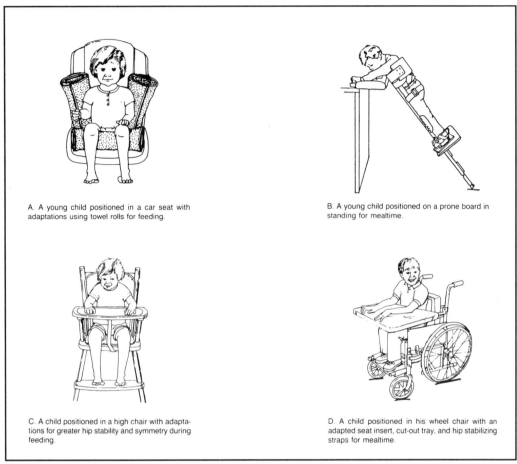

A. A young child positioned in a car seat with adaptations using towel rolls for feeding.

B. A young child positioned on a prone board in standing for mealtime.

C. A child positioned in a high chair with adaptations for greater hip stability and symmetry during feeding.

D. A child positioned in his wheel chair with an adapted seat insert, cut-out tray, and hip stabilizing straps for mealtime.

Figure 10-3. Examples of proper body positioning for improved oral-motor and respiratory functioning during mealtime.

ing, the abdominals actively stabilize the rib cage from below. This results in elongation of the musculature between each rib and between the ribs and spine. Thus, the rib cage can expand on inhalation and provide a foundation for longer controlled exhalation. This allows more adult type abdominal/thoracic respiratory function to occur. In addition, active shoulder girdle and rib cage mobility and stability, along with active abdominal musculature, provide a basis for coordinated oral-motor and oral-pharyngeal movements.

Modifying oral tactile sensitivity is another important aspect of treatment. Deep pressure tactile stimulation presented on the face and within the oral area can prepare the mouth for more normal sensory-motor activity. Deep pressure stroking on the face toward and through the lips helps to elongate check and lip musculature. The child then may be able to initiate more active cheek, lower lip, and upper lip movements. Subsequent presentation of cup drinking, bottle drinking, spoon feeding, or stimulation for bilabial sound production then is introduced.

A consistent program of deep pressure input through the biting surfaces of the gums or teeth can help reduce the occurrence of a tonic bite. A tonic bite may occur in response to the presentation of the spoon, cup, bottle, the child's own fingers, toys, and solid foods. Tonic biting does not occur in isolation and generally reflects problems in tolerating other tactile information on the body and extremities.

The strength of the gag response and the range and quality of tongue movements in sucking and suckling activities can be modified. One technique is the use of rhythmical, well-graded, moderate pressure stroking of the lateral aspects of the tongue body prior to feeding and sound production stimulation. As the child begins to respond positively to this stimulation, tactile input can be moved to include downward and slightly forward, moderate pressure stroking more directly on the superior surface of the tongue. This tactile input to the tongue also will have an influence on respiratory function as well as the development of more coordinated head flexion and neck elongation.

Treatment of oral-motor, feeding/swallowing, and respiratory-phonatory function must allow the child to develop functional skills based on knowledge of the motor components or sequences required for certain functional activities. Strategies for direct treatment and carryover activities must be well-coordinated if the child is to function effectively and efficiently in the oral-motor, feeding/swallowing, respiratory-phonatory, and speech areas.

Case Study #1: Jason

➤ Practice pattern 5C: Impaired Motor Function and Sensory Integrity Associated With Nonprogressive Disorders of the Central Nervous System—Congenital Origin or Acquired in Infancy or Childhood

➤ Medical diagnosis: Cerebral palsy, right hemiparesis

➤ Age: 24 months

Examination and Evaluation

A clinical evaluation of Jason's oral-motor, feeding/swallowing, and respiratory coordination function was conducted at his home. He was observed during play, communication, gross motor, and mealtime activities.

At rest, Jason exhibits subtle check/lip retraction on the right, an asymmetrical contour to his tongue, and a slight pull of his jaw laterally to the right. During play and gross motor activities, cheek/lip retraction and lateral jaw deviation to the right increase with some asymmetry of the tongue evident. Drooling, which increases with gross motor and upper extremity activities, is noted from the right side of the mouth.

Jason relies heavily on gestures and movement for communication. As with most children his age, he has a small number of real single words. His overall use of vocalizations and jargon with gestures for communication is limited, especially when he is ambulating. His vocalizations are nasal in quality and reveal minimal variety in intonation and inflectional patterns unlike what would be expected at his age.

Jason produces a variety of vowel sounds, while his consonants are limited in quantity and have some distortions. He is unable to produce good quality lip activity for bilabial productions (m, b, p, w) due to his cheek/lip retraction.

Jason eats a limited variety of foods. He chews easily dissolvable solids, such as cookies or crackers, only on the left side of his mouth and uses his hand to move pieces initially placed on the right to the left. His tongue lateralizes better to the left than the right. His lips surround the spoon for food removal, but he cannot clear all of the food from the spoon with his lips. Food remains on his lips, especially on the right, during spoon feeding. When cup drinking, Jason places the cup far back between his teeth and uses slight head/neck hyperextension to compensate for his cheek/lip retraction. He occasionally loses some liquid when the cup is removed.

Jason exhibits problems in his coordination of breathing with oral and pharyngeal activity. He gasps for breath after drinking a cup of liquid. His vocalizations are somewhat limited in length. He has some observable asymmetry of his rib cage with greater flattening of the upper anterior thoracic area on the right. Rib flaring is evident revealing his lack of good, consistent use of abdominal musculature.

FUNCTIONAL LIMITATIONS

Jason has difficulty using speech to communicate with others and relies more on gestures than other children his age. He is a "messy" eater, often leaving food on his lips and cheeks. He has difficulty eating foods with increased texture and often spits pieces out. He frequently gasps for breath and coughs after drinking several sips in a row from an open cup.

IMPAIRMENTS

Jason demonstrates poor sensory awareness on the right side of his body, on his face, and within his oral mechanism. He demonstrates poor lip closure with retraction of the cheeks and lips, greater on the right. He has difficulty moving his tongue laterally, especially to the right, and generally exhibits a thickened tongue contour. His jaw deviates to the right when the mouth is open and during closure. He has difficulty coordinating breathing with oral, pharyngeal, and some general movement activities.

GOALS

Treatment goals are for Jason to:

1. Increase sensory awareness of the right side of his body, face, and within the oral mechanism
2. Increase lip closure with reduced cheek and lip retraction during eating, drinking, sound/speech production, upper extremity, and gross motor activities
3. Increase use of up/down, forward/backward, and lateral tongue movements with thinning of the tongue contour during eating, drinking, sound/speech production, upper extremity, and gross motor activities
4. Increase use of graded jaw movements with reduced jaw deviation during eating, drinking, sound/speech production, upper extremity, and gross motor tasks
5. Improve the coordination of respiration with oral and pharyngeal activity during eating, drinking, and sound/speech production tasks

FUNCTIONAL OUTCOMES

Following 3 months of intervention, Jason will:

1. Take three to four sips of liquid from an open cup before pausing to breathe with no gasping or choking
2. Produce the consonant sounds for "b" and "m" spontaneously with good symmetrical lip closure
3. Maintain symmetrical lip closure on the cup rim while drinking 4 ounces of liquid
4. Eat soft meats using lateral tongue movements without losing food or saliva from his mouth
5. Remove food from the spoon using symmetrical lip closure and graded jaw opening

Intervention

In treatment, it is essential to combine movement facilitation with appropriate tactile and proprioceptive sensory input directed through the rib cage and shoulder girdle in order to assist Jason in establishing a more symmetrical foundation of postural control and alignment. This should be done prior to and in coordination with work presented more directly to the face and oral mechanism. Well-graded input to increase rib-to-spine and rib-to-sternum mobility within the rib cage must be combined with activities to encourage greater abdominal musculature activity, especially through the internal and external abdominal obliques. While on a movable surface (eg, ball, peanut roll), Jason is encouraged to play using transitional movements (eg, supine to sidelying to sitting or prone to sidelying to sitting), while tactile input is presented through the rib cage and abdominals directed toward the base of support. Longer and more varied sound productions, including vowel-consonant combinations, are stimulated through movement activities combined with singing and other sound play games.

Jason is given the opportunity to take sips of liquid by cup periodically during treatment as his respiration appears to be increasing in its depth and his sounds are longer in duration. When drinking, he is assisted in maintaining a symmetrical upright posture with his feet weight bearing on a stable surface.

Well-graded oral sensory stimulation directed at the cheeks and lips, through the biting surfaces of the teeth/gums, on the hard palate, and at the tongue may be presented in conjunction with general movement facilitation activities as well as prior to more specific sound production, eating, and drinking activities. Jason's caregivers have been instructed in oral sensory stimulation procedures so they can implement them as part of his daily tooth brushing routine and periodically during his day.

Following oral sensory stimulation, thickened liquid to be drawn into the mouth using the lips and cheeks is presented by cup. Pieces of crunchy cereal are placed on the biting surfaces of the teeth/gums, more often on the right, while encouraging active lateral tongue movements. Active symmetrical lip closure and jaw grading are stimulated with the presentation of yogurt by spoon. Jason's caregivers are encouraged to follow similar procedures for food presentation during meals at home.

Case Study #2: Jill

➤ Practice pattern 5C: Impaired Motor Function and Sensory Integrity Associated With Nonprogressive Disorders of the Central Nervous System—Congenital Origin or Acquired in Infancy or Childhood

➤ Medical diagnosis: Cerebral palsy, spastic quadriparesis, microcephaly, mental retardation, seizure disorder

➤ Age: 7 years

Examination and Evaluation

A clinical evaluation of Jill's oral-motor, feeding/swallowing, and respiratory coordination function was conducted. She was observed during activities both in and out of her wheelchair.

Jill uses head/neck hyperextension with shoulder girdle elevation and internal rotation, tongue retraction, severe cheek/lip retraction, and jaw thrusting with retraction in all her attempts to move, communicate, eat, and drink.

Her rib cage generally is immobile. The sternum is fixed in retraction by her shortened, tight rectus abdominus. Although the lower ribs appear flat in contour, the upper ribs appear rounded in the front and flat laterally. Jill has a shallow belly breathing pattern with retraction of the sternum and anterior ribs on inhalation. Greater retraction of the anterior rib cage with severe rib flaring is evident as she attempts to move, communicate, and eat.

Jill sits in a wheelchair with adaptations for feeding. She continues to exhibit asymmetry, head/neck hyperextension, humeral extension/adduction/internal rotation, hip extension/adduction/internal rotation, and significant problems with coordinating her respiratory function in this position. Therefore, her body alignment in her adapted wheelchair does not provide an optimal foundation for oral-motor, oral-pharyngeal, and respiratory functioning.

While feeding, Jill remains in some degree of head/neck hyperextension with humeral extension/adduction/internal rotation and shoulder girdle elevation. Her tongue is thick in contour and retracted, with only a small range of forward/backward movement noted during spoon feeding and cup drinking. Check/lip retraction is noted during all feeding activities, although she inconsistently attempts to compensate with lip pursing at the initiation of cup drinking. Initially when food is presented, jaw thrusting with retraction occurs. She uses some exaggerated jaw closure on the spoon and cup rim for stability. Small horizontal shifts of the tongue are noted to the left with solid food presentation. Generally, Jill uses her head/neck hyperextension and small-range, suckling movements of the tongue to move food and liquid back for swallowing. Respiratory coordination during cup drinking is poor with much coughing and choking.

Jill attempts to say a few words such as "bye," "hi," and "mom." However, her attempts to say these words are greatly restricted by the body hyperextension she uses to initiate sound.

Recommendations from the clinical evaluation included requests for additional medical evaluations in the areas of nutrition and pulmonary function. Jill's history of upper respiratory infections, coughing and choking during cup drinking, oral motor dysfunction, and poor postural alignment during eating and drinking tasks support the need for an instrumental evaluation of her swallowing process such as an oral-pharyngeal motility study (ie, videoswallow study, modified barium swallow). The study should provide more specific information related to her oral and pharyngeal function, especially in regard to her posterior tongue activity and her ability to protect her airway during swallowing. Prior to making any changes in her head/neck and body position during feeding, it will be important to have the information from the oral-pharyngeal motility study. Information from the study also will help in the further development of treatment goals and strategies.

Functional Limitations

Jill coughs and chokes often during feeding due to the poor coordination of her breathing with oral and pharyngeal function. She eats a very limited variety of food textures due to her poor oral motor function. Jill is resistant to tooth brushing which puts her at higher risk for dental problems, ear infections, and upper respiratory infections. Jill can produce only a few single syllable words using excessive hyperextension of her body. Her communication generally consists of vocalizations with some variations in loudness and intonation.

Impairments

Jill demonstrates overresponsiveness to oral tactile stimulation. Her rib cage lacks mobility and her respiratory pattern is shallow, asynchronous, and poorly coordinated with oral and pharyngeal function. She exhibits severe cheek/lip retraction, severe jaw thrusting with retraction, and severe tongue retraction with a thick tongue contour.

GOALS

Treatment goals are for Jill to:

1. Improve coordination of respiration with oral and pharyngeal activity during eating, drinking, sound/speech production, and gross motor tasks

2. Increase forward/backward, up/down, and lateral tongue movements with reduced tongue retraction and reduced thickness in tongue contour during feeding and sound/speech production tasks

3. Increase cheek and lip activity with reduced cheek/lip retraction during cup drinking, spoon feeding, sound/speech production, upper extremity, and gross motor tasks

4. Increase active jaw movements and graded jaw closure during feeding, sound/speech production, and gross motor tasks

5. Increase tolerance for oral tactile stimulation on her face, through her teeth/gums, and on her hard palate

FUNCTIONAL OUTCOMES

Following 3 months of intervention, Jill will:

1. Initiate the production of vowel sounds without hyperextension of her body

2. Close her lips on the cup rim upon presentation of the cup

3. Use forward/backward tongue movements with a thinner tongue contour to move pureed foods back in the oral cavity during spoon feeding

4. Tolerate having a toothbrush brought into her mouth, providing input through the biting surfaces of her teeth/gums and on her hard palate, without increased cheek/lip retraction

Intervention

In treatment, activities need to combine facilitation strategies directed toward increased mobility of the ribs at the spine and at the sternum with tactile and proprioceptive input to stimulate greater overall postural musculature activity and sensory readiness. In sitting, slowly graded lateral and rotational trunk movements are facilitated while providing moderate pressure inward and downward on a diagonal through the lateral rib cage toward the weight bearing hip to increase rib cage mobility and improve alignment of the rib cage within the trunk. As rib cage mobility increases, input is moved to the area at which the lower anterior-lateral rib cage meets the abdominal area to encourage abdominal musculature activity. Jill may sit on a bench or straddle a roll held between the legs of the therapist. Activities to stimulate mid-vowel sounds then can be presented.

In side-lying, facilitating slow, graded movements in and out of sidelying with moderate pressure inward and downward on a diagonal through the rib cage toward the base of support can assist in stimulating greater rib cage and scapulohumeral mobility, as well as prepare the trunk musculature for greater activity. This may be done on a mat or a large ball and followed by activities to stimulate longer mid-vowel sounds.

Well-graded moderate pressure combined with elongation through the musculature of the cheeks and lips helps to establish a better sensory-motor base for cheek and lip activity. This input can be combined with movement facilitation in sidelying and sitting in order to better organize Jill's cheek and lip activity with head, neck, and trunk activity. Other oral sensory activities within the oral mechanism are combined with well-graded body movements to assist Jill in tolerating tactile input using a soft brush through the biting surfaces of her teeth/gums and on her hard palate. Jill's caregivers have been shown procedures for oral sensory stimulation at home and are encouraged to provide input for brief periods of time throughout her day and prior to mealtimes, whenever possible.

Oral sensory input is followed by spoon feeding of a thickened pureed food encouraging more sustained closure of the lips on the spoon upon presentation. This also will encourage more rhythmical forward/backward tongue movements with a thinner tongue contour to move the food back for swallowing. Closure of the lips on the cup rim upon the presentation of the cup will help Jill generally organize her oral mechanism for cup drinking. (Please note: Goals and strategies directed toward feeding/swallowing activities will be modified in conjunction with additional instrumental evaluation information.)

Case Study #3: Taylor

➤ Practice pattern 5C: Impaired Motor Function and Sensory Integrity Associated With Nonprogressive Disorders of the Central Nervous System—Congenital Origin or Acquired in Infancy or Childhood
➤ Medical diagnosis: Myelomeningocele, repaired L1-2
➤ Age: 4 years

Examination and Evaluation

Taylor's oral motor activity during spoon feeding, cup drinking, and solid food intake appears to be within normal age limits. He uses a variety of communication modes including speech. His average sentence length of three to four words and the sounds he produces during spontaneous speech appear to be within normal age limits.

Taylor does not have adequate abdominal activity to support sustained exhalation and good respiratory coordination. He appears to run out of air after about three words and can sequence only about three sips from a cup before stopping to breathe.

Taylor should have a thorough evaluation of his language functioning by a qualified speech-language pathologist. Children with myelomeningocele and hydrocephalus often appear to have normal language functioning according to tests of intelligence and vocabulary comprehension which require specific verbal responses. Many speak excessively using clichés and phrases learned by rote. These children may be unable to identify words during testing that they produce in spontaneous speech. This suggests the existence of very specific expressive and receptive language deficits.

Functional Limitations

Taylor cannot speak in sentences over three to four words in length due to his inadequate breath support for sustained exhalation. He can sequence only up to three sips of liquid from a cup before he has to stop to breathe.

Impairments

Taylor exhibits generalized weakness through his upper extremities and trunk, especially in his abdominal musculature. Rib flaring is evident on inhalation due to abdominal musculature weakness. Limited sustaining of respiratory musculature activity impacts speech, endurance, and respiratory coordination with upper extremity activities.

GOALS

Treatment goals are for Taylor to:

1. Improve coordination of respiration with oral and pharyngeal activities during speech and other communication tasks
2. Improve coordination of respiration with oral and pharyngeal activities during cup drinking, straw drinking, and blow toy activities
3. Other goals will depend on results from an evaluation of Taylor's language function.

FUNCTIONAL OUTCOMES

Following 3 months of intervention, Taylor will:

1. Produce sentences of three to four words on one exhalation without running out of breath support
2. Drink three to four sips of liquid from a cup before stopping to breathe

Intervention

Increasing Taylor's respiratory support for speech and other oral/pharyngeal activities will require the incorporation of activities suggested by his physical and occupational therapists. These activities will focus on the stimulation and strengthening of the activity of the muscles of Taylor's upper extremities and trunk, especially his abdominals and back extensors. Tasks to encourage speech production on a more sustained exhalation can be incorporated into these activities.

While in supported sitting on a bench or roll, Taylor can come forward over his hips while pushing with extended arms and hands on the wall. While pushing through his arms, he is asked to repeat sentences of three to four words in length presented by the therapist on one exhalation. Subsequent to activities encouraging greater trunk and abdominal activity, Taylor will drink a sequence of four sips from a cup before lowering the cup from his lips to breathe.

Case Study #4: Ashley

➤ Practice pattern 5B: Impaired Neuromotor Development

➤ Medical diagnosis: Down syndrome

➤ Age: 15 months

Examination and Evaluation

A clinical evaluation of Ashley's oral motor, feeding/swallowing, and respiratory coordination function was conducted. She was observed during play, communication, gross motor, and mealtime activities.

According to her mother, Ashley had esophageal atresia and required a gastrostomy tube for feeding for the first 6 months of her life. She has a history of chronic otitis media with a mild conductive hearing loss. Pressure equalizing tubes were placed at the age of 12 months. Consultative speech services are provided as part of a mother-infant early intervention program that Ashley and her mother attend two times per week.

Ashley generally has low muscle tone providing a poor base for oral-motor and respiratory-phonatory functioning. A suckle pattern is used in all feeding activities. The tongue is thick in contour and always protrudes from the mouth. The hole in the nipple has been slightly enlarged to allow for greater liquid intake during bottle drinking. She has to pause frequently to breathe during bottle drinking.

Cup drinking has been introduced, but only during snack time. Ashley only accepts stage 2 baby foods by spoon. She has been given some solids (crackers, cookies), but her lack of positive response to them has not encouraged their consistent presentation. She takes a maximum of 3 to 4 ounces of food by spoon per meal.

Ashley's mother reported that Ashley spit up frequently when she was fed by G-tube. Since the tube was removed and her cardiac defect was repaired, she does not spit up during or after a meal.

During spoon feeding, it was noted that some food remains in her mouth between her gums and cheeks even after several swallows of one spoonful. If she is not presented with another spoon of food immediately, some of the remaining food residual drools out of her mouth. She shows no sensory awareness of the food remaining in her mouth.

Ashley's rib cage is flat, yet high in position. Retraction of the anterior rib cage, especially at the sternum, during belly breathing increases in severity with effortful crying, movement, and attempts at vocalization. Her vocalizations are breathy, nasal, soft, and short. She is a mouth-breather and struggles for breath if her mouth is held in a closed position. This is not unusual for children with Down syndrome. Their small oral mechanism size does not appear to provide enough space for the tongue to sit in the oral cavity without closing off the oropharyngeal and naso-pharyngeal areas when the mouth is closed.

A thorough prelinguistic/cognitive/language evaluation needs to be conducted because of Ashley's present lack of goal-directed play activities and her history of chronic otitis media with a mild conductive hearing loss. Additionally, she should have periodic reevaluations of her hearing status by a qualified audiologist.

Functional Limitations

Ashley takes limited amounts of food by spoon at a meal. She has shown no interest in crackers or cookies. She uses a suckle pattern with a thickened tongue contour and excessive tongue protrusion in all feeding activities. Liquid and food are lost from her mouth during all feeding activities. Her vocalizations are breathy, nasal, soft, and short in duration.

Impairments

Ashley demonstrates poor oral sensory awareness and poor oral-motor activity. Her tongue movements are limited to the forward/backward dimension. Poor lip closure is evident. She reveals no awareness of food remaining in her mouth after swallowing or when she drools. Problems in respiratory coordination with oral and pharyngeal activity are evident during bottle drinking, sound production, and general movement activities.

Goals

Treatment goals are for Ashley to:

1. Improve coordination of respiration with oral and pharyngeal activity during feeding and sound/speech production tasks

2. Increase active use of the cheeks and lips during feeding and sound/speech production tasks

3. Increase active up/down and lateral movements of the tongue during feeding and sound/speech production tasks

4. Increase oral sensory awareness during feeding and sound/speech production activities

FUNCTIONAL OUTCOMES

Following 3 months of intervention, Ashley will:

1. Bring her lower lip up and out stabilizing under the cup rim when the cup is presented for drinking
2. Move her tongue laterally to touch solids and objects placed on her side gums/teeth
3. Produce vocalizations of 3 to 5 seconds in length with reduced nasality and increased loudness
4. Position her tongue more within her oral cavity with reduced protrusion during non-feeding activities when in supported sitting and when supported in standing

Intervention

In treatment, it will be essential to combine appropriate somatosensory, vestibular, visual, and/or auditory sensory input with the facilitation of active movements that focus on greater trunk, shoulder girdle, and lip musculature activity. Combining moderate pressure through the lower rib cage and abdominals with the facilitation of transitional movement (eg, sidelying to sitting, sitting to quadruped, kneeling to standing) activities can assist Ashley in developing a postural foundation for improved breath support. Activities to stimulate louder and longer vocalizations can be presented in conjunction with these movement activities to engage Ashley in some vocal interaction.

At brief intervals during movement facilitation activities, provide well-graded oral sensory input to the cheeks and lips, through the biting surfaces of the gums/teeth, to the hard palate, and to the tongue. Once Ashley begins to exhibit greater postural activity and increased active responses to the oral sensory input, present some feeding experiences. Introduce cup drinking with a thickened liquid or pureed food, present easily dissolvable solids to the side-biting surfaces for chewing, or present food by spoon while encouraging active lip closure on the spoon for food removal.

Introduce different food textures (thick purees, cereal, crackers), tastes, and smells as part of play. While performing active transitional movements, hands, feet, trunk, face, and mouth can be brought in contact with different food textures to encourage increased tolerance for these new tactile experiences. Different smells and tastes can be introduced to determine those that elicit the most active and positive responses of the oral and pharyngeal mechanisms. These can be incorporated into Ashley's mealtime routine.

Strategies and procedures found successful in treatment may be incorporated into Ashley's daily routine as long as they have a positive impact on Ashley's nutritional intake. Ashley's caregivers will need to view such recommendations as beneficial if they are to be carried over by them into daily activities. This will be especially important when introducing new experiences with solid foods and cup drinking.

Case Study #5: John

➤ Practice pattern 5B: Impaired Neuromotor Development
➤ Medical diagnosis: Attention deficit hyperactivity disorder, developmental coordination disorder
➤ Age: 5 years

Examination and Evaluation

John's kindergarten teacher expressed concerns regarding his speech to the school's speech-language pathologist. The speech-language pathologist arranged to observe John in his kindergarten classroom to determine whether more formal testing needs to be scheduled.

Prior to this classroom observation, John's parents were contacted by telephone to obtain some background information related to his speech and language development and function.

John's mother reported that she and John's dad understand most things that he says, although other adults have trouble understanding him, especially when he is excited and talking quickly. He becomes frustrated when not completely understood. For a long while, he primarily communicated using facial expressions, gestures, pointing, and by producing grunts and some vowel sounds. His speech became more intelligible about a year ago. He still has problems sitting for long periods of time to play games or to color, although this has gotten better since he started taking Ritalin.

John's mother noted that he has always been a picky eater. He drank from a bottle until he was about 3 years old and still does best when drinking from his lidded sipper cup. He enjoys eating crackers, cold cereal without milk, peanut butter and jelly or grilled cheese sandwiches cut in quarters, cheese cubes, raisins, marshmallow treats, macaroni and cheese, and canned spaghetti. He only likes to drink milk, not juices or water. He refuses to open his mouth for fruits. He will eat French fries and mashed potatoes and has occasionally eaten some cooked carrots. John's mother assists him at dinner, which is when he appears to have more trouble feeding himself if he needs to use a spoon or fork. John's mother noted that he still puts some objects in his mouth for biting especially when he is very tired. Although she is pleased that the neuropsychologist said that John appears to have above normal intelligence, she is very concerned about his temper tantrums, his speech, and the diagnosis of DCD.

During the classroom observation, it was noted that John prefers to play with toys he has already experienced. He tends to be a loner and does not initiate conversations or play with other children in his class. He willingly interacts if another child initiates the activity.

John uses gestures to supplement his speech when communicating with others. He often takes an adult's arm to show them what he wants at the same time he is speaking. The other children in his class do not generally like it when he does this to them.

During snack time, he showed no interest in the juice that everyone else was drinking. He drank the milk that his mother sent along for him. He appears to initially bite on the sipper cup's spout when starting to drink. He ate graham crackers, exhibiting some rhythmical vertical jaw movements and tongue lateralization. He refused to try the jello and insisted on having more graham crackers instead.

His speech reveals expressive language delays. He often omits consonants, especially those in the middle or at the end of a word. It was noted that he also omitted words from sentences during his spontaneous speech productions. It was recommended that John be referred for a comprehensive speech and language evaluation. His parents will be contacted to obtain additional information related to nutrition, eating, and drinking.

FUNCTIONAL LIMITATIONS

The intelligibility of John's speech is variable, resulting in his consistent use of gestures and pointing to help communicate what he wants. When not understood, he may become extremely frustrated. He has problems attending to a task for an extended period of time. John is a picky eater and frequently refuses drinks and foods offered to him.

IMPAIRMENTS

John demonstrates difficulties coordinating and sustaining his jaw, tongue, and lip movements for consistently intelligible speech production. He exhibits problems in the somatosensory area as well as in his ability to modulate visual and auditory information in the environment. Respiratory coordination with oral and pharyngeal activities and with gross motor and upper extremity activities is restricted.

GOALS

Treatment goals are for John to:

1. Improve the coordination of respiration with oral and pharyngeal activity during eating, drinking, sound/speech production, blowing, upper extremity, and gross motor tasks

2. Improve coordination of lip, tongue, and jaw movements during speech, eating, and drinking tasks

3. Increase oral sensory awareness and sustained muscle activity of the tongue, lips, and jaw

These goals will be modified based upon the findings of the comprehensive speech and language evaluation.

FUNCTIONAL OUTCOMES

Following 3 months of intervention, John will:

1. Attend to an activity while sitting at a table without being distracted by other visual and auditory stimulation in the environment

2. Blow a toy horn or whistle, sustaining a sound for 3 to 5 seconds

3. Produce the consonants "t" and "d" when they appear at the end of a word in sentences of three to four words in length

Intervention

Before presenting activities that involve changes in oral and pharyngeal function, it is necessary to engage John in activities that prepare his overall sensory motor foundation. Activities that stimulate greater shoulder girdle/upper extremity and/or hip/lower extremity strength with sustained muscle activity will help establish a base for improved oral and pharyngeal activity. Activities that assist John in modulating and integrating somatosensory information generally in his body, as well as specifically within his oral and pharyngeal areas, also help to establish readiness for more specific speech/sound production tasks. A number of activities can be developed from which John and the speech-language pathologist can choose a few to do prior to focusing on more speech-specific tasks. These same sensory preparation activities can be used at home and at other times during school to keep John in a state that allows him to attend to tasks longer and to be able to handle more challenging tasks such as speech.

Activities that are more directly related to oral, pharyngeal, and respiratory coordination function must be related to John's motor planning, motor learning, and somatosensory issues. Practice of specific sounds and specific sound combinations subsequent to providing tactile, visual, and auditory cues will be essential. Repetition of these tasks will be required for John to maximize his potential for learning. Combining "t" and "d" with vowels into vowel-consonant combinations and then into single syllable words will provide a starting point from which further expansion into phrases and sentences can occur.

Finding the combinations of sensory cues that work best for John will be a primary initial focus so that the same framework can be used for the learning of other consonants and words for speech.

Blowing activities using musical instruments and blow toys will be useful in helping to increase John's respiratory depth, ability to sustain exhalation, and overall endurance. Focus should be on the length of the sounds rather than the loudness in order to increase support for exhalation. Provide cues prior to blowing into the toy that assist John in expanding his anterior chest wall on inhalation so that greater respiratory depth is stimulated. It may be necessary to start with some movement activities that encourage greater mobility within the rib cage in the lateral, diagonal, and rotational dimensions prior to presenting cues that focus on the expanding of the inhalation/exhalation process. Consistent practice as part of a daily routine will be an essential part of any intervention program in which John is expected to be successful.

References

1. Sander E. When are speech sounds learned? *J Speech Hear Disord.* 1972;37:55-63.
2. Netsell R. Speech motor control development. In: Reilly A, ed. *The Communication Game.* Somerville, NJ: Johnson & Johnson Baby Products; 1980:33-38.
3. Lass N, McReynolds L, Northern J, et al, eds. *Speech, Language and Hearing.* Vol 1. Philadelphia, Pa: WB Saunders; 1982.
4. Bloom L, Lahey M. *Language Development and Language Disorders.* New York, NY: John Wiley & Sons; 1978.
5. Alexander R, Boehme R, Cupps B. *Normal Development of Functional Motor Skills: The First Year of Life.* San Antonio, Tex: Therapy Skill Builders; 1993.
6. Bosma J. Introduction to the symposium. In: Bosma J, Showacre J, eds. *Symposium on Development of Upper Respiratory Anatomy and Function: Implications for the Sudden Infant Death Syndrome.* Washington, DC: US Government Printing Office; 1975:5-49.
7. Bosma J. Structure and function of the infant oral and pharyngeal mechanisms. In: Wilson J, ed. *Oral-Motor Function and Dysfunction in Children.* Chapel Hill, NC: University of North Carolina; 1978:33-65.
8. Kapandji I. *The Physiology of the Joints: The Trunk and the Vertebral Column.* Vol 3. 2nd ed. New York, NY: Churchill Livingstone; 1974.
9. Alexander R. Feeding and swallowing. In: Bigge J, Best S, Heller K, eds. *Teaching Individuals with Physical, Health, or Multiple Disabilities.* 4th ed. Upper Saddle River, NJ: Merrill Prentice Hall; 2001:504-535.
10. Arvedson JC, Brodsky L. *Pediatric Swallowing and Feeding: Assessment and Management.* 2nd ed. Albany, NY: Singular Publishing Group; 2002:283-340.
11. Girolami GL, Ryan DF, Gardner JM. Clinical assessment of the infant. In: Scherzer A, ed. *Early Diagnosis and Interventional Therapy in Cerebral Palsy: An Interdisciplinary Age-Focused Approach.* 3rd ed. New York, NY: Marcel Dekker; 2001:139-184.
12. Sheppard JJ. Clinical evaluation and treatment. In: Rosenthal SR, Sheppard JJ, Lotze M, eds. *Dysphagia and the Child with Developmental Disabilities: Medical, Clinical, and Family Interventions.* Albany, NY: Singular Publishing Group; 1995:37-75.
13. Arvedson JC, Lefton-Greif MA. *Pediatric Videofluoroscopic Swallow Studies: A Professional Manual with Caregiver Guidelines.* San Antonio, Tex: Communication Skill Builders; 1998.
14. Willging JP, Miller CK, Link DT, Rudolph CD. Use of FEES to assess and manage pediatric patients. In: Langmore SE, ed. *Endoscopic Evaluation Treatment of Swallowing Disorders.* New York, NY: Thieme; 2001:213-234.

15. Fee M, Charney E, Robertson W. Nutritional assessment of the young child with cerebral palsy. *Infants and Young Children*. 1988;1:33-40.

16. Putnam PE. Gastroesophageal reflux disease and dysphagia in children. In: Arvedson JC, Lefton-Greif MA, eds. *Pediatric Dysphagia II: A Team Approach for Assessment, Management, and Special Problems. Seminars in Speech and Language*. 1997;18(1):25-38.

17. Alexander R. Prespeech and feeding development. In: McDonald E, ed. *Treating Cerebral Palsy: For Clinicians By Clinicians*. Austin, Tex: Pro-Ed; 1987:133-152.

18. Alexander R. Oral-motor treatment for infants and young children with cerebral palsy. *Seminars in Speech and Language*. 1987;8(1):87-100.

19. Alexander R. *Pediatric Feeding and Swallowing: Assessment and Treatment Programming* [self study video and manual]. Rockville, Md: American Speech-Language-Hearing Association; 2002.

20. Alper BS, Manno CJ. Dysphagia in infants and children with oral-motor deficits: assessment and management. In: Arvedson JC, Lefton-Greif MA, eds. *Pediatric Dysphagia: Complex Medical, Health, and Developmental Issues. Seminars in Speech and Language*. 1996;17(4):283-310.

21. Lowman DK, Murphy SM, eds. *The Educator's Guide to Feeding Children with Disabilities*. Baltimore, Md: Paul H. Brookes; 1999.

22. Glass RP, Wolf LS. Feeding and oral-motor skills. In: Case-Smith J, ed. *Pediatric Occupational Therapy and Early Intervention*. Stoneham, Mass: Butterworth-Heinemann; 1993:225-288.

23. Morris SE, Klein MD. *Pre-Feeding Skills*. 2nd ed. San Antonio, Tex: Therapy Skill Builders; 2000.

24. Pinder GL, Faherty AS. Issues in pediatric feeding and swallowing. In: Caruso AJ, Strand EA, eds. *Clinical Management of Motor Speech Disorders in Children*. New York, NY: Thieme; 1999: 281-318.

25. Stamer M. *Posture and Movement of the Child with Cerebral Palsy*. San Antonio, Tex: Therapy Skill Builders; 2000.

26. Howle J. *Neuro-Developmental Treatment Approach: Theoretical Foundations and Principles of Clinical Practice*. Laguna Beach, Calif: NeuroDevelopmental Treatment Association; 2002.

DEVELOPING AMBULATION SKILLS

Judith C. Bierman, PT

When the parent of a child who is unable to walk independently is asked, "What are your goals for physical therapy?" the answer is inevitably " I want my child to walk." For a therapist, contributing to a child's ability to take the first steps is a source of great professional satisfaction. There also are fewer questions more challenging to a therapist than a parent's sincere question "Will my child walk?" Physicians and therapists strive to give objective and reliable answers to this question.[1] Walking is a valued milestone, an important functional skill, and an indicator of increased independence that is based on motor control. For all of these reasons, families and therapists frequently focus on ambulation as an outcome of therapeutic intervention. While it may be a simple task to identify some individuals who will be able to walk, it is far more difficult to identify the impairments that prevent walking, the factors that limit efficiency of gait, or the specific functional limitations that result from a child's ineffective gait pattern. It is even more difficult to establish an effective and efficient intervention plan that will help a child begin to walk or to increase the performance or expand the function of walking into a variety of meaningful contexts.

This chapter addresses these important and difficult questions. The basics of ambulation will be outlined using an enablement model to organize the problem-solving process and information. Developmental issues related to how and why gait changes across childhood will be reviewed; the impact of neuromuscular pathophysiology and related impairments to a child's ability to ambulate functionally will be discussed. Guidelines for examination, treatment planning, and treatment procedures then will be introduced. Finally, the guidelines will be applied in a series of case studies to demonstrate the clinical processes described.

Definitions and Basic Concepts

The terms "locomotion," "walking," "gait," and "ambulation" frequently are used interchangeably in the literature. In this chapter, however, the following definitions taken from *Dorland's Medical Dictionary*[2] will be used:

➤ *Locomotion* is the ability to move from one place to another

➤ *Walking* is progressing on foot

➤ *Gait* or *ambulation* is the manner or style of walking

These terms are more useful in the context of the enablement model and the various dimensions described in the World Health Organization (WHO) or Neurodevelopmental Treatment (NDT) models.[3,4] Locomotion is clearly a functional activity that influences an individual's ability to participate fully in society. It is necessary to be able to move within a room, within a school, or in the community. The specifics of how this is accomplished could vary from rolling or scooting on one's bottom across a room, to walking with a walker down the hall of a school, to driving a car, to propelling a wheelchair in the community. Walking specifies that the individual is upright against gravity and moving on the feet, but not necessarily able to move in a functional context, given limitations of time, direction, environmental distractions, or variations in surfaces. Gait describes the posture and movement of the individual and clarifies how a person walks. In the NDT enablement model this is in the dimension of "motor function."[4] In this framework a therapist might separate therapy outcomes or goals that address: 1) limited ability to move or use locomotion independently through space in a specific functional context, 2) limited ability to walk independently or with assistance, or 3) decreased energy efficient or effective gait. In this chapter, the focus will be on walking and gait as they lead to greater functional independence of the child.

Locomotion

Although developmental sequences vary, a child often begins the process of moving in space by the fourth month of age with rolling activities. This typically is followed at 5 to 6 months with pivoting in prone and pushing backward through space when prone. Belly crawling usually is the first form of forward mobility and emerges at about 7 months. Creeping on hands and knees follows at 8 to 9 months. These forms of locomotion are augmented by the development of walking followed by running, skipping, bicycling, and other age-appropriate motor skills as the child continues to develop. In the past, based on maturational theory, clinicians assumed that one form of locomotion prepares the child or leads the child to the next more mature level of locomotion. Based on this assumption, a therapist who is treating a child who is non-ambulatory would focus on the child's next "higher" or more mature level of locomotion prior to introducing walking and gait activities. Currently there are many questions that challenge this "developmental" assumption (see Chapter 3). Perhaps each pattern of locomotion is the functional solution at the time, given the constraints of the child's growth, body system interactions, environmental context, and individual need for movement. In this framework, patterns of locomotion would not be considered prerequisite developmental activities for the eventual emergence of walking as the mature form of locomotion.[4]

Walking

Typically developing children begin to take assisted steps in the eighth or ninth month. Near the first birthday a child begins to take independent steps and is able "to walk" by 13 to 15 months of age. The parent carefully supervises as the child learns to walk on a wider variety of surfaces and in more complex environments. The child must learn to ambulate in different directions; go up and down stairs; avoid obstacles in the pathway; stop, start, and change directions; carry items while walking; and walk and talk at the same time while coping with distractions in the environment. The emergence of these skills is well-documented in developmental charts and tests.[5-8] It is important for the clinician to consider carefully not only the presence or absence of walking, but also the impact of walking on functional abilities or limitations of the child and the changes this skill brings in participation in home, school, and community life.

Gait

Perry[9] defined gait as a repetitive sequence of stable upright postures in which the body weight is advanced over a constantly changing base of support. When gait is observed in typically functioning individuals it is seen as rhythmical, stable, predictable, and yet individualized. Gait varies within each individual as changes in the neural and body systems occur both in real time and developmental time. Gait also changes with the demands of complexities in the environment. Body systems organize to provide upright stability, forward progression with a forward propulsive force, shock absorption, and energy conservation. In addition to analysis of the body systems, therapists must consider biomechanical or physical contributions to an individual's gait. While gait can be broken down into different phases or cycles for examination or for basic understanding, it also is critical to realize that just as a symphony cannot be understood or appreciated by studying each note in isolation, gait cannot be understood by only studying the individual cycles or aspects. The following terms frequently are used to describe specific parameters of gait:

➤ *Step length*: The distance between the initial contact point of the two opposite feet. Therefore, right step length would be the longitudinal distance between the left heel strike to the right heel strike. The two step lengths can be added together to calculate the stride length

➤ *Stride*: One entire cycle in the gait process beginning when one foot contacts the ground and continuing until the same foot once again contacts the ground

➤ *Stance phase*: Stance phase refers to the period of time when the foot is contacting the ground. It occupies approximately 60% of the total cycle. It is critical in providing stability in gait. Stance is divided into five subphases. These are initial contact, loading response, mid-stance, terminal stance, and pre-swing

➤ *Swing*: Swing phase refers to the time when the foot is moving forward and is not contacting the ground. It occupies approximately 40% of the total time. It is critical for the advancement of the body and contributes to the efficiency of movement by the use of momentum. Swing is divided into three subphases. These are initial swing, mid-swing, and terminal swing

➤ *Velocity*: The rate or speed of gait is measured to determine the distance traversed in a specific time

➤ *Cadence*: The number of steps taken in a specific time. Cadence usually is measured in steps per minute

Growth and Development

Gait parameters change across the lifespan. The therapist considers these changes when evaluating and intervening with children of different ages. These parameters generally show greater variability with younger children. Across childhood, step and stride lengths increase with age. Cadence decreases as step and stride lengths increase. The base of support decreases with age.[10] The changes in these parameters reflect changes in many of the body systems and continual refinements of global neuronal maps. Changes also are based on overall physical growth (Table 11-1).

Changes in the Musculoskeletal System

In order for walking to develop, remarkable shifts in physical skeletal growth must occur. The relative size of the head compared to the trunk and limbs in early infancy

Table 11-1
Gait Parameters: Changes Associated With Growth

Age (years)	Mean Velocity (cm/sec)	Mean Cadence (steps/min)	Cycle Time (secs)	Step Length (cm)	Stride Length (cm)
1	64	176	0.68	22	43
2	72	156	0.78	28	55
3	86	154	0.77	33	67
4	100	152	0.78	39	78
5	108	154	0.77	42	84
6	109	146	0.82	44	89
7	114*	143†	0.83	48	97

* Variability nearly constant across all age groups
† 26% higher than adult mean value

Adapted from Sutherland DH, Olshen RA, Biden EN, et al. *The Development of Mature Walking*. Philadelphia, Pa: JB Lippincott; 1988.

makes independent walking impossible. After 12 months of age, trunk growth and the relative growth of the lower extremities provide a biomechanical advantage for walking. At the same time, there are changes in the shape of the bones that change the efficiency of gait. Specific examples include the decrease in the angle of inclination of the femur with the coexisting shift in the amount of femoral antetorsion. These two factors are key in decreasing the size of the base of support allowing the feet to be positioned closer to each other and, therefore, decreasing the energy cost associated with weight shift. The knees demonstrate a gradual increase in genu valgum until age 2.5 years and then a decrease until the age of 6 years. In addition, the growth of the long bones in the lower extremities can account for increased step and stride lengths.[11]

The growth of the long bones is associated with growth of and increased length of the muscles and soft tissue. In muscle, the increase in length is an adaptive response by adding sarcomeres. In addition to increasing length, strength also increases dramatically in the early years. The child gains extensor strength that eliminates the hyperflexion stance seen in the first year. The increase in strength of extensor muscles also provides power in push off for increasing step length and is critical in developing skills such as stair climbing, jumping, and running.[12] There is a shift in the proportion of fat to muscle with an increase in the proportion of muscle to fat in the early years.[13]

Changes in the Neuromuscular System

The neuromuscular system demonstrates changes in both control and coordination of muscle activity that are reflected in changes of gait parameters. During early walking, the child demonstrates increased co-contraction or "fixing."[14] This pattern of co-contraction diminishes with experience. There is a gradual increase in the recruitment of patterns of axial rotation with a period of hyper-rotation. The changes in control of trunk rotation occur simultaneously with increased isolated control both between and within the extremities.[15]

Changes in Sensory Systems

There is evidence of changes in sensory systems that are reflected in changes in gait. Children under the age of 3 years rely heavily on vision for postural alignment during stance. Between the ages of 4 to 6 years, the sensory systems apparently reorganize with vestibular, somatosensory, and visual integration.[15] Perceptual reorganization of a child's body image, body in space, and motor planning must occur following growth spurts.

Interaction of Systems

It is important for the clinician studying the development of gait in any child to consider all of the interacting systems. For example, it is not only increasing leg length that explains longer step lengths, but also the interaction of other variables including:

➤ Increasing range of motion

➤ Increasing strength of the extensor muscles

➤ Changes in postural control and movement coordination that allow greater trunk rotation and greater isolated movement between and within the limbs

➤ Refinement of modulation of forces of muscle synergies

➤ Integration of multiple sensory systems

➤ Increased interest, motivational drive, environmental, and functional demands

There are additional factors to consider in the analysis of gait based on the interaction of body systems. For example, balance, postural control, alignment, or mid-range control are analyzed based on contributions from multiple systems. Changes in all of these areas are evident as the child grows, matures, and develops.[4]

Implications of Pathology

In addition to the impact of growth and systems maturation discussed earlier, it also is important to consider the impact of pathology on the parameters of gait. Certainly not all children with developmental disabilities have the potential to walk independently. There are clearer indicators for eventual ambulation in children with myelodysplasia than there are in children with cerebral palsy, mental retardation, or specific syndromes that include significant sensorimotor impairments.

Myelodysplasia

Children with myelodysplasia with lesions above L4-L5 will ambulate only with orthoses, crutches, or walkers.[16-19] In a study of 68 children with myelodysplasia, DeSouza and Carroll[17] reported that none of the children with thoracic level lesions who also lacked power in the muscles crossing or distal to the hip joint were community ambulators. In children with high lumbar lesions, with power in the hip adductors or flexors or in the extensors of the knee, 10% were community ambulators. Thirty-three percent of children with low lumbar lesions, with power in the knee flexors, dorsiflexors of the ankles, or hip abductors, and 50% of children with sacral lesions, who had power in the plantarflexors of the ankle or toes or in the extensors of the hips, were community ambulators. While the eventual ambulatory status seemed to depend primarily on neurosegmental level, the extent and degree of orthopedic deformities also were significant factors.

Hoffer and colleagues[16] followed 56 children and reported that none of the children with thoracic level lesions walked, while all with sacral level lesions became community ambulators. In children with lesions at the lumbar level, 45% were functional ambulators. In addition, those who achieved functional ambulation did so prior to 9 years of age.

Mental Retardation

Uncomplicated mental retardation must be extremely severe to prevent ambulation. The mental age for walking has never been determined.[18,20] Shapiro and colleagues[21] reported that 92% of profoundly retarded children (IQ less than 25) walked if retardation was not accompanied by another neurological dysfunction. The median age of walking for this group was 20 months, while only 11% of a group with cerebral palsy and mental retardation walked. The median age of walking for the group with cerebral palsy and mental retardation was 63.5 months. Donoghue et al[22] reported on 36 children who were residing in institutions and who had severe mental retardation. They found that fewer children, about 9% in those cases complicated by cerebral palsy, walked at age of 5.4 years, while 80% of the children with Down syndrome walked at a mean age of 3.2 years. Seventy percent of the children in the group with uncomplicated mental retardation walked at a mean age of 4.2 years. The majority of children who succeeded in walking did so by 5 years of age, and nearly all of the remaining children walked by 7 years. Melyn and White[23] reported on children with Down syndrome who were noninstitutionalized. The average age of walking was 26 months for boys and 22.7 months for girls. The difference in the age of onset of walking in children with Down syndrome reported in these two studies probably is related to the samples under study. Donoghue et al[22] reported on children who were institutionalized and who experienced changing staff, high staff absence rates, and suboptimal conditions for development. The children examined by Melyn and White[23] remained at home and attended developmental day care programs.

Cerebral Palsy

Of all children with developmental disabilities, the most complicated group for prediction of independent walking potential is children with cerebral palsy. This group represents a very heterogeneous collection of individuals with varying pathophysiology, degrees of severity of primary and secondary impairments, and courses of intervention and recovery. Montgomery[24] reviewed seven studies across 25 years that attempted to identify predictors of ambulation in children with cerebral palsy. The studies considered the impact of the type of cerebral palsy, the timing of acquisition of other motor milestones, the presence or absence of primitive reflexes, impact of age/maturation, cognition, and finally interventions such as surgery and physical therapy. Montgomery noted that there was not a consistent definition of "ambulation" across studies. The results of the studies reviewed suggested that almost all children with hemiplegia ambulated independently without an assistive device by the age of 2 to 3 years. Most children with diplegia became independent ambulators either with or without an assistive device; while the majority of children with quadriplegia remained non-ambulatory, and those who became ambulatory required an assistive device. It also is of concern that even children with disabilities, who are independent ambulators with an assistive device, take fewer steps in a day than able-bodied peers. Davis[25] reported that a child with cerebral palsy in the sixth grade who was an independent community ambulator took, on average, only 6.1% of the number of steps of the average for able-bodied classmates during a school day.

Molnar and Gordon,[26] reporting on 233 children, found that 78% achieved some degree of functional walking. Children diagnosed with a hemiplegia walked by 2 to 3 years of age. Children with ataxia walked later, but all walked by 8 years of age. Children with spastic diplegia were found to have a favorable outcome for ambulation with 65% walking unassisted, 20% requiring assistive devices, and an additional 15% relying on wheelchairs (did not walk). However, of the children who ambulated, most walked by 3 years of age. Children with quadriplegia had the most variable outcome. Twenty-five percent never became ambulatory, 33% walked only with assistive devices, and only 30% ambulated independently. Children with athetosis had a favorable outcome with 75% becoming ambulatory with or without assistive devices. Of these children, 50% walked by the age of 3 years.

Largo and colleagues[27] found that the type of cerebral palsy and the severity of tonal abnormalities were correlated with the development of locomotion skills. The mean age for attaining all forms of locomotion (ie, crawling, creeping, cruising, and walking) was higher in a group of preterm infants with cerebral palsy than in either normal preterm or full-term infants. Badell-Ribera[28] reported that, in children with spastic diplegia related to prematurity, control of sitting and crawling between 1.5 to 2.5 years was predictive of the eventual level of ambulatory function. Molnar[29] also compared sitting and ambulation and found that sitting by 2 years of age was a good predictive sign for eventual ambulation in children with spastic diplegia, quadriplegia, and athetosis.

Bleck[30] and Molnar and Gordon[26] recommended using the persistence of primitive reflexes to predict walking. There are physicians who use this system to help predict the potential for ambulation in a specific child. However, this understanding of the underlying problems of control does little if anything to aid the therapist in planning or implementing intervention. The reflex model does not fit with current theories of motor control, such as neuronal group selection theory (NGST). Therapists now consider these stereotypic movements (ie, reflexes) to represent limited primary repertoires, which, if persistent, interfere with the ability to produce adaptive synergies needed for walking[4,31] (see Chapter 8).

Implications for Practice

In reviewing studies of ambulatory outcomes, especially of children with cerebral palsy, it quickly becomes evident that there is lack of consistency in definitions used by the authors, the types of intervention provided, service delivery models, and environmental influences. The problem is further complicated by the changes that have occurred in service delivery models used across those 25 years. While it is clear that it is extremely difficult to predict with confidence the potential for ambulation in a specific child, there are good reasons to continue to search for evidence to predict ambulation outcomes and to address these issues with families. It is very important for the child and the family to have realistic expectations related to ambulation. Families may perceive the failure to ambulate independently as an indicator of their own failure to work hard or long enough. The child or family may resent the hours spent in therapy if it only focused on an unreachable outcome of walking. A child's self-esteem may be damaged by unfounded hopes that if the child just worked harder that ambulation would be possible. However, the parent and child can just as likely resent a therapist or physician who does not do everything possible to reach this important goal. The family has the right to expect health care professionals to use all of the knowledge, skill, and resources available to aid in reaching this important milestone, while also considering available evidence to make realistic decisions.

It is critical for the therapist to establish appropriate long- and short-term functional outcomes to direct and assess the efficacy of the therapy process as it relates to walking.

It is important to identify those children with the potential to ambulate in order to develop the most efficient interventions to reach that outcome. It also is important to identify those children who may not be ambulators so that alternative interventions, such as acquiring needed assistive devices and making environmental modifications, can be implemented. In addition, it is important to provide non-ambulatory children with appropriate interventions to address the secondary impairments that can emerge due to a sedentary lifestyle, a decreased amount of time spent in the upright position, and a dependence on others for transitions in their environments (see Chapter 18).

Examination

General Considerations

A useful assessment of a child's gait includes gathering a wide variety of information and performing specific examinations. Several methods, including referral to a gait lab, use of video analysis, footprint analysis, and clinical observations, are options. The first step in any process, whether or not it includes these specific methods of examination, is an interview with the child and the child's family to determine the depth and focus of the examination process.

PARTICIPATION/PARTICIPATION RESTRICTIONS

The therapist can be most effective when beginning the process by obtaining a "big picture" of the child's life with observations of the child in various settings or by gathering this information from family and significant persons in the child's life. It is important to understand how the child's ambulation supports or interferes with full participation at home, at school, or in the community. The family can provide descriptions of how the child participates in family life. Examples of questions that will provide relevant information include:

➤ What, if any, are the concerns within family life?

➤ Can the child participate in age-appropriate activities that require walking, such as setting the table, picking up the bedroom, playing with siblings, or taking care of the family pets?

➤ Are there environmental barriers to full participation and have environmental modifications been made to allow full participation?

➤ Are there assistive devices that fit into the home to allow participation?

The participation assessment continues with a widening circle of focus. If the child is school-aged, assessment of participation in the school environment must be included. Examples of questions that will provide relevant information include:

➤ Can the child attend the neighborhood school?

➤ Is full participation in school activities possible?

➤ What are the restrictions that occur in school activities?

➤ Does the child move freely through the classrooms, the hallways, and the library at the same time that other children in the class do?

➤ Can the child participate in mealtimes with all other students?

➤ Can the child take part fully in physical education or recess activities?

➤ Does the child have access to restrooms that accommodate any special needs?

➤ What are the considerations for future schools? Does the middle school have stairs while the elementary school is on one level? Will the child be able to move to the same school with the current group of friends?

Finally, the therapist asks questions that focus on the child's ability to participate at the community level.

➤ Can the child participate in typical community activities, such as sports teams, recreational activities, church, synagogue, and social activities?

➤ Are there other key community environments that the child participates in on a regular basis?

The family needs to provide input as to the participation restrictions that the child and family are most vested in addressing. One child may want to be able to walk the long distances at the local mall with friends while another child may prefer to negotiate the narrow stacks in the public library to participate in a summer reading program.

FUNCTIONAL ABILITIES AND LIMITATIONS

Specific functional limitations or abilities directly related to the ability to walk should be identified. It is not a report of function to simply state that a child can walk a set distance. The examination must focus on the functional implications of walking that distance. For example:

➤ Can the child walk the distance from the bedroom to the bathroom and negotiate the turns required?

➤ Is it also possible for the same ability to be demonstrated at night with poor lighting?

➤ Can the child walk to the neighborhood school without an assistive device?

➤ Can the child walk the distances required in the cafeteria while carrying the tray of food?

➤ Can the adolescent walk through the crowded hallways of a middle school, carrying all required textbooks, and socialize with friends simultaneously?

It is through the combining of multiple functional skills that the individual demonstrates increased ability to participate in all of the roles associated with childhood. Once again, functioning must be explored in multiple environments. A child may walk independently in the home, but once in school be unable to demonstrate that same skill. Following intervention, a child may demonstrate progress by either acquiring a new functional ability or by generalizing a previously acquired skill in new, more complex environments.

The therapist gathers information from the family on which specific functional outcomes are most important to them. Functional outcomes/goals should be established with the family and child's input. It is at this point that the therapist may begin to educate and counsel the family as to the feasibility of the child reaching desired outcomes. The family cannot be expected to write functional outcomes, but can direct the course of the therapy intervention. For example, the family may indicate that it is most important to focus on in-home ambulation to increase independence in the bathroom and bedroom now that the family has a second child. In another situation, it may be more important that the adolescent walk longer distances (even if it is with an assistive device) in the school now that the child must change classes every hour.

Gait Analysis

The therapist also examines the child's posture and movement as related to gait. This portion of the examination usually is referred to as a "gait assessment." Perry[9] included the following areas in this part of the examination:

➤ Upright posture and stability against gravity

➤ Forward progression with forward propulsive force

➤ Shock absorption

➤ Energy conservation

GAIT LAB ASSESSMENT

This assessment may be performed either in a formal gait lab or in a clinical setting. An early decision for the therapist is to decide which alternative is the best one for this child at this time. Gait labs are available in many major cities across the country. Labs can produce a wealth of very specific and objective data. Obtaining this information, however, can be expensive for the family. In addition, gait labs may have specific prerequisites, such as an overall height or weight requirement, limb length requirement, or specific functional skill level. Therefore, there must be specific goals or questions that need to be answered and a careful review of the potential gait lab data to answer these questions to justify the cost. Analyses from a pediatric gait lab could provide:

➤ Motion analysis

➤ EMG studies during gait

➤ Force plate studies

➤ Measurement of basic gait parameters

➤ Measurement of energy consumption

Labs that include additional examinations by a pediatric orthopedist, physiatrist, or orthotist might add valuable interpretation of the data and recommendations to aid in planning intervention.

CLINICAL GAIT ASSESSMENT

Clinical examinations also can provide a wealth of information and obtain much of the same information as generated by a gait lab for significantly less cost. Only a few basic tools are needed. A stopwatch and tape measure are essential. Access to a videocamera and VCR that permits frame-by-frame viewing is extremely useful. A system for recording and measuring footprints also is important. Bleck[11] clearly outlined a system of analysis he referred to as "pedography." Therapists have used a wide variety of methods for this task including:

➤ Directing the child to walk down a length of shelf paper after stepping into tempra paints

➤ Dusting the feet with chalk powder and having to child walk across dark paper or mats

➤ Stepping on temporary mats to record steps

➤ Utilizing tri-fold carbon paper for a more permanent record with more clearly differentiated patterns of pressure display

The following aspects of gait analysis should be considered during clinical examinations.

Motion Studies

The therapist can observe the walking pattern of the child and do frame-by-frame analysis of joint positions if the child is recorded on video from the sagittal and frontal planes. The camera needs to be positioned at a 90-degree angle to the child for accurate observations to be made. It is useful to have a zoom option on the camera when the child is walking toward and away from the therapist. This type of analysis is time consuming for the therapist but useful in analyzing the gait of a child who walks quickly or with unpredictable patterns when observed clinically. It allows the therapist to focus on one joint or body part at a time and also allows the child to only have to do the task of walking once while providing multiple opportunities for review.

It is useful for the therapist during this process to think of the ABCs of examination:

➤ "A"lignment: Examine the alignment of the body in the upright posture. Is the alignment adequate for efficient antigravity control? Look at the entire body as well as specific joint relationships. At this point it may be more effective to begin looking from the base of support upward rather than the head-to-toe approach. Analyze the alignment of the foot, ankle, knee, hip, and spine including the neck and head. What is the impact of each joint on the body above and below? Look at the impact of the ground forces on alignment and movement. Frequently, an examination in both non-weight bearing and weight bearing positions is needed to determine if the observed deviation in alignment is a structural problem or a dynamic substitution

➤ "B"ase of support (BOS): Consider the size of the BOS and what portions of the body need to be included in establishing that BOS. Many children must have contact with the floor surface with the upper extremities (through an assistive device) to be stable. This means including the position of the upper extremities as part of the BOS. The larger the BOS, the more difficult it is to shift the center of mass (COM) over that base. For example, a child who walks with a scissoring style gait with the feet close together while in a posture walker still is demonstrating a large BOS. Even though the feet are close together, the size of the BOS is large. It also incorporates the upper extremity contacts with the walker and subsequently the BOS includes the entire area within the walker base

➤ "C"enter of mass: In assessing posture and alignment, the therapist considers the relationship of the child's COM to the BOS. Is the child increasing stability by lowering the COM in a crouched gait pattern? How is weight shifting of the COM achieved? Does the child shift weight only by shifting upper body weight over a more stable base and shortening on the weight bearing side or does the child control the weight shifting efficiently through the recruitment of patterns of rotation?

Westcott and coworkers[32] defined balancing as the process by which postural stability is maintained. Postural stability was defined as the ability to maintain or control the COM over the BOS to prevent falling and to complete desired movements. These authors outlined the need to develop valid and reliable measurement tools for balance in children. The focus during examination of variables contributing to balance included the sensory systems, the motor system, range of motion, and biomechanical factors. Kembhavi et al[33] found that the Berg Balance Scale was a useful clinical measure of balance for children with cerebral palsy. However, in a survey by Westcott et al[34] of pediatric physical therapists, 75% of the therapists indicated that they would prefer a nonstandardized test for evaluating balance. These findings indicated a decreased awareness and ability of clinicians to consistently and reliably assess complex concepts such as balance.

Force Plate Studies

The therapist can use a segment of Doc-U-Prints to gain information that is obtained with the force plates. Using Doc-U-Prints, it is possible to demonstrate what part of the foot is bearing most of the weight. It also is possible to record toe drag. It is clear if there is no heel contact or if more weight is put on the left foot than the right. While the actual amount of force exerted cannot be calculated without force plates, this method records the present pattern and changes across time.

Measurement of Basic Parameters

It is possible to record specific objective data including items such as step length, stride length, line of progression, angle of foot placement compared to line of progression, width of BOS, velocity, and cadence.[11] It is valuable to the clinician to have recorded data on gait parameters to document the impact of treatment. Changes then can be demonstrated pre- and post-surgery or botulinum toxin injections as well as following the provision of therapy services.

Energy Consumption

Although not all therapy centers have access to formal methods of testing energy consumption directly, there are several clinical methods that can produce useful data. If the child can walk for 6 minutes it is possible to calculate an energy efficiency index (EEI) that reflects specifically the health of the heart.[34,35] Rose et al[35] used these data to describe typical problems in several groups of children with developmental disabilities. Certainly, simple tests such as recording pre- and post-activity heart and respiratory rate are possible. If this information is coupled with measures such as recovery time from exercise and use of the Berg Perceived Exertion Scale, baseline data can be obtained.

Systems Analysis

SYSTEM EXAMINATION

If the previous steps have been followed, the clinician now has a good understanding of what the child can do related to walking and how it influences participation at home, in school, and in the community. Information on how the child walks (both qualitative and quantitative) has been gathered to describe and document the gait pattern. The next phase of the examination is to ask why these signs or symptoms appear, based on a careful analysis of the multiple systems within the individual. It is the interaction of the body systems within the child's environments that results in the observed gait deviations and functional limitations. The therapist evaluates each system to hypothesize its role in contributing to the overall clinical status of the child. The system integrities or impairments are identified.

MUSCULOSKELETAL

Many factors within the musculoskeletal system can significantly impact the child's ability to walk. Skeletal factors include the symmetry of leg length; the appropriate formation of the acetabulum and lower extremities, including factors such as angle of inclination, femoral antetorsion, and tibial torsion; and formation and alignment of the bones of the feet.

Muscles must not only have full passive range if elongated slowly, but also must be able to achieve full range quickly to be functionally useful. The soft tissue length must be adequate to allow for aligning the hips over the knees and the knees over the feet. Inadequate soft tissue length frequently is seen at the ankle preventing dorsiflexion, at the knee preventing full knee extension, and at the hip preventing full extension.

The child must have adequate strength to be able to walk. Many gait deviations can be attributed, at least in part, to a particular muscle weakness. An example is the gluteus medius "limp" that reflects decreased strength in the hip abductors. Muscle testing aimed specifically at the child with neuromuscular disorders focuses on testing each muscle both "in pattern," as well as with "conscious control." The two scores are important in determining the impact of weakness.[36] In addition this examination has been proposed as part of pre/post rhizotomy assessment.[37]

NEUROMOTOR

The clinician carefully assesses the child's ability to recruit, terminate, and grade motor unit activity as it relates to gait. The child must be able to selectively recruit postural muscles for stability in some areas while simultaneously recruiting other dynamic "movement" muscles to provide propulsive forces. It is especially important to consider the child's ability to control muscle contractions during gait with not only isometric or concentric contractions, but also eccentric control. A child with control of only isometric contractions may stand well, but be unable to move through space. A child with both concentric and isometric control may be able to walk, but be unable to stop without use of outside supports and, therefore, will constantly be bumping into other individuals, furniture, or walls.

The child must be able to shift between patterns of co-contraction or coactivation of agonists and antagonists for stability, to patterns that provide for both more ballistic wide-ranged movement and ramped or controlled mid-range movement. The child must be able to simultaneously isolate movements between the two lower extremities, allowing one leg to hold in extension for stance while the other flexes during swing. In addition, the child must be able to isolate activation within the limb so that one joint of the limb can flex while another extends. This is critical as the child swings the leg forward reaching for the ground with knee extension, but with ankle dorsiflexion.

One of the major factors contributing to inefficient gait is the recruitment of inefficient synergies.[15] Children with cerebral palsy demonstrated reversed, poorly timed, and dysfunctional synergies as compared to a matched group of peers when their COM unexpectedly was perturbed. It is important to review the strategies children use when the COM is perturbed over the BOS.

The child should be observed for the overall level, control, and coordination of dynamic muscle stiffness (change in force over change in length) during gait. Can the child intrinsically control stiffness or is it altered by changes in effort, emotion, or postural challenges? Can the child's lower extremities be stiff enough to hold the antigravity posture while allowing the upper extremities to be compliant enough to move through arm swing?

Are there extraneous movements that interfere with smooth gait? These extraneous movements can include clonus, tremor, or choreo-athetoid movements. How does the child manage or attempt to manage these signs of an under-damped system?

SENSORY

The sensory systems are evaluated for potential contributions to gait difficulties. While every sensory system may contribute to gait abnormalities, only those that frequently interfere will be discussed.

Vision

It has been demonstrated that for children under the age of 3 years, vision is the primary system used to provide for postural stability.[15] The therapist must determine if the child has reliable visual input for postural stability. In addition, is it possible for the child to utilize the visual flow that occurs with movement through space? Can the child scan the environment for obstacles and attend to or ignore specific visual features while maintaining postural stability with ambient vision and continue to walk? These are difficult tasks for the child with neuropathology even when the visual system is intact.

Somatosensory

Can the child register and integrate information from joint receptors, muscle receptors, skin, and soft tissues to provide accurate awareness of each limb and the body in space? Can the child use this information to anticipate changes that will be needed while walking by shortening or lengthening stride, increasing or decreasing speed, or changing direction to walk safely? Can the child perceive the lower body as the BOS and the source of postural security? Is the child also aware of and able to accommodate for small shifts in weight bearing during the phases of gait? Does the child demonstrate the ability to discriminate between noxious and non-noxious touch to the feet? A child with tactile hypersensitivity may refuse to allow bare feet to contact the surface, preferring to keep socks and shoes on at all times. A child may withdraw the feet from the surface rather than hold the body weight, not due to weakness, musculoskeletal issues, or control problems but for sensory reasons.

Vestibular

Does the child demonstrate difficulties with vestibular awareness? Is there a history of ear infections that might impair balance and, therefore, walking? Does the child demonstrate "postural insecurity" or fear of moving or being moved?

RESPIRATORY

There are many aspects of respiratory function that may affect gait. The child's resting and post-exercise rate should be determined. The patterns of breathing must be observed. Many children help to establish proximal postural stability via breath holding. While this strategy may be effective for short episodes (eg, picking up a heavy toy), it certainly is not effective for walking the length of a mall.

CARDIOVASCULAR

It also is important to consider the impact of the cardiovascular system on ambulation. It is evident that cardiovascular endurance is a critical component for many functional tasks. In addition, there are other cardiovascular factors that might influence a child's gait. If there is decreased circulation to the lower extremities, the child might hesitate to weight bear on the feet, experience claudication when walking long distances, or experience numbness and tingling when wearing orthotics.[12]

INTEGUMENTARY

The therapist must examine the condition of the skin. The skin reflects nutritional status as well as weight bearing history. If the child has very fragile skin across the foot or has developed calluses or areas of breakdown, the child may shift weight to avoid contact with that part of the body.

Evaluation

The evaluation process begins as the therapist hypothesizes about the relationships among the areas of concern noted during the examination. The strengths of the child, family, and environment are compared to areas of concern. Barriers the child may meet that may prevent functional walking will be considered; the posture and movement problems interfering with walking will be prioritized. Finally, the specific system impairments are listed, and the clinician then hypothesizes on the relationship of each of these factors to the critical functional limitations and participation restrictions. Specific functional outcomes and related impairment, posture, and movement objectives are identified for both long- and short-term periods.

Plan of Care

Based on the evaluation, a plan of care is established that includes:

➤ The frequency and duration of treatment

➤ The equipment that will be necessary

➤ Adjuncts to therapy that may speed progress

➤ A plan to educate the client and family

➤ The specific strategies to be used during therapy to improve performance as well as to lay the foundation for motor learning and a more permanent change in the child's functional abilities[38]

Intervention

The therapist will make decisions on specifics of intervention based on the *Guide to Physical Therapist Practice*[38] and anticipated outcomes from the Gross Motor Function Classification System (GMFCS).[39] According to the *Guide*, the intervention provided by the therapist can include three main components. These components include: 1) coordination, communication, and documentation; 2) patient/client education; and 3) direct intervention. As coordination, communication, and documentation and patient/client education are a part of every intervention, they will not be specifically addressed in this chapter. The therapist selects direct intervention strategies based on the examination, evaluation, and anticipated outcomes. Forms of direct intervention that are included when focusing on changes in walking or gait are:

➤ Therapeutic exercise

➤ Functional training in self-care and home management

➤ Functional training in community and work (job, school, play) integration

➤ Manual therapy

➤ Electrotherapeutic modalities

➤ Physical agents and mechanical modalities

➤ The prescription, application, and fabrication of assistive, adaptive, orthotic, protective, supportive, or prosthetic devices and equipment

Palisano and coworkers[39,40] provided an additional framework for problem solving with the GMFCS. Five levels of severity of gross motor functioning in children with cerebral palsy based on age-specific gross motor activities were described. The Levels I to V demonstrate increasingly compromised functional locomotive abilities. Each level reflects the highest level of mobility anticipated for a child between the ages of 6 to 12 years. Descriptions of locomotion abilities at earlier age ranges (birth to 2 years, 2 to 4 years of age, and 4 to 6 years of age) also are provided. In this classification system, Level I includes children who walk without restrictions and with limitations only being evident in more advanced gross motor skills (Figures 11-1 through 11-3). Level II includes children who

Figure 11-1. Level I: Emma walks well independently. Her difficulties in functional ambulation include walking while carrying items that require careful orientation, such as her cafeteria tray and ascending and descending stairs without a rail. Her personal goal is to be able to jump rope with friends at school. Here she is seen descending stairs.

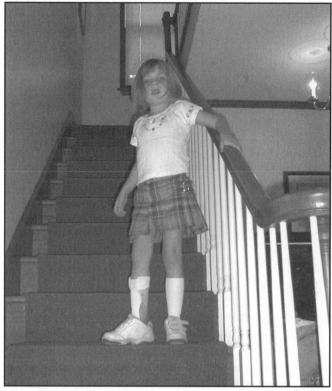

Figure 11-2. During ambulation on flat surfaces, asymmetry in the upper extremity is evident. She wears AFOs during ambulation and receives periodic injections of botulinum toxin.

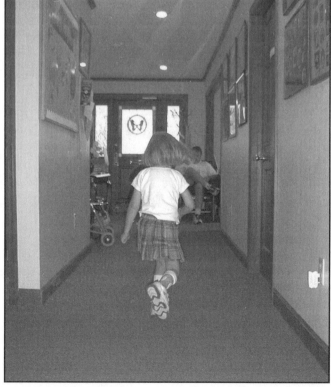

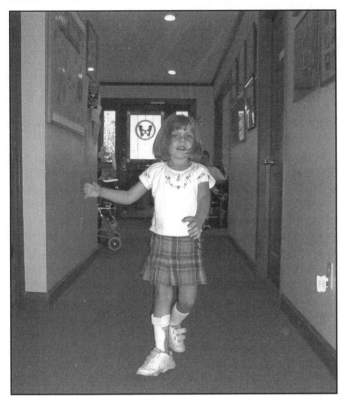

Figure 11-3. During running, posture and movement-related impairments become more evident.

walk without assistive devices but who demonstrate limitations in walking outdoors and in the community. The child in Level II might initially require an assistive device when very young and has more limitations in the ability to run and jump than children in Level I (Figures 11-4 and 11-5). Level III includes children who walk with assistive mobility devices and who have limitations in walking outdoors and in the community. These children typically will always require an assistive device and perhaps the use of orthotics (Figures 11-6 through 11-16). Level IV includes children who have self-mobility with limitations and who are usually transported or use power mobility outdoors and in the community. Children at this level typically function in sitting, usually with support. Independent mobility is very limited (Figures 11-17 and 11-18). Level V includes children whose self-mobility is severely limited even with the use of assistive technology. At this level the children have no means of independent mobility and are transported unless control of a powered wheelchair is mastered with extensive adaptations (Figures 11-19 through 11-21).

Descriptions of interventions will begin by addressing children who are in the most severely functionally limited groups (Levels IV and V) and proceed to those with less significant limitations. Although these functional levels were described for children with cerebral palsy, this chapter will focus on questions or general principles of practice for children with varying diagnoses to guide the clinician in establishing specific intervention plans. In addition, a brief discussion on the appropriate referral to other health care practitioners for additional interventions outside the scope of physical therapy will be presented. This will include implications for the therapist's plan of care or nontherapist interventions such as botulinum toxin or phenol injections, orthopedic surgeries, selective dorsal rhizotomy, and other procedures, such as insertion of a baclofen pump or stimulators.

Figure 11-4. Level II: This 19-year-old girl has walked independently since 4 years of age. However, due to significant visual impairments, decreased neuromuscular control and coordination, decreased range of motion at the ankles, and a scoliosis her functional abilities in novel situations in the community are restricted.

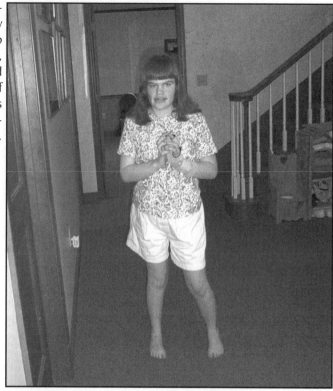

Figure 11-5. She now wears AFOs bilaterally and periodically has botulinum toxin and taping to her back and legs. She participates in a therapeutic horseback riding program and gymnastics.

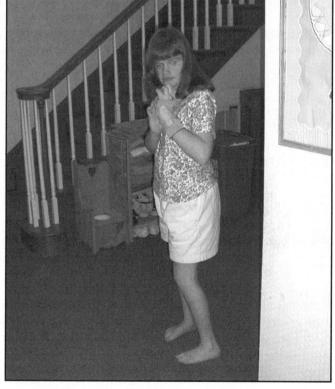

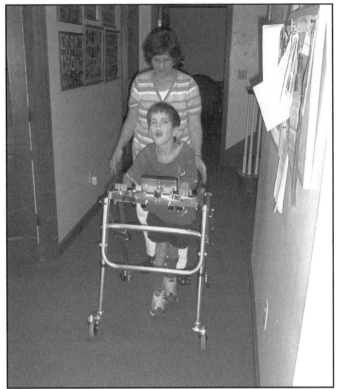

Figure 11-6. Level III: This 11-year-old boy moves independently by self-propelling a wheelchair and walking supported in a Pony (Snug Seat, Matthews, NC). He walks with stand by guarding at household levels and is developing basic skills at community distances.

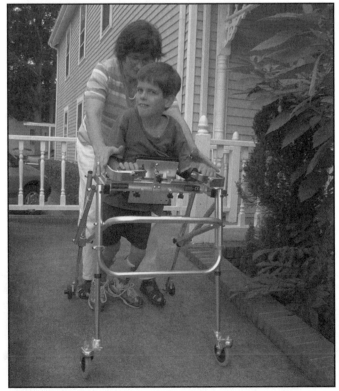

Figure 11-7. He requires physical assist to descend a ramp.

Figure 11-8. This 3-year-old child moves around the floor by "bunny hopping."

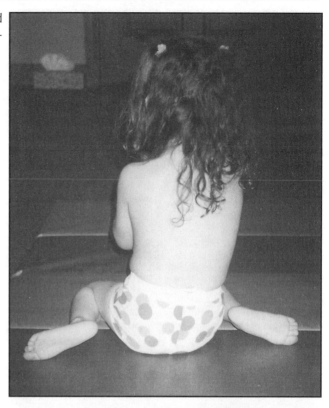

Figure 11-9. She pulls to stand and walks community distances with a posture walker.

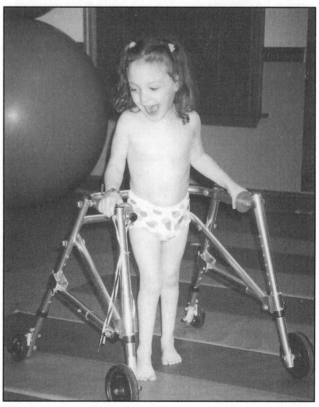

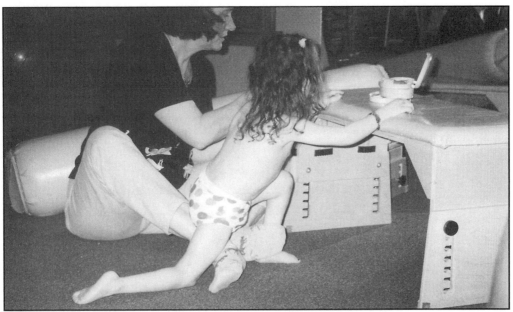

Figure 11-10. Transitions to and from the floor encourage a lower extremity isolated control (one leg flexed and one extended).

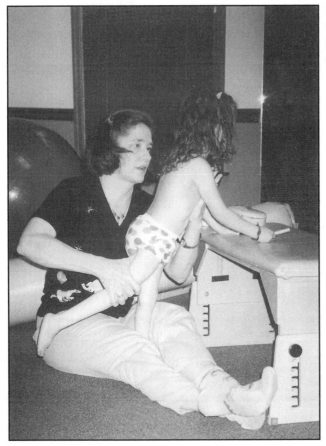

Figure 11-11. Transitions to and from the floor encourage a lower extremity isolated control (one leg flexed and one extended).

Figure 11-12. Gait is facilitated to increase hip and knee extension in terminal ranges to increase her step length.

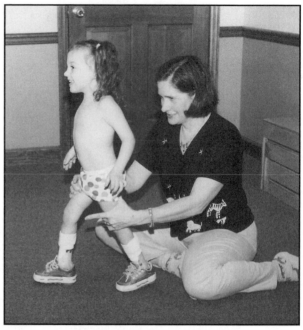

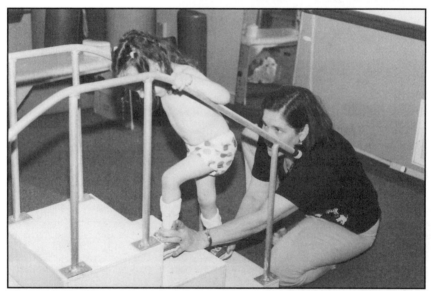

Figure 11-13. The muscles in the lower extremity are strengthened and ankle range of motion increased dynamically via a stair climbing activity.

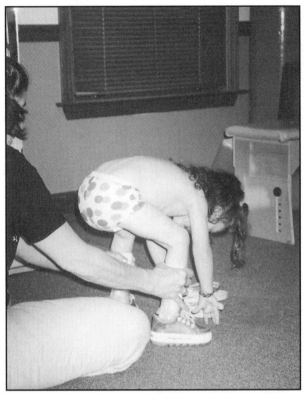

Figure 11-14. The child works in squatting activities to gain control of her COM over her BOS. Assistance is provided to minimize her tendency to adduct and internally rotate the lower extremities and to have a toe only contact.

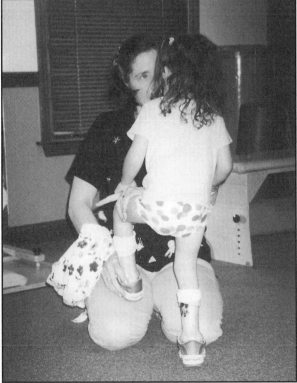

Figure 11-15. Another activity to promote motor learning is to teach the family about how she can assist in dressing in standing.

Figure 11-16. She is now able to stand and walk independently across the floor to give an object to a family member. This goal is important to the family as the child attends preschool and needs to walk from one area to the other carrying objects.

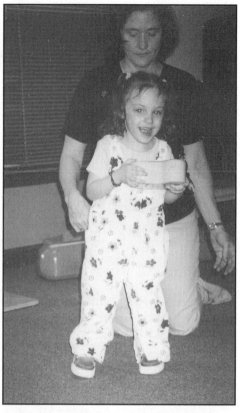

Figure 11-17. Level IV: This teenager was involved in a motor vehicle accident 3 years ago. He has a power wheelchair.

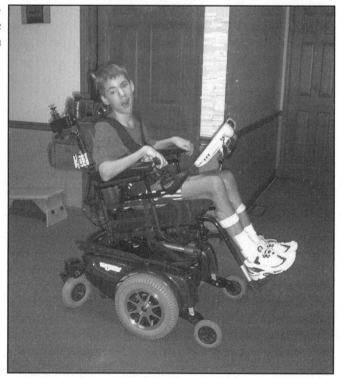

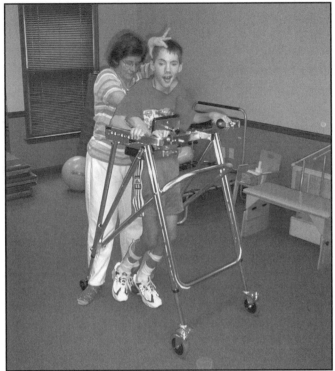

Figure 11-18. In recent months, he has demonstrated an increased ability to ambulate short distances with an assistive device. This makes it possible for him to walk from his bedroom to the bathroom or to walk into a restroom in the community that is not wheelchair accessible.

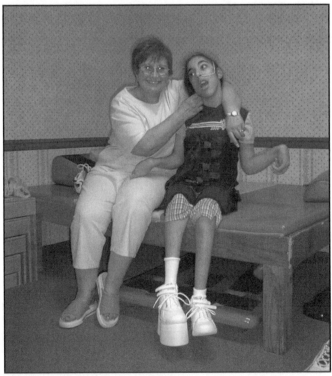

Figure 11-19. Level V: Michelle, at 16 years of age, is seen sitting with her mom. She has no independent mobility and is dependent on caregivers for all transfers. She has a dislocated hip and scoliosis.

Figure 11-20. Michelle loves standing in a partial body weight bearing (PBWB) device and can safely be positioned upright.

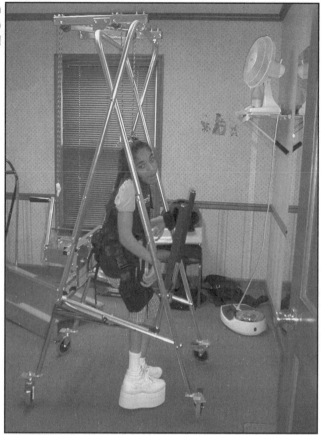

Figure 11-21. She enjoys ambulating on the treadmill with approximately 50% weight bearing. Her cardiopulmonary endurance has improved to 10-minute episodes of walking.

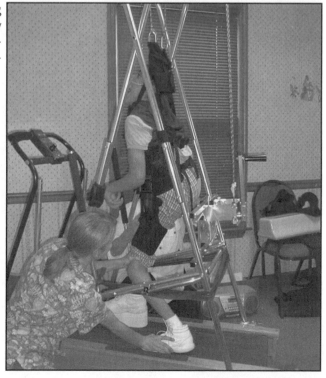

Intervention for Children at Level IV or V

Several questions must be asked in regard to therapeutic intervention for a child who will probably never be unable to walk in a functional manner to move through the environment independently. These include:

➤ Is there any reason to work toward goals of ambulation?

➤ Is there any value to this child or family in ambulation assisted by another person or by extensive assistive devices?

➤ Are the results or outcomes of this intervention worth the cost in terms of time, money, and effort?

These questions are very difficult to answer and require the careful consideration of the entire team. There is no one correct answer. Once the decision has been reached and specific outcome measures have been established, the clinician then develops specific strategies to address the impairments and motor component problems that interfere with successful performance of the desired outcomes.

The family and intervention team can begin by discussing the participation restrictions that result from the inability of the child to ambulate even with an assistive device. Mobility in a powered chair may increase participation at school and in the community as well as at home. Using powered mobility, the child may be able to go to a friend's or extended family member's home to spend the night or afternoon. The family may recognize that the ability to ambulate with the assistance of another person might allow the child to go out into the community more often. The child may be able to participate more in community activities if able to take steps with physical assistance into a restaurant or building that is not wheelchair accessible. The family and child may believe that the functional outcome of being able to take assisted steps to move in and out of the family bathroom or bedroom is worth the energy and financial cost of intervention.

Next the team must consider the potential risks of not providing the intervention.

➤ Are there secondary impairments that might emerge if no intervention is provided?

➤ What is the potential of developing complications secondary to a more sedentary lifestyle?

➤ Are there risks of increased cardiopulmonary impairments?

➤ Are there risks to the musculoskeletal system such as increased contractures, weakness, or osteoporosis?

➤ What are the implications for the child's self-esteem or sense of well-being?

➤ What will be the cost to the child or family if these complications occur?

If the answer to the questions posed above lead the team to decide that intervention is warranted, the intervention will include the use of extensive assistive technology as well as direct intervention. Activities in therapy will continue to have a focus on sitting function and on developing maximal skills for locomotion in the wheelchair. Additional equipment to aid the family in transport (eg, lifts or ramps for a van) may be indicated. The intervention may include:

➤ Using partial body weight bearing (PBWB) training over a treadmill to establish basic patterns of ambulation[41-44]

➤ Instructing caregivers in supported ambulation

➤ Training the child to control a powered wheelchair

➤ Focusing on cardiopulmonary fitness

➤ Monitoring and addressing musculoskeletal issues (eg, range of motion, strength)

➤ Addressing skeletal changes in bone mineral density

➤ Addressing issues related to self-esteem

The frequency and duration of intervention are established to: match proposed functional outcomes, address the prevention of secondary impairments or greater functional limitations, address new issues related to growth or changes in body systems, address changes in environmental demands, and meet the needs of the individual family. Frank discussions with the family are important to ensure that the therapist and family all anticipate the same outcomes. For example, the family should not hope for an outcome of independent ambulation because intervention is addressing supported walking.

Basic Treatment Principles

1. Explore all options of locomotion or mobility including independent wheelchair use, powered mobility, or modified battery-operated riding toys. Intervention strategies during direct services may include emphasis on sitting control with upper extremities free for use to control the mobility device

2. For upright posture and stability and forward propulsive force generation, the therapist can provide equipment to compensate for postural and movement control limitations. These options might include the use of PBWB device, a gait trainer, or a Pony (Snug Seat, Matthews, NC) type device. It may be possible to use an assistive device such as an anterior support walker for assisted household level ambulation. These devices can be important to aid the caregivers and prevent injury to their backs, even when the child cannot use it independent of standby assistance. During therapy sessions, intervention addresses increased postural control to hold the head and trunk upright with less assistance. Activities should be done in the upright posture as the impact of gravity is reduced as compared to work in lower positions against gravity, and the postural synergies require less isolated control. Trunk extension is coupled with hip and knee extension. Ambulation over a treadmill may be useful to initially develop the sense of forward progression with a forward propulsive force. It is important to work to obtain the correct alignment of the trunk over the extremities. The use of prone, supine, or vertical standers can be used to ensure this alignment. This is an important component of intervention if the child spends most of the day sitting. Orthotics are used to maintain biomechanical alignment and soft tissue mobility during other parts of the day when the child is not walking, However, the child may be more successful during ambulation if the orthotics are removed

3. Shock absorption concerns are addressed by supporting more appropriate alignment of the extremities and by limiting the amount of weight the child is expected to bear. A PBWB device can limit the amount of weight on an extremity and the use of orthotics may reduce the valgus or varus stress to a limb. Orthotics are monitored for indications of excessive weight-bearing and then modified to better distribute weight during ambulation

4. The therapist is not expecting energy conservation to be a goal in this limited, assisted ambulation. The purpose of the assisted ambulation can be to challenge the child's cardiac and respiratory systems. The child may be participating in the activity as a form of aerobic exercise to increase cardiopulmonary fitness. The therapist first may need to address these issues with careful supervision in the therapy setting, but later the activity might occur in a classroom or physical education program

without direct supervision of the therapist. It is important, however, to use caution during the decision-making process. Supported ambulation for these children involves risk both of immediate injury and the development of secondary impairments with additional functional limitations. While almost every child needs a standing program to address issues of bone mineral density, alignment, and soft tissue length, not every child needs to participate in a walking program

Intervention for Children at Level III

The therapist faces different questions with children at Level III. Most therapists and parents see the need for therapy for these children, but the challenge is to effectively focus therapy to have the greatest impact on the child's participation and function. The therapist begins by addressing participation of the child at home and in the community. The family identifies both specific participation restrictions and desired outcomes. The therapist then selects potential strategies for intervention. In addition, the therapist and family must review the potential devices and orthotics that might be used by the child within the key environments and then select and obtain the most appropriate ones. As these children typically use different forms of ambulation in different environments, the child may use a less cumbersome assistive device at home than in the community. The therapist must train the child with those specific devices and then allow practice with the device in the critical environments in order to ensure functional use.

The therapist, with the family, identifies specific functional outcomes to be achieved in therapy. Once these outcomes are established, the therapist identifies and plans strategies to address the impairments as well as posture and movement problems that are hypothesized to interfere with the desired functional outcomes. The therapist must search for efficient strategies to address each of the impairments or posture and movement problems. The therapist plans activities to nurture motor learning. In addition, the therapist treats with the goal of minimizing anticipated future impairments. The balance between striving to improve function immediately and the need to anticipate and manage impairments that might influence future functional abilities and participation is critical for these children.

Intervention frequently includes coordination of services from a wide variety of professionals including the possibility of orthopedic surgery, injections of botulinum toxin or phenol, use of medications, and considerations of neurosurgical or orthopedic interventions. The therapist is a resource for the family who is confronted with a wide array of possibilities for interventions from TV, magazines, the Internet, friends, and families (see Chapter 16).

Basic Treatment Principles

1. For upright posture and stability, the therapist can begin with the ABCs of posture described in the examination section. The therapist must treat to develop alignment for efficient upright posture. The ability to keep the head stable while scanning the environment during ambulation is critical. Activities to address alignment can include promoting soft tissue length throughout the body. Providing a BOS that is large enough for stability, but not so large as to limit mobility, will require both the careful selection of an assistive device as well as the selection of orthotics. It is critical for the child to develop strategies to control weight shifting of the COM. These strategies will lead to increased balance. Strengthening of the postural muscles should include isometric work in shortened ranges. Emphasis on strengthening the

extensors of the trunk and lower extremities is needed. Extended practice or experience in locomotion on the floor (eg, creeping, bunny hopping, or knee walking) may not carry over to the development of synergies required for upright postures. A child may use these methods of locomotion at home for increased independence. However, the relative cost and benefit of promoting these patterns of mobility for a child who is anticipated to have the potential for upright locomotion are part of the educational program both for the family and the child. The team will need to discuss the selection and use of assistive devices in different environments to allow the child immediate independent mobility without jeopardizing greater independence in the future

2. The development of smooth forward progression with forward propulsive forces is a complex motor control problem for the child and the therapist to address. Focus in therapy is on developing efficient forward progression of the COM with less lateral and/or up and down movement. This is promoted by facilitating increased proximal co-contraction or coactivation with axial rotation to decrease the excursion of the COM during the gait cycle. A prerequisite to this control is spinal and rib cage mobility in all planes (see Chapter 9). The forward propulsive forces include both phasic burst activity from the plantarflexors as well as hip extensors. These forces may be limited if the child wears orthotics to limit movement into plantarflexion. The therapist, therefore, should have the child work both in and out of the orthotics during direct services. Concentric burst work through the lower extremities is included as well as eccentric work to control the advancement of the COM. In addition, the child must develop isolated control both between and within the lower extremities. It is more effective to stress work in stride positions for mobility rather than in a static position as synergies, including isolated or fractionated control, are used. The use of supported ambulation over a treadmill can increase the speed of the child's gait through increased isolated control and reciprocity without compromising proximal control

3. A child at Level III frequently demonstrates difficulties related to shock absorption. These problems can decrease the efficiency of gait. There also are implications for long-term independent ambulation due to injury to the joints or soft tissues or an increased likelihood of the development of arthritic changes. The most critical factor for the therapist is to be diligent in the observation and modification of alignment. Modifications with orthotics, taping, shoes, and assistive devices can alter alignment significantly. Particular attention should be given to knee alignment as the knees are at the greatest jeopardy from forces from both above and below. This problem is complicated by the use of orthotics that may improve alignment, but can simultaneously decrease the inherent ability of the child to absorb shock because interactions within the foot or between the foot, ankle, knee, and hip are limited

4. Energy conservation is a key issue for the child at Level III. A child in this group may ambulate well in early childhood, but then rely more and more on wheelchair transport during adolescence or adult life due to the high-energy demands experienced during ambulation. The therapist needs to monitor and appropriately treat or manage the respiratory and cardiovascular impacts of ambulation. Treatment can include both addressing the patterns of respiration as well as issues of endurance particularly as the child matures into adolescence. Posture and movement problems also change the overall efficiency of gait. The therapist should address these problems to increase energy efficiency

Intervention for Children at Level I or II

When treating children who are at Level I or II, the therapist again is faced with questions about the necessity of direct therapy to address walking. These children can walk independently. However, it is now the inability to adapt walking to meet a wide variety of functional demands in different settings that creates problems for the child. Most of these children are functioning in classrooms in community schools. The expectation that, because they can walk, they will be able to participate in all areas of family and school life may create unrealistic demands on their walking abilities. Many of these children still have significant functional limitations and restrictions in participation. For example, children may be able to walk independently by using weight shifting from the upper body with lateral trunk flexion, but need assistance at school due to an inability to carry a lunchroom tray independently.

While the child at Level I or II is able to walk, intervention may be needed to modify the quality of the child's gait that limits function. The therapist now is responsible for gait training. The therapist may develop a plan to address parameters related to step length or line of progression to increase overall efficiency. It is very important for the therapist to address ambulation in varying environmental contexts as well as focusing on functional outcomes. The therapist must plan ahead for the anticipated functional and environmental challenges for the child. To meet these outcomes the therapist will need to address the specific impairments and atypical motor components that decrease the efficiency and effectiveness of gait.

An additional question or issue that can arise is the time to most effectively introduce independent ambulation as a therapy outcome or goal. For example, it can be assumed that the child with a hemiplegia will ambulate independently. However, if the child begins to ambulate very early, the gait often demonstrates marked asymmetries in both posture and movement that can have long-lasting impact. Would this child's gait be more functional and efficient in the long term if the onset of ambulation is delayed until greater postural control is developed? While it is not advisable to actively restrict a child's attempts to ambulate, it may be appropriate to focus initially on increasing control and coordination in creeping on the floor rather than encouraging upright independent ambulation. This is an unresolved issue, however, as it is not clear how much transfer there will be of postural control in one position to postural control in another position (see Chapter 3).

Therapy for children in Level I or II may include more involvement in community-based activities in addition to or in place of traditional direct services. Therapy may be more effective if performed in water, on horseback, or in a karate gym.[45] Group activities may reflect more accurately the functional demands encountered by the child. However, a singular "coaching" approach of therapy for this child may result in increasing secondary impairments and later functional limitations.

Basic Treatment Principles

PRINCIPLE 1

For upright posture and stability, the therapist performs an ongoing analysis and evaluation of the child's postural control while ambulating in different functional activities and environments. It is common for children functioning at this level to recruit the two joint, long muscles for postural stability even though these muscles are more typically used for movement. The implications are a reduction in the multifunctional tasks that require both postural stability and free use of the extremities during ambulation and a reduction of overall balance. For example, the child who uses the latissimus to increase stability in the trunk by stabilizing the upper extremity to the pelvis may be unable to walk and carry large items (eg, a large box or a tray) in front of the body with two upper extremities for support. In addition, the child may be unable to anticipate and respond to unexpected perturbations, such as remaining standing on a bus when it departs or walking across the uneven surface of the playground. The child often will return to less refined patterns for stability when postural control is challenged. Postural challenges can include complex tasks, the introduction of more complicated environments, or growth. A child may walk at home with good balance and be able to efficiently anticipate changes in floor surfaces, but when in the midst of the new kindergarten classroom, trip and fall over the edge of the carpet when moving to "circle time."

Therefore, the therapist facilitates and strengthens appropriate recruitment of the postural muscles and then adds the simultaneous recruitment of the movement muscles for tasks during ambulation. It is important to work in a variety of settings and with different associated functional demands. The therapist must provide the "just right" challenge both with tasks and environments. The parents and therapist also must be prepared for skills accomplished at one age to disappear after a major growth spurt. It may be necessary to return for an episode of more intense therapy. The therapist also carefully considers the use of orthotics and/or taping to simultaneously improve alignment but reduce the degrees of freedom available for postural adjustments. The therapist may consider the use of: therapeutic adjuncts such as therapeutic electrical stimulation (TES),[46,47] neuromuscular electrical stimulation (NMES),[48,49] serial casting,[50,51] referral to physicians for periodic injections of botulinum toxin or phenol,[52] or surgical interventions such as consideration of a selective dorsal rhizotomy or baclofen pump. However, it is important for the clinician to research both the evidence to support the practice as well as all contraindications or potential risks of the strategy before recommending an adjunct to therapy (see Chapter 16). Recommendations to the family to incorporate tasks on a daily basis provide motor learning opportunities.

Efficient and effective forward progression also can be a problem for the child. Key factors that contribute to this difficulty are:

➤ Inability to develop axial rotation for the management of weight shifting to aid in step length

➤ Inefficient use of eccentric control to manage the speed of progression

➤ The lack of precise timing and sequencing of muscles that adapt quickly to changes in the environment on a moment-to-moment basis

PRINCIPLE 2

The therapist focuses on the smooth forward progression of the child's COM in which the child controls the speed and direction of gait to match environmental constraints as well as functional demands. The child must be able to manage all typical environmental barriers encountered in daily life. The posture and movement impairments relating to balance and function and the individual system impairments that impede functional progress are addressed within functional activities. Specific attention is directed to increasing the child's ability to isolate movement both between and within the lower extremities. More complex activities such as running, jumping, stair climbing, bicycling, and rollerskating both challenge the child and aid in developing greater control and coordination. Orthotics must be reviewed on a regular basis for both fit and function. The orthotic that worked well for the elementary school-aged child may become ineffective in the middle school-aged child due to both growth and social issues. Shifts in the style of the orthotic and the wearing schedule can alter the impact of orthotic use for the child. In addition to focusing on proximal issues discussed earlier, the therapist also focuses on details of the three-rocker action of the foot as it promotes the smooth forward progression of the body mass over the alternating feet.

The therapist must address difficulties related to the child's ability to absorb shock. The child's decreased ability to isolate movement, particularly in the foot, and to time foot movement with movement throughout the rest of the body can lead to limited functional abilities related to decreased balance. The therapist also works on issues in the musculoskeletal system, such as range of motion and strengthening, as well as neuromuscular control and coordination. As the child grows and the biomechanics of upright posture change, revisions in the plans for orthotics, taping, or even the provision of direct services must be reconsidered.

PRINCIPLE 3

Many typically developing children in the United States demonstrate limited physical fitness and increased risk of obesity. Children with disabilities are at an even greater risk for a sedentary lifestyle and therefore changes in energy conservation during gait should be monitored. Inefficient gait patterns gradually may lead to functional limitations. The therapist should monitor heart and respiratory rates during gait training activities and during the introduction of new functional activities, such as stair climbing or running. A regular fitness program for the child including aspects of flexibility, conditioning, and strength can be done through a community program or within the school program.[53] The therapist may need to introduce the program, monitor it for initial safety, develop parameters or boundaries of the program, and then transfer responsibility for ongoing programming to the child and/or family.

Summary

Children with developmental disabilities have multiple issues that can limit their ability to functionally ambulate and, therefore, to participate fully in home, school, and community life. The therapist needs an understanding of the basics of gait and of the changes that occur across development. An evaluation that includes examination of functional abilities and limitations, posture and movement strengths and problems, as well as individual system integrities and impairments, provides a basis for formulating hypotheses for intervention planning. The intervention plan needs to account for the child's medical diagnosis and potential for ambulation as well as current status. The therapist then selects specific strategies for intervention to reach the anticipated outcomes. In the following case studies, the guidelines for evaluation and the principles for intervention presented in this chapter will be illustrated.

Case Study #1: Jason

➤ Practice pattern 5C: Impaired Motor Function and Sensory Integrity Associated With Nonprogressive Disorders of the Central Nervous System—Congenital Origin or Acquired in Infancy or Childhood

➤ Medical diagnosis: Cerebral palsy, right hemiparesis

➤ Age: 24 months

Examination

PARENTAL GOALS

The family is very interested in Jason being able to walk well at home while playing independently and to play outdoors on playgrounds with his brother and other children without falling.

FUNCTIONAL ABILITIES

The parents report that Jason can assume all fours and crawl short distances. He can get into sitting and standing independently. He began walking at 15 months of age. His most recent test scores revealed gross motor skills between 12 to 15 months. He has no assistive devices or adaptive equipment.

POSTURE AND MOVEMENT

In standing, Jason demonstrates an asymmetrical posture with anterior tilt of the pelvis and pelvic retraction on the right. He has an observable asymmetry in his rib cage. The right upper extremity usually is held in a posture of shoulder elevation, scapular adduction with humeral hyperextension and medial rotation, and elbow, wrist, and finger flexion. Weight is shifted to his left and the left lower extremity is in slight genu recurvatum with the right lower extremity in a posture of hip and knee flexion with the ankle in slight plantarflexion. He demonstrates decreased isolated control on the right in both the upper and lower extremity.

Jason can maintain an upright posture against gravity. In doing so he recruits and overuses muscles of movement for stability. This limits the freedom of movement of his trunk and upper extremity. He achieves forward propulsion through space but has difficulty with grading his speed. He does not manage the absorption of shock on the right side and is, therefore, at risk for injury to that side. He relies heavily on momentum to advance his body in space. His gait demonstrates a short swing phase on the right, short step length, with minimal right knee and ankle flexion at mid-swing. There is short stance on the right with genu recurvatum and a valgus position of the right foot at mid-stance. He always initiates steps with his left leg.

SYSTEMS EXAMINATION

Anthropometric Characteristics

Jason is noted to have a slightly smaller right upper extremity when compared to the left. His lower extremities currently measure the same in length and girth. He is scheduled to be evaluated by an orthopedist for a baseline study of limb length and hip stability.

Regulatory System

Jason is an active child and is able to follow directions and cooperate with the therapist.

Musculoskeletal System

Jason demonstrates tightness to passive stretch in the hip muscles and lateral trunk flexors on the right with limitation in trunk rotation. He has weakness in the right extremities.

Neuromuscular System

Jason can initiate, sustain, and terminate motor unit activity throughout the body. He relies most heavily on concentric and isometric contractions particularly on the right. He has difficulty in isolating muscle activation within both the upper and lower extremities. He demonstrates increased clonus at the right ankle when tested.

Sensory Systems

Jason demonstrates neglect of the right side of the body, upper extremity greater than lower extremity.

Respiratory System

Breath holding is noted during stressful activity, such as running or transitioning from the floor to standing.

Evaluation

Jason is developing gross motor skills as anticipated for a child with a hemiplegia. He is at Level I of the GMFCS. It is anticipated that he will be a community ambulator without an assistive device. He may have functional limitations related to complex environments or tasks that require precise balance and symmetrical use of the upper extremities. The slower acquisition of functional skills of ambulation is related to the complex interaction of posture and movement asymmetries; the interaction of his neuromuscular, sensory, and musculoskeletal impairments; and his growth. He already is demonstrating asymmetries and is at risk for developing secondary impairments, such as a scoliosis or a subluxing or dislocating hip on the right from increased femoral antetorsion. Although at this time his leg lengths measure the same, it is anticipated that with decreased weight bearing the bone growth on the right side might slow. It is assumed that intervention can minimize the appearance of these secondary impairments. Intervention will be most necessary during growth spurts and when there are new environmental or functional demands.

FUNCTIONAL LIMITATIONS

Jason creeps on his hands and knees, but occasionally collapses on his right arm. He falls frequently during the day. He attempts to run, but is clumsy and usually falls. When he falls, he is unable to catch himself with his right hand. He is unable to keep up with peers or sibling on the playground or when playing outside on uneven terrain.

IMPAIRMENTS

Based on the examination, several impairments that relate directly to ambulation were identified. These included: 1) tightness in the hip muscles and lateral trunk flexors on the right side, 2) difficulty in isolating muscle activation in the right lower extremity, and 3) neglect of the right side. Jason has an asymmetrical posture in standing and during ambulation. Specific gait deviations were a short swing phase on the right and short step length. Short stance on the right with genu recurvatum and a valgus position of the right foot at mid-stance also were observed.

GOALS

Treatment goals are for Jason to demonstrate:

1. Increased symmetry in his standing posture
2. Increased speed of achieving soft tissue mobility in the right lower extremity during active movement
3. Increased strength in the right extremities
4. Increased isolated control within the right upper and lower extremities
5. Longer and more equal step lengths

FUNCTIONAL OUTCOMES

Following 6 to 9 months of intervention, Jason will:

1. Ambulate on a community playground, mounting and dismounting from at least four pieces of equipment without falling

2. Walk in his playroom at home picking up and carrying items requiring two hands for support and then placing the items on a shelf at shoulder height

3. Propel a riding toy while sitting both forward and backward using both lower extremities

Intervention

Jason will continue to receive direct services from the physical therapist. A knee immobilizer and an orthosis for the right lower extremity to wear occasionally at night will be recommended. A shoe insert to aid in the alignment of the right foot during ambulation also will be recommended. An orthopedist will follow Jason for both hip integrity and spinal alignment. If, in the future, Jason develops tightness that cannot be addressed through therapeutic procedures, he can be referred to a physician for evaluation for botulinum toxin injections of the gastrocnemius and possibly hamstring muscles on the right. Another alternative would be serial casting. Coordination of services among the physical, occupational, and speech therapists will be achieved via telephone conversations and written communication.

Activities will focus on increasing skill in ambulation in a wider variety of environments with increasing demands for the upper body. Sessions may occur in the home, at community playgrounds, or at an outpatient facility to allow beginning work in PBWB over a treadmill. Soft tissue elongation using myofascial and mobilization strategies, strengthening activities, and activities to increase control and coordination of the right side will be emphasized along with increasing meaningful sensory input to the right side of the body. The parents will be instructed in activities to do at home to generalize functional use and to provide greater opportunities for motor learning.

Case Study #2: Jill

> Practice pattern 5C: Impaired Motor Function and Sensory Integrity Associated With Nonprogressive Disorders of the Central Nervous System—Congenital Origin or Acquired in Infancy or Childhood

> Medial diagnosis: Cerebral palsy, spastic quadriparesis, microcephaly, mental retardation, seizure disorder

> Age: 7 years

Examination

PARENTAL GOALS

The family reports increasing difficulty with transferring Jill. They have the most difficulty with transfers into the bathtub and into the family vehicle. While the current wheelchair will go into the bathroom there is little space to move once it is in the room. They also anticipate that the next sized wheelchair will not go through the door. The mother is worried that Jill will have a seizure while she is in the tub or in mid transfer and that she may be hurt.

FUNCTIONAL ABILITIES

Jill is able to lift her head briefly when prone and can roll from supine to sidelying. Jill will assist briefly with standing pivot transfers, but she does not maintain standing unless supported in a stander.

POSTURE AND MOVEMENT

Jill demonstrates a fixed kyphosis with an emerging scoliosis. These postural deviations are noted in all postures but are most evident in sitting. She has limited self-generated movement, preferring to keep her COM well within the BOS. Movement that occurs remains in the sagittal plane. Her upright stability against gravity is severely limited. She does not achieve any forward propulsion. She makes no attempts to manage shock absorption. All attempts to move independently through space are very costly in terms of energy conservation.

SYSTEMS EXAMINATION

Anthropometric Characteristics

Jill is below the 10th percentile for height and weight. She has a small head (microcephaly).

Regulatory System

Jill demonstrates a decreased ability to regulate arousal. She often is lethargic, which may be related to her seizure medications. However, when she is alert she is distractible and has poor selective attention. She responds to vestibular input with autonomic distress.

Musculoskeletal System

Jill demonstrates limited range of motion in the neck, spine, hips, and shoulders. Her strength is reduced throughout and the size of her muscles is small compared to her peers.

Neuromuscular System

Jill is able to initiate and sustain motor unit activity, but at times has difficulty with termination of the activity. Muscle contractions are limited to either concentric or isometric contractions. She, therefore, frequently demonstrates excessive co-contraction with resulting stiffness throughout the extremities. She has a very limited repertoire of movements available to her. She also has very little ability to isolate muscle activation and therefore recruits total patterns of flexion or extension. Her upper extremities demonstrate patterns of full flexion, while the lower extremities can flex or extend briefly when coupled with full body extension.

Sensory Systems

Jill has good vision by report but does have difficulty with oculomotor control. Hearing is normal. She demonstrates decreased somatosensory awareness throughout the body and especially in the lower body. However she is hyperresponsive to oral input. Her vestibular system is hyperresponsive to movement input.

Cardiopulmonary System

Jill demonstrates shallow respiration that is frequently asynchronous in nature. She does not always coordinate respiration with other functional activities. The shape of her rib cage makes it difficult for her to achieve chest expansion when positioned in prone or when in her prone stander. She does not always breathe regularly during transitions. She also demonstrates difficulties in the cardiovascular system with decreased distal blood supply. Her limbs become purplish when in dependent positions for long periods.

Integumentary

The skin is clear at this time but is at high risk for breakdown due to lack of active movement and prolonged positioning in sitting.

Evaluation

Jill is a young child with multiple and severe impairments that result in significant functional limitations. She functions at Level V in the GMFCS. It is anticipated that Jill will remain dependent on others for her locomotion. She may be able to learn to take assisted steps to aid in transfers and to move very short distances in the home when supported by an adult. She may have a wider range of living possibilities as an adult if she is able to transfer with the assist of one and able to take assisted steps. It is not anticipated that she will be an ambulator, but it is important that she achieve the ability to assist more with transfers. It may be possible for her to eventually be able to take a few assisted steps to assist during activities of daily living, such as bathing. It is important that she be positioned in standing on a regular basis to improve bone density, to position the soft tissues for elongation, and to improve circulation and respiration. Jill will require ongoing monitoring. If programming to address her positional changes is not integrated into her daily routines, it is anticipated that she may develop significant secondary impairments with severe medical implications. These problems could relate to her respiratory, digestive, or orthopedic status.

FUNCTIONAL LIMITATIONS

Jill has limited floor mobility and is unable to ambulate. She is dependent on others for mobility and self-cares.

IMPAIRMENTS

Based on the examination, several impairments were identified. The primary impairments related to her ambulatory status are her limited repertoire of movements and restricted range of motion in the trunk and lower extremities. She also has generally diminished strength, endurance, and respiratory function.

GOALS

Treatment goals are for Jill to demonstrate:
1. Improved soft tissue mobility and bone mineral density
2. Improved respiratory and cardiovascular endurance
3. Increased strength
4. Improved regulatory control
5. Increased postural control
6. Improved isolated control in the lower extremities to allow reciprocity for assisted step taking

FUNCTIONAL OUTCOMES

Following 6 to 9 months of intervention in her school program, Jill will:
1. Stand and transfer, with the assist of one adult supporting her around the upper chest area, from her wheelchair to a classroom chair of equal height requiring her to take two steps

2. Tolerate without signs of autonomic distress being transitioned from sit to stand when positioned in an EZ-Stand (EZ-Way, Clarinda, Iowa) at least twice daily with the assist of the classroom aide

3. Stand for a classroom activity for a minimum of 30 minutes while positioned in a standing device and while wearing her orthotics, at least three times per week

4. Participate in 20 minutes of aerobic exercise with her peers while positioned either in a PBWB device, a gait trainer, or a mobile stander and assisted by a classroom aide

Intervention

Physical therapy services for Jill will continue in the school setting for 30 minutes per week. Most sessions will be indirect, but it is anticipated that occasional periods of more intensive direct services will be necessary to introduce new skills to Jill and her classroom attendant. Instruction will be provided to the teacher as well as to the adaptive physical education instructor. The current stander will be exchanged for a EZ-Stand to allow introduction of more dynamic transfers. This stander will decrease weight bearing through her anterior chest, and, therefore, improve her depth of respiration and allow more frequent changes in her posture for circulatory stimulation. The correct positioning of Jill in her adaptive equipment, signs and symptoms of distress to be observed carefully, and the timing or scheduling of positional changes will be reviewed with the staff. This plan will be reviewed with the parents annually. It is suggested that the family arrange home-based services to assist in problem solving issues related to transferring Jill to and from the bathtub as well as in and out of the family car. This could be arranged over a summer break.

Case Study #3: Taylor

➤ Practice pattern 5C: Impaired Motor Function and Sensory Integrity Associated With Nonprogressive Disorders of the Central Nervous System—Congenital Origin or Acquire in Infancy or Childhood

➤ Medical diagnosis: Myelomeningocele, repaired L1-2

➤ Age: 4 years

Examination

PARENTAL GOALS

The family wants Taylor to be able both to self-propel his wheelchair long distances to keep up with his peers while out of doors and to walk using long leg braces and crutches in the house and the classroom.

FUNCTIONAL ABILITIES

Taylor is able to roll, assume and maintain sitting on the floor, and move to all fours. He can scoot around on the floor in sitting. He can walk with a swing-to gait using a parapodiuim and a walker. He can self-propel his wheelchair.

POSTURE AND MOVEMENT

Taylor demonstrates a marked lordosis related to his surgical repair. He compensates with increased kyphosis and slumps and hangs on the ligaments throughout his spine.

He prefers a very large BOS and keeps his COM low and well within the BOS. He has loss of motor function in his lower extremities.

Gait analysis reveals that Taylor ambulates with a swing-to gait using a parapodium and an anterior walker. He uses upper extremities effectively for both support and forward propulsion. He cannot adapt to changes in the floor surface. The activity is not yet energy efficient.

Systems Examination

Anthropometric Characteristics

Taylor has small lower extremities as compared to the rest of his body. In addition his head is slightly larger in proportion due to the hydrocephalus.

Musculoskeletal System

Range of motion is within normal limits in the upper body. He is somewhat tight at the hip in the hip flexors and adductors and can only bring the ankles to neutral (90 degrees of dorsiflexion). The plantar fascia is extremely tight. He has generalized weakness in the upper extremities and trunk, particularly in the abdominals. The lower extremities demonstrate 0 strength on a manual muscle test.

Neuromuscular System

Taylor demonstrates good control and coordination in the upper extremities. He has slightly decreased control of axial extension, with greater limitations in abdominal control. He demonstrates diminished control of lateral weight shifting as well as rotation.

Sensory Systems

Taylor has good vision and hearing. He has no somatosensory awareness below T-12. He demonstrates visual perceptual problems.

Integumentary System

Taylor has frequent skin breakdowns at the sacral area and in his feet and ankles.

Respiratory System

Taylor tends to hold his breath to increase proximal stability. He has inadequate abdominal strength for sustained exhalation. Overall pulmonary endurance is decreased as compared to his peers.

Evaluation

Taylor is a cooperative, engaging young man with many strengths and resources that make him an excellent candidate for habilitation. He will, however, always require an assistive device and use of orthotics to walk. He demonstrates the musculoskeletal impairments of decreased range of motion and strength in the lower extremities, along with decreased somatosensory awareness. He has limited respiratory support for gross motor activity. These impairments prevent him from locomotion at the speed of his peers, even in his wheelchair, and ambulation in his classroom and home, even with the use of assistive devices. He, however, is intrinsically motivated to ambulate with assistive devices and has support of his family and teachers to reach these goals. Without ongoing intervention, Taylor may be unable to achieve these reasonable goals. Developing an active lifestyle is important at this age to avoid the health risks associated with the more sedentary lifestyle of children who remain in wheelchairs for locomotion.

Functional Limitations

Taylor is unable to assume or maintain an upright position without assistance and the use of orthotics and a walker. His endurance for ambulation is limited and he moves slowly. He cannot propel his wheelchair fast enough to keep up with his peers, especially when playing outdoors.

IMPAIRMENTS

Based on the examination the most significant impairments that impact Taylor's ability to ambulate are the loss of muscle function and sensation in his lower extremities.

Muscle tightness and limited range of motion in the lower extremities may interfere with optimal use of orthotics. Taylor also has generalized weakness in the upper extremities and trunk, as well as poor respiratory function, all of which will adversely affect his use of ambulation aids and wheelchair.

GOALS

Treatment goals are for Taylor to:

1. Increase upper body and trunk strength

2. Improve respiratory support for gross motor activity

3. Improve control of lateral and diagonal weight shifting in the standing position

4. Increase range of motion in the lower extremities for proper alignment in standing

FUNCTIONAL OUTCOMES

Following 6 to 9 months of intervention, Taylor will:

1. Walk 25 feet to move from his bedroom to the living room or down the hall of his school to his classroom while wearing his hip-knee-ankle-foot orthoses (HKAFOs) with a walker and with supervision of an adult

2. Walk 10 steps in his classroom, while wearing his HKAFOs and using lofstrand crutches with standby guarding of an adult

3. Propel his wheelchair from his classroom to the cafeteria at the same speed of peers both while going to and returning from lunch

4. Move from bench sit to standing at his walker, lock his braces, and begin ambulating independently. He also will unlock his braces and lower himself from standing at the walker to sitting on a bench safely

Intervention

Taylor will continue to be seen twice weekly for physical therapy in his preschool program. Services will be coordinated with the parents, occupational therapist, and educators. An orthopedist will continue to follow Taylor annually. Gait training with bilateral long leg braces initially using a walker, but transitioning to crutches when possible, will be initiated to increase his functional use of walking. In addition, therapy will include activities to increase Taylor's skill in self-propelling the wheelchair at greater speeds and over more varied terrains. Strengthening for the upper body will be included as well as a positioning program to aid in soft tissue elongation. Taylor's father will begin a modified weight training program with Taylor at home. The adaptive physical education program will stress aerobic conditioning while Taylor is in the chair and will work to increase abilities in the wheelchair in modified sports such as T-ball or soccer.

Case Study #4: Ashley

➤ Practice pattern 5B: Impaired Neuromotor Development
➤ Medical diagnosis: Down syndrome
➤ Age: 15 months

Examination

PARENTAL GOALS

The parents are interested in having Ashley learn to walk.

FUNCTIONAL ABILITIES

Ashley is able to roll, assume and maintain sitting, move to all fours, kneel, and pull to stand at furniture. She can take steps with two hands held.

POSTURE AND MOVEMENT

Ashley can assume many antigravity positions up to standing with support. In all positions she uses a wide BOS and keeps the COM low and well within the middle of the base. She relies on ligamentous integrity for alignment rather than dynamic activation of her postural system. She moves more with phasic bursts of activity and then rests on ligaments for mechanical stability. She, therefore, has least stability in weight bearing postures such as all fours or standing with support. She does not demonstrate consistent balance in any anti-gravity posture. Movement is slow and tends to be in the sagittal plane with little to no spontaneous recruitment of patterns that include axial rotation.

SYSTEMS EXAMINATION

Anthropometric Characteristics

Ashley's height and weight are within ranges established for children with Down syndrome. She demonstrates the typical facial characteristics of children with Down syndrome. Although it has not yet been evaluated due to her young age, she is at risk for cervical instability due to orthopedic anomalies.

Regulatory System

Ashley is a passive child who requires a great deal of stimulation to attend to either motor or cognitive tasks.

Musculoskeletal System

Ashley demonstrates hypermobility and instability at all the joints in the body. She continues to overly stretch joint ligaments in her daily postures.

She has decreased strength throughout the body with poor muscle definition.

Neuromuscular System

Ashley is able to initiate, sustain, and terminate motor unit activity throughout her body. She has greatest difficulty sustaining postures, demonstrating more phasic burst activity. It is assumed she is using more of her fast twitch motor units than the slow twitch ones. She uses more concentric muscle contraction with almost no isometric or eccentric control being noted. She only can set the lower levels of dynamic stiffness and cannot control or coordinate the stiffness to meet the demands of functional tasks. She has difficulty in recruiting complex synergies that include abductor/adductor control or axial rotation. She does not demonstrate any extraneous movements.

Sensory Systems

Ashley has good vision. She has a mild hearing loss and signs of decreased somatosensory awareness throughout her body. She avoids movement-based activities, which suggests immaturity or deficits in vestibular function.

Respiratory System

Ashley demonstrates a decreased respiratory base for motor activity. The decreased control in the rib cage contributes to a decreased vital capacity. She has small nasal passages and is a mouth breather. She holds her breath during difficult movement transitions.

Cardiovascular System

Although the cardiologist reports that Ashley's heart function is within normal limits, she occasionally turns blue with breath holding. She uses this behavior effectively to avoid activities in which she does not want to participate.

Evaluation

Ashley is a child who demonstrates many of the musculoskeletal, neuromuscular, and sensory impairments associated with Down syndrome. She is demonstrating functional limitations based on these impairments. She should, however, be able to walk independently in the home and, eventually, for community distances. She will require regular services to establish these skills and may periodically require additional services to address changes based on her growth (ie, episodic care). While at this time indirect services are being provided, an episode of direct services could be considered to try to speed the development of ambulation. Without intervention it is anticipated that the onset of ambulation may be further delayed. Ashley is at high risk for injury to her joints. She also is at risk for an increasingly sedentary lifestyle with the associated cardiovascular risks.

Functional Limitations

Ashley does not cruise at furniture or walk without support. She does not shift her weight in standing to be able to reach for objects that are not close to her or to change her position.

Impairments

Primary impairments related to Ashley's limited ambulation skills are generalized weakness, joint hyperflexibility, limited balance and postural control, and sensory hypersensitivity, especially to movement.

Goals

Treatment goals are for Ashley to:

1. Improve postural stability with increased coactivation/co-contraction

2. Increase control of lateral and diagonal weight shifts in standing

3. Maintain postures with good alignment (eg, sitting, all fours, and standing)

Functional Outcomes

Following 6 to 9 months of intervention, Ashley will:

1. Cruise in both directions the length of a sofa in order to obtain desired toys placed on the opposite end

2. Take steps to walk 5 feet between her parents in play

3. Creep on hands and knees while holding a small toy in one hand and moving between rooms in the home or within the classroom

Intervention

Ashley will continue in the infant-mother early intervention program. Additional direct services provided in the home can be considered at the parents' discretion. The use of a small bench or chair for her to sit in during daily activities should be suggested to help decrease the size of her base of support. A small but heavy baby carriage or push toy would be beneficial to encourage ambulation. Therapy activities will include: strengthening, facilitation to recruit the postural muscles in higher positions against gravity, guarding of the joints during weight-bearing activities, and introduction of increased weight shifting laterally and in diagonal planes while in all positions, but especially in standing. The parent will be instructed in activities to increase somatosensory and vestibular input such as extra toweling after her bath and regular visits to a playground with play on a swing. Services will be coordinated with the occupational therapist and special educator as well as with her pediatrician. Education concerning sequelae of common impairments associated with Down syndrome will be provided for the family.

Case Study #5: John

➤ Practice pattern 5B: Impaired Neuromotor Development
➤ Medical diagnosis: Attention deficit hyperactivity disorder, developmental coordination disorder
➤ Age: 5 years

Examination

PARENTAL GOALS

The family wants John to be able to go with them to the mall, into other homes, and to playgrounds without falling or bumping into other people or objects.

FUNCTIONAL ABILITIES

John is able to walk and run. He can perform most basic gross motor skills and can gallop.

POSTURE AND MOVEMENT

John demonstrates decreased postural control with a tendency to recruit long two joint muscles in the limbs to substitute for proximal postural control. Therefore, his legs frequently stiffen and he walks on his toes. He achieves forward progression by leaning forward and relying on momentum. He does not demonstrate refined isolated or fractionated movements in the limbs. The coordination of muscles diminishes the higher up against gravity he moves, as well as the more stressful the task or environment becomes. He has difficulty modifying the movement to match the specific task or environment. He has the greatest difficulty with movements or tasks that require multisegmental coordination (ie, upper extremities with lower extremities or eyes with hands or feet). He also has difficulty in selection of movements that require axial rotation as a component. He walks with stiffened legs and with a decreased arm swing. Thus, he gallops instead of skips, throws without trunk rotation, and cannot walk a balance beam. He also has difficulty with tasks that require varying the speed of movement.

SYSTEMS EXAMINATION

Anthropometric Characteristics

Average height and weight for his age.

Regulatory System

John has difficulty with gradation of arousal and selectivity of attention for work. He easily becomes frustrated and throws temper tantrums frequently. His attention has improved since he began taking his medication.

Musculoskeletal System

John demonstrates full ROM. His strength is decreased in both the upper as well as lower body. The greatest deficits occur proximally. Endurance is decreased as compared to his peers.

Neuromuscular System

John can initiate, sustain, and terminate motor unit activity throughout his body. However, he has difficulty with the control and coordination of muscle activity to match functional tasks. He most commonly uses concentric or isometric muscle contraction with decreased eccentric control, especially in the lower body. He does not recruit patterns of coactivation or co-contraction proximally and instead uses sustained holding in the distal movement muscles for stability. He cannot, therefore, quickly and efficiently recruit these muscles for dynamic actions. He also demonstrates poor grading of movements. He cannot accurately recruit the appropriate level of stiffness for a task (eg, increased stiffness in the lower extremities during ambulation). He has poor coordination with increased stiffness in the upper extremities in addition to that in the lower extremities during ambulation activities. He does not demonstrate extraneous movements.

Sensory Systems

John has good vision and hearing. Testing indicates impairments related to tactile discrimination, kinesthesia, and stereognosis. He has limitations in motor planning.

Cardiopulmonary Systems

At this point John does not demonstrate impairments in these systems but is at risk for decreased overall fitness due to his avoidance of aerobic activities.

Evaluation

John is a 5-year-old child with complex and interacting impairments that significantly limit his ability to function in his environments. He is an independent ambulator. The combination of decreased somatosensory awareness, decreased kinesthetic awareness, and decreased control and coordination of the neuromuscular system has resulted in poor mid-range control and decreased dexterity and coordination. He is an excellent candidate for intervention. If intervention is not provided, it is anticipated that he may demonstrate increasingly limited functional skills, greater frustration, and therefore avoidance of these activities. This would be detrimental for general cardiovascular functioning as well as emotional health and well-being.

FUNCTIONAL LIMITATIONS

John has difficulty with age-appropriate gross motor skills, such as being able to skip. He has difficulty with ball skills, such as catching, throwing, and dribbling. He is less skilled in gross motor skills as compared to his peers and has difficulty participating in gross motor games. He is clumsy, often bumping into objects or other people.

IMPAIRMENTS

Primary impairments related to ambulatory skills are difficulties with motor planning, motor control, strength, and selective attention.

GOALS

Treatment goals are for John to demonstrate:

1. Increased strength

2. Improved eccentric control

3. Increased repertoire of synergies including those with control of lateral weight shift and rotation

4. Increased agility during gross motor activities with more refined timing and sequencing of motor activities

FUNCTIONAL OUTCOMES

Following 6 to 9 months of intervention, John will:

1. Participate in a group community sport such as soccer, T-ball, or a swim team on a regular basis and complete all of the basic skills required by the sport

2. Be able to play safely and appropriately on equipment in a local fast food restaurant playground with other children being present

3. Walk through a neighborhood store with parental supervision for 10 minutes without bumping into any of the displays or individuals in the store

Intervention

The parents are encouraged to have John wear more spandex type clothing to increase sensory organization. They also are encouraged to have him participate in either a therapeutic horseback riding program or swimming in the community. Therapy will focus on organizing sensory perceptual information during complex motor tasks as well as increasing motor control and coordination. Strengthening activities of postural muscles with increased somatosensory feedback will be included. Rapid alternating movement through full range, including both concentric and then eccentric work, in the limbs will follow. John and his family will select preferred activities for focus such as bicycling, gymnastics, soccer, or karate to increase John's participation. Sessions will be structured with repetitions to provide increased opportunities for motor learning. As performance improves, small group work with other boys with similar impairments and interests will be utilized to improve motor and social skills.

Acknowledgment

I would like to acknowledge the work of Janet Wilson Howle, MACT, PT, who authored the chapter on gait in the previous two editions. Some of her original material has been incorporated into this chapter for the third revision and her input regarding the content of this chapter is much appreciated.

References

1. Rosenbaum PL, Walter SD, Hanna SE, et al. Prognosis for gross motor function in cerebral palsy: creation of motor development curves. *JAMA*. 2002;11:1357-1363.

2. Dorland WA, ed. *Dorland's Medical Dictionary*. 30th ed. Philadelphia, Pa: WB Saunders; 2003.

3. World Health Organization. *ICIDH-2: International classification of functioning and disability*. [Beta-2 draft, short version.] Geneva, Switzerland: WHO; 1999.

4. Howle JM. *Neuro-Developmental Treatment Approach: Theoretical Foundations and Principles of Clinical Practice*. Laguna Beach, Calif: NeuroDevelopmental Treatment Association; 2002.

5. Bly L. *Motor Skills Acquisition in the First Year: An Illustrated Guide to Normal Development*. Tucson, Ariz: Therapy Skill Builders; 1994.

6. Alexander R, Boehme R, Cupps B. *Normal Development of Functional Motor Skills The First Year of Life*. Tucson, Ariz: Therapy Skill Builders; 1993.

7. Folio MR, Fewell RR. *Peabody Developmental Motor Scales*. Austin, Tex: Pro-Ed; 2000.

8. Russell D, Rosenbaum P, Gowland C, et al. *Gross Motor Function Measure Manual*. Hamilton, Canada: McMaster University; 1993.

9. Perry J. *Gait Analysis: Normal and Pathological Function*. Thorofare, NJ: SLACK Incorporated; 1992.

10. Sutherland DH, Olshen RA, Biden EN, et al. *The Development of Mature Walking*. London, England: Mac Keith Press; 1988.

11. Bleck EE. *Orthopedic Management in Cerebral Palsy*. London, England: Mac Keith Press; 1987.

12. Stout JL. Gait: development and analysis. In: Campbell SK, ed. *Physical Therapy for Children*. Philadelphia, Pa: WB Saunders; 1994:127-157.

13. Thelen E. Learning to walk: ecological demands and phylogenetic constraints. In: Lipsitt LP, ed. *Advances in Infancy Research*. Vol. 3. Norwood, NJ: Ablex; 1994:213-250.

14. Bernstein N. *Co-ordination and Regulation of Movements*. New York, NY: Pergamon Press; 1967.

15. Woollacott MH, Shumway-Cook A. *Development of Posture and Gait Across the Life Span*. Columbia, SC: University of South Carolina; 1989.

16. Hoffer MM, Fiewell E, Perry J, et al. Functional ambulation in patients with myelomeningocele. *J Bone Jt Surg*. 1973;55A:137-148.

17. DeSouza MB, Carroll N. Ambulation of the braced myelomeningocele patient. *J Bone Jt Surg*. 1976;58A:1112-1118.

18. Capute AJ, Shapiro BK, Palmer TB. Spectrum of developmental disabilities: continuum of motor dysfunction. *Ortho Clin North Am*. 1981;12:3-22.

19. Carlson SJ, Ramsey C. Assistive technology. In: Campbell SK, ed. *Physical Therapy for Children*. Philadelphia, Pa: WB Saunders; 1994.

20. Cratty B. *Motor Activities in the Education of Retardates*. 2nd ed. Philadelphia, Pa: Lea and Febiger; 1974.

21. Shapiro B, Accardo P, Capute A. Factors affecting walking in a profoundly retarded population. *Dev Med Child Neurol*. 1979;21:369-373.

22. Donoghue E, Kuman B, Bullmore GH. Some factors affecting age of walking in a mentally retarded population. *Dev Med Child Neurol*. 1970;12:781-792.

23. Melyn M, White D. Mental and developmental milestones of noninstitutionalized Down syndrome children. *Pediatrics*. 1973;52:542-545.

24. Montgomery PC. Predicting potential for ambulation in children with cerebral palsy. *Pediatr Phys Ther*. 1998;10:148-155.

25. Davis S. *Stepping Out: A Science Project*. 2003 (Personal Communication).

26. Molnar GE, Gordon SU. Cerebral palsy: predictive value of selected signs for early prognostication of motor function. *Arch Phys Med Rehabil*. 1976;57:153-158.

27. Largo RH, Molenari L, Weber M, et al. Early development of locomotion: significances of prematurity, cerebral palsy and sex. *Dev Med Child Neurol.* 1985;27:183-191.

28. Badell-Ribera A. Cerebral palsy: postural-locomotor prognosis in spastic diplegia. *Arch Phys Med Rehabil.* 1985;66:614-619.

29. Molnar GE. Cerebral palsy: prognosis and how to judge it. *Pediatric Annals.* 1979;8:596-604.

30. Bleck EE. Locomotor prognosis in cerebral palsy. *Dev Med Child Neurol.*1975;17:18-25.

31. Campbell SK. *Physical Therapy for Children.* Chicago, Ill: WB Saunders; 1994.

32. Westcott SL, Lowes LP, Richardson PK. Evaluation of postural stability in children: current theories and assessment tools. *Phys Ther.* 1977;6:629-645.

33. Kembhavi G, Darrah J, Magill-Evans J, et al. Using the Berg Balance Scale to distinguish balance abilities in children with cerebral palsy. *Pediatr Phys Ther.* 2002;14:92-99.

34. Westcott SL, Murray KH, Pence K. Survey of the preferences of pediatric physical therapists for assessment and treatment of balance dysfunction in children. *Pediatr Phys Ther.* 1998;10:48-61.

35. Rose J, Gamble JG, Medeiros J, et al. Energy cost of walking in normal children and in those with cerebral palsy: comparison of heart rate and oxygen uptake. *J Pediatr Orthop.* 1989;9:276-279.

36. Fragala M, Lewis C. Pediatric physical therapy. In: Dershewitz RA, ed. *Ambulatory Pediatric Care.* 3rd ed. Philadelphia, Pa: Lippincott-Raven; 1999:274-279.

37. Ross SA, Engsberg JR, Olcree KS, et al. Quadriceps and hamstring strength changes as a function of selective dorsal rhizotomy surgery and rehabilitation. *Pediatr Phys Ther.* 2001;13:2-9.

38. American Physical Therapy Association. Guide to physical therapist practice. 2nd ed. *Phys Ther.* 2001;81.

39. Palisano RJ, Rosenbaum PL, Walter S, et al. Development and reliability of a system to classify gross motor function in children with cerebral palsy. *Dev Med Child Neurol.* 1997;39:214-223.

40. Palisano RJ, Hanna SE, Rosenbaum PL, et al. Validation of a model of gross motor function for children with cerebral palsy. *Phys Ther.* 2000;80:975-983.

41. Leonard CT, Hirshfeld H, Forssberg H. The development of independent walking in children with cerebral palsy. *Dev Med Child Neurol.* 1991;33:567-577.

42. McNevin NH, Coraci L, Schafer J. Gait in adolescent cerebral palsy: the effect of partial unweighting. *Arch Phys Med Rehabil.* 2000;81:525-528.

43. Richards CL, Malouin F, Dumas F, et al. Early and intensive treadmill locomotor training for young children with cerebral palsy: a feasibility study. *Pediatr Phys Ther.* 1997;9:158-165.

44. Schindl MR, Forstner C, Kern H, et al. Treadmill training with partial body weight support in non-ambulatory patients with cerebral palsy. *Arch Phys Med Rehabil.* 2000;80:301-306.

45. Winchester P, Kendall K, Peters H, et al. The effect of therapeutic horseback riding on gross motor function and gait speed in children who are developmentally delayed. *Phys Occup Ther Pediatr.* 2002;22(3/4):37-50.

46. Pape KE. Therapeutic electrical stimulation (TES) or the treatment of disuse muscle atrophy in cerebral palsy. *Pediatr Phys Ther.* 1997;9:110-112.

47. Sommerfelt K, Markestad T, Berg K, et al. Therapeutic electrical stimulation in cerebral palsy: a randomized, controlled, crossover trial. *Dev Med Child Neurol.* 2001;43:609-613.

48. Carmick J. Clinical use of neuromuscular electrical stimulation for children with cerebral palsy, part 1: lower extremity. *Phys Ther.* 1993;73:21-29.

49. Carmick J. Guidelines for the clinical application of neuromuscular electrical stimulation (NMES) for children with cerebral palsy. *Pediatr Phys Ther.* 1997;9:128-135.

50. Cusick BD. *Progressive Casting and Splinting for Lower Extremity Deformities in Children with Neuromotor Dysfunction.* Tucson, Ariz: Therapy Skill Builders; 1990.

51. Phillips WE. Use of serial casting in the management of knee joint contractures in an adolescent with cerebral palsy. *Phys Ther.* 1990;70:66-68.

52. Dumas HE, O'Neil ME, Fragala MA. Expert consensus on physical therapist intervention after botulinum toxin A injection for children with cerebral palsy. *Pediatr Phys Ther.* 2001; 12:122-132.

53. Erson T. *Courageous Pacers: The Complete Guide to Running, Walking, & Fitness for Kids Ages 8-18.* Corpus Christi, Tex: Pro-Activ; 1993.

CHAPTER 12

Developing Hand Function

Regi Boehme, OTR/L

The ability to freely and safely weight shift through the trunk while moving the arms and using the hands relates to some of the most important life skills. These activities of daily living (ADL) include eating, dressing, and hygiene tasks. For children, as they mature, independence in self-care is strongly related to feelings of self-worth or self-respect. The self-care tasks of dressing or using the toilet seem like small issues with which to contend. However, all children compare themselves to their peers. For children who are physically challenged and need assistance or adaptations for dressing or using the toilet, they often view themselves as inferior when they apply this natural comparison process.

When children enter school there is a major focus on communicating through writing. The ability to function with handwriting means that children can communicate their thoughts, take phone messages, send cards to friends, and, as adults, sign checks from their checking account.[1] For children with disabilities, writing with the fewest adaptations means they can communicate with dignity. For some children with developmental disabilities, however, handwriting is not possible or is too labor intensive and using a computer is their best option. Rogers and Case-Smith[2] demonstrated, in typically developing sixth-grade students, that handwriting and keyboarding require distinctly different skills. Keyboarding offers an alternative strategy that may allow children with motor deficits to communicate effectively.

Comparison with a peer group may generalize into social skills. For example, how often do peers choose children with disabilities for games during recess? Are they always picked last? Do they have friends to play with at school and in the neighborhood? Each time they compare themselves to peers, children with disabilities may see themselves as "less than others" or "not as good as others."

Developing upper extremity control and hand function to the greatest extent possible to allow children with developmental disabilities to function optimally is a primary goal of therapists. This chapter will address the prerequisites for developing upper extremity function and provide suggestions for examination, evaluation, and intervention strategies.

Postural Alignment

For shoulder girdle mobility, stability, and alignment, the need for a balanced pelvis is critical. When children cannot sit on both hips equally, the contour of the thorax changes, often becoming shorter or rotated on one side. Since the shoulder girdle is a floating system, with only one stable bony attachment at the sternoclavicular joint, changes in the thorax directly impact on the shoulder's alignment and muscle action can be compromised. Problems with alignment place muscles at distorted lines of force, thus impacting on the action of the arm. This may cause children to use compensatory movements that, over time, are very difficult to retrain and often result in secondary problems. Consequently, evaluation of the upper extremities and hand function begins with an assessment of symmetry in the thorax and pelvis for equal and active sitting and standing alignment.

Case Study

The following case study demonstrates the influence of structural problems in the trunk on upper extremity function.

Reason for Referral

Hallie is a 12-year-old girl who has maintained the same degree of scoliosis (approximately 35 degrees) for the past year. One physician recommended several years of bracing for the scoliosis. The parents chose a second medical opinion, which was 6 months of bracing with therapy and activities designed to address the scoliosis.

History

Hallie's birth history was provided by her mother, who stated that labor was induced because she was 15 days past her due date. At 2 weeks of age, Hallie was diagnosed as a "failure to thrive" infant. Hallie's mother worked with a lactation specialist who identified swallowing difficulties. Her mother remembers many choking incidences with semi-solids and thin liquids. Hallie received oral motor therapy one time per week initially, followed by monthly treatment.

At 6 months of age, Hallie received a diagnosis of mild gross and fine motor delays. At 9 months of age, Hallie developed a torticollis with a new diagnosis of marked hypotonicity. She began attending outpatient physical and occupational therapy and her mother carried out home programming suggestions.

Hallie's developmental delays impacted her gross and fine motor development, respiration, and eventually expressive language. She sat at 18 months with little stability, meaning she would topple easily in all planes. She had so much laxity in her hips that, in ring sitting, she could fall completely forward with her head and trunk flush with the floor.

Hallie stood at 2 years of age holding onto a table. She used orthotics to stabilize her arches and to improve ankle alignment. She walked at 2 years of age, using a posterior control walker. She began walking independently at age 3 years with immature balance and equilibrium reactions. Once she was erect in standing, she gradually increased in strength, and her therapy focused on balance reactions in all planes.

Hallie only babbled up to 3 years of age and her speech could not be understood by anyone but her mother. Hallie's mother taught her simple sign language to indicate her needs and preferences. Even at age 8 years, after 5 years of speech therapy, her speech could not be understood, except by those who saw her routinely. Hallie's mother translated for her, which reduced Hallie's frustration level. Knowing what she was trying to say, yet not being understood, was a very isolating feeling and Hallie has expressed negative feelings about her self-worth.

At one point Hallie was evaluated at a children's hospital. During a sleep study, seizure activity was observed. After trying a course of Depakote (Abbott Laboratories, Abbott Park, Ill), which caused drowsiness that lasted an entire day, a neuromuscular specialist and a neurologist decided that no medication would be used since Hallie was not having

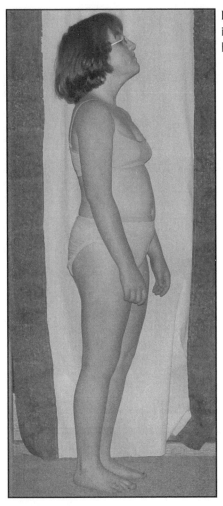

Figure 12-1. Full body assessment, side view. Hallie's weight is displaced forward, with neck hyperextension and a forward head position. This puts her vision in an upward orientation.

active, visible seizure activity. The neurologist gave Hallie a clear diagnosis of "hypotonia, resulting in a broad spectrum of developmental delays."

Hallie has received episodes of intervention throughout her childhood. She is being referred for a reevaluation to determine strategies that may minimize the impact of her scoliosis, which was diagnosed when she entered elementary school, on her upper extremity function and comfort.

EXAMINATION AND EVALUATION

Functional Limitations

Hallie tends to move with clumsiness and a lack of safety, in part due to the orientation of her vision, which has an upward displacement directly related to her neck hyperextension (Figure 12-1). This has impacted her self-care skills in dressing and undressing and her participation in leisure time activities, such as aerobics, yoga, and drama classes. However, at the initial therapy session Hallie had one chief complaint, neck pain.

Impairments

Due to the influence of the scoliosis on her spine and rib cage alignment, Hallie is unable to raise her arms above 90 degrees (Figures 12-2 and 12-3). As she attempts to raise

Figure 12-2. Full body assessment, posterior view. Hallie's rib cage on the left is shorter than the right. Because she displaces her weight primarily on her right leg, her right and left arms hang at different lengths. This indicates that the scoliosis has impacted her rib cage.

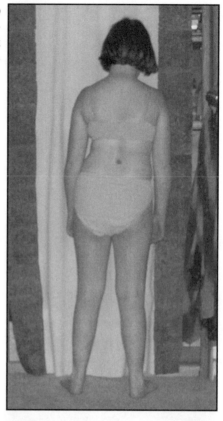

Figure 12-3. When asked to bring her arms above her head, her immobile rib cage, both between the ribs and at the attachment of the ribs to the spine, impedes her ability to raise her arms any further than 90 degrees.

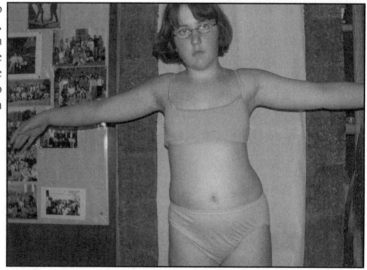

her arms further, the rib cage elevates, leaving the shoulder without stability, a prerequisite for above head reach.

Practice Pattern

Based on examination findings, Hallie is placed in practice pattern 4B: Impaired Posture.

Interventions

➤ Coordination, communication, and documentation
- With physician regarding plan of care
- With parent regarding home program
- With school staff regarding physical education
- With yoga instructor regarding appropriate activities

➤ Patient-client instructions
- Information to patient and parent regarding health, wellness, and fitness program
- Information to patient regarding self-management

➤ Procedural interventions
- Therapeutic exercise (posture awareness training, body mechanics training, flexibility exercises, relaxation techniques)
- Functional training in work, community, and leisure integration
- Manual therapy techniques

Treatment Session Goals

➤ In standing, with arms bearing weight on a treatment table, dynamic balance will be facilitated in the pelvis

➤ Scapular mobility on the thorax will be increased

➤ Mobility and symmetry in the rib cage and spine will be achieved by elongating her shortened side

➤ Ability to rotate her trunk will improve

➤ Visible tension in her axilla (an indication that her pectorals, internal rotators, and latissimus dorsi need more length for range of reach) will be decreased.

Appropriate structural alignment will put Hallie's musculature in a more advantageous position for graded muscle activity and muscle strengthening exercises. Scapular and clavicular rotation are prerequisites for above head reach. It is crucial to gain greater symmetry throughout her whole body to reduce her neck pain.

Home Program Exercises

While standing, Hallie will use above head reach and hold the position to the count of 10, three times per day (Figure 12-4). While standing, Hallie will use above head reach with lateral flexion to both sides, holding this position to the count of five, twice daily (Figure 12-5). A change in full body alignment before treatment (see Figure 12-1) and after treatment (Figure 12-6) can be observed.

Functional Objectives

In sitting, Hallie will use rotation five times a day during functional activities and as a part of her yoga class. Hallie will learn to use her downward gaze in activities she currently enjoys, such as using her computer, reading to her mother, doing crafts at camp, and collecting rocks for her rock garden.

Following a treatment session, the following question can be asked. How has function changed? In this case:

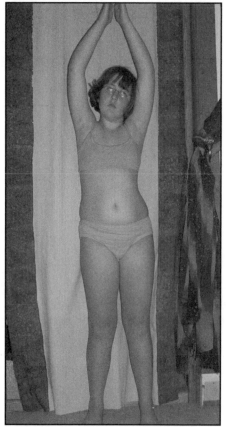 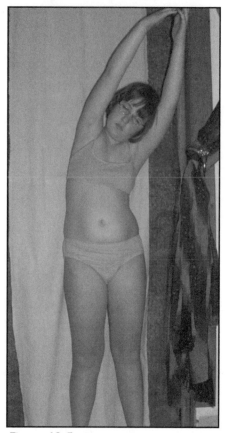

Figure 12-4. Home exercise program—arms over head.

Figure 12-5. Home exercise program—lateral flexion.

➤ Hallie's ability to don overhead clothes will be easier

➤ She has improved symmetry and mobility as a basis for movement of the arms in space

➤ As she becomes accustomed to using her downward gaze, movement in general will be safer

➤ These changes, as a whole, will result in more physical control and therefore improved performance and feelings of competence during dance, aerobics, and yoga

What is she missing that would expand her function further?

➤ Greater symmetry in the trunk

➤ Activation of abdominal obliques

➤ A more balanced pelvis—all bony landmarks should be aligned. Staying aligned would require elongation of her adductors, psoas, rectus abdominis, and hamstrings and strengthening of her abdominal obliques and gluteal muscles

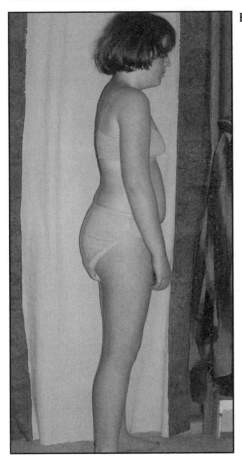

Figure 12-6. Full body alignment following treatment.

Postural Control

Hand function depends on many key proximal components. In order for children to use their hands efficiently in functional tasks, they need adequate postural control (see Chapter 8). The shoulder girdle is attached to the thorax and involves more than one joint. The shoulder girdle must have full flexibility to allow the arm to have full range of motion, thereby giving the hand access to a large range in space. At the same time, the shoulder girdle must have a variety of strong stable fixed points for actions specific to upper extremity function. When flexibility and stability are missing due to instability or immature postural control, compromised patterns of movement of the upper extremities result. From a developmental perspective, it has been hypothesized that the development of reaching is coordinated with the development of postural control.[3,4] Van der Fits and Hadders-Algra[3] documented in typically developing infants that, at 4 months of age when successful reaching emerges, reaching was accompanied by complex postural adjustments. Hopkins and Ronnqvist[5] studied infants at about 6 months of age who were not yet able to sit independently. They compared the infants' reaching performance when sitting in a commercially available chair to reaching when sitting in a chair designed to provide supplemental support for the pelvic region and upper legs. When provided with greater postural support, the infants demonstrated improved head stabilization and smoother reaching movements. The authors proposed that changes in postural control induce improvements in the control of reaching movements during infancy.

Figure 12-7. Shoulder girdle anatomy (adapted by John Boehme from Calais-Germain B. *Anatomy of Movement.* Seattle, Wash: Eastland Press; 1993).

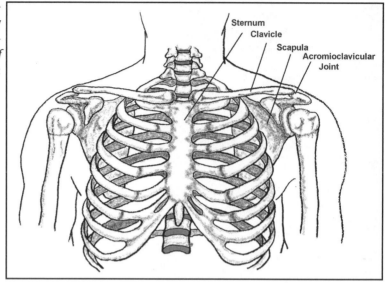

Figure 12-8. Clavicle (adapted by John Boehme from Calais-Germain B. *Anatomy of Movement.* Seattle, Wash: Eastland Press; 1993).

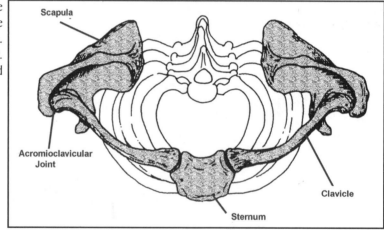

The Purpose of the Shoulder Girdle

The purpose of the shoulder girdle is to allow the arms and the hands to reach out in large ranges of space. Since the shoulder girdle is a floating system, it becomes one of the most complex units in the body (Figure 12-7). Each of the seven bones (scapula—2, humerus—2, clavicle—2, sternum—1) within the system has a unique way of moving and can contribute to the synergy of motion of the arm during function, as well as impede the interplay of motion. The anatomy of the shoulder girdle and associated musculature can be reviewed in many text books.[6,7]

The Clavicle

The clavicle is a flattened, elongated bone, roughly in the form of an S-shape (Figure 12-8). The clavicle has a rounded articular surface that is concave transversely and convex vertically creating a stable saddle joint with the sternum. This saddle joint allows flexion

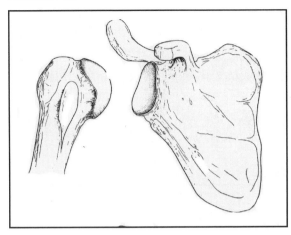

Figure 12-9. Acromioclavicular joint (adapted by John Boehme from Calais-Germain B. *Anatomy of Movement.* Seattle, Wash: Eastland Press; 1993).

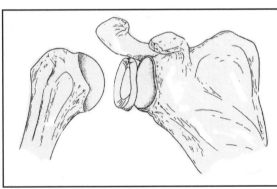

Figure 12-10. Glenohumeral joint (adapted by John Boehme from Calais-Germain B. *Anatomy of Movement.* Seattle, Wash: Eastland Press; 1993).

and extension, elevation and depression, and limited rotation. Most texts describe the movements of the clavicle as secondary to the movements of the scapula. But I have observed that when the clavicle's freedom of motion is impeded by short surrounding musculature, the clavicle can create a barrier to scapular motion. The acromion end of the clavicle is not a stable interlocking structure for the scapula. It relies heavily on ligaments for stability (ie, acromioclavicular joint) (Figure 12-9).

The Glenohumeral Joint

One of the primary joints of the shoulder is the glenohumeral joint. It lies between the head of the humerus and the glenoid cavity of the scapula. The glenoid fossa is small and flat in relation to the shape of the humeral head. On its own, the humeral head is not biomechanically stabilized by the glenoid fossa. There is a ridge at the lower border of the fossa that allows the humerus to safely drop down without subluxation as the arm reaches overhead (Figure 12-10). Without stability of the humerus within the glenoid fossa, the following childhood functions would be lost:

➤ Overhead reach

➤ Ability for palms touching over head

➤ Arms on head to comb or put barrettes in hair

➤ Pitching or catching a high ball

➤ Playing jump rope

Figure 12-11. Scapular attachments (adapted by John Boehme from Calais-Germain B. *Anatomy of Movement*. Seattle, Wash: Eastland Press; 1993).

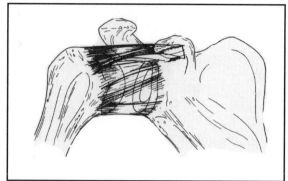

Figure 12-12. Shoulder abduction/protraction (adapted by John Boehme from Calais-Germain B. *Anatomy of Movement*. Seattle, Wash: Eastland Press; 1993).

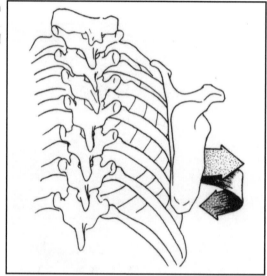

Scapular Movements

The scapula is a floating bone (ie, secured to the axial skeleton only by muscles) with a great deal of mobility (Figure 12-11). Its only bony attachment to the body is through the acromioclavicular joint, which articulates through the long narrow clavicle at the sternoclavicular joint. The shape of this articulating surface allows for some gliding movement. It also allows an opening and closing of the angle formed by the two bones.[6]

When the scapula adducts, the inferior angle of the scapula adducts and moves parallel to the spine. As it moves closer to the spine, the arm is free to abduct. This allows the hand to move through the sleeve of clothing. It also allows the arm and hand to produce lateral protective responses.

Scapular abduction (protraction) is coupled with humeral adduction in order for the hand to come to midline (Figure 12-12). The scapula must be free enough, yet stable enough, to allow the arm to cross the midline of the body. This freedom is coupled with an anterior displacement of the clavicle at the sternoclavicular joint. Depending on the position of the arm as it crosses midline (whether it moves above or below 90 degrees) the clavicle will accommodate either motion with rotation.

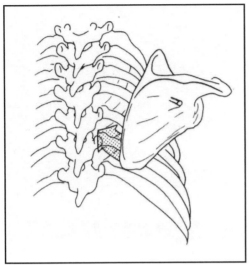

Figure 12-13. Downward rotation of the scapula (adapted by John Boehme from Calais-Germain B. *Anatomy of Movement.* Seattle, Wash: Eastland Press; 1993).

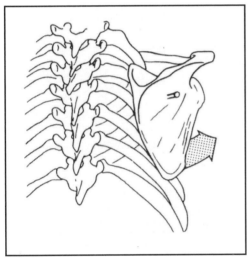

Figure 12-14. Scapular depression (adapted by John Boehme from Calais-Germain B. *Anatomy of Movement.* Seattle, Wash: Eastland Press; 1993).

Downward rotation is coupled with an anterior/superior displacement of the clavicle at the sternoclavicular joint (Figure 12-13). The inferior angle moves supra-medially, while the lateral angle moves inferior-laterally. Posturally, the spine flexes. This is important for donning and removing clothing and personal hygiene. This is called downward rotation because the glenoid cavity is moving downward. Upward rotation allows the arm and hand to reach and grasp overhead objects. Scapular depression is critical for weight bearing through the arm and hand, as well as pushing oneself out of a chair (Figure 12-14).

Elevation of the scapula (Figure 12-15) allows the top of the shoulder to come closer to the ears as in a shrug. Elevation of the scapula requires full clavicle and scapular mobility and requires multiple muscles between the neck and shoulder to coactivate. Because this motion moves the glenohumeral joint toward midline it allows the arm to reach, making greater use of postural stability.

Figure 12-15. Elevation of the scapula (adapted by John Boehme from Calais-Germain B. *Anatomy of Movement.* Seattle, Wash: Eastland Press; 1993).

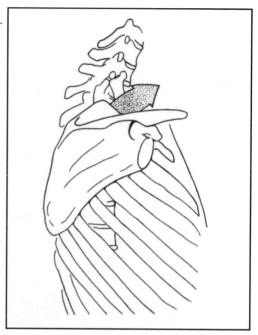

Figure 12-16. Depression of the scapula (adapted by John Boehme from Calais-Germain B. *Anatomy of Movement.* Seattle, Wash: Eastland Press; 1993).

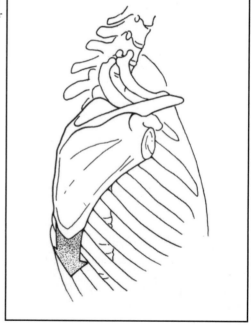

Depression of the scapula (Figure 12-16) allows the arms to push against a surface while bearing different amounts of body weight. Bearing weight requires downward rotation of the scapula. It also requires downward movement and rotation of the clavicle, active stability of the head on the neck, and adequate strength of the triceps as well as the latissimus dorsi.

The Functional Role of the Humerus

The upper arm is used primarily for reaching. Specifically, its job is to project the hand in a wide and varied range of space, to direct the hand to an object, or to place the hand on a surface for weight bearing. Functional humeral control means that the upper arm can reach, hold the reaching posture in mid-space, and correct or change the direction of reach during movement. As larger muscles move the humerus, smaller rotator cuff muscles hold the humeral head in the glenoid fossa and depress it slightly. These small rotator cuff muscles also alter the rotational component of the humerus during reach, making it possible for the large humeral head to clear the joint easily and comfortably.

The humerus needs stability and freedom in the glenoid fossa for controlled movement. When the joint capsule is not malleable or when the humeral head is poorly positioned in the joint, humeral range is restricted. Joint capsule tightness thus can result from a lack of active movement on the part of the child. A poorly aligned humeral head also may be due to an imbalance of muscle activity around the glenohumeral joint. When small rotator cuff muscles are shortened or tight, humeral range again is restricted. As the child attempts to reach, the humerus may pull the scapula away from the rib cage, creating lateral winging. This is described commonly as scapulohumeral tightness, but often is a combined problem of both shortened musculature and scapular-rib cage instability.

The Functional Role of the Elbow

The elbow allows the arm to become shorter or longer, bringing the hand either closer to or farther away from the body. The elbow can make the arm shorter or longer during reach and transitional movement patterns. Dynamic elbow control means that the elbow can move through its maximum range slowly, can stop and hold in mid-range, and is strong enough to make the arm longer or shorter as it is loaded with partial body weight. A child may be able to quickly flex or extend the elbow during reach, but lack the ability to make slow graded movement.

Generalized movement disorders that interfere with the experience of developmental transitional movements result in weak triceps. A child may be able to use the elbow for reaching out in space, but may not be able to use the elbow once the arm is loaded with body weight. Triceps weakness inevitably will interfere with gross motor skills and the child's ability to use ambulation aids. The development of elbow control depends on both glenohumeral activity and adequate hand placement for effective loading on extended arms. When positioned on extended arms, the child may compensate for lack of stability by locking the elbows into extension, which then interferes with dynamic weight shift. The child may fist the hands tightly to increase the stability in the arms in lieu of elbow control, but this compensation also will interfere with weight shift.

The ligaments and joint capsule at the elbow allow for flexion and extension, but block lateral motion. However, in many developmentally delayed children, ligamentus laxity is observed. Consequently, it is possible for these children to externally rotate their arms and bear weight using only elbow hyperextension. This, in turn, makes active muscular use of the shoulder girdle unnecessary.

Figure 12-17. Weight-bearing on knuckles.

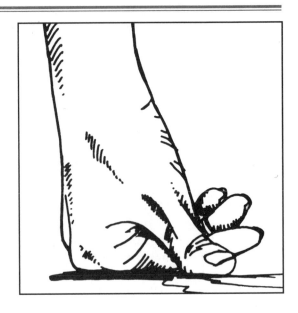

The Functional Role of the Forearm and Wrist

It is important to understand the structure of the proximal and distal joints of the forearm. At the proximal end, the ulna is much smaller than the head of the radius, and thus less stable. The radius slides on the distal end of the ulnar surface of the humerus. The ligaments act as pulleys in order to activate slow and controlled pronation. Strength is needed in radial deviation, to create space between the ulna and the lunate, allowing the ulna to rotate in synergy with the radius. Many children with developmental delays exhibit weak muscles with less than average endurance. Because of weakness, they may hold the wrist in ulnar deviation with a negative coupling pulling the thumb into the palm with eventual ulnar deviation of the fingers. With weight bearing on the arm and hand, the load forces misalignments and eventual deformities of the wrist and fingers.

The forearm and wrist orient the hand in space during reach and in preparation for weight bearing or weight shifting. Forearm rotation is critical for function and develops as a result of controlled humeral rotation, balanced elbow flexion and extension, and prone weight shifting experiences. Prone play experiences allow the child to isolate forearm movements while the humeral movements are restricted through the weight bearing posture. When any of these components are at risk, the development of forearm rotation may be blocked or functionally restricted. Limited freedom of forearm movement in either pronation or supination has a greater negative impact on hand function than it does on weight shifting.

The capability for wrist control depends on a balance of long finger flexion and extension across the wrist joint. When children lack range in wrist movement, hand placement is limited both in space and in weight bearing. As the child attempts to load the hand with body weight, compensations are evident. The child may bear weight on the knuckles or back of the hand when wrist extension is limited (Figures 12-17 and 12-18). When joint range is limited in either direction, the child will bear weight on the extreme radial or ulnar side of the hand. These compensations will impact the quality of weight shifting, but should not completely prevent movement transitions.

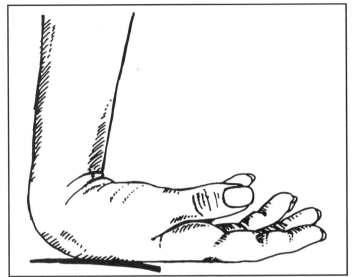

Figure 12-18. Weight bearing on back of hand.

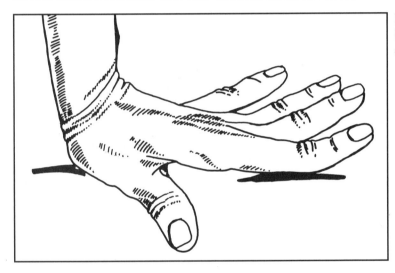

Figure 12-19. Weight bearing on palmar surface of metacarpal heads.

When wrist range is adequate, but muscle co-activation around the circumference of the wrist is poor, the child may feel unstable in weight bearing. Wrist instability creates the need for other compensations. The child may take weight on the palmar surface of the metacarpal heads, forming a modified tripod effect (Figure 12-19). This virtually locks the wrist joint so that it feels stable, but inevitably stretches out the metacarpalphalangeal tendons. Other children with wrist instability will opt to flex the fingers and adduct the thumb in an effort to gain distal stability in lieu of wrist control during weight shifting.

The Functional Role of the Hand

The development of the hand emerges through stages of sensory-motor experiences primarily during the first year of life. Familiarity with typical development, when working with children with developmental delays, is critical. It allows the therapist to recognize the glimpses of "typical movements" and try to build on them. It also allows the therapist to determine whether adaptations exhibited by children are functional or whether secondary problems may arise. This dynamic perspective is critical for the therapist working with children with developmental delays.

The hand has many functional and critical roles. Generally, it shapes itself around an object and accommodates its own shape to the shape to be held or the shape and contour of the weight bearing surface. In order to do this, it must be expandable enough to flatten out for weight bearing. It also must be malleable enough to shape itself around both large and small objects. The hand, at times, needs to be powerful and, at other times, delicate in its approach to grasp and manipulation. The ability of the hand to be functional in all of these situations depends on a variety of arching systems in the palm. The capability for arch development in the hand relies on balance of activity between the long finger flexors and extensors, the capability for neutral alignment between wrist and hand, mobility of the carpal and metacarpal bones, and activity of the intrinsic muscles of the hand.

Ongoing sensory-motor experiences prepare the hand for its long-term development of both simple and complex patterns of movement. The young child's hand-to-hand, hand-to-knee, and hand-to-foot play helps the hand to experience its accommodating potential. Ungraded pressure with the child's first attempts to grasp helps make the arches malleable. Early weight shifting experiences on extended arms help to expand the hand and develop balance reactions from the arches. The young child does not actually develop a controlled grasp until the hand is used in a neutral position at the wrist. Once this basic hand pattern is established, the fingers are able to develop more distal control for more refined function.

Dynamic function of the shoulder girdle has several important roles in the development of the hand. Enough proximal stability is needed for the hands to accept part of the body weight during transitional movements or from the impact of a fall. Function of the hand also requires a balance between:

➤ Mobility
➤ Stability
➤ Dynamic muscle activity
➤ Strength
➤ Sensory awareness

An Overview of Typical Development

During the first 6 months of life, shoulder girdle mobility, stability, and strength develop as infants, stimulated by vision, develop an increasing interest in the environment around them.[8,9] Their interest is reflected in the degree of work it requires to progressively push with their arms against the supporting surface. This is done first working prone on forearms, with eventual lateral weight shifts. Lateral weight shifts in prone propping positions lead them to isolate one side of the shoulder girdle from the other. Lateral weight shifting also prepares the forearm for rotation by elongating both the supinators and pronaters and provides increased sensory experiences throughout the hand.

This progression in prone occurs during the first 4 months of development. During this process, anterior trunk muscles become elongated, especially the pectoralis major, the muscles between each rib, and the rectus abdominis. By 6 months of age, children's elbow extensors have enough strength to allow play in prone on extended arms. This skill is key to preparation of the hand since it elongates the muscles that will become the arches of the hand.

One framework is to consider that children use the strength they gained in prone positions to bring their hands to midline in a supine position, initially using clothing for stability. An alternate view is to consider that infants may use clothing first for proprioceptive feedback. This awareness then would stimulate a primitive synergy of humeral flexion with internal rotation, progressively bringing their hands to their face and heads. Children would then take this a step further as they use a variety of arm movements to elongate their rotator cuff muscles, critical for future functional activities.

Reaching begins to develop around 4 months of age. Konczak and Dichgans[10] recorded reaching movements longitudinally from nine typically developing infants from 5 months to 3 years of age. They analyzed hand and proximal joint trajectories and temporal coordination between arm segments. The data suggested that: 1) most kinematic parameters did not assume adult-like levels before the age of 2 years, 2) infants appeared to strive to obtain velocity patterns with as few force reversals as possible at all three limb segments, and 3) a consistent interjoint synergy between shoulder and elbow movement was not achieved within the first year of life. Stable patterns of temporal coordination (among arm segments) emerged at 12 to 15 months and continued to develop up to 3 years of age.

Byl[11] discussed the connectivity of the corticospinal system, now studied in humans through transcranial magnetic stimulation, and stated that there appears to be an increase in density of neurons up to 10 years of age. Initially children use a highly variable and sequential coordination of the fingertips. An automatic coupling of grip and load forces is established, but this synergy is not fully mature until approximately 10 years of age. Kuhtz-Buschbeck and coworkers[12] analyzed the kinematics of prehension movements in 54 healthy children (ages 4 to 12 years). The children repeatedly reached for cylindrical target objects and grasped them with a precision grip of their dominant hand. The results of their study suggested that the development of prehensile skills lasts until the end of the first decade of life.

An Overview of Developmental Delay

Hand function and fine motor manipulation emerge as significant aspects of typical development. Even when children attempt to function with atypical development, as they reach their toddler years they continue to be driven to play and self-feed. Children want to rise above feelings of "What my body cannot do" and find a way "to do" and fashion a functional skill with the dignity of success. The pure joy that is created by a successful movement experience gives children increased motivation during therapy.

Children go through many phases of growth. As bones grow longer, muscles and tissues begin to shape and elongate and muscle fibers increase, and children grow stronger. During a growth phase there is a period of internal chaos. The dynamic systems begin to reorganize, gravitating toward greater stasis for the maturing child.

Children may feel a need for stability during times of growth. They may seek new ways to adapt and compensate for the changes going on in their bodies or return to using old compensations. Their bodies may feel unfamiliar to them, creating sensory and perceptual confusion. The shoulder girdle is one of the prime areas utilized to seek stability. Due to the structural complexity of the system, it offers a wide variety of fixation opportunities, since the attached muscles span C1 to T12. Visualize the muscles from the humerus to the sacrum and from the humerus to the scapula (both anterior and posterior). The muscles of the shoulder on the anterior trunk often are used by children with increased muscle tone to lower their center of gravity. This creates a feeling of safety since the relative difference between them and the supporting surface becomes smaller. In addition, children may fixate and reduce the excursion between inhalation and exhalation. They may have fear when separated from a parent and they may suddenly have more difficulty with being touched. When children's sensory systems "go into a tailspin" it may be related to an active growth period.

Many children with developmental disabilities have hypotonicity with excessively lax ligaments. This creates an increased weight to the body due to inactive musculature. These children often "fix" or tighten specific joints in an effort to find a source of stability. Other developmentally disabled children have impairments due to the influence of neurological injury, or prenatal or neonatal incidents, resulting in different levels of spasticity and stiffness.

Dynamic function of the shoulder girdle has several important roles in upper extremity control. Enough proximal stability is needed for the arms to accept part of the body weight during transitional movements. For example, proximal stability of the shoulder girdle is evident when the scapulas maintain their active connection with the rib cage as the body weight is shifted over the arms in any position. When the scapulas and rib cage separate, scapular winging is evident medially and inferiorally. Scapular winging is not, in and of itself, abnormal or atypical. Normal children and adults may exhibit scapular-rib cage separation during portions of upper extremity weight shifting. This scapular winging is created by changes in the center of gravity. The scapulas and rib cage may separate briefly, but they also are able to hold together during at least part of the movement pattern. When scapular instability on the rib cage is a problem, the child will compensate in a variety of ways. For example, in quadruped, the child may markedly internally or externally rotate the upper arms to achieve mechanical stability, or hip flexion may be used to keep most of the body weight on the legs instead of the arms. The child may move quickly between positions using momentum rather than postural control to shift weight. The child may "fixate" muscles on one side of the body for stability and direct movements asymmetrically, always moving one favorite side. The child may not feel secure enough to attempt transitional movements, thereby limiting his ability to move and explore the world. However, scapular instability is a problem only when it interferes with the child's ability to develop gross motor movement patterns.

Task Analysis

Therapists share a common goal in treatment, which is to guide children toward a life of independent function. The ability to tend to one's own needs is basic to the belief that we have control over our lives and ultimately our destinies. As we project specific functional goals for the children, we need to understand what we are asking them to do.

We can achieve the same functional outcomes in different ways. For example, there are a variety of methods for putting on a pair of shoes or a T-shirt. To determine the basic motor prerequisites for these tasks, move through the tasks yourself. An erroneous assumption is made if you think you understand the motor components, just because you do them automatically. Move through a task in slow motion and ask yourself what parts of your body are moving? What points of stability are you using to make your body move? Where do you feel yourself "holding" your position against gravity? What's preventing you from falling? When is breathing stressed?

Typically developing children may have developed many of the necessary motor prerequisites for movement and self-care by the age of 2 years. Yet, it takes many more years of practice to become graceful and controlled with movement and adept at dressing and other self-care skills. Independent, functional skills develop long after the motor components are available. Developing independence requires motor planning and sequencing, focused attention on the task, and goal-oriented behavior.

Examination and Evaluation

The first step in the examination is to identify the child's functional skills. Standardized tests, such as the Pediatric Evaluation of Disability Inventory (PEDI), can be used (see Chapter 2). Clinical observations also can be used. Regardless of the format, basic questions regarding functional skills should be asked. Examples are:

➤ Can the child use the upper extremities to help with movement in and out of positions?

➤ Can the child dress, use the toilet, and self-feed?

➤ Can the child use the hands for classroom learning?

➤ Can the child use the hands to explore and play with objects in the environment?

➤ Can the child use the arms and hands for mobility aids or transfers?

Secondly, questions also should be asked about how the child performs functional tasks. For example, does the child move the arms typically during activity? Is there an increase in muscle tone, atypical patterns, breath holding, or compensations? Identify those skills that the child is unable to perform. What consistent problems seem to interfere with function? Problems with functional independence may be due to a lack of mobility. The child may not have enough joint range to accomplish the functional task. There could be poor joint alignment. For example, the child may not be able to position the hips adequately to obtain a functional base of support for sitting. The child may have a lack of postural control against gravity. If this is the case, the child may not be able to maintain balance during the weight shift needed for a particular functional task.

If there is a lack of muscle activity, the child may not be able to organize the body and plan movements. Confusion about sensory input also may interfere with the child's motor abilities (see Chapter 7). Sensory organization contributes to the child's ability to plan movements and interact with the world. The inability to organize oneself and process sensory information may make learning frustrating. When describing the child's use of the arms and hands, use functional descriptions. For example, the upper arm can be described in terms of:

➤ Range of reach

➤ Holding the reaching posture against gravity

➤ Correcting the reach during movement

➤ Accepting weight on forearms

➤ Weight shifting on forearms

➤ Moving in and out of prone propping

➤ Demonstrating asymmetrical arm and hand use

> ➤ Demonstrating a bilateral approach
> ➤ Demonstrating unilateral control.

Functional descriptors for the elbow may include:

> ➤ Bringing the hand to the body, face, or foot
> ➤ Accepting weight on extended arms
> ➤ Moving in and out of extended arm weight bearing postures
> ➤ Demonstrating the ability to orient the lower arm and hand appropriately in space in preparation for grasp
> ➤ Using a variety of forearm positions or holding an object while moving the forearm and wrist

Evaluation of hand function may address the child's ability to:

> ➤ Bear weight on the hand
> ➤ Weight shift over an opened hand
> ➤ Grasp or immobilize an object in the hand
> ➤ Manipulate an object between two hands
> ➤ Manipulate an object inside one hand
> ➤ Release an object without having to fling it or flex the wrist to let it drop

Thirdly, the information gathered during the examination and evaluation process needs to be analyzed from a functional perspective.

> ➤ Why does the child move as he does?
> ➤ What motor components are present and which ones are missing?
> ➤ What atypical movements is the child using?
> ➤ How does he compensate for the limitations of his body?
> ➤ Do the compensations help or hinder the child's attempt at function?
> ➤ Can the child do a part of the functional task?
> ➤ Does the child have the cognitive/perceptual skills for the functional task?
> ➤ Is this an activity that the child is motivated to do?

It is easier to reach a functional goal that the child, the professional, and the parent(s) discuss and choose together. The child does not have to approach the task in the usual or the "culturally acceptable" way. Allow the child to try his own way. For example, a child may be able to undress while lying on the floor, but could not even begin to do the same task while sitting on a bench or chair.

Intervention

Many functional skills are learned cognitively and rely on initiating voluntary movement as compared to automatic movements used in response to loss of balance. Voluntary movements require effort and this may increase the atypical or less desirable muscle tone and poor postural control often observed in the child with cerebral palsy. Preparing the child before practicing a skill will make the task less effortful and will help the child to develop some of the motor components that may be missing. *Achieving scapulohumeral mobility*, for example, will give the child the potential for increased range of reach during functional movement. A typically developing infant acquires freedom of the humerus in the scapulohumeral joint while transitioning from supine to sidelying and rolling from supine to prone. As the weight of the trunk is loaded onto the upper arm in these transitional movement patterns, elongation of the musculature between humerus and scapula and between humerus and rib cage will give the child the freedom to initiate upper arm movements in a greater range. Reaching in prone then stimulates the child to use this new range. Scapulohumeral mobility develops in the typically developing baby between 3 and 6 months of age.

For the young child, *facilitating scapular-thoracic activity* will help develop stability needed for controlling reach in mid-ranges. Active thoracic extension is a prerequisite for medial scapular stability because it prevents excessive scapular winging. This initially is developed in prone play where the infant can work from the stability provided by the weight bearing surface. Appropriate prone play requires that the body weight be transferred off the shoulders and onto the abdomen and thighs (see Chapter 9). With the weight shifted posteriorally, the child can begin to push up on forearms and the spine extends. With volitional or accidental weight shifting the scapula begins to hold onto the rib cage. As the child develops endurance in spinal extension, reach can be added. Control of reach in space depends on scapular-rib cage stability that begins to develop as early as 2 months in the typically developing infant.

Increasing shoulder girdle and elbow strength is an important aspect of the child's ability to use the arms for transitional movements, functional transfers, and use of mobility aids. Facilitation of slow graded movements where the child uses the arms to push from one position to another is the way the typically developing infant develops strength and endurance in the shoulders and elbows. This developmental play begins with the 5-month-old's experience with prone on extended arms. But the quality of control is related to the child moving from propping on his side up to sitting, sitting to quadruped, and creeping in quadruped.

Developing isolated elbow movements is critical to self-care skills. Hand-to-body play emerges in supine in the 3-month-old, with hand-to-chest along with hand-to-mouth play, and is used functionally throughout life. The child continues to develop isolated elbow movement in prone play at 5 months of age by shifting weight from the forearms, back to the elbows where the lower arm is freed for elbow flexion/extension and the humeral movements are inhibited by the weight bearing position. The child then generalizes this sensory/motor experience in other positions, using the elbow movement to activate or explore a toy. The elbow movements are used again as the child attempts to hold his bottle at 6 to 7 months of age and in finger feeding at 8 to 9 months. Similar experiences can be used in treatment to assist the child in moving the elbow through the range of motion while grading movements.

Isolated control of the forearm and wrist is facilitated by prone on elbow play at 5 months of age. The mobility for forearm rotation at 4 months occurs by weight shifting prone on forearms. The child shifts weight back to the elbows and experiments with movements of the forearm and wrist. Movements of the forearm in supine and sitting occur first by holding the upper arm against the rib cage for stability. Active forearm rotation, however, is not used functionally until about 8 to 9 months. An important developmental experience that prepares the wrist for eventual control is active weight shifting on extended arms. This play elongates the muscles around the wrist. The young child generalizes the isolated wrist control during self-feeding and play at 8 to 9 months. For example, the child places a bread stick or toy in the mouth, stabilizes it with the jaw, and then plays with wrist movement. These varied experiences can be used in therapy to help the child use the forearm and wrist during functional activities.

Facilitating hand function requires a combination of therapeutic activities. Weight shifting on extended arms in quadruped and in transitional movements helps to expand the hand so that it will be malleable enough to actively arch during grasp and manipulation. Ongoing hand-to-body play provides the hand with a sensation of accommodation, where the hand shapes itself around objects. Helping the child grasp with the hand held in a neutral position at the wrist will facilitate an appropriate balance between flexion and extension over the wrist, through the palm, and over the metacarpal joints. The palm of the hand is the proximal point of control for the fingers. Digit activity is merely a reflection of palmar activity. The development of release is based on the child first learning to work long finger extensors from a point of stability. Experience with release begins with simple hand-to-hand play. The child then works on transferring objects from one hand to another, working from the stability provided by the first grasping hand. Children then let go of objects on a surface, the surface being the stable point. They also release objects to an adult who stabilizes the object. This process is generalized at 8 to 9 months of age, when the child has enough internal stability to release an object in space.

Simulating a skill through play helps the child use the movements and plan the sequence without the stress of the actual task. For example, pushing a large toy or therapy ball will give the child experience with elbow extension for crutch walking. Placing hoops on the feet will prepare the child for putting on socks, orthotic devices, and shoes.

Practicing the Skill

Children learn to develop skills through successive approximation with much repetition. Repetition brings the skill from a voluntary to a more automatic level. Preparing the child will not in itself create a functional skill. The skill must be practiced and the caregivers need to help the child cope with any problems that occur. Functional skills often are learned in small parts. If the child is not having success in the development of independence, the task may need to be broken down into smaller steps (refer to Chapter 3 regarding motor learning issues). Many verbal cues may be needed. The child can be coached as he practices in therapy, at home, or at school. He may not always know when he is being successful. He may not necessarily recognize improved skill or improved efficiency of movement. Temporary adaptations also may be helpful during a training program. Seating devices, for example, help the child work on upper extremity movements required in a task without demanding that he control his whole body at the same time. Temporary adaptations should be reevaluated frequently and removed when possible and when the child can function without them.

Carryover

Carryover is a critical concept. It allows the child valuable sensory repetition, which creates independence. A child with a disability may need even more repetition, especially if non-functional habits have developed. Carryover should be based on reasonable expectations that take into account individual and environmental factors. Expecting parents to work with their child on dressing in the morning when the child has to go to school may not be reasonable. It is reasonable to ask parents to work on dressing and undressing in the evening at bath time or in the family room after school when the child can practice in a leisurely manner. It may not be reasonable to ask a teacher to work on independent spoon-feeding during school lunch, when time is limited and many children need to be fed. It is reasonable, however, to ask a teacher to work with a child during snack time.

Additional examples of intervention strategies for developing upper extremity function and self-care skills are illustrated in the following case studies.

Case Study #1: Jason

➤ Practice pattern 5C: Impaired Motor Function and Sensory Integrity Associated With Nonprogressive Disorders of the Central Nervous System—Congenital Origin or Acquired in Infancy or Childhood
➤ Medical diagnosis: Cerebral palsy, right hemiparesis
➤ Age: 24 months

Examination and Evaluation

Jason exhibits sensory disregard on the right side. Sensory deficits in children with a hemiparesis are related to central nervous system (CNS) pathology, but a contributing factor may be lack of weight bearing and weight shifting experiences on the involved side of the body. Jason's inability to tolerate or interpret light touch and his hypersensitive palmar grasp also are consistent with a lack of weight bearing experiences. Loading the hand, arm, and shoulder girdle with weight during developmental activities provides sensory information into the joints, tendons, and muscles, as well as the skin.

Inactivity of the right shoulder girdle complex is consistent with a hemiparesis and puts the development of upper extremity function at risk. This inactivity of the right shoulder girdle prevents Jason from developing full symmetrical flexion and extension in the trunk for optimal anterior/posterior righting and diagonal control. The response of Jason's less involved shoulder is to increase activity to compensate for impairments on the involved side.

Inadequate shoulder girdle stability on the rib cage is a consequence of Jason's basic problem of inactivity. The most obvious instability is observed in scapular winging. Other subtle areas of instability are found in the glenohumeral joint, the clavicle, and the right side of the rib cage. Instability interferes with Jason's ability to support his weight through the right arm during transitional movements, such as moving from supine into sitting or quadruped to right side sitting.

As a consequence of his scapular/rib cage instability, Jason's reach is limited to 90 degrees of humeral abduction with internal rotation. There is poor scapulohumeral rhythm with his attempts at movement. Because the scapula pulls away from the ribs, rather than upwardly rotating as he reaches, the humerus mechanically cannot move above 90 degrees.

Atypical posturing of the right arm in humeral extension, adduction, internal rotation, and elbow flexion along with his associated reactions during effort may be Jason's attempt to control his posture and movements without the proximal control that should be present. His upper extremity posturing may be considered an adaptive movement strategy. Although a clinical description might indicate increased "tone," the underlying impairment may be more related to problems with motor control.

Weakness in elbow extension is due to several factors. Elbow flexion is used as a point of stability in lieu of proximal control, creating a situation where flexion dominates the posture of the arm. He can extend his elbow in space, but does not have the strength and endurance to extend his elbow when it is loaded with partial body weight.

Jason's lack of isolated forearm and wrist movements are reflected by his lack of symmetrical prone play experiences in combination with stiffness in the hand that occurs with efforts at movement against gravity. Jason's hand function is limited to a gross grasp with poor control of release. He lacks the hand expansion that normally occurs during extended arm weight bearing positions. He also lacks hand-to-body play that contributes to the ability to control and shape the hand for functional tasks.

FUNCTIONAL LIMITATIONS

Jason does not use his right arm and hand effectively for self-care tasks or for manipulation of toys during play. He does not protect himself adequately with his right upper extremity when falling backwards or to the right side in sitting or standing. He does not use the right arm well for transitions of movement such as moving from sitting on the floor onto hands and knees. He also does not bear weight symmetrically on his upper extremities for games that include handstands, "wheelbarrowing," or "leapfrog."

IMPAIRMENTS

Jason demonstrates poor sensory awareness on the right side of his body and sensory disregard of the right upper extremity. He has poor motor control of the right upper extremity for fine motor tasks. Jason has poor shoulder girdle stability with scapular/rib cage instability and active range of motion of the right upper extremity is limited.

GOALS

Treatment goals are for Jason to:
1. Improve sensory awareness in the right arm and hand
2. Increase symmetrical activity in the shoulder girdle
3. Increase range and variety of reaching patterns
4. Improve posture of the right upper extremity during ambulation
5. Increase active forearm rotation and wrist extension
5. Improve hand control

FUNCTIONAL OUTCOMES

Following 3 months of intervention, Jason will:
1. Demonstrate awareness of temperature differences in environmental objects with both hands (eg, warm oven surface vs cold metal surface)
2. Reach forward for a 12-inch diameter ball with both elbows extended, two of five trials
3. Grasp a hat with both hands and reach overhead with both arms to place it on his head
4. Walk and run with the right arm less flexed, using the right arm to attempt to break his fall when he loses his balance, one of four occurrences
5. Use both hands to take off socks
6. Begin to scribble and color with the right hand using large color markers

Intervention

Intervention strategies to increase sensory input and awareness to the right side of the body should be incorporated into his therapy sessions and home program (see Chapter 7).

Weight shifting over forearms and extended arms would be an important component of interventions designed to increase sensory awareness. Weight bearing on the upper extremities will increase shoulder girdle stability, elbow extension strength (with arms extended), and endurance. Games such as "wheelbarrowing" and "leapfrog" can be used as part of his home program. Symmetrical flexion and extension upper extremity movements can be facilitated through assisted weight-shifting in sitting or on hands and knees while on sofa cushions, bolsters, or balls. Playing in prone over a roll or wedge can facilitate increased range of reach of the right arm and facilitate a more extended and functional arm position. Playing with weight taken on the elbows, as in a prone on elbows position, can help free up the forearm and wrist for functional activities such as manipulating toys.

Finger feeding with the right hand will stimulate functional use, with the mouth serving as a point of stability. Sticker play will facilitate simultaneous use of two hands. Placing stickers on the left hand, forearm, and upper arm, for example, will require the stickers being removed with the right hand. Using both hands to manipulate toys appropriate for his cognitive level (eg, toy accordion, pull-apart toys) will challenge him to develop improved fine motor control and bilateral hand use.

Case Study #2: Jill

➤ Practice pattern 5C: Impaired Motor Function and Sensory Integrity Associated With Nonprogressive Disorders of the Central Nervous System—Congenital Origin or Acquired in Infancy or Childhood

➤ Medical diagnosis: Cerebral palsy, spastic quadriparesis, microcephaly, mental retardation, seizure disorder

➤ Age: 7 years

Examination and Evaluation

Jill's use of head and neck hyperextension with tongue retraction virtually "locks" the neck and upper body together. She responds to the head and neck hyperextension by pulling the shoulders forward. The shoulder elevation that she maintains helps to support her head but limits attempts at head movement contributing to her poor head control.

Jill's eye tracking is inadequate because she cannot visually scan her environment efficiently. Her lack of downward gaze is consistent with neck hyperextension. Her eyes and head may attempt to move together, but her head control is too poor to allow coordinated eye-head coordination.

Shoulder girdle immobility limits her reach to 60 degrees of humeral abduction. Limited spine and rib cage mobility result in a poor base of support for dynamic shoulder girdle function. Scapulohumeral and humeral-rib cage immobility limit her arm movements to humeral extension, adduction, and internal rotation. This prevents free and varied reach for play and environmental interactions.

Jill makes attempts to grasp, but her hand closes involuntarily prior to obtaining objects. This indicates that she has not yet developed voluntary control of her hands. Without a basic palmar grasp pattern, the development of release and manipulation is inhibited.

Functional Limitations

Jill has limited ability to use her upper extremities for functional activities, such as manipulating toys or self-feeding. She lacks enough upper extremity control to propel her wheelchair or use other mobility devices. She has limited ability to assist with dressing, such as consistently pushing her arm through a coat sleeve.

Impairments

Jill has generally decreased range of motion of the spine, rib cage, and shoulder girdle. She has poor motor control over her head, trunk, and upper extremities. Poor ocular control contributes to lack of eye-hand coordination. Jill has intellectual deficits that impact her ability to physically interact with her environment.

Goals

Treatment goals are for Jill to:

1. Demonstrate increased range of motion of the spine and upper extremities
2. Develop eye tracking with emphasis on downward gaze
3. Improve head control in sitting for eye-head coordination
4. Demonstrate improved controlled upper extremity movements
5. Demonstrate a gross grasp

Functional Outcomes

Following 3 months of intervention, Jill will:

1. Reach above 60 degrees, three of five attempts in supported sitting to touch a communication (eg, picture) board
2. In supported sitting, visually follow moving objects 30 degrees left and right from midline
3. Grasp an object placed in her hand five of 10 attempts in supported sitting
4. Release an object that is stabilized by an adult, one of five attempts in supported sitting
5. Use one upper extremity to bat at a joystick in preparation for a trial with a power mobility device
6. Maintain elbow extension while pushing her arm through a coat sleeve

Intervention

Activities should be incorporated into Jill's daily routine to facilitate relaxation and increased range of motion of her trunk and upper extremities. Slow, passive trunk rotation in supine or sitting will increase spinal and rib cage mobility. This will facilitate general relaxation and decreased stiffness. Slow oscillating movements of each glenohumeral joint also will facilitate relaxation and increase her potential range and variety of reach. Assisted movement in and out of sidelying will improve mobility between the scapula and humerus. These intervention strategies should be followed by opportunities to reach actively to accomplish functional or recreational tasks (eg, touch a communication board, bat at a joystick, bat a balloon). Assisted expansion of her hand in weight bearing or onto body parts (such as the pressure of her hand onto her knee) may assist her in developing body awareness and control of grasp and release.

Case Study #3: Taylor

➤ Practice pattern 5C: Impaired Motor Function and Sensory Integrity Associated With Nonprogressive Disorders of the Central Nervous System—Congenital Origin or Acquired in Infancy or Childhood

➤ Medical diagnosis: Myelomeningocele, repaired L1-2

➤ Age: 4 years

Examination and Evaluation

Taylor has developed basic grip, manipulation, and release skills in the upper extremities. Visual-motor integration delays are present that interfere with academic and self-care activities. Spatial perceptual problems may be negatively impacted by limitations in movement experiences. Taylor lacks upper extremity muscle strength and endurance necessary for prolonged ambulation with mobility aids.

FUNCTIONAL LIMITATIONS

During fine motor activities that also require balance (eg, playing with toys in unsupported sitting), Taylor demonstrates fatigue more quickly than his peers. He also has difficulty with tracing circles and squares and connecting dot-to-dot patterns with crayons (preschool academic activities), perhaps related to his visual-perceptual difficulties. Taylor has limited ability to assist with lower extremity dressing and undressing tasks, needing adult assistance and supervision. He propels his wheelchair independently, but cannot keep up with peers when long distances in the community are required.

IMPAIRMENTS

Taylor demonstrates generalized weakness and poor endurance in his upper extremities. He has loss of sensory integrity and motor control in his lower extremities related to the level of his myelomeningocele. He has visual-motor perceptual problems.

GOALS

Treatment goals are for Taylor to:

1. Improve visual-motor skills
2. Increase upper extremity strength and endurance
3. Develop independence in lower body dressing

FUNCTIONAL OUTCOMES

Following 3 months of intervention, Taylor will:

1. Maneuver through an obstacle course for 3 minutes while using the arms to push a scooter board (supported prone on the scooter board)
2. Put on and remove sweat pants with minimal assistance while sitting on the floor leaning against furniture or a wall
3. Successfully trace a circle and square with a large colored marker
4. Self-propel his wheelchair for 10 to 15 minutes during community outings with three brief rest breaks

Intervention

Negotiation of scooter board obstacle courses will improve visual-motor integration, spatial perception, and coordinated use of the arms for planned movements. This activity also will contribute to increased strength and endurance of the upper extremities. General strengthening activities such as prone push-ups, wheelchair push-ups, and "tug-of-war" games also would be appropriate. Hand strength can be improved by activities using pinch-type clothespins or a paper punch. Balloon "tennis" using a lightweight badminton or ping-pong racket will require eye-hand coordination. Direct practice of adapted dressing techniques on the floor, bench, toilet, or mat table should be incorporated into his daily routines. Clothing modifications that might be required, such as Velcro closures on shoes, should be explored.

Case Study # 4: Ashley

➤ Practice pattern 5B: Impaired Neuromotor Development
➤ Medical diagnosis: Down syndrome
➤ Age: 15 months

Examination and Evaluation

Ashley has a basic palmar grasp, but cannot release objects with control. She prefers to "fling" objects to dispose of them. She cannot pick up pellet-sized objects. Ashley has not yet developed goal-directed play, but does enjoy playing randomly with objects and toys. Ashley uses her upper extremities to help with movement transitions but locks her elbows into extension and externally rotates her humerus. This movement pattern may be used to compensate for poor scapulothoracic stability. Consistent use of extended elbows and external rotation at the shoulder limits her to the use of anterior and posterior movement transitions. She is unable to control movement patterns that require rotation of body weight over either arm.

FUNCTIONAL LIMITATIONS

Ashley is slow during movement transitions, especially if trunk rotation is required, contributing to her inability to keep up with her peers. She is limited in her play repertoire as compared to her preschool classmates. She prefers to bang toys on surfaces, rather than manipulate them. She is unable to pick up small objects, such as Cheerios, which limits her ability to practice self-feeding skills.

IMPAIRMENTS

Ashley is noted to have generalized hypotonia, weakness, and limited endurance for motor activities. She has poor balance (ie, impaired postural control). Ashley demonstrates sensitivity to movement-based activities and has a mild hearing loss. She has intellectual deficits associated with her diagnosis of Down syndrome.

GOALS

Treatment goals are for Ashley to:

1. Improve muscle coactivation (ie, stability) around major joints with emphasis on the shoulder girdle

2. Demonstrate varied positions of upper extremities during movement transitions on the floor

3. Develop voluntary controlled release and pinch

4. Demonstrate goal-directed play

FUNCTIONAL OUTCOMES

Following 3 months of intervention, Ashley will:

1. Move in and out of positions on the floor without locking her elbows, three of six movement transitions observed

2. Release an object on verbal request (without flinging it), five of 10 trials

3. Pick up a small pellet-sized object or Cheerio, without "raking," three of 10 times

4. Participate successfully in two goal-directed activities with adult encouragement during each preschool session

Intervention

Assisted bouncing on extended arms in a hands and knees position on a small trampoline or therapy ball will help increase muscle coactivation around joints and provide increased proprioceptive and vestibular input. Activities with assisted transitions in and out of side-sitting and hands and knees will provide Ashley with movement experiences requiring trunk rotation. The therapist should assist Ashley during these transitions and manually prevent her from locking her elbows. Playing in a quadruped position (eg, "horsey" or "doggie") with diagonal movements also requires improved motor control involving the shoulder girdle. Ashley should be provided with weighted, resistive toys to improve hand strength, increase sensory input, and upgrade prehension patterns. Sticker play and finger feeding, with facilitation of palmar arches, will help develop pinch. Tearing paper of different thickness will require bilateral hand use and facilitate increased hand strength. Goal-directed play should be emphasized during her preschool sessions to facilitate functional cognitive learning.

Case Study #5: John

➤ Practice pattern 5B: Impaired Neuromotor Development

➤ Medical diagnosis: Attention deficit hyperactivity disorder, developmental coordination disorder

➤ Age: 5 years

Examination and Evaluation

Although John demonstrates adequate motor control of his upper extremities, he appears to have generalized motor planning difficulties (ie, DCD) that interfere with age-appropriate fine motor skills. He also uses a less than optimal grip (eg, lateral pinch) for coloring and printing. Right/left hand dominance is not consistent.

FUNCTIONAL LIMITATIONS

John does not like to participate in age-appropriate games, such as catch, as he is unco-ordinated in relation to his peers. He is clumsy with utensils, such as silverware, and demonstrates poor coordination with paper and pencil tasks in his academic setting. John has difficulty with buttons, snaps, and zippers on clothing.

IMPAIRMENTS

John is noted to have a decreased attention span. He has upper extremity weakness and poor endurance for gross and fine motor activities. John has poorly coordinated movements for fine motor tasks associated with academic skills and self-cares. He has sensory processing problems in the areas of tactile discrimination, kinesthesia, and stereognosis.

GOALS

Treatment goals are for John to:

1. Demonstrate improved sensory processing of tactile information with decreased tactile defensiveness
2. Increase upper extremity strength and endurance
3. Improve upper extremity coordination for fine motor academic and self-care tasks
4. Improve fine motor planning skills

FUNCTIONAL OUTCOMES

Following 3 months of intervention, John will:

1. Use utensils during mealtime to stab food (fork) and butter bread (knife)
2. Demonstrate a three-finger grip on a pencil during printing tasks
3. Independently button and unbutton large buttons on a shirt
4. Independently zip and unzip the zipper on his jacket after being assisted to engage the zipper
5. Be able to identify a quarter, nickel, and penny in his pocket without using vision
6. Successfully cut out large, simple shapes (eg, circle, square) with scissors

Intervention

John will need repeated practice to develop fine motor skills. He should be encouraged to use a knife, fork, and spoon during mealtime. He can help make simple snacks, for example, using a knife to put peanut butter and jelly on bread. John can be supervised at the local playground with emphasis on climbing skills to develop upper extremity strength. An individualized exercise video ("starring John") using elastic tubing and small hand weights can be developed for John to exercise along with two to three times each week. His karate class also will provide opportunities to develop upper extremity strength. He will need to be assisted with proper grip positioning on pencils, crayons, and markers to develop a more efficient grip for academic activities. John's parents should purchase clothing that is easier for him to manage independently (eg, shirts with large buttons, jackets with large zippers) until his skill with clothing closures improves. Because tactile discrimination problems often are associated with motor planning problems, emphasis on tactile activities (eg, using water, playdough, sand) and games should be included in his therapy and home programs. If he expresses interest, John would benefit from piano lessons to improve fine motor control and planning.

Acknowledgments

In my 34 years as a pediatric therapist, I learned my most valuable lessons from the children, their parents, and the students participating in Boehme Workshops. To all of you, I am most grateful. Because we need a variety of vantage points to see the whole child with an ever-changing dynamic system, children, parents, and students created the challenges that continually enhanced my vision, sense of touch, and heartfelt connection to the children. I owe my deepest gratitude to my husband, John, for his work on figures and photos; to Mary Boehme for covering my office work while I worked on this chapter; to Trish Montgomery for her patience; and to Mari Lynn Young for her support with word processing.

References

1. Woodward S, Swinth Y. Multisensory approach to handwriting remediation. Perceptions of school-based occupational therapists. *Am J Occup Ther*. 2002;56:305-312.
2. Rogers J, Case-Smith J. Relationships between handwriting and keyboarding performance of sixth-grade students. *Am J Occup Ther*. 2002;56:34-39.
3. Van der Fits IBM, Hadders-Algra M. The development of postural response patterns during reaching in healthy infants. *Neurosci Biobehav Rev*. 1998;22:521-526.
4. Thelen E, Spencer JP. Postural control during reaching in young infants: a dynamic systems approach. *Neurosci Biobehav Rev*. 1998;22:507-514.
5. Hopkins B, Ronnqvist L. Facilitating postural control: effects on the reaching behavior of 6-month-old infants. *Dev Psychobiol*. 2002;40:168-182.
6. Calais-Germain B. *Anatomy of Movement*. Seattle, Wash: Eastland Press; 1993.
7. Kendall FP, McCreary EK, Provance PG. *Muscles: Testing and Function*. 4th ed. Baltimore, Md: Williams & Wilkins; 1993.
8. Bly L. *Motor Skills Acquisition in the First Year of Life: An Illustrated Guide to Normal Development*. Tucson, Ariz: Therapy Skill Builders; 1994.
9. Alexander R, Boehme R, Cupps B. *Normal Development of Functional Motor Skills: The First Year of Life*. Tucson, Ariz: Therapy Skill Builders; 1993.
10. Konczak J, Dichgans J. The development toward stereotypic arm kinematics during reaching in the first 3 years of life. *Exp Brain Res*. 1997;117:346-354.
11. Byl N. Neuroplasticity: applications to motor control. In: Montgomery PC, Connolly BH, eds. *Clinical Applications for Motor Control*. Thorofare, NJ: SLACK Incorporated; 2003:79-106.
12. Kuhtz-Buschbeck JP, Stolze H, Johnk K, et al. Development of prehension movements in children: a kinematic study. *Exp Brain Res*. 1998;122:424-432.

Suggested Reading

Bly L. *The Components of Normal Movement During the First Year of Life and Abnormal Motor Development*. Chicago, Ill: NeuroDevelopmental Treatment Association; 1983.

Boehme R. *Developing Mid-Range Control and Function in Children with Fluctuating Muscle Tone*. Tucson, Ariz: Therapy Skill Builders; 1990.

Boehme R. *Improving Upper Body Control: Approach to Assessment and Treatment of Tonal Dysfunction*. Tucson, Ariz: Therapy Skill Builders; 1988.

Boehme R. *The Hypotonic Child*. Tucson, Ariz: Therapy Skill Builders; 1990.

Charles J, Lavinder G, Gordon A. Effects of constraint-induced therapy on hand function in children with hemiplegic cerebral palsy. *Pediatr Phys Ther*. 2001;13:68-76.

Crocker MD, MacKay-Lyons M, McDonnell E. Forced use of the upper extremity in cerebral palsy: a single-case design. *Am J Occup Ther.* 1997;51:824-833.

Eliasson AC, Gordon AM, Forssberg H. Basic co-ordination of manipulative forces of children with cerebral palsy. *Dev Med Child Neurol.* 1991;22:661-670.

Erhardt RP. *Developmental Hand Dysfunction: Theory, Assessment, Treatment.* Laurel, Md: Ramsco; 1982.

Erhardt R. *Developmental Visual Dysfunction Models for Assessment and Management.* Tucson, Ariz: Therapy Skill Builders; 1990.

Johnston LM, Burns YR, Brauer SG, et al. Differences in postural control and movement performance during goal directed reaching in children with developmental coordination disorders. *Hum Mov Sci.* 2002;21:583-601.

Peloquin S. Reclaiming the vision of reaching for heart as well as hands. *Am J Occup Ther.* 2002;56:517-526.

Pereira HS, Eliasson AC, Forssberg H. Detrimental neural control of precision grip lifts in children with ADHD. *Dev Med Child Neurol.* 2000;42:545-553.

Savelsberg G, von Hofsten C, Jonsson B. The coupling of head, reach and grasp movements in nine month old infant prehension. *Scand J Psyc.* 1997;38:325-333.

Schieber MH, Poliakov AV. Partial inactivation of the primary cortex hand area: effects on individuated finger movements. *J Neurosci.* 1998;18:9038-9045.

Segal R, Mandich A, Polatajko H, et al. Stigma and its management. A pilot study of parental perceptions of the experiences of children with developmental coordination disorder. *Am J Occup Ther.* 2002;56:422-428.

Van der Fits IB, Otten E, Klip AW, et al. The development of postural adjustments during reaching in 6- to 18-month-old infants. Evidence for two transitions. *Exp Brain Res.* 1999;126:517-528.

Von Hofsten C, Vishton P, Spelke E, et al. Predictive action in infancy: tracking and reaching for moving objects. *Cognition.* 1998;67:255-285.

Withers GS, Greenough WT. Reach training selectively alters dendritic branching of sub-populations of layer II-III pryamidals in rat motor-somatosensory forelimb cortex. *Neuropsychologica.* 1989;27:61-69.

CHAPTER 13

SELECTION AND USE OF ASSISTED TECHNOLOGY DEVICES

Judith C. Bierman, PT
Janet M. Wilson Howle, MACT, PT

Assistive technology (AT) devices refer to a wide range of appliances or tools with a goal of ameliorating problems faced by individuals with disabilities. Public Law (PL)100-407[1] defined an AT device as, "any item, piece of equipment, or product system whether acquired commercially off the shelf, modified, or customized that is used to increase, maintain, or improve functional capabilities of individuals with disabilities." The AT device can vary from low to high technology and can target a wide range of functional domains.[2] This chapter specifically focuses on adaptive equipment (AE) (eg, low technology AT), which includes wheelchairs, ambulation aids, and positioning equipment. High technology AT, which includes computerized communication systems, electronic environmental control devices, and educational aids will not be addressed.

Public law in the United States mandates that children be included in the least restrictive environment and that all persons have reasonable accommodations to allow access to public settings. Basic requirements for least restrictive environments and accommodations were established in the Rehabilitation Act of 1973 with further amendments in 1998, which included specific provisions concerning AT.[3] The Individuals with Disabilities Education Act Amendments of 1997 (IDEA 97)[4] outlined the requirements of making public education available to all children and stated that AT needs of the child must be considered when selecting the appropriate environment and accommodations. In addition, the Assistive Technology Act of 1998[5] provided state grants to support AT programs, increased coordination of federal efforts related to AT, and added a requirement that the Secretary of Education award grants to states to share the cost of financing systems for AT for people with disabilities. The Americans with Disabilities Act of 1990[6] prevents discrimination of individuals with disabilities in employment, state and local government agencies, public transportation, public accommodations, and telecommunications.[7] Public laws emphasize the importance of including AT devices in the lives of individuals with disabilities to ensure their participation and increase their independent functional abilities in all meaningful environments.

The selection of AE and the integration of this equipment into the total plan of care are complicated and often time-consuming processes for the therapist and family. Historically, both families and professionals have included AE as an integral part of the treatment and management of the child with special needs. Parents often begin the process by selecting and using something as simple as a rolled up towel placed in a high chair to help position their infant during mealtime, or by using an infant style walker for a long period of time to allow a non-ambulatory child the freedom of moving around the room more easily. Therapists constantly search for AE to increase functional abilities, improve posture and movement, or promote carryover of intervention strategies.

The process begins with a comprehensive examination, based on a thorough understanding of AE and the purposes for its use. The team, including the family and professionals, navigates through the selection of the required item(s), seeks the approval for funding of the equipment, and then establishes a plan for the acquisition, use, modification, and monitoring of each piece of equipment selected. For the process to work smoothly, the client, family, therapists, physicians, educators, and durable medical equipment (DME) representative must work together consistently with a shared purpose and clearly stated goals and outcomes.

General Purposes of Using Adaptive Equipment

The purpose of using AE must be clear to all members of the team. There are times when a single piece of equipment can meet several different purposes, while in other situations several different devices will be needed to meet a postural need or functional objective. For example, the parents of a young infant can find a single device to safely and appropriately position the baby in the car, act as a seat in public settings, and act as a stroller when placed in a frame for mobility through the mall or in the neighborhood. However, the family of an older child may need to obtain nighttime positional devices, a support for standing, and a specialized chair at school, all with the same objective of positioning the lower extremities to address musculoskeletal impairments.

An "enablement" model provides a framework to relate various dimensions of disability with the objectives for using AT.[8] This chapter uses an enablement model, which is based on the International Classification of Function (ICF) model from the World Health Organization (WHO)[9] to explore four dimensions of disability. Selection and use of AE related to each of the four dimensions are discussed. This expanded model also includes a dimension of posture and movement that relates to multisystem concerns.[10]

The general purposes of AT for children include:

➤ Facilitating participation of the child into a wider variety of environments

➤ Increasing functional independence or functional skill level

➤ Improving the quality of postural control, alignment, and movement

➤ Minimizing, preventing, or managing system impairments

➤ Preventing the emergence of secondary impairments or additional pathophysiology

Facilitating Participation

AE often is used to increase a child's ability to participate in age-appropriate activities within the family or community. AE allows the child to direct his energies toward participation in educational or social programs rather than maintaining posture and gaining mobility. Hulme[11] assessed the benefits of adaptive equipment and found a significant (P=0.01) increase in the times the client left the bedroom or the home and an increase (but not significant) in places visited by the client in the community if AE was available. Burt-DuPont[12] described the use of AE as a key element in allowing children with developmental disabilities to participate in developmental dance programs with greater independence. McEwen[13] documented a relationship between position and social communicative interactions and positioning in students with profound multiple disabilities. The relationship was not an anticipated one, which suggests that therapists must carefully assess each child before making positioning decisions.

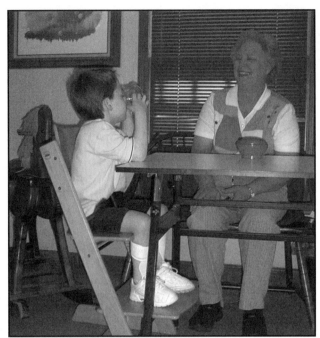

Figure 13-1. This young boy with Angelman's syndrome enjoys a snack with his grandmother while positioned in his Tripp Trapp chair. He is well positioned, safe, and the chair fits well into the family home.

A specific device may address a specific system or motor impairment or reduce a functional limitation, but if it is too complicated to use or too large to fit in the physical setting, its use is diminished in encouraging participation. For example, a freestanding prone stander with a tray top may ideally position an adolescent child in full hip extension and provide weight bearing to lessen the development of osteoporosis. However, if the prone stander consumes a large portion of a small classroom, breaks frequently, is not mobile, requires frequent readjusting, or requires two adults to safely transfer and position the child in the device, the overall impact may be to decrease the teen's participation in the class. In another example, if a device is perceived as less than aesthetically pleasing to either the child or to the child's peers it might result in decreasing rather than increasing participation. The child may find himself sitting well-positioned in a wheelchair inside the classroom at recess because he is embarrassed to be seen outside by his able-bodied peers in the chair. Many children have removed and discarded parts of AE, such as an abductor wedge on the wheelchair, if they considered it unacceptable in a particular social or functional setting. Most therapy centers have at least one closet or room filled with "pieces and parts" of equipment that have been removed by either a family member or staff member for some reason. Likewise, when a therapist suggests that an accessory may improve the child's positioning, it is not infrequent for the family member to recall having that particular piece "somewhere at home." The intervention team always must keep in mind what is acceptable to the child and family in order to expect AE to increase or at least not to limit participation by the child in appropriate settings.

Clinical Examples

In the home setting, a Tripp Trap seat (Stokke LLC, Kennesaw, NC) permits the child to sit at the family dinner table for meals and participate in family conversation and social mealtime activities (Figure 13-1). A bath or toilet seat may increase the independence of a teenager who does not want adult supervision in daily hygiene activities. Positional

Figure 13-2. These siblings are able to fish together using the posture walker with a seat modification for extra support. Participation in recreational activities is enhanced.

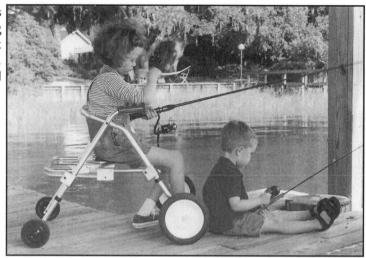

devices (eg, corner chairs or small chairs and tables) and switches to activate toys or computer games can increase independence in play activities for the young preschool or school-aged child. As the child moves outdoors, the use of walkers, crutches, adapted tricycles, or battery-operated riding toys increases participation in outdoor activities both with the family and with peers (Figures 13-2 and 13-3). Finally, for community activities or school-based activities, car seats, vans with lifts, powered chairs, walkers, crutches, sports equipment (eg, sport wheelchairs), augmentative communication devices, and specialized classroom seating can increase the participation of the child into a wider variety of settings and activities (Figures 13-4 through 13-6). An adapted stroller, even though it may not provide the best possible position, allows self-propulsion or independent transfers. It also allows a parent to include the child on short excursions such as a quick stop at the grocery store, library, or drug store when time is short or the weather is bad. The parent, otherwise, might be inclined to leave the child in the family's van if the only option is to unload and set up the child's wheelchair.

Increasing Functional Independence

As with all interventions, the objective is to increase the child's ability to function in all critical environments. Functional gains may be observed in multiple domains related to a single item of AE. Butler[14] evaluated the changes in frequency of self-initiated interactions with objects, spatial exploration, and communications with the caregiver and found that if children with cerebral palsy had independent powered mobility, they improved in all three behaviors. Haley and coworkers[15] in the Pediatric Evaluation and Disability Index (PEDI) described and tested changes in functioning in children including several different avenues of progress when they used AE. Examples of increasing functional independence are that:

➤ A child may be able to demonstrate a functional ability that was not possible without AE. For example, a child might use the toilet purposefully when provided with an adaptive toilet seat (Figure 13-7)

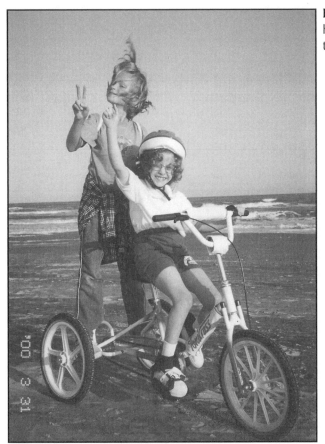

Figure 13-3. Bicycling on the beach with her sister is feasible with the modified three-wheeled bike.

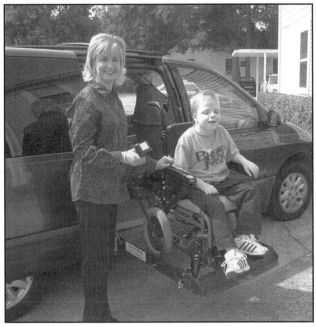

Figure 13-4. This youngster can be transferred into the family vehicle and transported to school, medical appointments, to the mall, and to friend's home alone by the mother who also has two younger children. Although he is still young, he is heavy and does not assist effectively with this difficult transfer into the family vehicle.

Figure 13-5. This teenager is now independent in his power wheelchair. He moves through the home and school well. He can now get home from school in the afternoons, let himself into the home, and start homework before the parents get home from work.

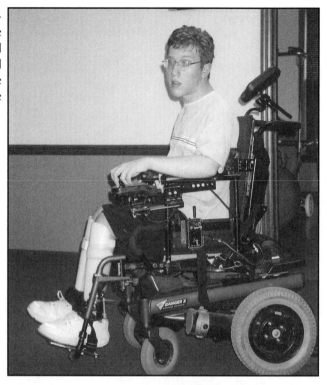

Figure 13-6. This young man uses a chair that has elements of a sports chair for participation in basketball and soccer and a more supportive higher backed chair for postural support during the school day.

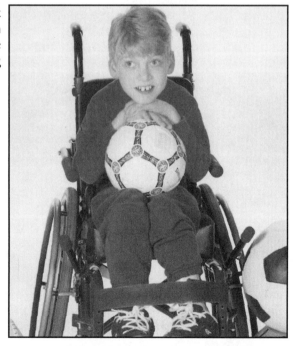

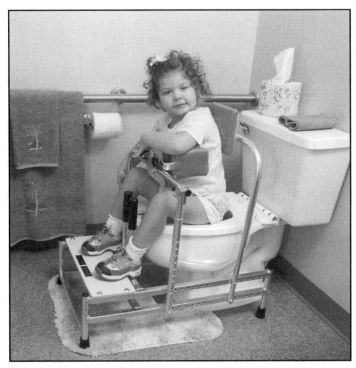

Figure 13-7. Increased independence in toileting will allow this young girl to participate in a school program more appropriately.

➤ A child may perform a task in broader contexts. The child who could sit on a bench at home while watching TV or listening to audiotapes now can bench sit safely in the family vehicle when positioned with an EZ Vest (EZ On Products, Jupiter, Fla) (Figure 13-8)

➤ A child may be able to perform a familiar task with less assistance. A bath seat may allow a child to bathe with assistance only for shampooing

➤ A child may be able to perform the same function with less assistive AE. A child may progress from ambulating with a walker to ambulating with forearm crutches and thus be able to move through a wider variety of environments and have equipment that is easier to transport

Changes in functional abilities may be viewed in five different domains: gross motor functions, fine motor functions, activities of daily living, work and play, and communication.

Gross Motor Functions

This domain includes activities such as the ability to move against gravity independently and through space. Logan[16] found improved upright posture as well as improvements in the parameters of gait when using a reverse posture control walker as opposed to a standard forward walker.

CLINICAL EXAMPLES

Gross motor functions include getting out of bed, rising from the classroom chair, crossing a room, going down the hall to the cafeteria, or moving across town using public or private transportation. At home, the family may use a mechanical lift to move the child from the bathtub or bed to a chair. A wheelchair or walker may increase mobility

Figure 13-8. This 11-year-old is safely transported in the family car with his special car seat. He is well-positioned with a five-point seat belt and the entire device is tethered to the car for safety.

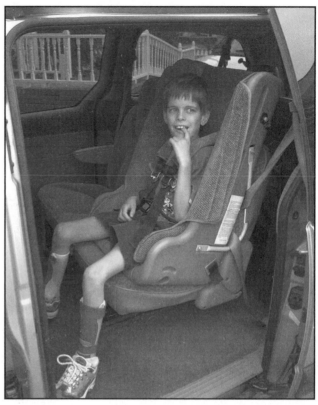

within the home. In school, a child may be able to move from sit to stand while positioned in an EZ-Stand (EZ Way, Clarinda, Iowa) with a hand pump lift mechanism (Figure 13-9). Another child may be able to move from the classroom to the cafeteria with peers and obtain lunch independently by using a walker modified with a tray holder. Finally, a teenager may be able to drive himself to school when the vehicle is modified with hand controls (Figure 13-10).

Fine Motor Functions

This domain includes activities such as managing tools or objects to solve environmental problems. Many investigators have explored the relationship between seating and upper extremity functioning. Nwaobi et al[17] reported that the angle of hip flexion had a positive effect on timed upper extremity movement. McClenaghan and colleagues[18] and Seeger et al[19] both investigated the impact of a slightly posterior tilt to the angle of seating to upper extremity use and found contradictory results.

CLINICAL EXAMPLES

At home, the child may use switches to activate battery-operated toys, household appliances, or environmental controls. Modified crayons may allow the child to color with a gross palmar grasp. Specialized clothing with Velcro (Manchester, NH) fasteners may permit independent dressing for a child with poor bilateral hand use. At school, a laptop computer may substitute for note taking in a classroom when handwriting is too slow. Adapted scissors may permit the child to complete projects independently, rather than depending on an attendant's assistance.

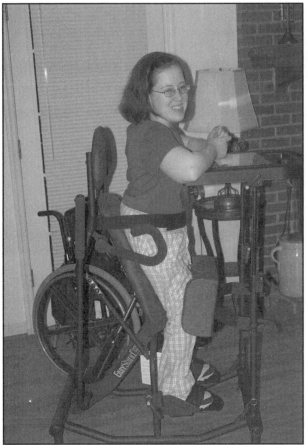

Figure 13-9. Joan can transfer from her wheelchair to the EZ-Stand independently. She is able to use the pump mechanism to raise herself to a standing posture without assistance.

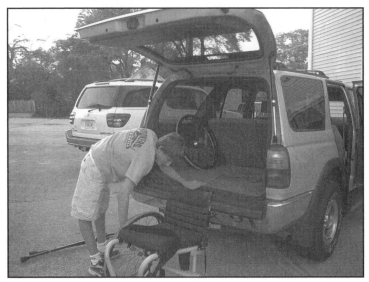

Figure 13-10. This 15-year old has learned to load and unload his wheelchair and crutches in order to drive using specialized hand controls. His goal is to have his driver's license like his peers at school.

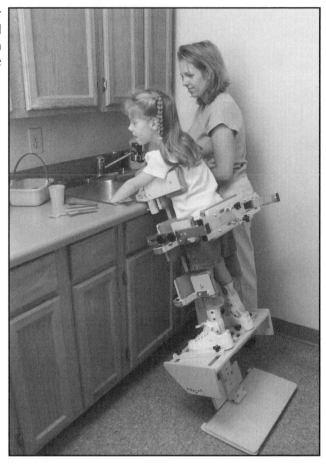

Figure 13-11. This mom and daughter work on washing dishes while the child is positioned in a prone stander. Both mother and daughter are free for the task while the child is well-aligned.

Activities of Daily Living

This domain includes activities such as performing daily hygiene, preparing and consuming meals, and dressing and undressing. Typically these activities require the individual to participate in "multitasking" or doing a fine motor task while simultaneously completing a gross motor activity (Figure 13-11).

CLINICAL EXAMPLES

At home, the child may use devices such as bath seats or adapted toilet seats to increase independence in personal hygiene. Adapted spoons, forks, cups, or plates can increase independence during mealtimes. At school, a bathroom modified with grab bars can increase the child's independence and safety during toileting. An electronic feeder and cup holder may allow the child to eat independently, rather than relying on an adult to assist in feeding (Figure 13-12).

Work and Play

This domain includes activities that form the foundation of work and play skills and support independent exploration, learning, and recreational activities.

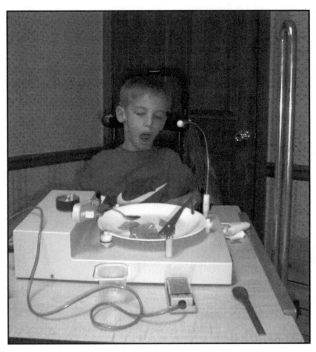

Figure 13-12. Justin can feed himself using this electronic feeder.

CLINICAL EXAMPLES

At home, the child may use a computer with specialized software, such as voice-activated programs, to play with or to call friends. An adapted chair may provide the postural support that allows a child to operate a computer mouse (Figure 13-13). Battery-operated riding toys and adapted bicycles or tricycles can increase leisure or recreational activity options. In the community, sport wheelchairs and modified aquatic, horseback riding, or ski gear can increase opportunities to participate in individual or group sports and recreational activities.[20]

Communication

This domain includes the ability to both receive and express ideas, thoughts, wants, and needs.

CLINICAL EXAMPLES

At home, a child may use a simple communication board to make choices during daily life. The mother may wear a "communication bib" during meals to allow the child to select whether or not he wants to eat another bite of food, have a swallow of his drink, or stop eating all together. In the community, a child can use a DynaVox (DynaVox Systems, Pittsburgh, Pa) to communicate meal selection in a restaurant or to share an answer in a timely fashion within a classroom.

Improving Postural Control, Alignment, and Movement

AE frequently is used to increase a child's postural control and improve efficiency of movement. Postural control and the efficiency and effectiveness of movement are determined by the interaction of multiple systems. As a result, integrative analyses by the cli-

Figure 13-13. The Kinder Chair (Kaye Products, Hillsborough, NC) positions the child well to use the computer with a standard mouse.

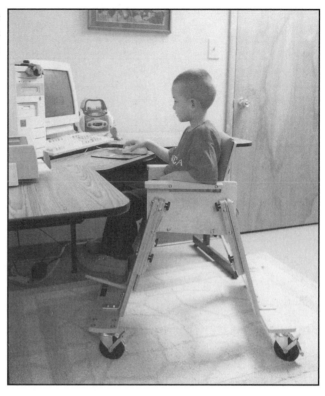

nician are required. Through a careful analysis of the child's posture and movement control and coordination, the therapist can identify critical contributions to functional abilities and limitations and hypothesize the relationship to specific underlying impairments. It is this dimension in the enablement model that is frequently referred to as the "quality of movement" by therapists.

Impairments in Alignment

AE is used to align single or multisegmental joints or the whole body. AE might be selected to support, assist, or require a specific alignment needed for a functional activity.[21] Gibson and associates[22] found that incorporating a lumbar support, as well as lateral supports, in wheelchairs of children with Duchenne's muscular dystrophy decreased the severity of their scoliosis. For those individuals with more significant postural or spinal deformities, the use of total contact systems such as contoured foam systems can provide more complete support and therefore improve proximal alignment.[23]

In seating, the angle of the seat cushion and back has been found to impact overall posture and movement. Nwaobi et al[24] evaluated tonic myoelectric activity of the low back extensors of children with spastic cerebral palsy and found changes in response to seat inclination. They also reported less extensor muscle activity when the seat was at 0 degrees and the backrest at 90 degrees. Reid and Sochaniwskyj[25] found that an anteriorly tipped seat facilitated extension of the spine and decreased deviation from midline. Miedaner[26] found that sitting on an anteriorly tipped seat facilitated trunk extension. Reid[27] compared the sitting posture of school-aged children with spastic cerebral palsy on a flat bench vs saddle-bench seating and stated that the saddle bench appeared to allow improved postural control. Cristarella[28] compared the sitting posture of a child with cerebral palsy when seated on a child's chair and when seated on a bolster seat. She found a more vertical pelvis and hip and knee flexion of 90 degrees when the child straddled a bolster. Posture and spinal curves approximated the posture of a typically developing child. Hulme and colleagues[29] reported significant improvement in sitting posture (P=0.01), head control (P=0.01), and grasp (P= 0.003) in children with multiple handicaps when fitted with adaptive seating devices. These somewhat conflicting reports suggest that therapists must carefully analyze the impact of seating components on the individual child.

Relationship of the Child's Center of Mass and the Base of Support

The most efficient relationship of the center of mass (COM) to the base of support (BOS) in any posture is one that minimizes the amount of force required to hold the posture.[30] A goal of AE is to support this efficiency while providing the fewest restraints to free, active, dynamic functional movement. The therapist also must consider the dichotomy of providing adequate stability while permitting necessary mobility. A walker might provide greater stability because it increases the size of the BOS and therefore immediately increases function for a child beginning to take assisted steps. Yet this same factor eliminates the need for the child to practice control of lateral weight shift of the COM over the BOS and reciprocity in the lower extremities. The walker, then, might slow the development of unsupported ambulation.

Movement Synergies

The design, placement, and use of AE also can modify movement patterns. The selection and use of AE can have an impact on symmetry, and increase or reduce activation of specific muscles for function. For example, poor placement of a head control system for a powered wheelchair might increase the tendency for the child to push backwards into cervical extension. This pattern of mass extensor muscle recruitment is a movement that is frequently discouraged during intervention because it may decrease the ability of the child to separate movements of the eyes from head movement, focus the eyes in midline, bring the hands together in midline, and achieve lip closure. Using a contoured head support system, or altering the place where the system contacts the occiput, can ensure that the time the child spends in the chair facilitates, rather than opposes, the posture and movement goals. In another example, a child who uses a PBWB device during early gait training activities may be able to practice task-specific movements, recruit the appropriate muscles, and reduce coactivation of the leg muscles to compensate for decreased strength.[31,32]

System Impairments

It is possible to address individual system impairments using AT. AT is a nonintrusive method to manage impairments that are not possible to treat or eliminate with other forms of intervention. For example, a child may wear corrective lenses to manage a visual impairment. Likewise, a child might be positioned prone over a wedge to manage a decrease in soft tissue length of the hip flexors, a common musculoskeletal impairment. Non-intrusive methods often are preferred over casting or surgery.

Common system impairments of the child that may be addressed via the use of AE include the following.

Musculoskeletal Impairments

Musculoskeletal impairments can be successfully addressed by AE. Placing a child in positions he cannot assume or maintain independently can minimize the development of bony deformities and contractures or tightnesses in the soft tissue. AE is used to position a child in order to counter the deforming forces of gravity or unbalanced muscle groups due to the child's habitual or stereotypical postures and movements. Professionals carefully examine positioning in neonatal intensive care units in order to impact the shaping of the infant's head and rib cage. As outlined in Wolff's Law, the altered shape (structure) influences the biomechanical basis for muscle activation and therefore the functional abilities of the individual.[33]

All the forces acting on the musculoskeletal system influence bone integrity, growth, and shape. Stuberg[34] demonstrated that with the regular use of standers with nonambulating school-aged children, bone mineral density could be increased. This impact reversed in periods of no equipment use. The use of orthotics in children with myelodysplasia who are unable to hold the foot and lower leg in proper alignment while standing can help prevent additional bony deformities in the foot and lower extremity.[35] The lower extremity position of hip adduction and internal rotation in children with spastic diplegia or quadriplegia is associated with an increase in femoral antetorsion and increased probability of hip dislocation. This position can be managed partially with AE. For example, the use of a solid seat in a wheelchair rather than a sling seat helps minimize the contributing posture throughout the day. In addition, the use of small benches or bolster chairs during circle time or play can decrease the amount of time spent "W" sitting (partial knee-sitting with bilateral hip internal rotation and knee flexion) and thus impact muscle length as well as the bony deformities.

Muscle length, growth, and use also are influenced by positional factors. Tardieu et al[36] showed that keeping muscles in a lengthened state requires 6 hours per day in the lengthened position. This fact certainly argues for careful positioning in bed and in school activities using devices such as orthotics, knee immobilizers, special chairs, sidelyers, and serial casting.[37]

Limitations in muscle strength also can be addressed via AT. Some children do not have the strength to lift the head from a fully prone position. Positioning on a prone stander, just 10 degrees off the vertical, allows the child to lift and hold the head while using hands in an activity. A child who has had a selective dorsal rhizotomy and is temporarily weak might use a PBWB mobility device to ambulate either on a treadmill or over ground, to develop specific lower extremity coordination strategies, and simultaneously strengthen weak muscles.[38]

Neuromuscular Impairments

In most children with developmental disabilities, neuromuscular impairments are primary contributors to functional limitations and participation restrictions. Impairments include deficits in the appropriate recruitment and activation of muscles and muscle types. Control and coordination of muscles to provide posture and movements that are both reliable and variable are limited. Both control and coordination factors can be impacted directly by AE. The tilt of the seat of a chair can be altered to more specifically recruit trunk flexors or extensors. An antithrust cushion combined with a subanterior superior iliac spine (ASIS) bar can be included to decrease active hip extension while the child is seated in a wheelchair. A child can control a powered chair by movement of any body part in any specified manner. Therefore, desired movements can be encouraged and undesirable ones limited by the placement of control switches. A posture walker may be used to increase thoracic extension during ambulation in a child who typically overuses the pectoral muscles for postural stability.

Sensory Impairments

Impairments in sensory systems that are treated, managed, or compensated for by AT include problems in registration, modulation, or discrimination of sensory information. Sensory aids can augment (magnify) input to a system or substitute for a limited system by providing input to an alternative system. For example, a swing may be recommended to a family to aid in a child's modulation of vestibular input. A NUK brush (Gerber, Parsippany, NJ) may be used to decrease oral hypersensitivity prior to a meal. Children may wear specialized prism glasses to accommodate for atypical visual perception or field deficits. A slanted easel top for the desk can compensate for poor downward visual gaze. A ball with a beeper can allow children with visual impairments to participate in ball games. Hearing aids or auditory filters can address hearing or auditory perceptual deficits. Specialized cushions with gels imbedded in them can dissipate pressure in sitting when somatosensory awareness is decreased in the lower body and children are at risk for skin breakdown.

Cardiopulmonary System Impairments

Nwaobi and Smith[39] examined changes in pulmonary function in children with cerebral palsy when seated in a sling-type wheelchair vs an adaptive seating system. Improved vital capacity and forced expiratory volume were found when the children were properly seated and positioned. The authors hypothesized this was related to improved alignment of the neck, thorax, and abdomen while in the adapted seating system. Stallard and colleagues[40] reported that heart rate decreased and speed of ambulation increased when children with spina bifida used orthoses. Bard and Ralston[41] evaluated gait in children with cerebral palsy using ambulation aids and found that the closer the gait pattern was to normal gait, the less energy was expended. Decisions on the progression from one type of assistive device to another must consider cardiopulmonary factors. Forearm crutches may be more appropriate in a small cluttered environment such as a classroom, but the higher energy requirements may make it necessary for the child to use a walker for long distance ambulation in the school hallways, playground, or cafeteria.

At this time it is very evident that there is a clear relationship in positioning for cardiopulmonary reasons and the impact on posture movement and eventual function. The American Academy of Pediatrics strongly encourages parents to have all infants sleep in a supine position to decrease the risk of sudden infant death syndrome (SIDS) from compromised respiration during sleep. Data suggest that the incidence of SIDS is decreasing in families who follow this advice. However, it also is evident that the children are rolling later and tend to develop a flattened shape to the back of the skull. A typically developing child adapts well to this variation in handling and positioning and the delays in typical milestone acquisition disappear by the end of the first year.[42] A child with impairments in other systems may have longer lasting deficits.

Integumentary System Impairments

Impairments in the integumentary system are frequent in children with developmental disabilities. Skin changes can be due to poor nutrition or hydration, atypical or sustained pressure or weight bearing, or atypical exposure to moisture due to excessive drooling, incontinence, or trauma due to biting or sucking on the skin. Appropriate AT can include, but is not limited to, use of specialized cushions or mattresses, orthotics, chairs, gloves, and taping in combination with a program to monitor the devices and alter the child's position throughout the day. The intervention method used will vary according to the specific needs of the individual. One child may need a communication device to request a positional shift while another child may need a G-tube to improve nutrition. A tilt-in-space chair may be needed to provide an upright position of the head and mouth to decrease drooling.

AT offers strategies to address most system impairments. However, even when the therapist is confident that AT devices address system impairments, functional and environmental constraints must be considered to ensure that AT devices are included in the overall intervention plan. The therapist must address the child's comfort. In addition, convenience and acceptance to the caregivers must be determined as these factors often determine the ultimate use of the device.

Pathophysiology

AE does not address the underlying central nervous system (CNS) pathophysiology that leads to developmental disabilities. The roles for AE are aimed at symptoms that present secondary to the underlying pathology. However, there is a preventative role in avoiding the emergence of secondary or associated pathophysiology. For example, positioning in weight bearing postures with AE might make it possible to minimize the emergence of osteoporosis as a secondary problem for the child[34] (see Chapter 18). Careful positioning during and after feedings might assist with avoiding aspiration pneumonia.

Environmental Constraints

In order to fully address participation, functional needs, posture and movement problems, and impairments of a child, the key environments also must be considered. Palisano[43] demonstrated that children use different amounts of both adult support and assistance, as well as AT devices, based on the environmental conditions. He found that children who are independent ambulators in the home environment and use only walls or furniture for support frequently require adults, walkers, or crutches for support when outdoors or in community settings. Likewise, children communicate with familiar adults with less augmentative communication devices. However, children may require a communication device when moving into different environments with different listeners.

In addition, equipment that is functional in one setting may be nonfunctional in another. A power wheelchair may appear to be a perfect solution for a child in a school with wide halls and doorways built on a single level with access to appropriate bus services. If, however, that child lives in a tri-level home with multiple staircases and with access to only a small family vehicle, this same solution will not be appropriate. The therapist must consider all of the key environments. This analysis includes the immediate home as well as the homes of extended family members. If the child spends weekends at the grandparents' home or is in the home of an aunt each afternoon after school, the characteristics of those environments and the persons in them must be considered. The therapist must review schools, day care centers, or community sites that the child frequently visits. The therapist must consider if the AE will stay at the family home or if it must be able to be regularly transported to a babysitter's, and if so, how it is going to be transported. Finally, a long-term view of the child and various environments is important. If the child is now in a preschool that is totally accessible, but the neighborhood elementary school is not, the therapist considers both environments when selecting equipment if it is expected to meet the needs of the child during this entire time frame.

Examination, Evaluation, and Intervention

These general guidelines allow therapists to analyze each child's AT needs. The problem-solving process includes examination and evaluation, a review of potential methods for providing equipment, determining key factors in selection of equipment, the acquisition process, and the development of a plan of care for equipment use, monitoring, and reevaluation. The family, the child, and direct service professionals are key members of the habilitation or rehabilitation team. Lee et al[44] found that consumer feedback was a key to the development of an adapted toileting system for children with neuropathology and emphasized the importation of consumer involvement. Family trials provided the means to develop and evaluate the product they developed and the experience of patients and rehabilitation professionals guided design decisions and evaluation. Additional therapists, teachers, or caregivers at school or in the private sector who are involved in the child's care should be included as indicated. Other persons also may have useful information, input, or questions related to the child and the potential use of equipment.

Examination

Assessment is always child focused or oriented. A comprehensive examination includes data collection or history of the key information related to medical, social, and educational background as related to AT. An accurate medical diagnosis and an understanding of the implications of that diagnosis have a direct bearing on the decisions related to AT. Does the child have a progressive disorder with a limited life expectancy? Is the current condition temporary with spontaneous recovery anticipated within 6 months? Is this a chronic condition that is expected to impact, with little change, on the child's life across the lifespan? Has an event, such as a surgery or a growth spurt, caused a temporary change in the child's health condition?

The therapist then examines the child's participation, functional activities and limitations, posture and movement concerns, and system integrities and impairments. The child's age and history of growth and development are recorded. It is critical to examine all of the relevant body systems as well as typical postures and movements that will have an impact on the child's use of AT devices. In addition, it is important to consider other contextual factors such as the child's ability to adapt to change. For example, how easily is the child frustrated? While physically capable, a child who is easily frustrated may not be willing to use a feeding device he must wait for an adult to set up, as it slows down the mealtime process. These contextual issues can dramatically affect the acceptance and use of AT.

In addition to determining the needs of the child, the therapist must determine caregivers needs regarding their ability to understand and use AE. Caregivers must be able to understand the purpose of AE in the child's life and find it convenient to use. Caregivers might include parents, siblings, teachers, personal care attendants, babysitters, grandparents, or volunteers. The therapist evaluates the caregiver's understanding of the child's abilities and acceptance of AE to meet some of the child's needs. The therapist assesses the physical ability of the caregiver to handle the child and the equipment. An older parent with a history of back pain may find it difficult to manage a large piece of equipment requiring transport in the family car. A grandparent may not be able to lift and position a child onto a prone stander. While the parent or therapist may be able to independently transfer a child from the wheelchair to the toilet, the attendant at school may find that a two-man transfer is needed.

The therapist also examines the key environmental constraints. Where does this child spend each day? Does the child go to school? How is the child transported? What are other settings in which the child regularly functions? Does the child attend a day care center, go to a babysitter's home, or stay at a relative's home? What changes in these environments will occur? Will the child change from home-based to school-based therapy? Is an upcoming surgery going to result in an inpatient rehabilitation stay? Will the child transition to a group home in the future? Equipment used in schools and day care centers frequently must meet different standards for safety and durability. Space available for use as well as for storage of equipment will be different based on the size and type of home or school. Will the equipment be shared with other children or be used around other children? Will there be other individuals, such as siblings, who might assist the child in the use of the equipment?

Evaluation

The team, including the child, family, the DME dealer, and therapists establish functional outcomes for the use of AT devices both for long-term as well as for short-term timelines. For example, the long-term outcome for a 4-year-old child may be to become independently mobile in the home using a power wheelchair. The short-term objective is to drive the power chair the length of the hallway without scraping the walls. Because this is a growing child who will use the chair in indoor environments, an appropriate choice for the team is a chair that is very maneuverable, rather than one that is durable in all terrains. A second chair, when the child has outgrown this one, may be one that can manage terrains around the home, school, and community. The specific choices are made based on these anticipated outcomes. Hypotheses are developed that relate the information in the examination to equipment options. For example, based on the examination, the team hypothesizes that a 4-year-old-child who has limited upper extremity control will be able to operate a power wheelchair in the home and preschool environment. It also is hypothesized that the child's visual-perceptual impairments and impulsive behaviors currently will prevent use of a wheelchair in outside environments without close adult supervision.

In addition to establishing these outcome measures, the therapist also evaluates the caregiver's understanding of the use and potential abuse of equipment as the child grows and develops. Adaptive equipment needs may change across time. The equipment will need to be monitored for fit and for continued need. The equipment may need adjustment due to growth or changes in functional ability. It may require different adjustments in different environments or for different tasks. For example, a child may require a head support system on the wheelchair with a harness while being transported on the bus, but may need to have times during the day to work on developing head control without use of these optional supports.

Finally, it is important for the therapist to have a clear picture of the caregiver's lifestyle before selecting equipment. It is very important to some families to be able to include the child in as many outings as possible and, therefore, lightweight strollers are more convenient and appropriate. Other families tend to leave the child at home with an adult and the focus is more on positioning devices that do not need to be as portable. As much as possible the equipment should meet the needs of the caregiver's lifestyle and make care easier while still meeting the child's needs. The therapist must understand that families come from a wide range of cultures, with varying priorities, values, interests, and ethics. With these differences come marked differences in the need, use, and acceptance of AE.

The evaluation also focuses on the specific objectives for each piece of recommended equipment, the costs of equipment, and available funding sources. The team must agree on the specific objectives that any piece of equipment is expected to meet. Options for renting, buying, constructing, or borrowing should be explored based on the needs and resources of the child and family. The funding may come from the family directly, from insurance companies, from state agencies, from Medicare or Medicaid, or from service organizations or groups. At this time, the role of the DME dealer becomes increasingly more important. This person often is knowledgeable about options in equipment, measurement of equipment, and the eligibility of equipment for payment under different systems. For example, in some states Medicaid may routinely pay for one type of stander and deny another one based on cost. It is important that the therapist be well-informed as to equipment options as well as to the DME representative's skills and biases.

DETERMINING SPECIFIC DURABLE MEDICAL EQUIPMENT

➤ The first decision is to select the method of positioning or assistance. Ward[44] described three options to enhance a child's functional abilities. The first option is using an adult's body to hold or position the child. Parents, therapists, and teachers universally use this system. It has many advantages including being dynamic and being the only system that includes sensory feedback and cognitive problem solving. The biggest disadvantage is that it requires the presence of an adult and limits both the child's and the adult's independence

➤ The second option is the use of standard furniture. Many ideas for adaptive equipment have originated from families modifying a standard piece of equipment. The advantage is that the device is more readily available from more sources and may fit into a wider variety of settings. The disadvantage is that the nonspecific nature of household items may not entirely meet the needs of the child

➤ A third option is to construct or purchase a specialized product. If there is a team member who is capable of constructing a device, the equipment may be specifically tailored to meet the needs of the child. While material costs may be less expensive, construction of a "one of a kind" generally involves intensive labor costs. Family members, neighbors, church, and social organizations who volunteer often find constructing a chair or stander a rewarding experience. The end product, however, is clearly based on the skill of the individuals fabricating the device. The time taken to complete a project is subject to the fabricator's other commitments. It is not possible to pressure volunteers to hurry the construction. This type of construction may not be acceptable in various public settings due to fire or safety requirements. Another disadvantage is that the device may be less adaptable to growth of the child and therefore may need to be reconstructed frequently

➤ If equipment is purchased there are different advantages and disadvantages. One advantage is that purchased equipment often is more adaptable to growth and to use by a wider variety of children. Therefore, one chair may be ordered for a classroom and can be used with several different children throughout the day as well as across the years. The equipment tends to be more durable and carries with it manufacturer's guarantees, such as being crash tested if the device is used in transportation. In addition, the equipment is more likely to be funded through third party payers. A disadvantage is the need to go through the approval process that can be both time-consuming, labor intensive, and frustrating. Finally, while the equipment may be able to be used for several different children and accommodate to greater growth, it may be more difficult to get a specific fit to accommodate one child's needs or body[45]

Intervention (Plan of Care)

The plan of care includes an outline of the intervention provided, personnel involved, and timelines in terms of frequency and duration of the use of the AT device in direct services and home programs. In addition, specific strategies to be used, equipment to be used, and instruction to be provided to the family, caregivers, or client are determined. A specific plan for AT is included in the overall plan of care. A sample intervention would be that the child will use a corner chair during mealtimes to aid symmetry of trunk and head and facilitate head and oral posture for eating and drinking. The chair will be adjusted with the seat elevated so that the knees are flexed at 90 degrees with the child's feet flat on the footrests. This will aid in achieving vertical pelvic position and normal spinal curves. The tray should be attached so the back of the chair inhibits scapular adduction as the child actively reaches forward and places the hands on the tray. The child then has the postural alignment and positioning of the upper extremities to pick up finger foods or to hold a cup in midline (functional outcomes). In addition to mealtimes, the child should use the corner chair for 30-minute periods several times during the day to use the same posture while playing with toys on the tray. The child should not be placed in the corner chair for more than a total of 4 hours during any given day and always should be supervised directly by an adult. The fit of the chair and its use will be evaluated in 6 months as part of the reexamination.

Acquisition

The team now must acquire the selected AE. If the family has a third party payer involved it is necessary to write a letter of medical necessity. The more specific the justification, the more effective the request will be. It is not adequate to write that the child requires a wheelchair because he has cerebral palsy. It is necessary to write that the child needs an ultra lightweight frame with removable armrest and footrests and a solid seat and back with a sub-ASIS bar to position the pelvis in a vertical symmetrical position. This position will help prevent further hip joint asymmetry and a possible scoliosis. The removable footrests and armrests will make it easier for the child to transfer into the chair from a walker and will make it feasible to be transported in the family vehicle. The lightweight frame will make it possible for the child with compromised cardiopulmonary support to propel the chair independently. This chair should meet the child's needs for the next 3 years or until substantial growth occurs. Remember, the equipment must be "medically necessary" for the child and not just make care easier for the caregivers. Typically both the therapist and the physician must sign the letter prior to submittal for approval. It is frequently very beneficial to contact the child's case manager with the third party payer if one has been assigned. This person should know if additional information is required or would be helpful. The appropriate information can be submitted with the original request rather than waiting for a denial and a subsequent resubmittal.

The time to obtain approval for DME may be lengthy. If the therapist can inform the family prior to the process of expected timetables it can be less frustrating to all. It is not unusual for the process to take many months and, therefore, it may be beneficial to develop a follow-up checklist with the DME representative to avoid unnecessary lapses.

Direct Use

Once the AE has been ordered, received, and assembled, the therapist or DME dealer fits the equipment to the child. At this time the therapist provides the caregivers with detailed instructions in the use and care of the devices. This includes specific use schedules. The therapist provides a schedule to monitor the fit and continued need for the equipment. A chair well-adjusted for a child in January may need adjusting again in July if a major growth spurt has occurred. The therapist should include in annual reevaluations and quarterly summaries a report from the caregivers on equipment use, fit, and, whenever possible, view the child while using the equipment in the typical environments for which it was selected.

Summary

When included in comprehensive examination, evaluation, and intervention, AT devices can play an important role in increasing the functional independence of many children with special needs. To assist the therapist in making knowledgeable decisions in selecting equipment for the children he or she serves, the Appendix on page 531 provides a list of manufacturers and distributors for AT devices. The list is not all-inclusive but is representative of the types of commercial products available as of this writing. In addition, several references and resources are provided concerning the funding, fabrication, and modification of equipment.

In summary, the therapist evaluates the child, the caregivers, and the environments in which daily life occurs for the child and considers possible solutions that AT devices can offer. Based on familiarity with the strengths and limitations of many AT devices and the options for obtaining the devices, therapists can make decisions whether to include AT as an intervention strategy. AT may address objectives in various dimensions of disability and enhance the overall quality of the child's life.

A brief review of the functional limitations, impairments, treatment goals, and functional outcomes related to the use of AT for children in the five case studies will provide additional clinical examples.

Case Study #1: Jason

➤ Practice pattern 5C: Impaired Motor Function and Sensory Integrity Associated With Nonprogressive Disorders of the Central Nervous System—Congenital Origin or Acquired in Infancy or Childhood

➤ Medical diagnosis: Cerebral palsy, right hemiparesis

➤ Age: 24 months

Functional Limitations

Jason's family is very interested in having him walk well at home while playing independently. He has difficulty playing outdoors on playgrounds with his brother and other children without falling. His family also wants him to be able to participate more in self-help skills, such as dressing, toileting, and self-feeding.

IMPAIRMENTS

Jason is demonstrating postural asymmetries and is at risk for developing secondary orthopedic impairments, such as a scoliosis, as well as asymmetrical limb lengths (upper and lower extremities). Limitations in bilateral upper extremity use and balance skills adversely affect his self-care skills, such as dressing and undressing.

GOALS

Treatment goals are for Jason to:

1. Achieve increased flexibility in the right lower extremity
2. Demonstrate improved symmetry in sitting and standing postures
3. Use his thumb in opposition to his fingers during gross grasp and release
4. Participate in bilateral upper extremity activities in several different sitting positions

FUNCTIONAL OUTCOMES

Following 3 to 6 months of intervention, Jason will:

1. Stand with both heels flat on the floor surface and not fall over when bumped or pushed by another child
2. Grasp 1-inch diameter pegs with the right hand and place them in a peg board
3. Sit on a bench and assist with removing a T-shirt

Intervention

An orthotic and a knee immobilizer to wear occasionally at night for the right lower extremity may be indicated to maintain range of motion. A shoe insert to aid in alignment of the right foot also is an option. In addition, Jason may benefit from a small neoprene or other type hand splint on the right hand to position the thumb in opposition for more effective grasp and release. These items could be ordered through a vendor with the necessary prescriptions and letters of medical necessity. As Jason is interested in toileting, it is suggested that the family obtain a small potty seat with an attached tray to encourage him to stay on the toilet for an adequate length of time. He also could benefit from sitting at the table to encourage greater symmetry and stability at the hips. A Tripp Trapp chair could be used for both Jason and his brother. Finally, a small bench or chair for play, TV time, and dressing activities could be obtained. These positioning alternatives would encourage increased symmetry by getting Jason up off the floor. These items could be acquired commercially, through yard sales, or from friends or relatives.

Case Study #2: Jill

➤ Practice pattern 5C: Impaired Motor Function and Sensory Integrity Associated With Nonprogressive Disorders of the Central Nervous System—Congenital Origin or Acquired in Infancy or Childhood

➤ Medical diagnosis: Cerebral palsy, spastic quadriparesis, microcephaly, mental retardation, seizure disorder

➤ Age: 7 years

Functional Limitations

The family reports increasing difficulty with transferring Jill. They have the most difficulty with transfers into the bathtub and into the family vehicle. While the current wheelchair will go into the bathroom, there is little space to move once it is in the room. They anticipate that the next wheelchair will not go through the door. The mother is worried that Jill will have a seizure while she is in the bathtub or in mid-transfer and that she may be hurt. The family also realizes that it is time to order a new car seat as Jill has outgrown the one they currently use. The family would like additional options, other than her chair, stander, or floor for safe positioning when Jill is at home in the afternoons and on weekends. Jill does not have any form of floor mobility and cannot sit without support. While she will assist briefly with standing pivot transfers, she does not maintain standing unless supported in a stander or by an adult.

IMPAIRMENTS

Jill has significant neuromotor deficits with little voluntary motor control. Her seizure activity and medication, as well as intellectual deficits, adversely affect her ability to communicate and participate in self-cares.

GOALS

Treatment goals are for Jill to:

1. Maintain or increase range of motion in the trunk and extremities
2. Tolerate a variety of positions, including prone on a wedge and standing in a stander
3. Improve ability to bear weight in standing

FUNCTIONAL OUTCOMES

Following 3 to 6 months of intervention, Jill will:

1. Stand in her stander twice daily (once at school and once at home) while attempting to touch objects on the tray
2. Assist with standing pivot transfers by maintaining weight-bearing for 5 to 10 seconds
3. Assist during transfers into the bathtub by maintaining head control

Intervention

At school, the current stander will be exchanged for an Easy Stand to allow introduction of more dynamic transfers. This stander also will decrease the weight bearing through her anterior chest, and therefore, improve depth of respiration. Correct positioning of Jill in her adaptive equipment and signs and symptoms of distress will need to be observed carefully. The therapist will recommend timing and scheduling of positional changes in conjunction with the school staff.

At home, the family will need to acquire a bathseat, a new car seat or EZ Vest, a lift, and a small bench for use in transfers to and from the family vehicle. When she outgrows her current prone stander at home, a vertical type stander will be recommended to capitalize on Jill's improved head control in the upright position. In addition, Jill could benefit from an additional activity chair for positioning for play activities. This chair should have a tray with the option to suspend toys for reach and activation. The therapist can request the local equipment vendor to bring several different types of lifts into the home for a trial. A lift for bathtub and other transfers would need to be tried in the home setting to make sure it will fit into all of the appropriate rooms (eg, bathroom). The car seat, bathseat, lift, and stander may be purchased with preapproval from the third party payer. The intervention team, after trials with several items, will recommend the best options. The activity chair could be a gift from both sets of grandparents. The parents can purchase a lightweight plastic bench the height of Jill's wheelchair footrests to ease the transfer in and out of their vehicle. The bench can be stored in the car under Jill's feet during travel.

Case Study #3: Taylor

➤ Practice pattern 5C: Impaired Motor Function and Sensory Integrity Associated With Nonprogressive Disorders of the Central Nervous System—Congenital Origin or Acquired in Infancy or Childhood

➤ Medial diagnosis: Myelomeningocele, repaired L1-2

➤ Age: 4 years

Functional Limitations

The family wants Taylor to be able to self-propel his wheelchair long distances to keep up with his peers while outdoors and to be able to walk using long leg braces and crutches in the house and the classroom. They would like him to be able to play more with neighborhood friends, and, in the future, they want him to be able to attend regular education classes.

IMPAIRMENTS

Taylor demonstrates the musculoskeletal impairments of decreased range of motion and strength in the lower extremities, along with decreased sensory awareness in the lower body related to his L1-2 myelomeningocele. He has limited respiratory support for gross motor activities.

GOALS

Treatment goals are for Taylor to:
1. Increase upper extremity strength and endurance for motor activities
2. Improve balance skills in standing with long leg braces and crutches
3. Demonstrate improved spatial skills in motor planning during gross motor activities

FUNCTIONAL OUTCOMES

Following 3 to 6 months of intervention, Taylor will:
1. Self-propel his wheelchair for two city blocks with one brief rest period
2. Self-propel a riding toy using his upper extremities for 10 to 15 minutes with frequent rest breaks
3. Stand independently with long leg braces while leaning against a classroom table
4. Participate in a group activity

Intervention

Taylor will continue to use his manual wheelchair. When a new wheelchair needs to be ordered, the family should consider one with a power assist to increase his ability to self-propel at higher speeds. The chair needs to be as light as possible, as the mother usually transports him and she is a small woman. Another option, if a heavier chair is required, is to purchase a portable ramp to be used for the family van and a tie-down system so the wheelchair and Taylor can be transported easily. Taylor recently received long leg braces. He is using an anterior support walker, but also has bilateral forearm crutches to use with his new braces. A tricycle that is propelled with the upper extremities may be obtained for Taylor through a local philanthropic group. In addition, his extended family could purchase a battery-powered hand-controlled riding toy for him so he can ride with neighborhood friends.

Case Study #4: Ashley

➤ Practice pattern 5B: Impaired Neuromotor Development

➤ Medical diagnosis: Down syndrome

➤ Age: 15 months

Functional Limitations

The parents are interested in having Ashley learn to walk, to talk, and to play more appropriately with toys. Ashley is not cruising independently at furniture and cannot walk without support. She does not play independently with toys, usually throwing them. She does not interact often with other children. Ashley does not assist in ADL, except with feeding.

IMPAIRMENTS

Ashley has poor balance in all positions. She has intellectual deficits related to her medical diagnosis. Ashley demonstrates decreased muscle tone and joint hyperflexibility. She also appears to be "posturally insecure," avoiding movement activities.

GOALS

Treatment goals are for Ashley to:

1. Assist with self-care skills

2. Improve balance skills in all positions (eg, sitting, kneeling, standing)

3. Use a greater variety of play schemes with developmentally appropriate toys

FUNCTIONAL OUTCOMES

Following 3 to 6 months of intervention, Ashley will:

1. Sit independently on a small bench and bat a suspended balloon without falling

2. While sitting on the floor, take off her shoes (laces undone) independently

3. Push a push toy in standing for 10 to 15 foot with stand-by assistance for safety

Intervention

While AE can be useful in aiding Ashley to reach her functional potential and minimizing the development of secondary impairments, the family is hesitant to incorporate dramatic changes in their home. Therefore, most recommendations will be for standard furniture or toys commercially available. Education will be provided to the family on other options that are available if, in the future, they would like to explore additional modifications or equipment.

A small bench or chair for Ashley to sit in during daily activities should be purchased to help decrease the size of her BOS. If a tray top is available, it would help limit the throwing of toys. A small, but heavy, baby carriage or push toy would be beneficial to encourage ambulation. Ashley also may benefit from a small swing to increase vestibular input. A swing could be obtained from a local toy store or the family could make frequent visits to a neighborhood park. Specific recommendations for a NUK toothbrush and adaptive spoon, plates, and cups to increase independence also can be made. The therapists and school staff providing intervention will continue to assess the family's interest in using AE at home.

Case Study #5: John

➤ Practice pattern 5B: Impaired Neuromotor Development

➤ Medical diagnosis: Attention deficit hyperactivity disorder, developmental coordination disorder

➤ Age: 5 years

Functional Limitations

The family wants John to be able to go with them to the mall, into other homes, and to playgrounds without falling or knocking down other people or objects. They want him to be able to attend regular education classes as he matures. However, they would rather he develop good self-esteem while attending a resource or self-contained class than struggle in a regular classroom with increasing frustration. John avoids physical activity and group sports. He has difficulty with ball skills and cannot ride a bike without training wheels. He has poor handwriting/printing. He also has difficulty using utensils during meals and is not totally independent in ADL.

IMPAIRMENTS

John demonstrates decreased motor control, coordination, and adaptability. He has decreased somatosensory and kinesthetic awareness.

GOALS

Treatment goals are for John to:

1. Demonstrate improved gross and fine motor skills
2. Complete self-care skills with verbal cues only
3. Participate with peers in age-appropriate gross motor activities

FUNCTIONAL OUTCOMES

Following 3 to 6 months of intervention, John will:

1. Use utensils during meals and not use his fingers to manipulate food items
2. Independently brush his teeth with parental supervision
3. Interact with other children at the neighborhood playground

Intervention

John can benefit from careful selection of equipment that is available in standard toy or department stores. There are many games or toys that would promote improved eye-hand coordination. It would be helpful for the therapist to accompany John and his parents to a local store to select appropriate items. In addition, the family may find that John's behavior will improve if more consistent sensory cues are provided in his environment. John could try more spandex type clothing to increase sensory input. Eating utensils that are heavier and provide more tactile feedback might improve his fine motor control during mealtime. A standard bright colored placemat to indicate his place at the table, combined with a small patch of nonskid material in his seat cushion, may improve his participation during meals. An electric toothbrush may increase his proficiency and interest in toothbrushing; a bath mitt could be used during bathing. Electric scissors, a squiggle or vibrating pencil, and writing with his paper positioned over a screen may be strategies that will improve his fine motor academic skills.

References

1. Technology-Related Assistance for Individuals with Disabilities Act: Public Law 100-407, 1988; reauthorized 1994.

2. Cook AM, Hussey SM. *Assistive Technologies.* St. Louis, Mo: Mosby; 2002.

3. Rehabilitation Act of 1973 and Amendments of 1998 PL 105-220, Sect.508, 29 USC Sec 794 d.

4. Individuals with Disabilities Education Act Amendments of 1997, Public Law (20 USC, SEC 1400 et.seq.) 1997; 105-117.

5. Assistive Technology Act of 1988: PL 105-394, codified at-Title 29 of United States Code at Section 3001 and following (29 USC Sec. 3001 et seq.), amending PL 103-218 (1994) and PL 100-407 (1998).

6. Americans with Disabilities Act of 1990: PL 101-336 Title 42 USC 12101 et seq.

7. Olson DA, Deruyler F. *Clinicians Guide to Assistive Technology.* St. Louis, Mo: Mosby; 2002.

8. Steiner WA. Use of the ICF model as a clinical problem-solving tool in physical therapy and rehabilitation medicine. *Phys Ther.* 2002;82:1098-1107.

9. World Health Organization. *International Classification of Functioning, Disability and Health-ICF.* Geneva, WHO; 2001.

10. Howle J. *NeuroDevelopmental Treatment Approach: Theoretical Foundations and Principles of Clinical Practice.* Laguna Beach, Calif: NeuroDevelopmental Treatment Association; 2003.

11. Hulme JB, Poor R, Schillein M. Perceived behavioral changes observed with adaptive seating devices and training programs for multi-handicapped developmentally disabled individuals. *Phys Ther.* 1983;63:204-208.

12. Burt-DuPont B. Developmental dance therapy. *Clinical Management: Magazine of the American Physical Therapy Association.* 1985;5:20-25.

13. McEwen IR. Assistive positioning as a control parameter of social-communicative interactions between students with profound multiple disabilities and classroom staff. *Phys Ther.* 1992;72:634-644.

14. Butler C. Effects of powered mobility on self-initiated behaviors of very young children with locomotor disability. *Dev Med Child Neurol.* 1986;28:325-332.

15. Haley SM, Costner J, Ludlow LH, et al. *Pediatric Evaluation of Disability Inventory (PEDI) Development, Standardization and Administration Manual.* Boston, Mass: New England Medical Center Hospitals and PEDI Research Group; 1992.

16. Logan L, Byers-Hinkley K, Ciccone C. Anterior versus posterior walkers for children with cerebral palsy: a gait analysis study. *Dev Med Child Neurol.* 1990;32:1044-1048.

17. Nwaobi OM, Hobson DA, Trefler E. Mechanical and anatomic flexion angles on seating children with cerebral palsy. *Arch Phys Med Rehabil.* 1988;69:265-267.

18. McClenaghan BA, Thombs L, Miner M. Effects of seat surface inclination on postural stability and function of the upper extremities of children with cerebral palsy. *Dev Med Child Neurol.* 1992;34:40-48.

19. Seeger BA, Caudrey DJ, O'Mara NA. Hand function in cerebral palsy: the effect of hip flexion angle. *Dev Med Child Neurol.* 1984;26:601-606.

20. Lawton J. Can real sports opportunities make a difference: how does participation in an adapted sports program influence the identity formation of a physically challenged athlete? A dissertation. University of Sarasota; Sarasota, Fla; 2002.

21. Bergan AF, Presperin J, Tallman T. *Positioning for Function: Wheelchairs and Other Assistive Technologies.* Valhalla, NY: Valhalla Rehab Publications; 1990.

22. Gibson DA, Koreska J, Robertson D, et al. The management of spinal deformities in Duchenne muscular dystrophy. *Orthop Clin North Am.* 1978;9:437-450.

23. Hobson DA. Seating and mobility for the severely disabled. In: Smith RV, Leslie JH, eds. *Rehabilitation Engineering.* Boca Raton, Fla: CRC Press; 1990.

24. Nwaobi OM, Brubaker CE, Cusick B, et al. Electromyographic investigation of extensor activity in cerebral palsied children in different seating positions. *Dev Med Child Neurol*. 1983;25:175-183.

25. Reid DT, Sochaniwskyj A. Effects of anterior-tipped seating on respiratory function of normal children and children with cerebral palsy. *Int J Rehabil Res*. 1991;14:203-212.

26. Miedaner JA. The effects of sitting positions on trunk extension for children with motor impairment. *Pediatr Phys Ther*. 1990;2:11-14.

27. Reid DT. The effects of the saddle seat on seated postural control and upper-extremity movement in children with cerebral palsy. *Dev Med Child Neurol*. 1996;38:805-815.

28. Cristarella M. Comparison of straddling and sitting apparatus for the spastic cerebral palsied child. *AJOT*. 1975;29:273-276.

29. Hulme JB, Poor R, Schillein M, et al. Perceived behavioral changes observed with adaptive seating devices and training programs for multihandicapped developmentally disabled individuals. *Phys Ther*. 1983;63:204-208.

30. Adrian MJ, Cooper JM. *Biomechanics of Human Movement*. Indianapolis, Ind: Benchmark Press; 1989.

31. Richards CL, Malouin F, Dumas F, et al. Early intensive treadmill locomotion training with cerebral palsy: feasibility study. *Pediatr Phys Ther*. 1997;9:158-165.

32. Schindl MR, Forstner KH, Hesse S. Treadmill training with partial body weight support in non weight bearing patient with CP. *Arch Phys Med Rehabil*. 2000;81:301-306.

33. LeVeau BF, Bernhardt DB. Developmental biomechanics effects of forces on the growth, development, and maintenance of the human body. *Phys Ther*. 1982;64:1874-1882.

34. Stuberg WA. Considerations related to weight-bearing programs in children with developmental disabilities. *Phys Ther*. 1992;72:35-40.

35. Knutson LM, Clark DE. Orthotic devices for ambulation in children with cerebral palsy and myelomeningocele. *Phys Ther*. 1991;71:947-960.

36. Tardieu C, Huet de la Tour E, Bret MD, et al. Muscle hypoextensibility in children with cerebral palsy: clinical and experimental observations. *Arch Phys Med Rehabil*. 1982;63:97-102.

37. Cusick BD. *Progressive Casting and Splinting for Lower Extremity Deformities in Children with Neuromotor Dysfunction*. Tucson, Ariz: Therapy Skill Builders; 1990.

38. Leonard CT, Hirschfield H, Forssberg H. The development of independent walking in children with cerebral palsy. *Dev Med Child Neurol*. 1991;33:567-577.

39. Nwaobi OM, Smith P. Effect of adaptive seating on pulmonary function of children with cerebral palsy. *Dev Med Child Neurol*. 1986;28:24-25.

40. Stallard J, Rose GK, Tart J, et al. Assessment of orthoses by means of speed and heart rate. *J Med Engineering Tech*. 1978;2:22-24.

41. Bard G, Ralston HJ. Measurement of energy expenditures during ambulation with special references to evaluation of assistive devices. *Arch Phy Med Rehabil*. 1959;40:415-420.

42. Dewey C, Fleming P, Golding J, et al. Does the supine sleeping position have any adverse effects on the Child? II. Development in the first 18 months. *Pediatrics*. 1998;101:E5-10.

43. Palisano R, Tieman B, Walter S, et al. Effect of environmental setting on mobility methods of children with cerebral palsy. *Dev Med Child Neurol*. 2003;45:113-120.

44. Lee DF, Ryan S, Polar JM, et al. Consumer based approaches used in the development of an adaptive toileting system for children with positioning problems. *Phys Occup Ther Pediatr*. 2002;22:5-24.

45. Ward D. *Positioning the Handicapped Child for Function*. 2nd ed. Chicago, Ill: Phoenix Press; 1984.

CHAPTER 14

Physical Therapy in the Educational Environment

Joanell A. Bohmert, MS, PT

The goal of education is to prepare all children for adult life. The role of the physical therapist in the educational setting is to assist children with disabilities to attain this goal. Children fulfill many roles—that of son/daughter, sibling, friend, student, and worker. Their jobs are to play, learn, and work. Their work sites include home, day care, parks, stores, shopping centers, job sites, and school. The physical therapist working with these children is not only a pediatric therapist, but also an industrial therapist. The physical therapist's primary purpose is to assist children with disabilities to function at their "work."

The purpose of public education is to provide a free and appropriate education for all children. Federal and state laws and regulations establish minimum standards for general education and special education. It is a challenge to provide an education that will prepare children with disabilities for their adult life. This challenge is significant in that the percentage of youth with disabilities who have not graduated from high school (20% vs 9%)[1], percentage of youth who pursue postsecondary education in the first 2 years following graduation (19% vs 56%),[2] and the percentage of adults with disabilities who work (29% vs 79%)[1] is significantly less than that of youth and adults without disabilities. Many children with disabilities complete their high school program with a certificate of completion vs a diploma, making it more difficult for them to pursue competitive employment.[3-5] Children with disabilities not only need to attain the ability to complete academic components of education but also the functional skills necessary for post-secondary education, jobs and job training, independent living, and social competence for adult life.[3-6]

The purpose of this chapter is to discuss the role of the physical therapist in the educational environment. Aspects of federal laws most pertinent to the school physical therapist will be highlighted. Types of physical therapy services in the educational environment and the roles and functions of the school physical therapist will be discussed. Special emphasis will be placed on the relevance of physical therapy services to educational goals in light of professional standards and evidence-based practice. The chapter will conclude by addressing the role of the physical therapist in an educational environment for children in the case studies.

Education Laws

Education laws are the bases for the provision of services for children with disabilities in public schools. To understand the role and function of the physical therapist in an educational setting, we must understand the contents and implications of the laws. We also must understand the history of educational law, interaction between federal and state laws, and the interaction between physical therapy practice laws and professional standards and educational laws.

Historical Overview

In 1965, Congress passed the Elementary and Secondary Education Act (ESEA). This act established funding and minimum standards for public education for children. In 1975, Congress passed Public Law 94-142, the Education for All Handicapped Children Act (EHA). By mandating a free and appropriate public school education for all school-aged children with disabilities, PL 94-142 opened schools' doors to children with severe disabilities who had not been served previously. As stated by Congress, the purposes of PL 94-142 are: 1) to ensure that all handicapped children have available to them a free and appropriate public education, 2) to ensure that the rights of handicapped children and their parents are protected, 3) to assist states and localities to provide for the education of all handicapped children, and 4) to assess and ensure the effectiveness of all efforts to educate such children.[7]

In 1986, EHA again was amended through enactment of Public Law 99-457, significantly changing services for infants and young children. Congress stated there was an urgent and substantial need to: 1) enhance the development of handicapped infants and toddlers and to minimize their potential for developmental delay; 2) reduce the educational costs to our society, including our nation's schools, by minimizing the need for special education and related services after handicapped infants and toddlers reach school age; 3) minimize the likelihood of institutionalization of handicapped individuals and maximize the potential for their independent living in society; and 4) enhance the capacity of families to meet the special needs of their infants and toddlers with handicaps.[8]

Through PL 99-457 Congress established a policy to financially assist states to: 1) develop and implement a statewide, comprehensive, coordinated, multidisciplinary, interagency program of early intervention services for handicapped infants and toddlers and their families; 2) facilitate the coordination of payment for early intervention services from federal, state, local, and private sources (including public and private insurance coverage); and 3) enhance its capacity to provide quality early intervention services and expand and improve existing early intervention services being provided to handicapped infants and toddlers and their families.[8] PL 99-457 did not mandate services for infants and toddlers, but provided financial support for states that chose to provide services for these children.

A major revision and reauthorization of EHA occurred in 1990 when the act was renamed the Individuals With Disabilities Education Act (IDEA).[9] IDEA was reauthorized and amended in 1997[10] with federal regulations finalized in 1999.[11] IDEA was to be reauthorized in 2002 by Congress but hearings were delayed until 2003. At the time this chapter was written, IDEA was still being debated in Congress. Readers are encouraged to check the Office of Special Education Programs (OSEP) web site (http://www.ed.gov/offices/OSERS) for current information on IDEA law and regulations.

EHA, PL 94-142, and PL 99-457 established the foundation and framework for special education, and while amended several times, their essential components still remain a part of IDEA today.

Current Education Laws

No Child Left Behind Act

From the initial enactment of the ESEA in 1965, it has been reauthorized and amended over the years. In 2001, Congress reauthorized and renamed the ESEA as the No Child Left Behind Act 2001 (NCLB).[12] The US Department of Education states this law "represents a sweeping overhaul of federal efforts to support elementary and secondary education in the United States. It is built on four common-sense pillars: *accountability for results, an emphasis on doing what works based on scientific research, expanded parental options, and expanded local control and flexibility.*"[12] The major thrust of NCLB is to ensure that all children will read and demonstrate progress in reading, math, and science as measured by statewide assessments. This law has significant impact for students with disabilities as it requires special education students to participate in testing and demonstrate progress in academic areas. The constructs of the four pillars also are being carried over into the reauthorization of IDEA in 2003, especially as related to additions regarding "doing what works based on scientific research." There also is the expectation that students of minority background, who have traditionally been overrepresented in special education, will be supported through NCLB rather than IDEA.

Individuals With Disabilities Education Act

The last major revision of IDEA occurred in 1997. Significant revision is anticipated in the reauthorization of IDEA in 2003, however, the core constructs and provisions appear to remain. The following is a description of IDEA as reauthorized in 1997[10] and defined in the final federal regulations of 1999.[11] The OSEP web site has the most current information on IDEA law and regulations (http://www.ed.gov/offices/OSERS/OSEP).

CONTENTS

IDEA contains four parts: Part A—General Provisions; Part B—Assistance for Education of All Children With Disabilities (addresses special education for children 3 through 21 years); Part C—Infants and Toddlers With Disabilities (addresses special education for children birth through 2 years); and Part D—National Activities to Improve Education of Children With Disabilities (addresses grants, research, personnel preparation, technical assistance, and dissemination of information). Part B and Part C are the sections most often referred to for the provision of services.

PURPOSE

Congress stated the purposes of the IDEA Amendments of 1997 as being:

➤ (1) (A) To ensure that all children with disabilities have available to them a free appropriate public education that emphasizes special education and related services designed to meet their unique needs and prepare them for employment and independent living; (B) to ensure that the rights of children with disabilities and parents of such children are protected; and (C) to assist states, localities, educational service agencies, and federal agencies to provide for the education of all children with disabilities

➤ (2) To assist states in the implementation of a statewide, comprehensive, coordinated, multidisciplinary, interagency system of early intervention services for infants and toddlers with disabilities and their families

➤ (3) To ensure that educators and parents have the necessary tools to improve educational results of children with disabilities by supporting systemic-change activities; coordinated research and personnel preparation; coordinated technical assistance, dissemination, and support; and technology development and media services

➤ (4) To assess and ensure the effectiveness of efforts to educate children with disabilities[10]

CONSTRUCTS

To implement the purposes of IDEA, Congress imbedded several constructs within the law. These included: a whole-child approach, a family-focused approach for infants and toddlers, use of the least restrictive environment (LRE), obligation to provide a free appropriate public education (FAPE), collaboration of services at all levels, and due process procedures.

Whole-Child

IDEA requires that all aspects of the child be addressed in all aspects of education. The whole-child approach means the evaluation and individualized education plan (IEP) must address all areas of development and the skills needed to work and live independently as an adult. This includes the ability to access general education curriculum, transition activities, and the preparation for employment and independent living. NCLB and IDEA stress the need to prepare children and youth for the work force and adult life.[11,12]

Family Focus

A significant difference in Part C (Infants and Toddlers) is the move from child-focused service to family-focused service. Family-focused means the assessment and present level of performance and needs must address not only the child but also the family. The parents, while being part of the focus, also are a part of the team. Parents need, and want, to be involved in the entire process, especially before decisions are made.[13,14] The focus on the family is needed as the parents are the child's primary caregivers and, as such, the child's primary teachers.[15] To empower the parents, to recognize the knowledge they have regarding their child, and to acknowledge their ability to become the child's "teachers" are important aspects of intervention.[16-19]

Least Restrictive Environment

The law requires that children with disabilities are educated in the LRE with children without disabilities. The intent of LRE is that all children should try to function in the regular classroom, first without support or modifications, and then with support or modifications. If this does not work, then other alternatives for instruction should be attempted.

➤ Part B—"To the maximum extent appropriate, children with disabilities, including children in public or private institutions or other care facilities, are educated with children who are not disabled, and special classes, separate schooling, or other removal of children with disabilities from the regular educational environment occurs only when the nature or severity of the disability of a child is such that education in regular classes with the use of supplementary aids and services cannot be achieved satisfactorily" (US 612[a][5][A])

➤ Part C—Natural Environments—"Settings that are natural or normal for the child's age peers who have no disabilities" (303.18). Services to meet the needs of infants and toddlers with disabilities and their families should be provided in natural environments as much as possible with children without disabilities. For most infants and toddlers this would be their home, however, it also may include day care or pre-school settings

Free Appropriate Public Education

When EHA was first enacted, states were required to provide students with disabilities the same resources as students without disabilities. To ensure equal treatment, Congress specifically stated that all children with disabilities are to receive a "free appropriate education which includes special education and related services."[20] It was not intended that education assume all of the health costs incurred by these children but that other agencies would continue providing health and/or medical services. There has been confusion as to the extent the schools are responsible for providing health-related services. Congress amended the EHA and the IDEA to provide clarification so that states may use "whatever state, local, federal, and private sources of support are available in the state"[11] and that funds for Part C may not be used to "satisfy a financial commitment for services that would have been paid for from another public or private source."[11] States also may not "reduce medical or other assistance available or to alter eligibility under Title V of the Social Security Act (relating to maternal and child health) or Title XIX of the Social Security Act (relating to Medicaid for infants and toddlers with disabilities) within the State."[11] The law further states that education is the payer of last resort if funding from private or public sources would have paid for the same service. However, educational services cannot be delayed or denied pending reimbursement from an agency.

Collaboration of Services

The IDEA recognizes the complex and varied needs of families of children with disabilities. It also recognizes that one agency cannot meet all these needs. To meet the needs of families, collaboration of services is required from multiple agencies. The designated agency for services for children ages 3 through 21 years is education, however, each state must designate a lead agency (education or other) to manage the implementation of services for infants and toddlers. States also must establish collaborative relationships to aid in the transition from education to adult services.

The construct of collaboration also applies to the educational team. The physical therapist must perform coordination, communication, and documentation for each child. This activity in the educational setting is consistent with the *Guide to Physical Therapist Practice (Guide)* definition of coordination, communication, and documentation that is a required component of all physical therapist intervention.[21] Therapists employed in educational settings are responsible for coordinating care and services with physicians and outside providers as well as other school personnel. Private physical therapists who provide services in the community or in educational settings also need to coordinate and communicate their services with educational personnel.

Due Process

IDEA requires documentation of due process and the plan for special education. Due process consists of procedural safeguards to ensure that the rights of parents and children with disabilities are maintained in the educational setting. Due process includes:

➤ Informed consent

➤ Confidentiality

➤ Timelines for assessment, placement, and service

➤ Procedures for the development and implementation of individualized programs

➤ Procedures for the resolution of conflicts

Part B and Part C include due process requirements but vary in the specific requirements and timelines.

DEFINITIONS

The following definitions form the basis for special education programs and services. As a result of public comments, court decisions, and amendments, IDEA has been refined to better address the needs of children with disabilities. For the most current definitions, please refer to current federal law (http://www.ed.gov/offices/OSERS/OSEP).

Child With a Disability

The definition of "child with a disability" in the law is virtually unprecedented in its inclusiveness. The terms included in the definitions are different for Part B and Part C and are considered educational categories of disability based on specific eligibility criteria. To be defined as a child with a disability in the educational setting, a child must meet the eligibility criteria for one of the disability categories defined by the law. These are:

➤ Part B—Mental retardation, hearing impairment including deafness, speech or language impairment, visual impairment including blindness, serious emotional disturbance (hereafter referred to as emotional disturbance), orthopedic impairment, autism, traumatic brain injury, other health impairment, specific learning disability, deaf-blindness, or multiple disabilities—who needs special education and related services (300.7[a][1]). The term also includes "children age 3 through 9 experiencing developmental delays" at the discretion of the State Educational Agency (SEA) and Local Educational Agency (LEA) (300.7[b])

➤ Part C—Cognitive development, physical development including vision and hearing, communication development, social or emotional development, adaptive development, or have a diagnosed physical or mental condition that has a high probability of resulting in developmental delay—who is birth through age 2 years and needs early intervention services. " The term may also include, at a state's discretion, children birth through age 2 who are at risk of having substantial developmental delays if early intervention services are not provided" (IDEA FR 99)

Eligibility

Eligibility identifies the requirements children must meet to receive special education services. There are four main requirements: 1) appropriate age, 2) complete an educational evaluation, 3) meet eligibility criteria, and 4) demonstrate a need for services. Parts B and C have different age and disability categories with associated eligibility criteria. Children in either part must complete an evaluation and demonstrate a need for services. It is not enough to have a medical diagnosis, as this does not equate to an educational disability. For example, a child may have a diagnosis of cerebral palsy but may not meet the eligibility criteria for an educational disability. By law, a child must meet the eligibility criteria for a disability category and demonstrate a need for special education. In addition, a child may have needs for physical therapy, but IDEA, Section 300.7(2)(i), specifically states that even though the child may meet the eligibility criteria for a disability category, "but only needs a related service and not special education, the child is not a child with a disability under this part" unless the related service being considered is a special education service.

➤ Part B—Children age 3 through 21 years, must complete a full and individual initial evaluation, must meet the eligibility criteria for the above listed disability categories, must also demonstrate a need for special education and related services (300.7)

➤ Part C—Children birth through age 2, must complete an initial evaluation, must meet eligibility criteria for one of the areas of delay or have a diagnosed physical or mental condition that has a high probability of resulting in developmental delay, must also demonstrate a need for early intervention services (300.7)

Special Education/Early Intervention Services

Special education is the program available to children with disabilities in the educational setting. It includes primary program areas based on the disability categories, such as specific learning disability (SLD), mental retardation including mild to moderate impairment (MMI) and moderate to severe impairment (MSI), physical impairment (PI), and other health impairment (OHI). Individual states use the disability categories identified in IDEA and may define their own specific disability categories and change the terms as they see appropriate to provide services in their state.

Special education services are mandated for children eligible under Part B. Services for children eligible for Part C are permissive at the federal level, allowing individual states to determine if they will provide services to this age group. Check your state's education laws to see if and how children, birth through 2 years of age, are provided services.

➤ Part B—Specially designed instruction, at no cost to the parents, to meet the unique needs of a child with a disability, including instruction conducted in the classroom, home, hospital, and institution, and in other settings and instruction in physical education. The term also includes speech-language pathology services, travel training, and vocational education (300.26)

➤ Part C—The term *early intervention services* is used in Part C to mean "special education, related services, free appropriate public education, free public education or education" (303.5[b][2]). It is defined as "services designed to meet the developmental needs of each child eligible under this part and the needs of the family related to enhancing the child's development"(303.12). These services are provided at no cost, in natural environments, and provide training for family. Early intervention services are defined as developmental services and may include: family training, counseling, and home visits; special instruction; occupational therapy; physical therapy; speech and language therapy; psychological services; medical services for diagnostic or evaluation purposes; health services; case management services; and early identification, screening, and assessment services

Related Services

Related services are those services required for the student to benefit from special education. While Part B provides a listing of related services, Part C includes the term in the definition of early intervention service.

➤ Part B—"Transportation and such developmental, corrective, and other supportive services as are required to assist a child with a disability to benefit from special education, and includes speech-language pathology and audiology services, psychological services, physical and occupational therapy, recreation, including therapeutic recreation, early identification and assessment of disabilities in children, counseling services, including rehabilitation counseling, orientation and mobility services, and medical services for diagnostic or evaluation purposes. The term includes school health services, social work services in schools, and parent counseling and training" (300.24)

➤ Part C—Includes related services in the term "early intervention services" where physical therapy is included as a primary provider. Federal law allows physical therapy to be a primary early intervention service, however, states may define this differently, requiring the infant or toddler also to receive services from an early intervention teacher

Physical Therapy

Physical therapy is defined differently in Part B and Part C. In addition to the stated definitions, physical therapists must meet the definition of "qualified personnel" that includes meeting "SEA-approved or SEA-recognized certification, licensing, registration, or other comparable requirements that apply to the area in which the individuals are providing special education or related services" (300.23). This requires physical therapists to review their state education law, as most states only require licensure as a physical therapist. Some states, however, require additional certification of the physical therapist to work in a school district.

> Part B—"Physical therapy means services provided by a qualified physical therapist" (300.24[b][8])

> Part C—"Physical therapy includes services to address the promotion of sensorimotor function through enhancement of musculoskeletal status, neurobehavioral organization, perceptual and motor development, cardiopulmonary status, and effective environmental adaptation. These services include:

   (i) Screening, evaluation, and assessment of infants and toddlers to identify movement dysfunction

   (ii) Obtaining, interpreting, and integrating information appropriate to program planning to prevent, alleviate, or compensate for movement dysfunction and related functional problems

   (iii) Providing individual and group services or treatment to prevent, alleviate, or compensate for movement dysfunction and related functional problems" (303.12[d][9])

Individualized Programs

A separate individualized program must be written for each child that qualifies for special education. The child's parent(s), and when appropriate the child, must be involved in the development of the program. Under Part B the program is the IEP while under Part C it is the IFSP (individual family service plan).

> Part B—IEP for all children age 3 to 21 years; for children 3 to 5 years an IFSP can be used. An IEP is a written statement that describes the abilities and needs of a child with the goals and objectives to address these identified needs. The IEP and IFSP are developed by the child's team which includes the parent(s) and when appropriate the child. Table 14-1 lists the components of the IEP

> Part C—IFSP for infants and toddlers ages birth through 2 years. The IFSP is a written statement of the family's resources, priorities, and concerns and the child's present developmental levels and expected outcomes (303.344). The IFSP is developed by the child's team which includes the parent(s), and if requested, providers from outside agencies. Table 14-2 lists the components of the IFSP

Travel Training

Travel training was added to IDEA as a special education service when IDEA was reauthorized in 1997. It is different than orientation and mobility training and applies to any student with a disability who demonstrates needs for training. Services may be an integral part of special education and are necessary for the student to prepare for transition to adult programs.[22]

The general definition of travel training "means providing instruction, as appropriate, to children with significant cognitive disabilities, and any other child with a disability, who require this instruction, to enable them to: (i) develop an awareness of the environment in which they live; and (ii) learn the skills necessary to move effectively and safely from place to place within that environment (eg, in school, in the home, at work, and in the community" (300.26[b][4]).

Table 14-1
Individualized Education Plan

Components of the IEP include:

➤ A statement of the child's present levels of educational performance

➤ A statement of annual goals, including short-term objectives

➤ A statement of specific education and related services and supplementary aids and services to be provided to the child and a statement of the programs, modifications, or supports for school personnel that will be provided

➤ An explanation of the extent, if any, to which the child will not participate with non-disabled children in the regular class

➤ A statement of any individual modification in the administration of state or district-wide assessments

➤ The projected date for initiation of services and modifications and the anticipated frequency, location, and duration of those services

➤ A statement of how the child's progress toward annual goals will be measured and how parents will be informed of progress at least as often as parents of nondisabled

➤ At age 14 or earlier, a statement of transition needs

Adapted from Individuals With Disabilities Education Act Amendments of 1997. 20 U.S.C. 1400.

Table 14-2
Individual Family Service Plan

Components of the IFSP include:

➤ A statement of the infant's or toddler's present levels of physical development, cognitive development, communication development, social or emotional development, and adaptive development

➤ A statment of the family's resources, priorities, and concerns

➤ A statement of the major outcomes expected to be achieved for the infant and toddler and family

➤ A statement of specific early intervention services

➤ A statement of the natural environments in which early intervention services shall appropriately be provided

➤ The projected dates for initiation of services and the anticipated duration of such services

➤ The name of the service coordinator

➤ The steps to be taken to support the transition of the infant and toddler to services provided under Part B (school-aged services)

Adapted from Individuals With Disabilities Education Act Amendments of 1997. 20 U.S.C. 1400.

Assistive Technology

Assistive technology devices and services are included in both Part B and Part C. IDEA mandates that assistive technology be considered by the IEP/IFSP team as a method to meet the child's needs. Assistive technology devices and services must be provided at no cost to the child if the IEP/IFSP team determines they are necessary to ensure FAPE. Assistive technology can be considered a related service or a supplementary aid and service.

➤ Assistive technology device—Any item, piece of equipment, or product system, whether acquired commercially off the shelf, modified, or customized, that is used to increase, maintain, or improve the functional capabilities of children with disabilities (300.5, 303.12[d][1])

➤ Assistive technology service—A service that directly assists a child with a disability in the selection, acquisition, or use of an assistive technology device (300.6, 303.12[d][1])

Transition Services

Transition services are defined differently in Part B and Part C. While both definitions address the need to plan for the transition of the child from one type of service or program to another, Part B specifically addresses areas of transition.

➤ Part B—"Coordinated set of activities" that "is designed within an outcome-oriented process, that promotes movement from school to post-school activities, including post-secondary education, vocational training, integrated employment (including supported employment), continuing and adult education, adult services, independent living, or community participation" is based "on individual student's needs, taking into account the student's preferences and interests," and includes instruction, related services, community experiences, employment and other post-school objectives, and acquisition of daily living skills and functional vocational evaluation. (300.29) Transition services are required for all students beginning at age 14 years, or earlier, if appropriate

➤ Part C—Activities used "to ensure a smooth transition for children receiving early intervention services under this part to preschool or other appropriate services" (303.148)

Extended School Year

ESY services are available to children under Part B, who may experience a loss of skills or regression and will not be able to recoup the skills in a reasonable amount of time.[18,22] Services are generally provided over the summer, however, they could also be provided over long breaks in the school calendar. ESY may be considered for children that turn 3 years old over the summer.

➤ Part B—ESY services are determined on an individual basis by the child's IEP team. A State or LEA may not limit the services to a specific disability category or limit the amount, type, or duration of services (300.309 [a]). Defined as "special education and related services provided to a child with a disability, beyond the normal school year, in accordance with the child's IEP, at no cost to the parents, and meet the standards of the SEA" (300.309 [b])

➤ Part C—ESY services may be considered for a child who turns 3 years old during the summer if the child has been receiving Part C services[22]

Table 14-3
Laws That Impact Individual With Disabilities

Act	Application
Section 504 of the Rehabilitation Act of 1973	Protects rights in programs that receive federal financial assistance from the US Department of Education. Must provide reasonable accommodations.
Americans With Disabilities Act (ADA)	Protects rights in public and private programs. Must provide reasonable accommodations.
The Assistive Technology Act of 1998 (ATA)	Requires states to provide programs and training for assistive technology.
The Family Educational Rights and Privacy Act (FERPA)	Protects rights regarding confidential health and education information.
The Health Insurance Portability and Accountability Act (HIPAA)	Protects rights for health insurance coverage and standards for privacy of individually identifiable health information. Rule does not apply to records covered by FERPA but may apply if information is used for outside billing or for research.

Other Laws That Impact Educational Settings

In addition to understanding education laws, physical therapists need to be familiar with other laws that impact children with disabilities in the educational setting. All of these acts are designed to protect the rights of individuals with disabilities in a variety of settings. These laws address civil rights not only in the educational setting, but also in community, health, and work settings in the real world. Table 14-3 provides an overview of federal laws that impact individuals with disabilities. See the Resources at the end of the chapter for web sites that address disability.

Section 504 of the Rehabilitation Act[23] has the most impact in the educational setting. Section 504 can be used if a child does not qualify or demonstrate a need for special education service but has an identified disability. This law requires that schools provide reasonable accommodations for any individual who is defined by the Act's definition as a person with a disability. The Act defines a person with a disability as "any person who has a physical or mental impairment which substantially limits one or more of the major life activities, has a record of such impairment, or is regarded as having such impairment" (34 CFR 104.3[j][1]). Schools or LEAs should have a process by which to identify and implement services for individuals, students and staff, who meet the criteria for a 504 plan. Physical therapists may be involved in the process to identify and implement a 504 plan, however this would not be considered a special education or related service.

Physical Therapy Practice Acts

Physical therapists and administrators need to be knowledgeable of their state's physical therapy practice act and its impact on educational services. Physical therapists are obligated to meet the requirements of their practice act, regardless of the setting in which they practice. Physical therapist assistants may or may not be regulated by their state. Additionally, state rules and regulations may or may not address the way a physical therapist should interact with the physical therapist assistant.

Physical therapist assistants may work in an educational setting, but must function under the direction and supervision of a physical therapist. Based on professional standards and education, physical therapist assistants cannot perform an evaluation or diagnosis but can assist the physical therapist in the implementation of selected interventions.[24] A physical therapist assistant cannot work independently of a physical therapist and should never be the only provider of physical therapy. It is important to review the regulations that apply to your state before providing service.

In addition to physical therapy practice regulations, states may have regulations that apply to all health care providers. It is important to review all the regulations that apply to health care providers in addition to those that specifically apply to physical therapy.

Roles and Functions of Physical Therapists in the Schools

The *Guide* states that the role of the physical therapist is to:

➤ Diagnose and manage movement dysfunction and enhance physical and functional abilities

➤ Restore, maintain, and promote not only optimal physical function but optimal wellness and fitness and optimal quality of life as it relates to movement and health

➤ Prevent the onset, symptoms, and progression of impairments, functional limitations, and disabilities that may result from diseases, disorders, conditions, or injuries[21]

This is the physical therapist's role regardless of the setting or patient population. The role of the physical therapist in the educational setting, as defined by IDEA, is to assist the child with a disability to benefit from special education. The challenge for the physical therapist is to determine the roles of the child in the educational setting, then with the child's educational (IEP/IFSP) team determine if the identified needs impact the educational program and if the expertise of a physical therapist is necessary to assist the child to meet those needs. The emphasis of therapy will depend on the special education and general education program in which the child is participating as well as the goals and objectives developed by the IEP or IFSP team. The primary focus for the physical therapist in the educational setting is to assist the child in the development of functional mobility, to assist the child to access the educational environment, and to assist the child to understand his or her disability and its impact on wellness and fitness.

The models of service in an educational setting are unlike those in the typical medical setting where direct one-to-one services are provided to each patient. Physical therapists in the schools need to adjust and redefine their intervention programs and objectives to assist the child to benefit from special education.[18,19,25,26] Physical therapists are considered a member of the child's IEP or IFSP team whose members jointly identify needs, develop goals and objectives, and determine programs and services.

General Functions

TEAMING

A critical aspect of working in an educational setting is the ability to function effectively on a team. The basic constructs of IDEA require that the child participate in the LRE and natural setting. The purpose of teaming is to bring a group of "experts" together to address the "whole-child" and what that child needs to be successful throughout the educational day. For each child, the team needs to be familiar with the age-appropriate general education curriculum, the daily classroom routine, and the typical expectations for same-age peers so they may determine how that specific child's disability and identified needs interfere with the ability to participate and learn in general education. For any child with a disability to be successful in the educational environment, the team must be able to work together. Collaboration is essential throughout due process from the identification and prioritization of needs through the development and implementation of the IEP/IFSP.[27] Teaming is considered a dynamic process, each member bringing a different perspective and expertise. Utley and Rapport[28] identified four elements which special education teachers and related service providers identified as essential to effective teaming. These were problem solving, willingness to share and combine intervention methods, importance of assessment data, and decision making. The ability of the team to problem solve is reported to be the highest value of teaming.[27,28]

Basic components for an effective team include: defined purpose for the team; clearly established team goals; high communication among team members; high commitment from team members; understanding of own and other professional's roles; respect and value for each others profession; equal participation, power, and influence; participation by all members; defined decision-making and conflict resolution process; and encouragement of differing opinions.[26-29] For effective teaming, adequate time must be committed to and provided on a regular basis by the administration and team members.[27,30] There are a number of references that further describe the process of effective teaming and factors that can interfere.[26-29,31-35]

Teaming in the educational setting generally is viewed as interdisciplinary or transdisciplinary. Both models require regular communication and a team approach to the development and implementation of the IEP/IFSP. Transdisciplinary teaming requires members of the team to teach others aspects of their own discipline and to learn aspects of the other team members' disciplines.[36,37] While this is defined as role release, many believe they are "giving away their profession" and are threatened by this process.[38] York, Rainforth, and Giangreco[38] attempted to clarify some of the misconceptions of transdisciplinary teamwork and integrated therapy. They stated that loss of direct student contact is not a result of released professional skills, but rather is a cooperation among team members to enhance the child's ability to function in natural settings. Rainforth[39] addressed the legal and ethical concerns of role release by physical therapists and found that the activities can be both legal and ethical. An important aspect of working in an educational setting is teaching others how to set up the environment and then practicing the skills when the child needs to use those skills. The *Guide* includes teachers and paraprofessionals in the definition of caregivers, not only physical therapy aides or support personnel, and allows for instruction and training of those individuals as part of patient/client-related instruction.[21]

Caution must be used so that the concept of the transdisciplinary approach is not used to limit the availability of or access to any discipline. It is critical in this discussion to remember that physical therapy can only be performed by a physical therapist or a physical therapist assistant under the direction and supervision of a physical therapist.[24] When activities or techniques are taught to other individuals, they are performing the activities, not physical therapy, and it should be documented as such on the child's IEP/IFSP.

Medical vs Educational Services

For many years administrators, legislators, parents, physicians, and even physical therapists have been trying to define the difference between medial and educational physical therapy services.[25] Many believe it is critical to define the difference since education is responsible to pay only for educational services and many private and public insurers will only pay for medically necessary services. With the passage and amendments to educational laws and PL 100-360, Section 411(k)(13), educational agencies have been allowed to seek reimbursement for "medically necessary" health-related services provided as part of a child's special education program (IEP/IFSP). These changes have added to the confusion because "medical" services can now be provided and reimbursed in an "educational" setting.

Overlaps also exist in the provision of medical and educational services. Education now encompasses teaching children in a variety of settings that include the home, classroom, playground, lunchroom, bus, community, and work sites. At the same time, the medical model has changed from the hospital setting to the home, community, and work site. Another overlap is the philosophical basis for practice of the physical therapist. The *Guide*, as described in Chapter 4, describes the practice of the physical therapist, which is the same, regardless of setting. Based on this, the physical therapist in either the educational or medical setting needs to base practice on the three concepts of the *Guide—the disablement model, a continuum of service,* and *the five elements of patient/client management.*[21] This results in the physical therapist in both settings addressing the "whole-child," the child's functional skills, and the roles of the child.

Perhaps one way to differentiate medical and educational services is to address the regulations and purpose of the service. Physical therapists in both settings are obligated to follow their state physical therapy practice act. In the medical setting, the additional regulations that oversee the service would be that of either federal and state health care laws, public or private insurers' policies, or, in cases of direct reimbursement, the desires of the patient/client. The purpose of physical therapy in the medical setting is to assist the patient/client to be as functionally independent as possible. This is done by addressing the patient's/client's pathology, impairments, functional limitations, disabilities, risk factors, and fitness and health/wellness needs. In other words, medical necessity may be defined as services needed to impact the process of disablement or enablement.

In the educational setting, the additional regulations that oversee the service are federal and state education laws. The purpose of physical therapy in the educational setting is to assist the identified special education student to be as functionally independent as possible to benefit from the educational program. Like the medical model, this is done by addressing the student's pathology, impairments, functional limitations, disability, risk factors, and fitness and health/wellness needs, however, it is only in relation to how these needs interfere with the student's ability to participate in the educational program. In other words, educational necessity may be defined as services needed to allow the student to benefit from education.

One major difference between medical and educational services is the process for accessing the service. In the medical model, any child can receive physical therapy service. In the educational model, the child must meet a minimum of two conditions before physical therapy services can be considered. First, the child must be identified as having an educational disability, as defined by federal and state laws. Second, the child must demonstrate a need for special education and related services. For children ages 3 through 21 years, only when these first two conditions are met can physical therapy be considered to assist in meeting the child's identified special education needs. Infants and toddlers also must be identified with an educational disability and in need of early intervention services. However, federal law allows physical therapy to be the primary early intervention service for these children.

Deciding whether therapy services are medically or educationally necessary is up to the individual states, school districts, and individual IEP/IFSP teams. The law requires that physical therapy must be provided when it is necessary to "assist the child to benefit from special education."[10] IEP/IFSP teams that include the physical therapist must determine what is educationally necessary for that specific child and provide the appropriate services.

Role in Due Process

The physical therapist plays a vital role throughout educational due process. Figure 14-1 identifies one state's model of the therapist's role and responsibilities at the various stages of due process. While the physical therapist participates in all the aspects of due process, it is not until the step involving the development of the IEP/IFSP, step 7 of 9, that the team discusses the need for the expertise of the physical therapist and services are determined.

IDENTIFICATION

Identification is used to identify children birth through 21 years who may have need for special education and related services. Activities may include screening, interagency activities, and prereferral activities including consultation and education of staff. Districts need to have a plan for identifying children within the community, including children attending private schools. Therapists in educational settings may participate in any of the identification activities. Therapists in other settings need to be familiar with their state's identification process and the role of the LEA so that children and families with suspected educational needs may be referred for evaluation.

REFERRAL

Referral is the process of recommending children who are suspected of having a disability for review and possible evaluation by an educational team. There are many sources of referrals including parents, teachers, physicians, physical therapists, and other professionals. Physical therapists may participate in the referral process by recommending a child for an educational evaluation and by consulting with educational staff regarding prereferral strategies to address motor concerns expressed by staff.

The process for referral is different for Part B and Part C. Therapists will need to review the requirements in law as well as SEA and LEA requirements.

EVALUATION

An evaluation is conducted "to determine whether a child is a child with a disability and to determine educational needs."(300.320) The information from the evaluation is used to determine if the child is eligible for a disability category and if the child qualifies for special education. This information also may be used in the development of the IEP/IFSP for the child. IDEA identifies a specific process for evaluation for Part B and Part C. Both parts require that all areas of a child are reviewed and assessed if further data

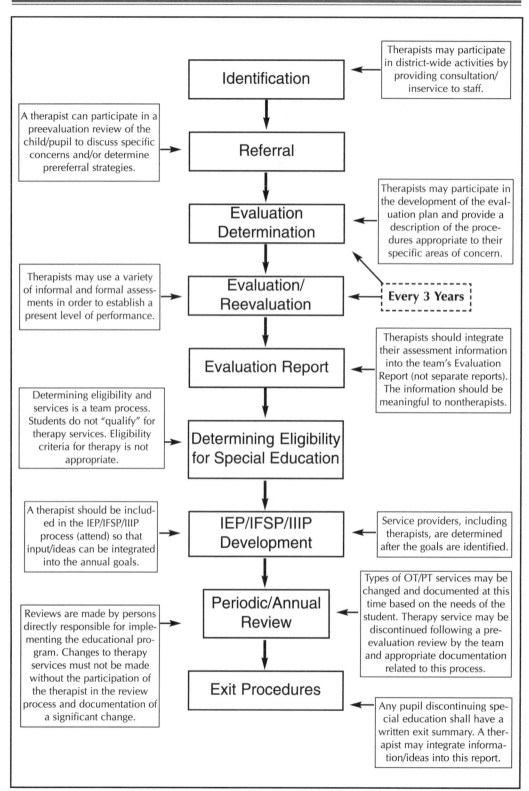

Figure 14-1. Therapist's role and responsibilities in due process.

are needed. The tools and materials selected must be culturally appropriate and valid for the purpose they are to be used. Information from the parent and general education staff must be included in the evaluation. Parents must give informed consent to perform an initial evaluation and also must provide consent to obtain or release information from other providers. Parents may refuse to have the evaluation performed and may refuse to release information. The LEA may choose to pursue due process to obtain the ability to have an evaluation performed.

Therapists need to work in collaboration with the entire team to determine the areas that need assessment and the tools and materials to be used. Procedures used by the physical therapist in performing an evaluation include administration of standardized tests, informal assessment, observation, interview, and review of records. As in the medical setting, the therapist must determine what is interfering with the student's ability to perform appropriate roles. Tests addressing functional skills, such as the School Function Assessment (SFA)[40] and the Pediatric Evaluation of Disability Inventory (PEDI),[41] are helpful in identifying needs and establishing a baseline of function. Impairments also are assessed, but evaluated in relation to how they impact the student's ability to function in the educational setting.

DETERMINING ELIGIBILITY FOR SPECIAL EDUCATION

Following the evaluation, the team must determine if the child qualifies for one or more disability categories. Generally, the disability categories require:

➤ That the student perform at or below a specific level on a standardized test

➤ Demonstrate through observation difficulty managing academic activities, difficulty with organization, or difficulties as a result of an identified condition (eg, cerebral palsy, deaf or hard of hearing, attention deficit)

➤ Demonstrate a need for special education

The only criteria for receiving physical therapy is that the child qualify for special education and demonstrate a need for special education and related services. Individual states or school districts should not have additional criteria for physical therapy. The need for physical therapy is not determined at the time of evaluation or determination of eligibility but at the end of the development of the IEP or IFSP.

Children who qualify for special education must be reevaluated every 3 years to determine if they still need special education. The physical therapist should participate in the reevaluation of children for which they are a part of the IEP/IFSP team. They may also participate in the reevaluation for any child whose team determines needs the expertise of the physical therapist to determine the needs of the child.

An integrated team report must be written by the team that summarizes the child's present level of performance and needs. This information then is the basis for the development of the child's IEP/IFSP.

IEP/IFSP DEVELOPMENT

The IEP and IFSP are legal contracts between the school district and the child and the child's family. They establish the framework for the child's special education program and any support or related services. Tables 14-1 and 14-2 list the components of the IEP and IFSP respectively.

The process for development of the IEP/IFSP begins by identifying the child's present level of function within the areas appropriate to the child's age. The information from the evaluation summary report, as well as information from the child when appropriate, child's parent(s), staff, and other appropriate individuals including outside providers is used as the basis for identifying the child's strengths, abilities and needs, and the family's concerns and priorities. From the statements of needs, the team prioritizes and develops goals and objectives that address these needs. It is important to address the identified needs as they relate to the educational program and recognize that not all identified needs have to be implemented in the IEP/IFSP. The team should prioritize which identified needs are important for the child for this IEP/IFSP and develop goals and objectives. In the development of the IFSP, the family's priorities and needs should be addressed before establishing expected outcomes or goals and objectives.[15,16,42] Once the goals and objectives are established they should not be considered static, but rather changing and evolving.[13] For those identified needs that team determines will not be included, a statement should be made regarding why they will not be addressed. Following the selection of the goals and objectives, the team determines which services are necessary for the child to achieve the identified goals and objectives. The team must determine if the expertise of the physical therapist is needed for the child to benefit from the identified educational program.

The goals and objectives form the basis for measuring change in the child's abilities and determining effectiveness of the selected program and services. As in the medical setting, the goals and objectives should be child focused, measurable, and context specific.[42,43] In the educational setting, the physical therapist works with the team to develop the child's goals and objectives. While the physical therapist may have more responsibility to develop and monitor a goal related to mobility, the entire team is responsible to implement the goal. Just as the physical therapist incorporates the child's communication and cognitive goals into activities and interactions with the child, the teacher incorporates the child's mobility goals into the classroom activities. The goals need to reflect what the child can attain within 1 year, how the child's condition impacts educational abilities, and have a direct link to the identified needs statements.[30]

Periodic Review

IDEA requires that the team review the child's progress at least as frequently as that done for the child's peers in general education. This means that the child's progress would be provided when reports are sent home for general education students, such as midterm reports and end of the quarter reports. Data need to be obtained throughout the year to determine progress and need for modification or development of new goals. NCLB legislation requires that all children will make progress. It is important that teams establish reasonable, attainable goals and objectives so that the child can demonstrate progress.

Periodic review is the time at which the team can decide to change goals and services including physical therapy services. A reevaluation is required to provide data to support the change in services. The physical therapist needs to be involved in the process to add, change, or discontinue physical therapy services.

Exit Procedures

Exit procedures generally apply to the discontinuation of special education. States define the procedures for determining if a student continues to qualify and have needs for special education. The procedures that allow for discontinuation of physical therapy are incorporated into the IEP/IFSP development and progress review as well as the reevaluation process. The physical therapist needs to be involved in the process to add, change, or discontinue physical therapy services.

Reimbursement of Therapy Services

Individual states have determined if and how they will coordinate state agencies and reimbursement from public and private sources. Following passage of EHA some private and public payers changed their policies to reduce or deny coverage of covered services for children if they received covered services through their school system. To address this, Congress passed the Medicare Catastrophic Coverage Act, PL 100-360. Section 411 (k)[13] specifically states that states cannot deny payment for Medicaid services "…because such services are included in the child's individual education program established pursuant to Part B of the Education of the Handicapped Act or furnished to a handicapped infant or toddler because such services are included in the child's individualized family service plan adopted pursuant to Part H of such Act."[26] Because this amendment was a technical amendment to Medicaid law, it has no impact on Medicare or private insurers unless they are involved in the state Medicaid program. To address private insurers, the IDEA was amended to allow states to seek reimbursement by having education be the payer of last resort, however, private payers are not required to participate and may deny payment. IDEA, Section 300.142(f), specifically states that when accessing a private payer parents must provide informed consent each time the district wishes to access the payer and that parental refusal to access private insurance does not "relieve the responsibility to provide all required services at no cost to the parent."[10]

Rogers[44] discussed "dangers to the family" that exist when schools access the family's private insurance. These include: "depletion of available lifetime coverage, depletion of annual or service charge, loss of future insurability, premium increase, or discontinuation of coverage."[44] LEAs also have expressed concerns regarding the use of private insurance as they are obligated to provide a "free" and appropriate public education. Their concerns include: payment of copays, request to pay increased premiums as a result of using the insurance, and the potential litigation resulting from the depletion of lifetime caps and the child, now an adult, who no longer has use of services.

The impact to school therapists may include additional documentation to meet the standards of the insurer, preauthorization, and denial with possible appeal. Each state determines the laws and rules and regulations that LEAs and therapists must follow. An important point is that the LEA cannot delay or deny any service that the child's IEP or IFSP team determines is necessary to meet the child's needs just because the service may or may not be reimbursed.[12]

Provision of Service

INTERVENTION OPTIONS

IDEA does not specify the types of intervention options that must be available to children with disabilities leaving it to states to define the types of services in their education laws. Generally two types of service that apply to special education and related or support services are defined. These are direct and indirect. Direct service usually is defined as those services provided directly to the child. The focus of direct service is to instruct the child. Indirect service may be defined as those services provided to the child, staff, and parents when appropriate. The focus of indirect service is to train the student and those working with the student throughout the day to incorporate activities that address the student's needs into the daily routine. An assumption should not be made that one type of service is better or worse than the other.[26,39] The service the child receives will depend on the individual child's identified needs, goals, and objectives as well as the specific educational program and setting.

The role of the physical therapist in the educational setting is to examine and evaluate the child (impairments/functional limitations/disabilities/fitness), the work environment (home/school/community/job), and the job (play/learn/work) expectations then determine how the child's condition impacts his or her ability to function and learn. Intervention *should* include adaptation or modification of the environment, task, and expectations; provision of assistive technology; training and instruction of the child, staff, and family; coordination and communication with appropriate providers; and interaction with the child. The specific type of interaction with the child will vary based on a multitude of factors,[21,45,46] but the focus for the physical therapist must always be on improving function in the educational setting, not fixing the impairments.[30]

When determining the type of service necessary to assist the child to benefit from special education, the physical therapist may wish to think in terms of what type of interaction is necessary, then apply the appropriate label. To assume that direct, one-to-one or pull-out service is the only way to have the physical therapist involved is erroneous.[26] Indirect service allows and frequently requires the physical therapist to be actively involved with the child and the team. In many cases it may be the preferred interaction as it embodies the principles of motor learning theory (see Chapter 3) and the educational constructs of a whole-child approach within the natural environment or LRE.

When making service delivery decisions, physical therapists must consider the following:

➤ Personal beliefs for how the brain learns, organizes, and uses information

➤ Role of environment in learning

➤ Role of family and social/emotional factors on learning

➤ Evidence-based practice that includes literature, self-experiences/knowledge, and patient/client preferences

➤ Purpose of education

➤ Impact of life-long condition on learning

➤ Management of life-long condition across the life span

➤ Continuum of service

➤ Models of service

➤ Timing and frequency of service that considers typical brain and body maturation, typical development for that specific condition, readiness of brain and child to learn the task, and level of expertise needed to assist the child to accomplish the goal

Evidence-based practice, that incorporates research, therapist experience, and desires of the child and family, forms the basis for making service delivery decisions.[47-49] Therapists need to evaluate their own beliefs and how those beliefs relate to current evidence.[45] Should the normal motor developmental sequence be used as the basis for pediatric therapy? While this may be a method to determine eligibility for special education, many believe that there is a need to address functional abilities using a motor learning approach emphasizing the interaction of the child with the task and the environment.[50-56] Studies have examined predictors of motor skills[51,57-59] and the frequency of intervention[60,61] and determined that it is important to address functional abilities and that the ideal frequency of intervention is unknown. Understanding of brain-based research and motor learning theory is essential for the physical therapist.[45] In order to impact learning, the child must be motivated to perform the task and must be able to repeatedly practice the task as it occurs within the natural setting.[53,62] Based on motor learning theory, Byl[63] stated that therapists would be unable to provide the amount of practice needed to impact learning and that our task should be to "mentor, guide, motivate, and teach our patients about the potential of their nervous system to adapt."[63]

Another important aspect to consider is that children who qualify for special education and related services generally have pathologies or conditions that are life-long. One of the physical therapist's roles is to help the family and child understand the condition and how to manage it as the child ages. It is important for the child and family to be aware of the implications of the condition, not only as they relate to the educational program, but how they may impact the child's ability to be independent as an adult and obtain post-secondary education, employment, health insurance, and a positive quality of life.[3-6] It should be expected that the involvement of the physical therapist will vary as the child's needs, priorities, and educational program changes. An "episode of care" in the educational setting should not be birth through 21 years, but rather there should be multiple episodes of care where the therapist moves in and out of service. The *Guide* provides information related to developing a plan of care and establishing appropriate anticipated goals and expected outcomes within the text and specific patterns.[21] Therapists also should consider factors that may modify the plan when considering the frequency and duration of service.[21,46]

Questions to consider when determining if the service to be provided is educationally necessary include:

➤ What role(s) does the child perform?

➤ What are the expectations for typically developing peers?

➤ How is the child functioning in the educational environments (home, school/community/work)?

➤ What is interfering with the child's ability to perform his/her role?

➤ Is the environment facilitating or interfering with the child's ability to perform his/her role?

➤ Is there assistive technology and how is it facilitating or interfering with the child's ability to perform his/her role?[64]

➤ Is this something that can be remediated, accommodated, or modified?

➤ Is this a priority to the child and/or family?

➤ Is this an educational priority as determined by the child's IEP/IFSP team?

➤ Is there a need to provide accommodations or modifications to the environment?

➤ Is there a need to provide assistive technology?

➤ Is the expertise of a physical therapist necessary to educate or train the child, family, or educational team?

➤ Is the expertise of a physical therapist necessary to address the identified needs, goals, and objectives?

➤ Is the expertise of a physical therapist necessary to assist the child to meet his/her educational goals?

SERVICE DELIVERY MODELS

The models for delivery of service have changed with the understanding of motor learning and the acceptance of children with disabilities in all educational settings. Evidence-based practice is not only a standard for the practice of physical therapy but also a requirement for education under NCLB legislation and the proposed 2003 revisions to IDEA. It is because of the evidence for learning in natural environments, doing real tasks and activities, and the legislative push to have all children benefit or be a part of general education that models for delivery of all educational services have changed.

Models can range from a more traditional "pull-out" service, to a full inclusion model with teachers and therapists providing services in the classroom, to a cooperative model with teachers and therapists providing consultation to classroom staff.[26,65] Massey-Sekerak et al[26] describes an integrated model of service delivery in which there is a continuum of service delivery models that the therapist can select based on the specific needs of the child. They note that consultation, working with the child's team, is a critical component of each model. As a result of their study, Massey-Sekerak et al[26] developed guidelines for integrating physical therapy services into preschool classrooms and identifying key components for successful integration. While these guidelines were based on interviews with therapists in preschool settings, the components easily can be applied to children in all settings.

The key to the provision of physical therapy is not what it is called, but rather how well it is integrated into the child's educational program. In an integrated model, the physical therapist has the option of providing service in or out of the classroom; working with the classroom staff, caregivers, and families; and providing patient/client-related instruction and coordination, communication, and documentation as needed to those in the educational program as well as outside providers and agencies.

In the integrated model, the therapist does not have separate goals, but the goals are the child's goals and are developed and implemented by the team.[18] When developing goals that are child- or family-focused it may be helpful to ask the child and family what is important to them, what is their lifestyle, and what is important in the future.[29,43] When working with families, therapists need to recognize and acknowledge that each family is different. Each family has a different value system which may be different from that of the therapist.[15,66,67] Cultural differences need to be addressed in the evaluation, identification of expected outcomes, and in materials and techniques used in intervention. The family's level of acceptance of the child and assistance from outsiders will impact their ability to participate in the IEP/IFSP process. The responsibility of the team is to determine which model and tools will address the individual family's needs appropriately.

Additional Roles of the Physical Therapist in Educational Settings

The *Guide* describes a number of roles of the physical therapist in addition to that of working with children with disabilities. These roles include consultation, education, critical inquiry, and administration. The physical therapist in the educational setting has the opportunity to participate in these roles in addition to his or her primary role of working with students, families, and staff. Listed below are the roles that may apply to the educational setting as adapted from the *Guide*,[21] the 1990 edition of the American Physical Therapy Association's (APTA's) guidelines and policies for *Physical Therapy Practice in Educational Environments*,[68] and the *Occupational Therapy and Physical Therapy in Educational Settings: A Manual for Minnesota Practitioners*.[30]

CONSULTATION

The *Guide* defines consultation as "the rendering of professional or expert opinion or advice by a physical therapist."[21] In the educational setting this includes interaction with teachers, administrators, parents, physicians, outside providers, community members, and other professionals or agencies. Activities may include classroom program development, general educational programming and long-range planning for children with disabilities, review of architectural plans or specific sites for accessibility, development of forms for documentation, providing peer review, and serving as a resource to administration. Due to educational and data privacy law, child-specific consultation only would occur if the physical therapist was a part of that specific child's evaluation process or a member of that child's IEP/IFSP team.

EDUCATION

The Guide defines education as "the process of imparting information or skills and instructing by precept, example, and experience so that individuals acquire knowledge, master skills, or develop competence."[21] Activities include planning and conducting general education inservice for staff, students, and parents about specific disabilities, body mechanics and lifting, evacuation for individuals with disabilities, general handling and positioning principles, and other topics that would complement the teacher-directed educational program. Physical therapists also can provide information regarding removal of architectural barriers, transportation needs, evacuation plans, special equipment needs, transition planning, prevocational and vocational planning, travel training, job site analysis, health/wellness and fitness plans, and long-range planning for students with disabilities. Again, due to educational and data privacy laws, patient/client-related education/instruction would occur only if the physical therapist was a part of that specific student's evaluation process or a member of that student's IEP/IFSP team.

CRITICAL INQUIRY

Critical inquiry, as defined in the *Guide*, is the "process of applying the principles of scientific methods to read and interpret professional literature; participate in, plan, and conduct research; evaluate outcomes data; and assess new concepts and technologies."[21] Activities include review of literature, evidence-based practice, collaborative research with physical therapist educational programs, outcomes data collection and analysis, and participation in study groups.

ADMINISTRATION

The *Guide* defined administration as the "skilled process of planning, directing, organizing, and managing human, technical, environmental, and financial resources effectively and efficiently."[21] Activities include coordination and implementation of services in a manner consistent with district, state, and federal educational and physical therapy practice regulations; purchase of equipment and supplies; staffing considerations; employment options; work and office space considerations; direction and supervision of physical therapist assistants; performance reviews; and clinical education of physical therapy students.

Employment Options

Physical therapists generally have two employment options, direct hire or contracting. In the direct hire option, the physical therapist is hired directly by a LEA or by a cooperative agency that serves several LEAs. Through this system, the therapist is placed on a teacher's contract and receives the same benefits as a teacher. The advantages of being an employee of the LEA are more direct contact with other staff, availability, flexibility in scheduling, and inclusion in the LEA "system" that includes professional liability insurance and health and disability benefits. The disadvantages may include supervision by an educational administrator, requirement to perform educational-related duties such as bus supervision, and limited contact with other therapists.[68]

When contracting, the therapist does not receive any of the "system" benefits of the LEA and must show proof of professional liability insurance. The advantages of contracting for the therapist may be in having more independence in determining the amount of time spent in the LEA and the case load. Generally, contracting is advantageous to the LEA when there are few students that require physical therapy service. Disadvantages include limited availability for additional meetings and interaction with staff and a payment system that frequently results in the LEA requesting therapist involvement only for direct student contact time and essential meetings. The *Minnesota State Manual* for occupational and physical therapists in the educational environment advises therapists that a contract should include the following: "purpose of the agreement, evidence of appropriate licensure of the therapist, availability of replacement therapists from agency, working conditions, documentation of expectations, identification of supervisory relationships and evaluation of staff performance, identification of how parties will resolve differences, payment schedule, cost of service and travel, effective dates, renewal conditions, and liability."[30]

Therapists should investigate all alternatives before deciding which option is best for them. Additional information may be available to the therapist by checking with the state's education department regarding any guidelines for school-based therapists and from each state's APTA chapter.

Staffing Considerations

When determining needs for staff, consideration must be given not only for student-related time, but also for the time needed for administrative tasks such as program development and planning; documentation requirements including development and writing of evaluations, IEPs, IFSPs, classroom programs, and third-party billing; student-related meetings including evaluation determination planning meetings, and IEPs/IFSPs; and staff training activities including general training and specific student training.

The need for physical therapy services is determined on an individual basis during the IEP or IFSP meeting. The law does not address case load limits for physical therapy. Each therapist needs to work with administration to ensure that the needs of students as well as the therapist are being addressed.

Performance Review

As in all physical therapy settings, performance review is an essential component to assure quality services. However, unlike most physical therapy practice settings, where the evaluating supervisor is a physical therapist, school physical therapists often are responsible to educational personnel, such as the school principal or the special education director. Performance standards such as professionalism, communication skills, organizational abilities, and adaptability and flexibility should be addressed in addition to the abilities of the therapist to perform specific examination or intervention techniques. If you are an employee of the school district, you may be required to participate in their performance appraisal process.

Peer review is a "system by which peers with similar areas of expertise assess the quality of physical therapy provided, using accepted practice standards and guidelines"[69] and may be used as a method of performance review. This process can include internal peer review by which therapists within the same setting evaluate their services and external peer review by which therapists outside the setting evaluate the services. In either review, peers use recognized professional standards and guidelines to determine the quality of service provided. The core documents for peer review include the APTA's *Standards of Practice and the Criteria*,[24] the *Guide*,[21] and *APTA Guidelines for Documentation*.[24] These and other professional documents can be accessed through APTA's web site, www.apta.org.

Conclusion

The purpose of education is to prepare children for adult life. The role of the physical therapist is to assist children with disabilities with that preparation. Physical therapists play an important role in the educational environment. As integral members of an educational team, physical therapists work to ensure the most appropriate education for children with disabilities. The physical therapist's unique skills in the understanding and implementation of motor learning and the impact of disease/conditions on function assist teachers, parents, administrators, and other educational staff in addressing the needs of children with disabilities.

Physical therapists in the educational setting have an ideal job—they practice in the actual setting that their clients need to perform. They have an excellent opportunity to implement strategies that facilitate motor learning and directly impact function. They can make a difference in the long-range life outcomes of a child by addressing the challenges of living with a disability. Theses challenges include employment, independence, relationships, and self-determination.[1-6,70-72] To do this the goals of the child need to be in terms of safe and efficient mobility, rather than "walking"; working on task for 1 to 2 hours, rather than developing head control; and health and wellness to have the physical capacity to work and play, rather than improving range of motion. We need to focus on the functional component of life not the impairments of the condition. We need to educate the child and family as to the lifelong implications of the condition and how to manage the condition so that the child can be as independent and self-reliant as possible. What an exciting challenge!

This chapter has provided an overview of the laws, roles, and functions of the physical therapist in the educational setting. Application of these topics will now be addressed in the case studies.

Case Study #1: Jason

➤ Practice pattern 5C: Impaired Motor Function and Sensory Integrity Associated With Nonprogressive Disorders of the Central Nervous System—Congenital Origin or Acquired in Infancy or Childhood (at age 24 months)

➤ Practice pattern 4C: Impaired Muscle Performance (at age 16 years)

➤ Medical diagnosis: Cerebral palsy, right hemiparesis

Jason initially was referred to his county interagency by his physician based on his birth history and medical diagnosis. Following an evaluation by the local school district an interagency team meeting was held with the family to discuss the results of the evaluation and determine eligibility for special education. Based on the evaluation, Jason met the eligibility criteria for early intervention services, having a diagnosed physical condition that has a high probability of resulting in developmental delay, and demonstrated a need for services in the areas of communication, adaptive development, and motor development. Jason's team developed an IFSP with the school, addressing needs in the areas of communication and self-help skills, and the family, through a private physical therapist, addressing the needs related to mobility. Through the school district, Jason received home-based services weekly, alternating visits from an early intervention teacher and an occupational therapist. He also received consultative services from the school physical therapist to coordinate services provided by his private physical therapist and to assist with transition to a school-based program when he was 3 years of age. Jason also participated in a center-based family support and play group once every other week. Through a private provider, Jason received private physical therapy for 3 months, one time a week, focusing on mobility in the home and community, as well as family education for his home program. Private physical therapy was to decrease to one time every 2 weeks with the private therapist coordinating services with the school physical therapist.

At age 3 years, Jason was eligible to participate in a community-based preschool program with support from special education. Jason's IFSP team began the transition to a center-based program that offered a model of inclusion with typically developing peers and coordination of special education and related services.

Depending on how Jason's impairments impact his ability to participate in his educational program, he may or may not continue to demonstrate a need for special education. He may continue to demonstrate a need for special education in elementary school but may not need the expertise of a physical therapist. Some states provide additional services in the area of developmental/adapted physical education, from which Jason's general motor skills and fitness needs may be addressed. It is appropriate for the physical therapist to be involved in Jason's 3-year reevaluations as a part of the evaluation team.

Jason is now 16 and a sophomore in high school. As a part of his comprehensive three-year reevaluation, the physical therapist and occupational therapist determine the impact of his disability on the transition areas. His parents have requested assistance in obtaining an evaluation to determine modifications or adaptations for driving. Jason states he would like to be able to drive as well as shoot baskets with both hands. As a result of growth and avoidance of use, Jason's right arm has become contracted so that he is unable to shake hands and has difficulty steering a car for driving. The team determines that Jason continues to meet the eligibility criteria for category (physically impaired) and demonstrates needs in the transition area for driving a car (travel training), ability to shake hands (jobs and job training, community participation), and fitness (overlies all transition areas) as related to flexibility, strength, and endurance of right arm and hand. Jason's IEP is developed with goals for driving, appropriate interaction with individuals in the community or on the job, and development of an individualized fitness plan. Jason's program includes a driving evaluation at a center for individuals with disabilities (interagency agreement with agency allows school district to send students to facility for evaluation and training) and participation in strength training classes at school. To facilitate attainment of his goals in strength training, a paraprofessional with additional training in high intensity strength training is assigned to work with Jason daily and a physical therapist is placed on indirect service with a burst of service three to four times per week for the first 3 weeks then weekly for the remaining 7 weeks. The physical therapist's role is to work with the strength training teacher and paraprofessional to develop, implement, and modify a high intensity strength training program for Jason that addresses his specific condition and needs (Figure 14-2).

Case Study #2: Jill

➤ Practice pattern 5C: Impaired Motor Function and Sensory Integrity Associated With Nonprogressive Disorders of the Central Nervous System—Congenital Origin or Acquired in Infancy or Childhood (at age 7)

➤ Medical diagnosis: Cerebral palsy, spastic quadriparesis, microcephaly, mental retardation, seizure disorder

➤ Age: 17 years

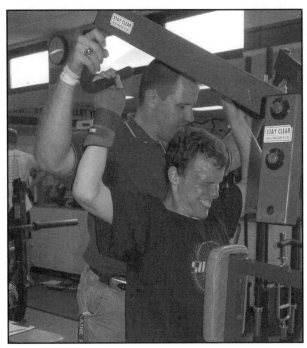

Figure 14-2. Strength training program for adolescent child with special needs.

Jill is now a senior in high school. She participates in a functional curriculum in the moderate-severe impairment (MSI) program, attends music class four times per week, and attends developmental/adapted physical education three times per week. As a part of her functional curriculum, Jill participates in a community outing one time per week, prevocational training two times per week, and apartment living 1 day per week. Jill's IEP team has exempted her from the statewide academic testing and has completed the alternative assessment. Jill's needs are addressed as they relate to the state's five areas of transition: jobs and job training, postsecondary education, recreation-leisure, community participation, and home-living.[70,71]

Jill has a tilt-in-space wheelchair with custom seating system. She is not able to propel her wheelchair, however, she is able to assist with cares by relaxing and assisting with movement and can perform a standing pivot transfer with minimal to moderate assistance. Jill never developed maintained head control but she is able to lift and control her head when motivated by the activity and is able to stay focused on a task for 5 to 10 minutes at a time. Her needs related to fitness include maintaining flexibility, functional strength, and endurance to participate in her educational program. She communicates through vocalizations and a simple augmentative device. She uses switches to interact with her environment. To participate in off-site community and work activities, Jill needs to tolerate sitting for 3 to 4 hours and be on task for a 10- to 15-minute period of time. She also needs to be able to manage cares with one staff person to assist and requires a private area with changing table.

The focus of Jill's program is on providing her with assistive technology that addresses her needs and facilitates her participation in her educational program. The physical therapist participates on Jill's IEP team to assist with problem solving for positions and equipment that will enhance her ability to participate in school and work activities. A hydraulic sit-to-stand upright stander is used at her work site to allow Jill to work while standing, take a break sitting, and resume standing to finish her work. Jill uses a supported gait trainer as part of her fitness plan in developmental/adapted physical education class. The physical therapist also has trained staff to incorporate movements into her daily routine and cares to address her flexibility. The physical therapist is able to assist with evaluation of community and potential work sites for accessibility and need for evacuation plans.

A major focus of Jill's program is on transition from high school. Jill's parents have decided that they would like Jill to continue in the district in the 18- to 21-year-old transition program. As a result, Jill is able to go through graduation ceremonies but will not accept her diploma. Jill's parents have been advised as to their need to address guardianship, as Jill will become her own guardian at age 18.[72] The physical therapist provides consultation regarding transition of medical providers from pediatric services to adult services and implications for future equipment needs.

Case Study #3: Taylor

➤ Practice pattern 5C: Impaired Motor Function and Sensory Integrity Associated With Nonprogressive Disorders of the Central Nervous System—Congenital Origin or Acquired in Infancy or Childhood (at age 4)

➤ Practice pattern 4C: Impaired Muscle Performance (at age 12)

➤ Medical diagnosis: Myelomeningocele, repaired L1-2

Taylor is now in seventh grade attending his neighborhood middle school. Taylor's middle school is a two-story building serving grades 6 to 8 with an average of 250 students per grade level. There are seven class periods, each 45 minutes, and a daily advisory period of 15 minutes, with a 5-minute passing time between classes and 30 minutes for lunch. He rides a regular bus route, using a regular bus equipped with a lift. Taylor has classes on the first and second floors, but his locker is located on first floor. Taylor decided in sixth grade to only use his manual wheelchair at school because of the amount of energy and time it took to walk between classes and because he was self-conscious of his body image (eg, less developed legs) when standing. He is independent in mobility within the building but has difficulty wheeling outside on the nature paths for science class and fields for physical education class. He is able to access all his learning stations in the classrooms either by transferring to a desk or wheeling under an adjustable height table. Taylor is independent in use of the elevator and opening inside and outside doors from his wheelchair. Taylor's evacuation plan when on the second floor for fire situations is to report to the fire rescue room. His method of evacuation is for the staff to lift and carry him in his solid frame wheelchair down the stairs. Taylor has a sling that he carries on his wheelchair in case there is a situation when staff are unable to lift him and his wheelchair. Taylor reports he sometimes has difficulty transferring into his friends' parents' cars. His parents report that they have a family membership at the YMCA and would like to have a specific program for Taylor to use when there.

Taylor demonstrates needs in the area of fitness as related to outside mobility and transfers. Taylor and his family also need education in how his condition impacts his ability to train and improve his fitness, as well as how Taylor can manage his condition as he ages. The physical therapist participates on Taylor's IEP to assist with developing, implementing, and monitoring his evacuation plan; his ability to access educational areas; and his mobility. The physical therapist works with the physical education and developmental/adapted physical education teacher to address Taylor's fitness plan. The physical therapist also works with Taylor's family to develop a training program at the YMCA and provides education to Taylor and his family regarding how his condition changes with age and what Taylor needs to do to manage his condition.

Case Study #4: Ashley

➤ Practice pattern 5B: Impaired Neuromotor Development (at age 15 months)
➤ Medical diagnosis: Down syndrome
➤ Age: 8 years

Ashley attends her neighborhood school in the third grade. Ashley's IEP team identified needs in preacademics (number and letter recognition, matching), social skills (turn taking, waiting in line, play, initiating interactions, independence), communication skills (conversation skills, written expression), motor skills (general endurance, ball skills, game skills, use of classroom tools), and functional skills (staying on task, following classroom routines, functional words, awareness of safety). Ashley's parents would like her to be able to play with children her age and be aware of what's gong on around her, especially when they are out in the community. The team prioritized the needs and developed goals and objectives and determined that Ashley would benefit from a program that included participation in the general education third grade classroom with a combination of in-class and out-of-class time to address her needs. The team prioritized safety areas and functional words that all staff would incorporate into their activities with Ashley. The general education and special education teacher agreed to collaborate on instruction of safety in the community as the classroom works on bus safety and general traffic and stranger safety as part of the general curriculum. The physical education teacher and the developmental/adapted physical education teacher agreed to collaborate on instruction of game and motor skills as well as general fitness.

To address Ashley's needs for improving her general endurance, following directions and classroom routines, and the parents' desire for Ashley to be able to play with her peers, the physical therapist proposed that the classroom participate in the Courageous Pacers[73] program as it addresses general fitness for kids and is an activity that Ashley could participate in with the whole class. The team agreed and the physical therapist worked with the classroom teacher to understand and incorporate the program into the classroom routine. Physical therapy services on the IEP were indirect, weekly for the first 4 weeks then monthly for the remainder of the IEP. The physical therapist put the following statement in the accommodations section of the IEP: "The physical therapist is available for consultation in the areas of fitness, mobility, and accessing educational activities and areas as needed by the team. The physical therapist will contact the IEP team a minimum of one time per month to monitor Ashley's program."

Case Study #5: John

➤ Practice pattern 5B: Impaired Neuromotor Development
➤ Medical diagnosis: Attention deficit hyperactivity disorder, developmental coordination disorder
➤ Age: 5 years

John's parents requested an educational evaluation following his medical work up that resulted in the dual diagnoses of ADHD and DCD. As a result of the parent request, the school referred John for an evaluation. An evaluation plan determination meeting was held at John's school and included the parental, kindergarten teacher, special education teacher, speech and language pathologist, school psychologist, principal, and a representative from the district's motor team (occupational therapist, physical therapist, and developmental/adapted physical education teacher). The team reviewed the medical reports and parent concerns. John's teacher provided information on how John was functioning in the classroom. An evaluation plan was developed with the developmental/ adapted physical education teacher assessing the motor skills and the physical therapist and occupational therapist assessing the motor abilities and functional skills.

Following the evaluation the team met with the parents to discuss the results and determine if John met any of the eligibility criteria for special education. Upon review of the evaluation results, John demonstrated difficulty with some tasks and activities, however, he did not meet the criteria for special education. The team discussed John's educational needs and it was determined that he did not need special education but would benefit from a 504 plan that addressed simple modifications and strategies for motor activities and behavior. The physical therapist, occupational therapist, and special education teacher are available to assist with the development and training of strategies for the teacher.

References

1. National Organization on Disability. 1998 N.O.D./Harris Survey of Americans with Disabilities. Available at www.nod.org/presssurvey. Accessed June 7, 2004.
2. Blackorby J, Wagner M. Longitudinal postschool outcomes of youth with disabilities: findings from the National Longitudinal Transition Study. *Exceptional Children.* 1996;62:399-413.
3. Johnson DR, Stodden RA, Emanuel EJ, et al. Current challenges facing secondary education and transition services: what research tells us. *Exceptional Children.* 2002;68:519-531.
4. Benz MR, Lindstrom L, Yovanoff P. Improving graduation and employment outcomes of students with disabilities: predictive factors and student perspectives. *Exceptional Children.* 2000; 66:509-529.
5. Babitt BC, White CM. "R U ready?" Helping students assess their readiness for postsecondary education. *Teaching Exceptional Children.* 2002;35:62-66.
6. Test DW, Browder DM, Karvone M, et al. Writing lesson plans for promoting self-determination. *Teaching Exceptional Children.* 2002;35:8-14.
7. Education for All Handicapped Children Act of 1975. 20 U.S.C. 1401.
8. Education of the Handicapped Act Amendments of 1986. 20 U.S.C. 1400.
9. Individuals With Disabilities Education Act of 1990. 20 U.S.C. 1400.
10. Individuals With Disabilities Education Act Amendments of 1997. 20 U.S.C. 1400.
11. Assistance to states for the education of children with disabilities and the early intervention program for infants and toddlers with disabilities; final regulations, Appendix A to Part 300. *Federal Register.* 1999;64(Suppl 48).
12. No Child Left Behind Act of 2001. Official US Department of Education Web site. Available at www.nclb.gov. Accessed June 7, 2004.
13. Able-Boone H, Sandall SR, Loughry A, et al. An informed, family-centered approach to Public Law 99-457: parental views. *Topics in Early Childhood Spec Educ.* 1990;10:100-111.
14. Cone J, Delawyer D, Wolf B. Assessing parent participation: the parent/family involvement index. *Exceptional Children.* 1985;51:417-424.
15. Bailey DB Jr, Simeonsson RJ. Critical issues underlying research and intervention with families of young handicapped children. *J Division Early Childhood.* 1984;8:38-48.

16. Dunst CJ, Trivette CM, Davis M, et al. Enabling and empowering families of children with health impairments. *CHC.* 1988;17:71-81.

17. Blackman JA. Early intervention: a global perspective. *Infants Young Children.* 2002;15:11-19.

18. McEwen I. *Providing Physical Therapy Services Under Parts B & C of the Individuals with Disabilities Education Act (IDEA).* Alexandria, Va: Section on Pediatrics, American Physical Therapy Association; 2000.

19. O'Neil ME, Palisano RJ. Attitudes toward family-centered care and clinical decision making in early intervention among physical therapists. *Pediatr Phys Ther.* 2000;12:173-182.

20. Code of Federal Regulations 300.550(b)(1-2), July 1988.

21. American Physical Therapy Association. *Guide to Physical Therapist Practice.* 2nd ed. Alexandria, Va: Author; 2001.

22. Assistance to states for the education of children with disabilities and the early intervention program for infants and toddlers with disabilities; final regulations, analysis of comments and changes. *Federal Register.* 1999;64(Suppl 48).

23. Rehabilitation Act of 1973 Section 504, 29 U.S.C. 794.

24. APTA. *House of Delegates Standards, Policies, Positions and Guidelines.* Alexandria, Va: American Physical Therapy Association; 2003.

25. McEwen I, Sheldon M. Pediatric therapy in the 1990s: the demise of the educational versus medical dichotomy. *Phys Occup Ther Pediatr.* 1995;15:33-45.

26. Massey-Sekerak D, Kirkpatrick DB, Nelson KC, et al. Physical therapy in preschool classrooms: successful integration of therapy into classroom routines. *Pediatr Phys Ther.* 2003;15:93-104.

27. Snell ME, Janney RE. Teachers' problem-solving about children with moderate and severe disabilities in elementary classrooms. *Exceptional Children.* 2000;66:472-490.

28. Utley BL, Rapport MJK. Essential elements of effective teamwork: shared understanding and differences between special educators and related service providers. *Physical Disabilities: Education and Related Services.* 2002;20:9-47.

29. Ovland Pilkington K, Malinowski M. The natural environment II: Uncovering deeper responsibilities with relationship-based services. *Infants Young Children.* 2002;15:78-84.

30. Bathke L, Bohmert J, Lillie L, et al. *Occupational Therapy and Physical Therapy in Educational Settings: A Manual for Minnesota Practitioners.* Roseville, Minn: Minnesota Department of Children, Families, & Learning; 2002.

31. Abelson MA, Woodman RW. Review of research on team effectiveness: implications for teams in schools. *School Psychology Review.* 1983;12:125-136.

32. Albano ML, Cox B, York J, et al. Educational teams for students with severe and multiple handicaps. In: York R, Schofield D, Donder D, et al, eds. *Organizing and Implementing Services for Students with Severe and Multiple Handicaps.* Springfield, Ill: Illinois Board of Education; 1981:23-34.

33. Bailey DB Jr. A triaxial model of the interdisciplinary team and group process. *Exceptional Children.* 1984;51:17-25.

34. Lyon S, Lyon G. Team functioning and staff development: a role release approach to providing integrated educational services for severely handicapped students. *J Assoc Severely Handicapped.* 1980;5:250-263.

35. Orelove FP, Sobsey D. Designing transdisciplinary services. In: Orelove FP, Sobsery D, eds. *Educating Children with Multiple Disabilities.* Baltimore, Md: Paul Brooks; 1987:1-24.

36. Sears CJ. The transdisciplinary approach: a process for compliance with Public Law 94-142. *TASH J.* 1981;6:22-29.

37. Harris SR. Transdisciplinary therapy model for the infant with Down syndrome. *Phys Ther.* 1980;60:420-423.

38. York J, Rainforth B, Giangreco MF. Transdisciplinary teamwork and integrated therapy: clarifying the misconceptions. *Pediatr Phys Ther.* 1990;2:73-79.

39. Rainforth B. Analysis of physical therapy practice acts: implications for role release in educational environments. *Pediatr Phys Ther*. 1997;9:54-61.

40. Coster W, Deeney T, Haltiwanger J, et al. *School Function Assessment*. San Antonio, Tex: Psychological Corporation; 1998.

41. Haley SM, Coster WJ, Ludlow LH, et al. *Pediatric Evaluation of Disability Inventory*. San Antonio, Tex: The Psychological Corporation; 1992.

42. Dole RL, Arvidson K, Byrne E, et al. Consensus among experts in pediatric occupational and physical therapy on elements of individualized education programs. *Pediatr Phys Ther*. 2003; 15:159-166.

43. Randall KE, McEwen IR. Writing patient-centered functional goals. *Phys Ther*. 2000;80:1197-1203.

44. Rogers JJ. Schools, insurance, and your family's financial security. *Exceptional Parent*. 1991;76-78.

45. Starks Hayes M, McEwen IR, Lovett D, et al. Next step: survey of pediatric physical therapists' educational needs and perceptions of motor control, motor development and motor learning as they relate to services for children with developmental disabilities. *Pediatr Phys Ther*. 1999;11:164-182.

46. Montgomery PC. Pediatric PT. *PT*. 1994;2(3):42-47,88-89.

47. Sackett DL, Straus SE, Richardson WS, et al. *Evidence-Based Medicine*. New York, NY: Churchill Livingston; 2000.

48. Law M. Strategies for implementing evidence-based practice in early intervention. *Infants Young Children*. 2000;13:32-40.

49. Dorling J, Salt A. Assessing developmental delay. *BMJ*. 2001;323:148-149.

50. Atwater SW. Should the normal motor developmental sequence be used as a theoretical model in pediatric physical therapy? In: Lister MJ, ed. *Contemporary Management of Motor Control Problems. Proceedings of the II Step Conference*. Fairfax, Va: Foundation for Physical Therapy; 1991:89-93.

51. VanSant AF. Motor control, motor learning, and motor development. In: Montgomery PC, Connolly BH, eds. *Clinical Applications for Motor Control*. Thorofare, NJ: SLACK Incorporated; 2003:79-106.

52. Attermeir S. Should the normal motor developmental sequence be used as theoretical model in patient treatment? In: Lister MJ, ed. *Contemporary Management of Motor Control Problems. Proceedings of the II Step Conference*. Fairfax, Va: Foundation for Physical Therapy; 1991:85-87.

53. Kamm K, Thelen E, Jenson JL. A dynamical systems approach to motor development. *Phys Ther*. 1990;70:763-775.

54. VanSant AF. Life-span motor development. In: Lister MJ, ed. *Contemporary Management of Motor Control Problems. Proceedings of the II Step Conference*. Fairfax, Va: Foundation for Physical Therapy; 1991:77-83.

55. Heriza C. Motor development: traditional and contemporary theories. In: Lister MJ, ed. *Contemporary Management of Motor Control Problems. Proceedings of the II Step Conference*. Fairfax, Va: Foundation for Physical Therapy; 1991:99-126.

56. Higgins S. Motor skill acquisition. *Phys Ther*. 1991;71:123-129.

57. Beals R. Cited in: Bleck EE. Cerebral palsy. In: Bleck EE, Nagel DA, eds. *Physically Handicapped Children: A Medical Atlas for Teachers*. 2nd ed. New York, NY: Grune & Stratton; 1982:59-132.

58. Bleck EE. Cerebral palsy. In: Bleck EE, Nagel DA, eds. *Physically Handicapped Children: A Medical Atlas for Teachers*. 2nd ed. New York, NY: Grune & Stratton; 1982:59-132.

59. Montgomery P. Predicting potential for ambulation in children with cerebral palsy. *Pediatr Phys Ther*. 1998;10:148-155.

60. Jenkins JR, Sells CJ, Brady D, et al. Effects of developmental therapy on motor impaired children. *Phys Occup Ther Pediatr*. 1982;2:19-28.

61. Law M, Cadman D, Rosenbaum P, et al. Neurodevelopmental therapy and upper-extremity inhibitive casting for children with cerebral palsy. *Dev Med Child Neurol.* 1991;33:379-387.

62. Hanft B, Pilkington K. Therapy in natural environment: the means or end goal for early intervention? *Infants Young Child.* 2000;12(Suppl 4):1-13.

63. Byl NN. Neuroplasticity: applications to motor control. In: Montgomery PC, Connolly BH, eds. *Clinical Applications for Motor Control.* Thorofare, NJ: SLACK Incorporated; 2003:79-106.

64. Morgan RL, Ellerd DA, Gerity BP, et al. That's the job I want! How technology helps young people in transition. *Teaching Exceptional Children.* 2000;32:50-55.

65. Cole KN, Harris SR, Eland SF, et al. Comparison of two service delivery models: in-class and out-of-class therapy approaches. *Pediatr Phys Ther.* 1989;1:49-54.

66. Bailey DB. Collaborative goal-setting with families: resolving differences in values and priorities for services. *Topics Early Childhood Spec Educ.* 1987;7:59-71.

67. Hanson M, Lynch E, Wayman K. Honoring the cultural diversity of families when gathering data. *Topics Early Childhood Spec Educ.* 1990;10:112-131.

68. American Physical Therapy Association. *Physical Therapy Practice in Educational Environments: Policies, Guidelines.* Alexandria, Va: Author; 1990.

69. American Physical Therapy Association. Guidelines for peer review training. In: *APTA Board of Directors Professional and Societal Policies, Positions and Guidelines.* Alexandria, Va: Author; 2003.

70. Demchak MA, Greenfield RG. A transition portfolio for Jeff, a student with multiple disabilities. *Teaching Exceptional Children.* 2000;32:44-49.

71. Modell SJ, Valdez LA. Beyond bowling transition planning for students with disabilities. *Teaching Exceptional Children.* 2002;34:46-52.

72. Squatrito Millar D, Renzaglia A. Factors affecting guardianship practices for young adults with disabilities. *Exceptional Children.* 2002;68:465-484.

73. Erson T. *Courageous Pacers.* Corpus Christi, Tex: Pro-Activ Publications; 1993.

Resources

American Physical Therapy Association: www.apta.org

APTA Section on Pediatrics: www.pediatricapta.org

Individuals With Disabilities Education Act Practices: www.ideapractices.org

National Organization on Disability: www.nod.org

National Youth Leadership Network: www.nyln.org

US Department of Education, No Child Left Behind: www.nclb.gov

US Department of Education, Office of Special Education Programs, Office of Special Education and Rehabilitation Services: www.ed.gov/offices/OSERS/OSEP

chapter 15

THE CHILDREN: PHYSICAL THERAPY MANAGEMENT

Patricia C. Montgomery, PhD, PT, FAPTA
Barbara H. Connolly, EdD, PT, FAPTA

A major focus of this text has been to move away from conceptualizing issues relevant to physical therapists as being based on the medical diagnoses of children with developmental disabilities. Instead, the authors of the various chapters have emphasized use of the disablement model, which focuses on functional limitations and related impairments. Physical therapists typically do not address underlying pathology, such as occurs with genetic syndromes, destruction of brain tissue associated with anoxia, or cardiac defects. Emphasis in physical therapy is on the sequelae of pathology and the relationship to functional limitations.

The purpose of this chapter is to summarize the primary functional limitations for each of the children in the five case studies. We also hypothesize about the primary impairments that are contributing to functional limitations. Although for teaching purposes, examination, evaluation, and intervention strategies related to specific problem areas have been presented in separate chapters, physical therapists must address the "big picture" and attempt to identify the primary issues related to intervention for children who demonstrate a variety of multiple interacting variables.

We also have taken the position that physical therapists are engaging more in prediction and management of physical therapy needs for children with developmental disabilities. In that regard, we have hypothesized about future considerations for intervention and periodic episodes of care.

Case Study #1: Jason

➤ Practice pattern 5C: Impaired Motor Function and Sensory Integrity Associated With Nonprogressive Disorders of the Central Nervous System—Congenital Origin or Acquired in Infancy or Childhood
➤ Medial diagnosis: Cerebral palsy, right hemiparesis
➤ Age: 24 months

Primary Functional Limitations

➤ Unable to use right arm and hand effectively for self-care tasks or manipulation of toys
➤ Does not protect himself adequately with loss of balance
➤ Falls frequently, especially when attempting to move quickly or run

➤ Unable to keep up with peers in play situations, especially outdoors

➤ Demonstrates difficulty eating textured food, often losing food out of his mouth or choking

➤ Does not communicate well using speech, relying more on gestures

Primary Impairments

➤ Poor sensory awareness on the right side of the body/mild disregard

➤ Motor control deficits on right side of body

➤ Sensory and motor deficits in oral-motor musculature

➤ Immature balance reactions and postural control

➤ Generalized weakness of right extremities

➤ Limited flexibility of muscles on right side of body

➤ Poor respiratory control

Primary Goals

➤ Improve sensory awareness on right side of body, as well as in oral-motor structures

➤ Improve balance reactions and postural control, especially in standing

➤ Improve coordination and speed during gross motor tasks, such as running

➤ Improve coordination during bilateral fine motor tasks

➤ Increase strength of right trunk and extremities

➤ Increase range of motion of right extremities and trunk

➤ Improve coordination of respiration with eating, drinking, sound/speech production tasks, and during gross motor skills

➤ Increase symmetry during sitting, standing, and fine motor activities

Primary Functional Outcomes

SELF-CARE

Jason will:

➤ Use both hands to take off socks

➤ Eat soft meats without losing food out of his mouth

➤ Take three to four sips of liquid from an open cup before pausing to breathe with no gasping or choking

➤ Maintain symmetrical lip closure on a cup rim without losing liquid

➤ Remove food from spoon without losing food out of mouth

➤ Sit on a bench and assist with removing a t-shirt

COMMUNICATION

Jason will:

➤ Sustain the volume of vocal sounds for simple songs and noises

GROSS AND FINE MOTOR SKILLS

Jason will:

➤ Use both hands to catch and throw a 12-inch diameter ball

➤ Reach forward for a 12-inch diameter ball with both elbows extended

➤ Grasp a hat with both hands and reach overhead with both arms to place it on his head

➤ Begin to "scribble" and "color" with the right hand using large color markers

➤ Run 10 to 20 feet and keep up with peers

➤ Be able to play "leapfrog" bearing weight on both extremities for several seconds

➤ Spontaneously position toys at midline or slightly to the right side of the body during play, two of five trials

➤ Independently bench-sit with symmetrical weight-bearing

➤ Climb on and off furniture using reciprocal movements in upper and lower extremities

➤ Ambulate on a community playground, mounting and dismounting from at least four pieces of equipment without falling

AMBULATION

Jason will:

➤ Walk up and down three to five steps, holding on to a railing, using a reciprocal pattern

➤ Demonstrate ability when walking to change direction quickly without falling, two of three attempts

➤ Walk in his playroom at home picking up and carrying items requiring two hands for support, then placing the items on a shelf at shoulder height

SAFETY

Jason will:

➤ Fall fewer than three times a day

➤ Use his arms to catch himself when he falls

➤ Demonstrate awareness of temperature differences in environmental objects with both hands

➤ When standing not fall over when bumped or pushed by another child

Additional Considerations/Prognosis

Although age-appropriate gross motor skills, such as balancing on one foot or walking a balance beam, may never be accomplished at the same level as his peers, Jason's physical therapy prognosis for functional gross motor skills (eg, walking up and down curbs, ramps, stairs) is excellent. Studies of potential for ambulation indicate that almost all children with spastic hemiparesis become independent ambulators.[1-3] When Jason's current level of motor performance is examined in relation to the Gross Motor Function Classification System (GMFCS),[4-6] he is classified at Level I, or the highest level of independent mobility in children with cerebral palsy.

In predicting and managing Jason's physical therapy needs, the physical therapist will want to emphasize intervention directed to the upper extremity. Lack of upper extremity dexterity and hand function presents the greatest potential for difficulties with fine motor and activities of daily living (ADL) tasks as Jason matures. Peterson and Peterson[7] stated that a direct therapeutic focus on the involved upper extremity in children with hemiplegia may result in frustration and withdrawal from the activity. They recommended an indirect strategy of adapting activities and toys in such a way that the two hands must be used to successfully complete the activity. The challenge for the physical therapist is to collaborate with the family, school staff, and others involved with Jason to determine appropriate activities and toys during various episodes of care that will promote bilateral upper extremity use and improved functional skills.

Several case studies of children with hemiplegia[8-11] suggest that constraint-induced therapy may be of benefit in improving function of the involved upper extremity and this treatment strategy should be explored with Jason and his family. Neuroplasticity is present throughout the life span. Functional magnetic resonance imaging has been used to measure cortical plasticity.[12] In one study, a 15-year-old girl with right hemiplegia demonstrated that motor tasks were associated with bilateral cortical activation, and language function was "rewired" to the contralateral hemisphere.[13] Cortical reorganization also has been reported in other individuals with hemiplegia.[14,15]

Children with spastic quadriparesis often have intellectual impairments, while approximately half the children with hemiparesis have IQs in the average range.[16,17] The presence of a seizure disorder in children with hemiplegia markedly increases the risk for cognitive deficits.[18] Frampton and coworkers[19] studied a sample of 149 children with hemiplegia between 6 to 10 years of age. Fifty-nine of these children had cognitive and predicted academic abilities within the average range. However, 36% were determined to have at least one specific learning difficulty (SLD). Those children with a SLD had more severe neurological impairments and a significantly higher rate of emotional and behavioral difficulties than the other children with hemiplegia who did not demonstrate a SLD.

Although Jason's cognitive abilities are difficult to predict at 2 years of age, he appears to have age-appropriate play skills and does not have a seizure disorder. It is likely that Jason will be able to attend the neighborhood elementary and high school with his peer group. He may not demonstrate intellectual difficulties as he matures, but if SLD should become evident, he would qualify for special education services.

Jason's motor needs may be addressed sufficiently through school and community-based programs. Private physical therapy services, however, may be indicated on an episodic basis to monitor the need for and fit of a lower extremity orthosis. There is evidence that lower extremity orthotics improve some gait parameters in children with cerebral palsy.[20,21] However, one study of children with cerebral palsy did not reveal improved ambulation and balance in a functional context when wearing orthoses, although many of the children noted increased feelings of stability and comfort.[22]

Antispasticity intervention also may be considered in the future for Jason. He may be a candidate for injections of Botox (Allergan, Irvine, Calif) to either the lower or upper extremity. Although some gait parameters in children with cerebral palsy are reported to improve with Botox injections,[23,24] there is some question as to whether lower extremity function improves.[25] Similarly, Correy et al[26] studied the effect of botulinum toxin type A on the upper extremities of children with hemiplegia. The children demonstrated increased maximal active elbow and thumb extension and improved grasp and release scores. However, fine motor function did not improve and, in some cases, temporarily decreased.

Jason and his family should be encouraged to explore community resources as his motor skill level increases and his interest in sports or fitness-related activities become evident.

As an adolescent and adult, Jason should be able to manage his care in relation to his hemiparesis. Periodic consultation with a physical therapist may be helpful to problem solve any difficulties he may encounter at home or work or to address home program or fitness needs.

Case Study #2: Jill

➤ Practice pattern 5C: Impaired Motor Function and Sensory Integrity Associated With Nonprogressive Disorders of the Central Nervous System—Congenital Origin or Acquired in Infancy or Childhood

➤ Medical diagnosis: Cerebral palsy, spastic quadriparesis, microcephaly, mental retardation, seizure disorder

➤ Age: 7 years

Primary Functional Limitations

➤ Nonambulatory
➤ Unable to maintain balance in any position
➤ Limited floor mobility
➤ Poor voluntary grasp and release for fine motor skills
➤ Problems eating and drinking
➤ Problems with visual tracking and focusing
➤ Requires maximal support in all positions
➤ Limited communication skills
➤ Inability to perform self-care skills

Primary Impairments

➤ Lack of motor control
➤ Limited cognitive ability
➤ Limited range of motion of trunk and extremities
➤ Generalized weakness
➤ Sensory hypersensitivity
➤ Seizure disorder
➤ Limited respiratory function
➤ Poor ocular control

Primary Goals

➤ Increase attention to visual and auditory stimuli
➤ Increase strength
➤ Improve motor control
➤ Improve ability to tolerate sensory input

➤ Maintain or improve range of motion

➤ Improve ability to bear weight in standing

➤ Improve coordination of respiration with oral and pharyngeal activity during eating, drinking, and sound/speech production

➤ Demonstrate a gross grasp

➤ Improve ocular control with emphasis on downward gaze

Primary Functional Outcomes

SELF-CARE

Jill will:

➤ Tolerate being lifted from her wheelchair and carried during movement transitions without signs of distress

➤ When positioned in her adapted wheelchair, maintain lip and jaw closure during feeding and appropriately close lips and jaw on the rim of a drinking glass

➤ Tolerate having a toothbrush brought into her mouth for oral hygiene, without increased cheek/lip retraction

➤ Maintain elbow extension while she pushes her arm through a coat sleeve

COMMUNICATION

Jill will:

➤ Produce a vowel sound for 2 to 3 seconds to communicate that she wants an adult's attention

➤ Reach above 60 degrees, three of five attempts in supported sitting, to touch a communication (eg, picture) board

GROSS AND FINE MOTOR SKILLS

Jill will:

➤ Hold head erect for 5 minutes when positioned in her vertical stander to watch a classroom activity or video

➤ Maintain range of motion to be comfortable in her wheelchair and stander and while positioned prone on the floor

➤ Roll from prone to supine, one of five attempts

➤ Lift her head in prone on elbows position and maintain the position for 5 seconds to visually locate a toy placed in front of her

➤ Participate in 20 minutes of aerobic exercise with her peers while positioned either in a partial body weight-bearing device, a gait trainer, or a mobile stander and assisted by an adult

➤ Grasp an object placed in her hand, five of 10 attempts in supported sitting

➤ Release an object that is stabilized by an adult, one of five attempts in supported sitting

➤ Use one upper extremity to bat at a joystick in preparation for a trial with a power wheelchair

AMBULATION

Jill will:

➤ Maintain assisted standing balance for 3 to 5 seconds during standing pivot transfers

➤ Stand and transfer, with the assist of one adult supporting her around the upper chest area, from her wheelchair to a classroom chair of equal height, requiring her to take two steps

SAFETY

Jill will:

➤ Right and maintain her head in vertical when being lifted or carried as part of her daily care at home and school

Additional Considerations/Prognosis

Jill's prognosis for independent motor function is poor. She has multiple severe impairments that interfere with her ability to develop gross motor and functional skills. Epilepsy is estimated to occur in approximately one-third of children with cerebral palsy and is more common in children with hemiplegia or quadriplegia than in children with diplegia.[27] Seizure disorders may be related to cortical involvement and severity of brain damage in children with hemiplegia and quadriplegia compared to brain damage that is more periventricular (ie, children with diplegia). It is likely that Jill will require moderate to maximal assist for ADLs as she matures. She is classified at Level V of the GMFCS,[4-6] representing children with cerebral palsy with the most limited independent function and mobility. Emphasis in physical therapy management will be on minimizing the development of secondary impairments and maximizing Jill's ability to assist with her care, thereby minimizing the level of assistance required of her caregivers while increasing her independence. Additional resources should be directed at developing a functional communication system for Jill so she will be able to express her needs to her caregivers to the greatest extent possible.

An ongoing maintenance program (administered by caregivers as part of Jill's daily routine) to maintain range of motion would be an important component of intervention for Jill. A pilot study of the effects of lower extremity passive stretching on children and youth with severe limitations in self-mobility suggested that, for this sample of subjects, nonintervention periods lasting greater than 5 weeks may result in loss of passive range of motion.[28] If Jill's limited range of motion in her trunk and extremities increases, antispasticity interventions may be considered. Intervention in this area would have to be considered carefully. The least invasive procedures (eg, serial casting or botulinum toxin injections) should be considered before surgical type interventions. Because Jill can assist with standing pivot transfers and has some head control, it would be important to preserve these functions. In that regard, insertion of a baclofen pump would be preferable to a selective dorsal rhizotomy. If there are negative functional sequelae (due to loss of stiffness and ability to bear weight), the dosage can be adjusted or the pump removed. Selective dorsal rhizotomy, however, would be a permanent, nonreversible procedure. Latash and Anson stated "we cannot agree, however, with the advocacy of destructive surgical procedures and blockades which may be effective in correcting some motor patterns but are also likely to create an additional source of disorders. These procedures may be used temporarily, until a better nondestructive treatment is available. For example, introducing intrathecal baclofen for treatment of spasticity of spinal origin has made destructive procedures for this disorder obsolete."[29]

As she ages, Jill's scoliosis may increase and she is at risk for hip subluxation or dislocation. Bleck[30] stated that dislocation of the hip is most prevalent in nonambulatory children with cerebral palsy who demonstrate total body involvement. He reviewed various orthopedic procedures to address hip dislocation based on the age of the child and potential for ambulation. It would be important for the physical therapist to review empirical studies in regard to the necessity for and expected outcomes of surgery. Pritchett[31] compared similar groups of adult patients with severe cerebral palsy and unstable hips to determine whether orthopedic surgery assisted with their care. Level of pain, sitting ability, pelvic obliquity, scoliosis, difficulty with nursing care, and complications such as decubitus ulcers and fractures did not differ between 50 treated and 50 untreated individuals. There also were no differences in frequency of complications between those who had stable hips following surgery (N=29) and those whose hips were still dislocated (N=21).

Because of her limited motor abilities and limited amount of weight bearing, Jill is at risk for osteoporosis and fractures. Skeletal maturation also may be delayed. In one study of children with cerebral palsy, skeletal maturation frequently was delayed and was present in early infancy with or without malnutrition or growth retardation. The authors speculated "that the cause of bone maturation delay might be deviated or disrupted embryonic bone maturation potentials."[32] With maturation the negative neuropathic effects of the central nervous system damage, severity and type of motor impairments, and nutritional deficiencies may have an additive effect on prenatally disturbed skeletal maturation potentials.

Episodic physical therapy care may be indicated to: periodically review Jill's status and her equipment, update her home program, and train her caregivers.

Case Study #3: Taylor

➤ Practice pattern 5C: Impaired Motor Function and Sensory Integrity Associated With Nonprogressive Disorders of Central Nervous System—Congenital Origin or Acquired in Infancy or Childhood

➤ Medical diagnosis: Myleomeningocele, repaired L1-2

➤ Age: 4 years

Primary Functional Limitations

➤ Requires external support to stand and ambulate

➤ Has difficulty maintaining balance in sitting and on hands and knees when reaching outside his base of support

➤ Requires assistance for lower body dressing

➤ Demonstrates limited independent transitions during floor mobility

➤ Requires assistance for wheelchair and toilet transfers

➤ Cannot keep up with peers when walking with an assistive device or propelling wheelchair

➤ Communication often limited to sentences three to four words in length

➤ Has difficulty with fine motor preschool activities such as tracing

Primary Impairments

➤ Loss of cutaneous and proprioceptive sensation below T-12
➤ Loss of motor function below T-12
➤ Problems with visual processing, especially figure-ground discrimination
➤ Inadequate balance reactions
➤ Generalized muscle weakness
➤ Limited endurance for motor activities
➤ Limited range of motion in hip musculature
➤ Poor respiratory function

Primary Goals

➤ Improve visual perceptual skills, especially figure-ground discrimination
➤ Improve balance reactions in all positions
➤ Increase strength of upper extremity and trunk muscles
➤ Decrease frequency of skin breakdown
➤ Increase independence in transfers
➤ Decrease sensitivity to head bending in standing
➤ Increase endurance for ambulation and propelling wheelchair
➤ Improve protective reactions in standing
➤ Increase speed of ambulation
➤ Improve coordination of respiration with oral and pharyngeal activities during speech and feeding activities
➤ Increase range of motion in lower extremities for proper alignment in orthotics
➤ Improve independence in self-care skills

Primary Functional Outcomes

SELF-CARE

Taylor will:
➤ Transfer in and out of his wheelchair to a classroom chair with minimal assist
➤ Drink three to four sips of liquid from a cup before stopping to breathe
➤ Put on and remove sweatpants with minimal assistance while sitting on the floor leaning against furniture or a wall

COMMUNICATION

Taylor will:
➤ Be able to walk with his walker, wheel his wheelchair, and make movement transitions while producing coordinated sounds such as in singing, yelling, or counting for up to 30 seconds
➤ Produce sentences of three to four words on one exhalation without running out of breath support

Gross and Fine Motor Skills

Taylor will:

➤ Independently lift his body weight with his arms during transfers

➤ Actively participate in movement games and activities for 30 minutes daily without needing a rest

➤ Propel his wheelchair from the classroom to the cafeteria at the same speed of his peers

➤ Self-propel his wheelchair for 10 to 15 minutes during community outings with three brief rest breaks

Ambulation

Taylor will:

➤ Maintain standing balance in his new orthotics for 15 seconds with his eyes closed (with crutches)

➤ Maintain standing balance in his new orthotics for 1 minute while moving his head up, down, right, and left (with crutches)

➤ Use his walker and follow a visual pattern (trail) on the floor without becoming unsteady or losing his balance

Safety

Taylor will:

➤ Correctly put on shoes and socks eliminating potential pressure areas every time

➤ From standing, actively fall forward on a 3-inch thick mat and catch himself with his arms, without hitting his head on the mat

Additional Considerations/Prognosis

Taylor has an L1-2 or high lumbar myelomeningocele. Studies comparing the level of lesion to ambulatory outcomes[33,34] suggest that Taylor has a guarded prognosis for independent ambulation (with orthoses and assistive devices). Williams et al[35] examined age-related walking in children with spina bifida. In the sample of children they followed, there were 10 children with high lumbar level lesions. Five of these children walked at an average age of 5 years, 2 months, but three ceased walking at an average age of 6 years, 11 months. Therefore, by 7 years of age, only two of the 10 children were ambulating. In two separate 25-year follow-up studies of individuals with spina bifida,[36,37] none of the participants with sensory or motor levels above L3 used ambulation for the majority of mobility, being primarily wheelchair dependent. This was in contrast to all but a few of the individuals with sacral level lesions who were community ambulators.

The increased energy expenditure required to ambulate often is excessive for the child when combined with energy requirements to perform other ADL and academic tasks.[38] Additional variables that adversely affect reaching an expected level of ambulation in children with myelomeningocele have been documented[39] to include: balance disturbances, occurrence of spasticity in knee and hip movement, an increased number of shunt revisions, and lack of motivation.

Physical therapists should provide education to children with spina bifida and their families regarding warning signs of tethering of the spinal cord and latex allergies. Tethering of the spinal cord is a complication associated with spina bifida.[40-42] It occurs as a result of pathological fixation of the spinal cord, resulting in traction on neural tissue. Ischemia and progressive neurological deterioration will occur unless there is a surgical intervention. In one 25-year follow-up study of 71 patients with myelomeningocele, a tethered cord requiring surgical release occurred in 23 individuals and the average age of symptoms was 10.9 years.[37] Symptoms can include: increased scoliosis, gait changes, increased spasticity in the lower extremities, back and leg pain, decreased muscle strength, lower extremity contractures, urinary bladder changes, and changes in motor or sensory level in extremities.[37,40,41] In the same 25-year follow-up study, latex allergy occurred in 32% of the individuals at an average age of 12.5 years. In several cases, the latex allergy was severe with life-threatening anaphylactic reactions.

Children with spina bifida and hydrocephalus are at risk for learning disabilities due to malformations of the CNS (neural tube defect). Yeates et al[43] examined verbal and learning memory in 41 children with myelomeningocele (33 with a history of shunted hydrocephalus). The children were between 8 to 15 years of age and demonstrated delayed recall of words compared to a control group of children. The children without shunts demonstrated better long-delay free recall than children with shunts but the differences in performance were not significant. Dennis and Barnes[44] studied 31 young adults with spina bifida and hydrocephalus who, as children, demonstrated poor math problem-solving skills. As a group, these young adults demonstrated poor problem solving and limited functional numeracy. Adult functional numeracy (but not functional literacy) was predictive of a higher level of social, personal, and community independence. In the 25-year follow-up study by Bowman and coworkers,[37] 85% of the children attended high school or college. Sixty-three percent of the children attended regular education classes, 14% needed additional assistance, and 23% were in special education. Taylor's perceptual-motor difficulties and academic performance will need to be monitored throughout his school years and intervention strategies and goals individualized to enhance his motor, cognitive, and social skills. It is likely that Taylor will need some level of special education services throughout his academic career.

As Taylor matures, he may wish to explore a combination of mobility devices, including a sports wheelchair and/or powered mobility. As an adult, he may develop the ability to live independently, but will need many architectural adaptations to accommodate his functional limitations and his primary use of a wheelchair for mobility. He also may need some level of support services in an independent living situation. Bowman and coworkers[37] found that 77% of the 71 individuals they followed continued to live at home with parents while 4% lived in residential homes and only 15% lived independently in the community.

Taylor's physical therapist (private and/or school-based) should work with him to improve his transfer, mobility, self-care skills, and fitness level as he matures. Physical therapy would not be provided continuously, but would be episodic as new needs or issues arise.

Case Study #4: Ashley

➤ Practice pattern 5B: Impaired Neuromotor Development
➤ Medical diagnosis: Down syndrome
➤ Age: 15 months

Primary Functional Limitations

➤ Avoids movement
➤ Moves slowly, cannot keep up with peers
➤ Does not attempt to cruise at furniture
➤ Falls over easily in all positions
➤ Does not assist in self-cares
➤ Does not interact with peers in play activities
➤ Loses liquid and food from her mouth during feeding
➤ Cannot pick up small objects

Primary Impairments

➤ Hypermobile joints
➤ Low muscle tone
➤ Mild conductive hearing loss
➤ Intellectual deficits
➤ Poor balance reactions and postural control
➤ Generalized weakness
➤ Poor endurance
➤ Poor oral sensory awareness
➤ Poor motor control

Primary Goals

➤ Increase stability in all positions
➤ Increase strength and endurance for motor activities
➤ Decrease apprehension regarding movement activities
➤ Improve balance reactions and postural control in all positions
➤ Improve oral-motor skills for feeding and sound/speech production tasks
➤ Develop voluntary controlled release and pinch
➤ Demonstrate goal-directed play
➤ Assist with self-cares

Primary Functional Outcomes

Self-Care

Ashley will:
➤ Use her lower lip to stabilize under a cup rim when cup is presented for drinking with minimal loss of fluid
➤ Lose only a minimal amount of food out of her mouth during snack time
➤ Pick up Cheerios independently during snack time
➤ While sitting on the floor, take off her shoes (laces undone) independently

COMMUNICATION

Ashley will:

➤ Smile or produce sounds during movement activities such as swinging in a swing, rocking in a chair, or propelling a small riding toy

GROSS AND FINE MOTOR SKILLS

Ashley will:

➤ Move from standing to sitting to all-fours position with minimal assist with no indications of apprehension

➤ Move around her parent-infant classroom (any method) to obtain a toy without prompting or assist from an adult

➤ Release objects into containers independently during play

AMBULATION

Ashley will:

➤ Begin to cruise at a support surface, three to four steps in either direction, to obtain a toy

➤ Take steps to "walk" 5 feet between her parents in play

➤ Push a push toy in standing for 10 to 15 feet with stand-by assistance for safety

SAFETY

Ashley will:

➤ Be able to reach laterally for a toy while sitting without loss of balance

➤ Catch herself 50% of the time with loss of balance in all fours

Additional Considerations/Prognosis

Children with Down syndrome have a good prognosis for developing motor skills and the average age for achieving independent ambulation is around 2 years of age.[45]

Physical therapists should be aware of the possibility of atlantoaxial instability that is estimated to occur in 12% to 20% of individuals with Down syndrome.[46,47] Radiographs are recommended at 2 years of age and periodically administered in childhood and adolescence. Children with asymptomatic instability typically do not require surgery, but should not engage in contact sports, gymnastics, diving, or other activities that might result in injury to the cervical spine. After the early intervention and preschool period, Ashley may not require motor-based services other than consultative physical therapy through her school district and adaptive physical education. Ashley's physical therapist should encourage the family to participate in school and community-based motor programs that will address fitness and life-long leisure skills for Ashley.

Spano and coworkers[48] studied perceptual motor competence in school-age children with Down syndrome between 4.5 and 14 years. Some aspects of gross motor function showed delayed development, but regular acquisitions. All aspects of fine motor skills assessed were more severely impaired and did not show similar development with age. In this sample of children, accuracy and timing of tasks requiring bimanual coordination were most impaired as compared to balance and ball skills, which showed more variability. Because of the cognitive deficits associated with Down syndrome, Ashley will be eligible for special education services throughout her school years. Individualized education plan (IEP) goals during her academic career and eventual vocational goals and training will need to be matched to Ashley's individual profile of motor abilities.

It is anticipated that, as an adult, Ashley will be able to function in a group home situation unless she remains at home with her parents. She also will be able to attend vocational training and work in a supervised setting within the community or through a work program for adults with developmental disabilities.

Unfortunately, recent studies have documented that many individuals with Down syndrome begin to develop dementia as they reach middle-age. Cognitive changes in about one-third of individuals with Down syndrome after age 35 years have been noted.[49] These cognitive changes have been associated with neuropathological changes in the brain of individuals with Down syndrome and with signs similar to patterns seen with Alzheimer's disease. Wisniewski et al[49] identified loss of vocabulary, recent memory loss, impaired short-term visual retention, difficulty in object identification, and loss of interest in surroundings as early cognitive changes. Dalton and Crapper[50] described memory loss in persons with Down syndrome ages 39 to 58 years over a 3-year period of time. Four of the 11 subjects deteriorated over the 3 years to the point that they could no longer learn a simple discrimination task. Fenner et al[51] found that the greatest decline in function was in a 45- to 49-year-old group. Physical therapists and occupational therapists should be aware of early signs of dementia in persons with Down syndrome and be prepared to intervene as necessary to retain as much adaptive functioning as possible.

Case Study #5: John

➤ Practice pattern 5B: Impaired Neuromotor Development
➤ Medical diagnosis: Attention deficit hyperactivity disorder, developmental coordination disorder
➤ Age: 5 years

Primary Functional Limitations

➤ Avoids physical activity
➤ Has difficulty performing age-appropriate fine and gross motor skills
➤ Limits interaction with peers during motor activities
➤ Demonstrates general "clumsiness" during daily activities, falling or bumping into objects
➤ Intelligibility in speech is variable
➤ Limits variety of drinks and food he will accept
➤ Has decreased attention span for motor tasks
➤ Poor handwriting and printing skills are evident in academic environment

Primary Impairments

➤ Attention deficit
➤ Expressive language delay
➤ Poor motor control and motor planning
➤ Weakness in upper extremities

➤ Limited endurance

➤ Difficulties with sensory processing, especially tactile discrimination and kinesthesia

Primary Goals

➤ Improve motor planning skills

➤ Increase upper body strength

➤ Increase endurance for gross motor activities

➤ Improve balance reactions and postural control

➤ Increase frequency of practice of self-selected motor activities

➤ Improve speech/sound production skills

➤ Complete self-cares independently

➤ Participate with peers in age-appropriate gross motor activities

Primary Functional Outcomes

SELF-CARE

John will:

➤ Use utensils during mealtime to stab food (fork) and butter bread (knife)

➤ Independently button and unbutton large buttons on a shirt

➤ Independently zip and unzip the zipper on his jacket after being assisted to engage the zipper

COMMUNICATION

John will:

➤ Produce the consonants "t" and "d" when they appear at the end of a word in sentences of three to four words in length

➤ Speak intelligibly enough to be understood by peers in a play situation

GROSS AND FINE MOTOR SKILLS

John will:

➤ Use both hands to throw and catch a 10-inch diameter ball

➤ Participate in physical activity with peers for 15 to 20 minutes without undue fatigue

➤ Ride his bike (with training wheels) for 5 miles during family bike trips

AMBULATION

John will:

➤ Walk independently, changing speeds and directions as needed on even and uneven terrain without falling

SAFETY

John will:

➤ Walk in a crowded environment, such as the mall, without bumping into objects or people

➤ Play safely and appropriately on equipment in a local fast food restaurant playground with other children present

Additional Considerations/Prognosis

John's medical diagnosis includes attention deficit hyperactivity disorder (ADHD) and developmental coordination disorder (DCD). Barnhart et al[52] reviewed the general parameters of DCD, which is considered a chronic, usually permanent, condition in children that is characterized by motor impairment significant enough to interfere with ADL. To be diagnosed with DCD children must not have abnormal muscle tone or movements or sensory loss. In addition, children should have an IQ greater than 70 and not meet criteria for a diagnosis of pervasive developmental disorder. Apraxia and dyspraxia often have been equated with DCD. Ayres[53] defined developmental dyspraxia as a motor planning disorder and as a "disorder of sensory integration interfering with the ability to plan and execute skilled or non-habitual tasks." Ayres discussed the lack of homogeneity of observations among children with dyspraxia. She also recommended criteria for using the diagnosis of development dyspraxia, which included a meaningful constellation of low scores on tests of praxis, normal IQ, and normal conventional neurological examination. Miyahara and Mobs[54] suggested that apraxia and dyspraxia primarily refer to problems in motor sequencing and selection, which not all children with DCD exhibit. They proposed various criteria to distinguish among these conditions.

John's prognosis for independent motor function is good. He may not develop motor skills adequate for athletic competition, but should have motor skills sufficient to enable him to participate in social recreational activities with peers (eg, bowling, swimming). Children with John's motor problems generally improve with maturation and practice of specific skills. In one follow-up study of "clumsy" children, those children with mild to moderate degrees of clumsiness improved to "normality" with maturation.[55] Children with severe degrees of clumsiness had a less favorable outcome in regard to motor proficiency, but their motor problems did not appear to affect social class or pursuit of sporting activities. However, more recent studies suggested that children with DCD do not outgrow clumsiness and that, without intervention, they do not improve.[56,57]

It would be important for John to develop competence in an area of interest to improve his self-image. Noncompetitive sports, such as karate, may be selected initially and would improve John's motor control while providing an outlet for his high energy level. Physical therapy services would be primarily consultative for John and his family. Emphasis would be on providing suggestions for home-based activities and community programs that would meet his individual needs as his motor abilities improve and interest in motor-related activities increases.

Conclusion

Although children with developmental disabilities may need physical therapy on an episodic basis throughout their life span, the goal is not life-long physical therapy. Rather, the goal of the physical therapist is to enable independence and self-management in the child and family. Physical therapists should strive to consider the "whole" child and emphasize appropriate goals related to the child's participation in societal roles.

Not all possible examination, evaluation, and intervention strategies for each of the children were addressed in this text. However, the examples provided should assist clinicians without experience in pediatrics and student physical therapists to assess their own level of knowledge and identify additional resources that may be necessary to ensure competence in the pediatric arena. It should be emphasized that establishing functional outcomes and hypothesizing about related underlying impairments is essential in establishing a framework for determining intervention strategies. A variety of treatment techniques often can be used to meet the same therapeutic objective or several objectives simultaneously. Although repetition is important in treatment, using a variety of activities contributes to making intervention enjoyable and motivating for the child and the therapist. Creativity, therefore, is the art of pediatric therapy.

References

1. Bleck EE. Locomotor prognosis in cerebral palsy. *Dev Med Child Neurol.* 1975;17:18-25.

2. Molnar GE, Gordon SU. Cerebral palsy: predictive value of selected clinical signs for early prognostication of motor function. *Arch Phys Med Rehabil.* 1976;57:153-158.

3. Watt JM, Robertson CMT, Grace MGA. Early prognosis for ambulation of neonatal intensive care survivors with cerebral palsy. *Dev Med Child Neurol.* 1989;32:755-773.

4. Palisano RJ, Rosenbaum PL, Walter SD, et al. Development and reliability of a system to classify gross motor function in children with cerebral palsy. *Dev Med Child Neurol.* 1997;39:214-223.

5. Palisano RJ, Hanna SE, Rosenbaum PL, et al. Validation of a model of gross motor function for children with cerebral palsy. *Phys Ther.* 2000;80:974-985.

6. Rosenbaum PL, Walter SD, Hanna SE, et al. Prognosis for gross motor function in cerebral palsy: creation of motor development curves. *JAMA.* 2002;288:1399-1400.

7. Peterson P, Peterson CE. Bilateral hand skills in children with hemiplegia. *Phys Occup Ther Pediatr.* 1984;41:77-87.

8. Crocker MD, MacKay-Lyons M, McDonnell E. Forced use of the upper extremity in cerebral palsy: a single case design. *Am J Occup Ther.* 1997;51:824-833.

9. Pierce SR, Daly K, Gallagher KG, et al. Constraint-induced therapy for a child with hemiplegic cerebral palsy: a case report. *Arch Phys Med Rehabil.* 2002;83:1462-1463.

10. Willis JK, Morello A, Davie A. Forced use treatment of childhood hemiparesis. *Pediatrics.* 2002;110:94-96.

11. DeLuca SC, Echols K, Ramey SL, et al. Pediatric constraint-induced movement therapy for a young child with cerebral palsy: two episodes of care. *Phys Ther.* 2003;83:1003-1013.

12. Poldrack R. Imaging brain plasticity: conceptual and methodological issues—a theoretical review. *Neuroimage.* 2000;12:1-13.

13. Briellmann RS, Abbott DF, Caflisch U, et al. Brain reorganization in cerebral palsy: a high-field functional MRS Study. *Neuropediatrics.* 2002;33:162-165.

14. Staudt M, Pieper T, Grodd W, et al. Functional MRI in a 6 year old boy with unilateral cortical malformation: concordant representation of both hands in the unaffected hemisphere. *Neuropediatrics.* 2001;32:159-160.

15. Stuadt M, Lidzba K, Grodd W, et al. Right hemisphere organization of language followed by early left-sided brain lesion: functional MRI topography. *Neuroimage.* 2002;16:954-967.

16. Nelson KB, Ellenberg JH. Children who "outgrew" cerebral palsy. *Pediatrics.* 1982;69:529-536.

17. Fennell EB, Dikel TN. Cognitive and neuropsychological functioning in children with cerebral palsy. *J Child Neurol.* 2001:16:58-63.

18. Vargha-Khadem F, Isaacs E, Vander WS, et al. Development of intelligence and memory in children with hemiplegic cerebral palsy: the deleterious consequences of early seizures. *Brain.* 1992;115:315-329.

19. Frampton I, Yude C, Goodman R. The prevalence and correlates of specific learning difficulties in a representative sample of children with hemiplegia. *Br J Educ Psychol.* 1998;68:39-51.

20. Radtka SA, Skinner SR, Dixon DM, et al. A comparison of gait with solid, dynamic, and no ankle-foot orthoses in children in spastic cerebral palsy. *Phys Ther.* 1997;77:395-409.
21. Rethlesfsen S, Kay R, Dennis S, et al. The effects of fixed and articulated ankle-foot orthoses on gait patterns in children with cerebral palsy. *J Pediatr Orthop.* 1999;19:470-474.
22. Knott KM, Held SL. Effects of orthoses on upright functional skills of children and adolescents with cerebral palsy. *Pediatr Phys Ther.* 2002;14:199-207.
23. Sutherland DH, Kaufman KR, Wyatt MP, et al. Injection of botulinum toxin A into the gastrocnemius muscle of patients with cerebral palsy: a 3-dimensional motion analysis study. *Gait Posture.* 1996;4:269-279.
24. Koman KA, Mooney JR III, Smith BP, et al. Botulinum toxin type A neuromuscular blockade in the treatment of lower extremity spasticity in cerebral palsy. A randomized, double-blind, placebo-controlled trial. Botox Study Group. *J Pediatr Orthop.* 2000;20:108-115.
25. Reddihough JA, King GJ, Coleman A, et al. Functional outcome of botulinum toxin A injections to the lower limbs in cerebral palsy. *Dev Med Child Neurol.* 2002;44:820-827.
26. Correy IS, Cosgrove AP, Walsh EG, et al. Botulinum toxin A in the hemiplegic upper limb. A double-blind trial. *Dev Med Child Neurol.* 1997;39:185-193.
27. Singhi P, Jagirdar S. Khandelwal N, et al. Epilepsy in children with cerebral palsy. *J Child Neurol.* 2003;18:174-179.
28. Fragala MA, Goodgold S, Dumas HM. Effects of lower extremity passive stretching: pilot study of children and youth with severe limitations in self-mobility. *Pediatr Phys Ther.* 2003; 15:167-175.
29. Latash ML, Anson JG. What are "normal movements" in atypical populations? *Behavioral and Brain Sciences.* 1996;19:55-106.
30. Bleck EE. Total body involvement. In: Bleck EE. *Orthopaedic Management in Cerebral Palsy.* Philadelphia, Pa: JB Lippincott; 1987:392-480.
31. Pritchett JW. Treated and untreated unstable hips in severe cerebral palsy. *Dev Med Child Neurol.* 1990;32:3-6.
32. Ilikkan DY, Yzlcin E. Changes in skeletal maturation and mineralization in children with cerebral palsy and evaluation of related factors. *J Child Neurol.* 2001;16:425-430.
33. DeSouza M, Carroll N. Ambulation of the braced myelomeningocele patient. *J Bone Jt Surg.* 1973;58:137-148.
34. Hoffer MM, Fiewell E, Peryr J, et al. Functional ambulation in patients with myelomeningocele. *J Bone Jt Surg.* 1973;55:137-148.
35. Williams EN, Broughton NS, Menelaus MB. Age-related walking in children with spina bifida. *Dev Med Child Neurol.* 1999;41:446-449.
36. Hunt GM, Poulton A. Open spina bifida: a complete cohort reviewed 25 years after closure. *Dev Med Child Neurol.* 1995;37:19-29.
37. Bowman EM, McLone DG, Grant T, et al. Spina bifida outcome: a 25-year perspective. *Pediatr Neurosurg.* 2001;34:114-120.
38. Franks CA, Palisano RJ, Darbee JC. The effect of walking with an assistive device and using a wheelchair on school performance in students with myelomeningocele. *Phys Ther.* 1991;71: 570-579.
39. Bartonek A, Saraste H. Factors influencing ambulation in myelomeningocele: a cross-sectional study. *Dev Med Child Neurol.* 2001;43:253-260.
40. Stiefee D, Stribata T, Meuli M, et al. Tethering of the spinal cord in mouse fetuses and neonates with spina bifida. *J Neurosurg.* 2003;99:206-213.
41. Sharif S, Allcutt D, Marks C, et al. "Tethered cord syndrome"—recent clinical experience. *Br J Neurosurg.* 1997;11:49-51.
42. Sarwark JF, Weber DT, Gabrieli AP, et al. Tethered cord syndrome in low motor level children with myelomeningocele. *Pediatr Neurosurg.* 1996;25:295-301.

43. Yeates KO, Enrile BG, Loss N, et al. Verbal learning and memory in children with myelomeningocele. *J Pediatr Psychol.* 1995;20:801-815.

44. Dennis M, Barnes M. Math and numeracy in young adults with spina bifida and hydrocephalus. *Dev Neuropsychol.* 2002;21:141-155.

45. Pueschel SM. The child with Down syndrome. In: Levine MD, Carey W. Crocker AC, et al, eds. *Developmental-Behavioral Pediatrics.* Philadelphia, Pa: WB Saunders; 1983:353-362.

46. Shea AM. Motor attainments in Down syndrome. In: Lister E, ed. *Proceedings of the II Step Conference; Contemporary Management of Motor Control Problems.* Alexandria, Va: Foundation for Physical Therapy; 1991:225-236.

47. Pueschel SM, Siola PH, Perry CD, et al. Atlantoaxial instability in children with Down syndrome. *Pediatr Radiol.* 1981;10:129-132.

48. Spano M, Meruri E, Rando T, et al. Motor and perceptual-motor competence in children with Down syndrome: variation in performance with age. *Eur J Paediatr Neurol.* 1999;3:7-13.

49. Wisniewski KE, Wisniewski HM, Wen GY. Occurrence of neuropathological changes and dementia of Alzheimer's disease in Down syndrome. *Annals of Neurology.* 1985;17:278-282.

50. Dalton AJ, Crapper DR. Down syndrome and aging of the brain. In: Mittler P, ed. *Research to Practice in Mental Retardation: Biomedical Aspects.* Vol. III. Baltimore, Md: University Park Press; 1977.

51. Fenner ME, Hewitt KE, Torpy DM. Down syndrome: intellectual and behavioral functioning during adulthood. *J Ment Defic Res.* 1987;31:241-249.

52. Barnhart RC, Davenport MJ, Epps SB, et al. Developmental coordination disorder. *Phys Ther.* 2003;83:722-731.

53. Ayres AJ. *Developmental Dyspraxia and Adult-Onset Apraxia.* Torrance, Calif: Sensory Integration International; 1985:8-9,58.

54. Miyahara M, Mobs I. Developmental dyspraxia and developmental coordination disorder. *Neuropsychol Rev.* 1995;5:245-268.

55. Knuckey NW, Gubbay SS. Clumsy children: a prognostic study. *Aust Paediatr J.* 1983;19:9-13.

56. Surden DA, Chambers ME. Intervention approaches and children with developmental coordination disorder. *Pediatr Rehabil.* 1998;2:139-147.

57. Coleman R, Piek JP, Livesey DJ. A longitudinal study of motor ability and kinaesthetic acuity in young children at risk of developmental coordination disorder. *Hum Mov Sci.* 2001;20:95-110.

CHAPTER 16

Research in the Era of Evidence-Based Practice

Meg Barry Michaels, PhD, PT

Therapists face ever-increasing pressure to provide evidence to support their approaches to patient examination and intervention. More and more frequently, third party reimbursement may be refused for treatments lacking evidence of efficacy. Families investigate new interventions on the Internet and they expect clinicians to be familiar with these treatments and the related research. As clinicians strive to provide the best possible care, they want to know which interventions are most likely to provide the greatest gains for their pediatric patients. The current buzz phrase is "evidence-based practice," but there are misunderstandings regarding the definition and its implications.[1] Sackett and colleagues defined evidence-based medicine as "the integration of best research evidence with clinical expertise and patient values."[2] This definition clarifies the concept of evidence-based practice. In addition to using the best research evidence, two other critical factors are included: the clinician's expertise and the individual patient. Knowledge of the patient's history, lifestyle, and values aid the clinician in making a determination as to whether the evidence applies to the patient.

This chapter promotes evidence-based practice in several ways. The primary goal is to assist therapists in understanding processes for obtaining and utilizing evidence and available resources. An explanation of fundamental research terms and methodology provides the necessary background to begin to critically appraise journal articles. Another goal is to provide ideas for clinicians interested in contributing to the available evidence through clinical research. The case studies demonstrate the use of the evidence as well as examples of participation in clinical research at a basic level. Ultimately, therapists must make a decision whether or not to contribute to the evidence and whether or not to follow the evidence in their practice.

Resources for Evidence-Based Practice

The American Physical Therapy Association (APTA) supports the concept of evidence-based practice through several avenues. The APTA has developed a clinical research agenda to guide research priorities within the profession.[3] The Foundation for Physical Therapy funds physical therapy research using this clinical research agenda as a basis for prioritizing funding of projects. Another way the APTA promotes evidence-based practice is through its publications. The APTA journal, *Physical Therapy*, has published a series of articles entitled "Evidence in Practice" demonstrating how to answer clinical questions using the evidence. One article in this series addressed the question of differential diagnosis in a 12-year-old child with back pain.[4] This article, as well as the others in the series, demonstrated the details of the process of answering a specific clinical question using the available evidence. The APTA also supports a means of gathering evidence on physical therapy interventions from the literature. The APTA Hooked on Evidence web site (www.apta.org) houses a database that provides a means of accessing information abstracted from research articles in physical therapy and related fields. However, Hooked on Evidence is available only to APTA members. Eventually it is anticipated that the project will provide complete data on all current citations on a topic and will expand to rate the quality of the research evidence. Sections of the APTA, including the Section on Pediatrics, provide their members with opportunities to apply for small research grants to allow members to contribute to the available evidence. The Section on Pediatrics and the APTA recognize outstanding researchers who make significant contributions to the body of physical therapy evidence.

Another organization that supports evidence-based practice is the American Academy of Cerebral Palsy and Developmental Medicine (AACPDM). The AACPDM has taken another approach to evaluating the evidence.[5] Rather than searching for the answer to a clinical question, the treatment outcomes committee performs systematic reviews of the relevant research for a specific treatment. Their reviews are available on the AACPDM web site at www.aacpdm.org. One of these reviews assessed the level of evidence for neurodevelopmental treatment (NDT) for children with cerebral palsy.[6] Although the authors concluded that there was a lack of strong evidence to support NDT, the lack of evidence does not mean that the treatment is not beneficial; the lack of evidence may indicate that the effects of NDT are not yet fully known.

A systematic review should follow a structured protocol for evaluating the evidence. This protocol involves gathering all the relevant research articles according to a set of standard criteria, following clear guidelines for the review of each article to make judgments as to the scientific rigor, and then compiling the results. The systematic review should be presented in a clinically useful format.

Importance of Evidence-Based Practice

Pediatric therapists benefit from knowledge regarding research in three arenas: as researchers, as educators, and as clinicians. Later in this chapter, suggestions for becoming involved in research will be offered, given the constraints of time and resources available in clinical practice. As educators, therapists are involved in teaching in a number of different roles. As clinical or academic instructors, therapists teach students about pediatric therapy. Students often ask why a particular assessment tool or intervention was chosen. Now, in many cases, there is evidence to support clinicians' choices. Working with patients, parents, and caregivers, therapists often serve in another educational role. Clients trust their therapists to provide current accurate information. Families often explore treatment options on their own and then ask therapists to interpret their findings. Parents want the therapist who is most familiar with their child to aid in determining if a particular treatment would be beneficial. Clinicians also may be in the position of educating colleagues (therapists as well as other professionals) regarding specific examination tools and interventions. Arranging an in-service to share strong evidence regarding the usefulness of a specific standardized test may convince colleagues to adopt the test.

In making clinical decisions, therapists also are consumers of research. In order to interpret the evidence, therapists need a background in research including familiarity with the terms and methods. Table 16-1 provides a refresher on the definitions of terms related to the psychometric properties of tests, such as different types of reliability and validity.

Table 16-1
Research Terminology

Term	Meaning
Reliability	Consistency or repeatability of measurements[50]
Intratester reliability	Indicates agreement in measurements over time[50] (for one person)
Intertester reliability	Indicates agreement of measurements taken by different examiners[50]
Test-retest reliability	Indicates stability over time[50]; there is no change in test score when there is no change in the condition
Validity	"Degree to which a useful (meaningful) interpretation can be inferred from a measurement"[50]
Construct	The conceptual or theoretical basis for using a measurement to make an interpretation[50]
Content	The extent to which a measurement reflects the meaningful elements of a construct—only the relevant elements[50]
Criterion-related	The correctness of an inferred interpretation can be tested by comparing a measurement with another measurement; concurrent and predictive validity are forms of criterion-related validity[50]
Concurrent	A measurement is compared with supporting evidence obtained at the same time as the measurement being validated[50]
Predictive	A measurement is compared with supporting evidence obtained at a later point in time; examines the justification for using the measurement to say something about future events or conditions[50]
Responsiveness	The ability of the measurement to detect a minimally clinically important change[7]
Diagnostic Testing Terms	
Likelihood ratio	"Likelihood that a given test result would be expected in a patient with the target disorder when compared with the likelihood that the same result would be expected in a patient without the target disorder"[2]
Sensitivity	Proportion with the target disorder with a positive test[2]
Specificity	Proportion without the target disorder with a negative test[2]
Positive predictive value	Proportion with a positive test with the target disorder[2]
Negative predictive value	Proportion with a negative test without the target disorder[2]

Evidence-Based Pediatric Practice: Examination

When performing patient examinations, therapists choose assessment tools based on a variety of factors including ease of administration and the psychometric properties of the test (as discussed in Chapter 2). Therapists choose tools with demonstrated reliability to ensure measurements are accurate and consistent. They also choose tools with demonstrated validity depending on the purpose of the testing and the testing situation. Researchers have investigated different types of reliability and validity for many pediatric assessment tools. The purpose of an assessment tool is important in choosing the tool, and there are three categories to consider: discriminative, evaluative, and prognostic.[7] A discriminative tool used by pediatric therapists most often is designed to distinguish between typical and atypical development. For example, the Peabody Developmental Motor Scales (PMDS-2)[8] may be used to identify children whose motor skills fall outside the typical range of motor development for their age. An evaluative tool, on the other hand, is designed to assess change after an intervention. One such measure is the Gross Motor Function Measure (GMFM), designed to evaluate change in children with cerebral palsy after interventions, such as physical therapy.[9] The GMFM was not designed to discriminate between children who have cerebral palsy and those who do not.

In some cases, assessment tools are chosen to aid in prognosis such as the Test of Infant Motor Performance (TIMP) which was designed to identify children at risk for poor long-term motor performance.[10] In addition to research demonstrating the reliability of this tool,[11] there is research to support its predictive validity.[12-14] Identifying infants at risk for continuing motor problems is critical in making decisions regarding early intervention for infants.[12] Table 16-1 defines additional terms that are important in certain diagnostic testing: sensitivity, specificity, positive and negative predictive values, and likelihood ratios. These definitions may be helpful in understanding the research related to diagnostic tests, such as the TIMP. For a test with high sensitivity, such as tests for tuberculosis, the test will be positive for nearly all of those who have the condition.[2] Persons with the condition are not likely to be missed by the test, consequently a negative result virtually rules out the condition. For a test with high specificity such as tests for tuberculosis, the test will be negative for nearly all of those who do not have the condition. People who do not have the condition are not likely to be diagnosed with the condition; therefore a positive test result is likely to be correct. However, few tests used by physical therapists have high sensitivity and high specificity. Therefore, in choosing a prognostic test, therapists face a difficult decision. Is high sensitivity critical due to the high cost or risks of providing treatment to a person without the disorder or is specificity of greater importance since the cost of missing a person with the disorder is very high? Therapists need to keep the psychometric properties and the purpose of the assessment in mind in choosing assessment tools, using the available research to make decisions.

Evidence-Based Pediatric Practice: Intervention

Learning about the properties of assessment tools is not only important in making decisions regarding the patient examination, but also in making decisions for patient intervention. The most common reason clinicians use research evidence is to justify their choice of intervention strategies. Therapists need to be able to interpret treatment outcomes. Knowledge of research and assessment tools is critical in performing meaningful interpretation. For instance, if researchers used a discriminative measure to assess the effects of an intervention rather than an evaluative measure, then the true difference due to the intervention may be missed.[15] The evidence to support an intervention may be useful in making a clinical decision or in persuading insurance companies to pay for a specific intervention.

Frameworks provide an organized approach to evaluating the evidence. One such framework is the disablement model used in this text and in the *Guide to Physical Therapist Practice*.[16] This model was developed by the National Advisory Board[17] and includes five dimensions: pathophysiology, impairments, functional limitations, disability, and societal limitations. The importance of using the disablement model in the evaluation of research studies is the inclusion of a broad range of outcomes. In the past, research often emphasized the impairments by studying the effects of interventions on variables such as range of motion, strength, and pain. In addition to studying the effects of interventions on impairments, the inclusion of functional activities and social roles is now considered critical in research design. For example, the effect of a treatment is important to a patient in terms of how life is different or not different if knee range of motion increases by 10 degrees; the effect of treatment may be important if it means a child can participate in T-ball. Therefore, in evaluating the supportive evidence for an intervention, the dimensions of the disablement model are important to keep in mind.

Perhaps the most common framework for evaluating research evidence is Sackett's levels of evidence.[18] These five levels designate the intensity of the scientific evidence based on the research design and implementation of the research study. Table 16-2 describes the types of studies included for each level.

The highest level of evidence, Level 1, refers to large, randomized controlled trials.[18] In these studies, subjects are assigned in a random manner to one or more treatment groups. A power analysis determines the number of subjects needed to detect a statistical difference between groups.[19] This estimate of the number of subjects needed is based on an estimate of the expected effect of the treatment. If the expected treatment effect is small, a greater number of subjects will be needed to show a difference between groups. In reviewing studies, more credence is given to studies that describe what has happened to every person enrolled in the study. Ideally, researchers analyze the data for all of the subjects based on the group to which they were randomly assigned, which is called "intention-to-treat" analysis.[2] Another consideration is the length of follow-up and whether the time is sufficient to assess the effects of the treatment. To reduce bias, neither the investigators nor the subjects should be aware of the treatment being received. In therapy, this blinding or masking of treatment status is not always possible; patients know if they are exercising or not. But masking the person assessing outcomes is one way to reduce bias; the person performing the assessments does not need to know which treatment has been administered. Groups should be treated in a similar manner, other than the treatment variable being studied. And although randomization attempts to form groups of patients who are similar, at times the randomization process results in substantial differences between groups before the intervention is implemented. The inherent differences between groups may impact the outcome of the study. All of these factors are important to consider, in addition to a consideration of the outcome measures chosen by the researchers, as previously discussed. Measures with sound psychometric properties matched to the appropriate purpose of assessment provide the best scientific evidence. Systematic reviews of Level 1 research provide the best compilation of evidence. Single-subject design research repeated over a number of subjects may be included in Level 1.[5]

If a study randomizes subjects but falls short in one or more of the areas mentioned above, the study is considered Level 2 evidence. Studies comparing two or more cohorts (groups) not randomly assigned to receive different treatments also are categorized as Level 2. For instance, one second grade class may participate in a strengthening program

Table 16-2
Levels of Evidence for Therapy Interventions

Levels of Evidence	Type of Study Design

Level 1	Randomized controlled trials
	    Systematic review
	    Individual studies

Level 2	Cohort studies
	    Systematic review
	    Individual studies
	        Including low quality randomized controlled trials
	Single subject design ABABA studies

Level 3	Case-control studies
	    Systematic review
	    Individual studies
	    Single subject design ABA studies

Level 4	Case series (no control group) Poor quality cohort and case-control studies Single subject design AB studies
Level 5	Case report Expert opinion

Adapted from Sackett D. Rules of evidence and clinical recommendations on the use of antithrombotic agents. *Chest.* 1986;89(Suppl):2S; and Butler C, Chambers H, Goldstein M, et al. Evaluating research in developmental disabilities: a conceptual framework for reviewing treatment outcomes. *Dev Med Child Neurol.* 1999;41:55-59.

and another class may be the control group. There may be differences between the groups that are not due to the strengthening program. There is less confidence in the results of Level 2 studies, and it is more difficult to generalize the results of these studies to other patients. Under the Level 3 category are case-control studies which are widely used in epidemiology (ie, the study of disease or injury in a population).[20] Case-control studies are useful in areas where a condition cannot be imposed on a group of subjects, such as a study of the effects of smoking. A group of smokers may be compared to a control group of non-smokers to document the incidence of lung cancer. However, case-control studies are not widely used in therapy research. Level 4 includes series of cases reported without control groups and lower quality studies of the previous designs. In much of medicine, the available evidence is based on reports of the before and after status for groups of patients treated in a similar manner. Level 5 evidence consists of case reports and expert opinion that may be based on evidence from the basic sciences not yet applied to patient populations.

Table 16-3
Database Information

Hooked on Evidence (created by the American Physical Therapy Association)
Scope: Physical therapy and related literature—under development
Access: APTA members only on web site: www.apta.org

PEDro: Physiotherapy Evidence Database (created by the Australian Centre for Evidence-Based Physiotherapy)
Scope: Physical therapy randomized controlled clinical trials and systematic reviews
Access: http://www.pedro.fhs.usyd.edu.au

MEDLINE (created by the National Library of Medicine)
Scope: More than 4600 biomedical journals
Timeline: 1966 to present
Access: Free searches: www.ncbi.nlm.nih.gov/PubMed and http://biomednet.com; fee for services such as OVID (www.ovid.com), EBSCO—available without charge at many academic institutions

CINAHL: Cumulative Index to Nursing and Allied Health Literature
Scope: More than 1600 nursing and allied health journals
Timeline: 1982 to present
Access: Fee for services such as OVID (www.ovid.com), EBSCO—available without charge at many academic institutions

SPORTDiscus (provided by the Sport Information Resource Centre)
Scope: More than 500,000 records on sports and fitness literature
Timeline: 1975 to present (journals); 1949 to present (monographs)
Access: Services such as OVID (www.ovid.com), EBSCO

PsycINFO
Scope: More than 1700 periodicals in the field of psychology and related fields
Timeline: 1887 to present
Access: Fee for services such as OVID (www.ovid.com), EBSCO—available without charge at many academic institutions

Evidence-Based Pediatric Practice: Implementation

There are steps to follow in evidence-based practice.[2] The first step is to ask an answerable question. To ask the question, the type of patient needs to be clarified as well as the specifics of what you want to know. The case studies provide examples of the process. Once the question is clearly defined, then the search for available evidence begins. This step may involve using a variety of tools, including the databases presented in Table 16-3. The APTA Hooked on Evidence database has already been mentioned. Another database was developed by the Australian Centre for Evidence-Based Physiotherapy; their Physiotherapy Evidence Database (PEDro) is available online free of charge at www.pedro.fhs.usyd.edu.au. This database provides ratings for systematic reviews and clinical trials. At this point, the database has limited information available for pediatric therapists. The Cochrane library is another resource that may be accessed on the Internet at http://www.updateusa.com. The Cochrane collaboration provides systematic reviews with a focus on medical interventions, but the scope of these reviews continues to expand. Other databases that may be searched for systematic reviews and individual articles are MEDLINE, Cumulative Index of Nursing and Allied Health Literature (CINAHL), SPORTDiscus and PsycINFO. The case studies provide specific information on the use of these databases in addition to the information provided in Table 16-3.

Once the evidence is gathered, then it must be critically appraised. This is Step 3. The disablement model provides a reminder to consider all aspects of a disease. The levels of evidence provide a framework for assessing the scientific rigor of the studies that have been gathered. Again, the cases will illustrate how to critically appraise the evidence. Finally, the most important step is to apply the evidence to the clinical situation. The evidence is applied at the discretion of the clinician based on the best available research, the expertise of the individual clinician, and the individual patient's values and goals.[2] Without the clinician, there is no evidence-based practice.

In providing direct intervention, the therapist's clinical skills also are part of the equation. If the evidence suggests that a technique produced the desired outcome in patients similar to the patient under consideration but the clinician does not have expertise in that technique, then the evidence may not apply. In that situation, the clinician may better serve the client by providing an alternate treatment also supported by the evidence or referring the client to an expert in the desired treatment technique.

Clinical Research

As professionals, therapists have an obligation to contribute to the body of knowledge pertaining to physical therapy. Clinicians are in the ideal situation to write case reports describing an aspect of clinical practice.[21] The case report may serve as the basis for the development of future research directions. The case report may be retrospective, meaning that existing data are used. With the inception of the Health Insurance Portability and Accountability Act (HIPAA), therapists must follow these regulations regarding the use of patient data. The APTA Government Affairs office provides information to therapists on HIPAA and its implications. The group that regulates human research at an institution, such as a hospital or university, is known as the institutional review board or the human subjects review board.[20] There are regulations to protect human rights which apply to all types of clinical research and must be addressed before a study may begin. In the case of a prospective study where new data are collected, the regulations include approved consent forms for subjects to sign before the study may begin. For studies involving children, they may sign an approved assent form describing the study and their rights in age-appropriate language and their parents must sign a consent form.

Clinicians with an interest in clinical research may be in a good position to perform single subject design research (see Chapter 17). In the clinic, this research may be more practical than trying to recruit large numbers of similar subjects. A single subject design follows many of the same procedures as other types of experimental design. A hypothesis defines the research question. The inclusion and exclusion criteria define the subjects who would be eligible to participate in the study. The treatment introduced by the investigator is the independent variable. The methods for the research include the use of measurements with appropriate reliability and validity. The outcome measure supplies the dependent variable, which is used to measure the effects of the independent or treatment variable.[20] This type of design allows subjects to act as their own controls through multiple measurements in the baseline and treatment phases. Typically a subject would be measured repeatedly, at least three or four times, before the introduction of the treatment. This baseline would be considered the A-phase of the study. Measurements then are taken during the treatment phase, which is the B-phase. A baseline followed by a treatment would be an AB design. This type of research falls into Level 4 evidence.[6] If another phase is added where measurements are taken after the treatment is withdrawn, the design would be ABA. This study design is stronger, and if well-executed, the evidence is Level 3. To be more convincing, an ABABA design would demonstrate the differences in the outcome variable when the treatment is repeatedly implemented and withdrawn. This design provides Level 2 evidence. For many treatments, the effects may be maintained into the second A-phase making comparisons difficult. In order to provide Level 1 evidence, the single subject design, also called an n-of-1 trial, is repeated over numerous subjects with the treatment phase introduced in a randomized manner.[6] If more than one treatment is compared, the second treatment would be introduced in a C phase. For populations that are heterogeneous, such as children with disabilities, there are difficulties in studying large numbers of similar children, so the single subject design is a valuable tool. These studies provide information that may be helpful in directing future trials, but the generalizability of the results is not known. Case Study #5 demonstrates a single subject design study.

Clinicians are in the best position to develop clinically relevant questions for research hypotheses. Some clinicians may choose to participate in large randomized controlled trials. In a perspective in *Physical Therapy*, Fitzgerald and Delitto outlined considerations for planning and conducting clinical research.[20] One way to facilitate this process is through the development of collaborative relationships with academicians. Relationships between universities and groups of clinicians allow research expertise to be matched with clinical expertise and resources. The Section on Pediatrics offers opportunities for the development of collaborative projects and opportunities for networking at the two annual APTA meetings as well as at regional events. The Section also has an online listserve that allows for informal communication between Section members through ongoing email discussions. Members of the Section may join the listserve to post questions for other members to answer, share knowledge, and develop professional relationships. Another avenue for assistance is the Members Mentoring Members program available for APTA members through the Web site. All of these resources facilitate the involvement of clinicians in clinical research. The following case studies illustrate evidence-based practice and clinical research that is intended for the clinician.

Case Study #1: Jason

➤ Practice pattern 5C: Impaired Motor Function and Sensory Integrity Associated With Nonprogressive Disorders of the Central Nervous System—Congenital Origin or Acquired in Infancy or Childhood

➤ Medical diagnosis: Cerebral palsy, right hemiparesis

➤ Age: 24 months

Jason's family is interested in a hippotherapy program which uses a horse as a treatment modality administered by a licensed therapist.[22,23] Hippotherapy differs from therapeutic horseback riding. Therapeutic horseback riding promotes people with disabilities learning to ride horses, whereas hippotherapy involves the use of the horse to attain therapy goals.[22,23] The family has heard from friends that hippotherapy may help Jason walk better. They looked for more information on the Internet and found the American

Hippotherapy Association, a section of the North American Riding for the Handicapped Association (NARHA) at www.narha.org. Jason's parents asked their insurance company if hippotherapy would be covered under their policy, and they were told that there is not supportive evidence for this treatment, therefore it is not covered. The family plans to appeal the insurance company's regulations. They would like to know what research evidence is available to support the effectiveness of hippotherapy in improving the ability to walk in children with cerebral palsy. They need help finding the answer.

Step 1: Develop the Clinical Question

Does hippotherapy improve gait characteristics in young children with cerebral palsy?

Step 2: Gather the Evidence

The decision was made to include only English-language systematic reviews and clinical trials of hippotherapy or therapeutic horseback riding published in peer-reviewed journals. To begin the search, the APTA Hooked on Evidence database was used at www.apta.org. There were no records found with the keyword *hippotherapy*. There were no records found with the keyword *horseback riding*. All records with the keyword *cerebral palsy* then were reviewed, but none of the study titles indicated that horses were involved. The process was repeated using the PEDro database at www.pedro.fhs.usyd.edu.au and the web site for the AACPDM was accessed at www.aacpdm.org. No studies were found that related to hippotherapy. Under the Treatment Outcomes committee page, there were no systematic reviews related to hippotherapy.

Since these resources failed to find any articles of interest, MEDLINE was searched. MEDLINE was accessed through the local university but also is available to anyone free of charge at www.ncbi.nlm.nih.gov/PubMed. The keyword *hippotherapy* found two records. One study was related to severe traumatic brain injury,[24] but the other article addressed children with spastic cerebral palsy.[22] The abstract of the study involving children with cerebral palsy indicated that gait outcomes were included so the article was put on a list of articles to be obtained. Next the keyword *horseback riding* was entered, and there were 37 records available. The titles of many of the studies were related to injuries due to horseback riding and did not involve the use of a horse for therapy. Titles of nine studies appeared to be relevant and those abstracts were chosen for closer review. Based on the abstracts, three articles were added to the list of articles to be obtained.[25-27]

Since allied health professionals perform hippotherapy, the CINAHL database was important to search. The search procedure utilized for MEDLINE was repeated in CINAHL. The keyword *hippotherapy* revealed 12 records. Only two of the records indicated clinical trials in peer-reviewed journals, therefore those abstracts were chosen for review.[22,23] One of these studies was already identified by the MEDLINE search, and the other was added to the list of articles to be obtained. The keyword *horseback riding* resulted in 67 hits. Rather than review all of these records, *horseback riding* and *cerebral palsy* were typed in for another search. A review of these abstracts resulted in one additional article being added to the list of articles to be obtained.[28] The other database that seemed likely to contain potential records was SPORTDiscus. The same search procedure resulted in a number of hits, but no new clinical trials were found. The search was completed, and the six articles on the list were obtained from the university library.[22,23,25-28] From the articles' reference lists, two additional studies were identified and obtained for review.[29,30]

Table 16-4
Hippotherapy: Evidence Regarding Improvements in Gait

	Bertoti[30]	McGibbon et al[22]	Haehl et al[23]
Research Design	Case report (not a single subject design, but measurements ABA)	Case series (not a single subject design, but measurements AB)	Case series (not a single subject design, but measurements AB)
Subject(s)	2.5-year-old with hemiplegia	5 children: 4 with diplegia and 1 with hemiplegia with mean age of 9.6 years	2 children: 9.5-year-old girl with quadri-plegia and 4-year-old boy with diplegia
Treatment Frequency	Once/week for 6 weeks	Twice/week for 8 weeks	Once/week for 12 weeks
Positive Outcomes	*Impairment*: Extrem-ity weight bearing *Functional limitation*: Anecdotal reports of gait improvements	*Impairment*: Energy expenditure index *Functional limitation*: GMFM	*Impairment*: Kine-matics *Functional limitation*: PEDI mobility scores improved for one child
Measurements	Baseline, after 6-week treatment program, and 6 weeks later	Baseline 1, baseline 2: 8 weeks later, and then after 8-week hippotherapy program	Kinematics: during 3 hippotherapy sessions; PEDI: Baseline and after 12-week program
Level of Evidence	5	4	4

Step 3: Critically Appraise the Evidence

For this step of the process, the eight articles were read and the evidence was appraised. There were no randomized controlled trials and no systematic reviews. Two of the studies did not specifically assess gait and were not included in the evidence summary.[27,29] Three articles were studies of therapeutic horseback riding studies and also were eliminated.[25,26,28] Although one of the remaining articles had therapeutic horseback riding in the title, the description of the treatment fit with hippotherapy.[30] The remaining three studies of hippotherapy had gait outcomes for children with cerebral palsy which are summarized in Table 16-4.[22,23,30]

Step 4: Apply the Evidence

The available evidence needs to be applied to the clinical question: Does hippotherapy improve gait characteristics in children with cerebral palsy? In this situation, the level of evidence to support hippotherapy as a treatment for improving gait characteristics in children with cerebral palsy was Level 4. The other factors involved in evidence-based practice are the clinician's expertise and the values and expectations of the individual patient. Thus, the clinician must determine if the evidence applies to this patient. For

Jason, the family's goal was walking better and specifically falling less frequently. The case report[30] involved a child with hemiplegia close to Jason's age. The outcome measure was extremity weight-bearing measured with a digital scale, which became more symmetrical immediately after the 6-week program but was not maintained 6 weeks later. The reliability of these measurements was not established. Anecdotal reports were positive, but since it was a case report, the results are only suggestive, not conclusive. The other two studies[22,23] used repeated measures but did not strictly meet the criteria for single subject design research of multiple measures in the baseline and the treatment phases. Overall, the evidence for improvements in gait due to hippotherapy was only suggestive, and the information was shared with the family for their appeal to the insurance company. The results also were shared with the APTA Section on Pediatrics listserve, the local Pediatric Special Interest Group, and as an in-service at the early intervention program.

Case Study #2: Jill

> Practice pattern 5C: Impaired Motor Function and Sensory Integrity Associated With Nonprogressive Disorders of the Central Nervous System—Congenital Origin or Acquired in Infancy or Childhood

> Medical diagnosis: Cerebral palsy, spastic quadraparesis, microcephaly, mental retardation, seizure disorder

> Age: 7 years

Jill already was participating in hippotherapy, but there had not been any consistent measurement associated with the program. As a new session of hippotherapy began, the therapist concentrated on setting goals and assessing functional outcomes. The therapist worked with several children like Jill who also were categorized as Gross Motor Function Classification Level V—the most severely physically limited children who do not have a means of independent mobility.[31] The outcome of interest for these children was improved postural control in sitting. For this population, the assessment of postural control presents a challenge. The therapist decided to try three different measures to assess sitting posture. Each child was assessed before the 8-week hippotherapy session, after 4 weeks of hippotherapy, and again after 8 weeks of hippotherapy. After looking at the results, the therapist found that one of the measures was clearly more responsive to change than the other measures.

The therapist realized that many other clinicians face these same challenges and decided to write a case report to submit to a journal. The first step was obtaining permission to use the patient's records from the institutional review board at the local university where the therapist was adjunct faculty. The board protects the human rights of research subjects, including the right to privacy and confidentiality. Although a case report has not always been perceived as a research study in the past, the use of existing medical records now requires patient permission. The therapist followed the required procedures, including obtaining informed consent from the parents and assent from the children.

The therapist purchased a copy of the book *Writing Case Reports: A How-to Manual for Clinicians*[21] from the APTA. The book provided step-by-step instructions for writing a case report. Although most case reports are related to intervention, writing a case report on patient examination also is very useful. The main components of this case report were the introduction, a description of the patients, a description of the assessment tools used (including a review of the published reliability and validity studies), a brief description of the intervention, the results for each subject for each of the assessment tools, the discussion, conclusion, and references. Using the manual,[21] the therapist followed the instructions for each component of the case report. Faculty at the local university reviewed the manuscript and provided suggestions before the manuscript was submitted for publication. The therapist also prepared a poster submission for the state physical therapy association annual meeting.

Case Study #3: Taylor

➤ Practice pattern 5C: Impaired Motor Function and Sensory Integrity Associated With Nonprogressive Disorders of the Central Nervous System—Congenital Origin or Acquired in Infancy or Childhood

➤ Medical diagnosis: Myelomeningocele, repaired L1-2

➤ Age: 4 years

Taylor is currently enrolled in a Saturday karate class that includes children who are disabled and children who are nondisabled. The family has a disagreement regarding the class. Taylor's father wants him to continue the class because Taylor has the opportunity to interact with children his own age and participate in a sport. He feels that Taylor will develop greater confidence, self-esteem, and social skills. Taylor's mother would prefer that Taylor take piano lessons. The parents ask the physical therapist who is a consultant in the karate program to help them settle their disagreement. The therapist does not want to interfere but agrees to search for research on the effects of karate in children with disabilities.

Step 1: Develop the Clinical Question

Does karate have positive effects for children with developmental disabilities?

Step 2: Gather the Evidence

Searching the Hooked on Evidence and PEDro databases did not reveal any articles on karate or martial arts, other than one article in PEDro related to exercise in patients with Parkinson's disease.[32] MEDLINE was the next database explored. The keyword *karate* produced 154 records which was too many to review. The keywords *karate* and *child* produced 17 records but none of those records seemed to relate to children with developmental disabilities. The search was repeated with the CINAHL database. *Karate* produced 29 hits, but only two of the titles seemed relevant and they were published in magazines, not peer-reviewed journals.[33,34] The keywords *martial arts* and *child* resulted in 39 hits; none of those titles seemed relevant. The SPORTDiscus database was searched next. The keyword *karate* found 1927 articles, so *karate* and *child* were entered and 48 titles were found. A quick review of the titles revealed nothing relevant. The keyword *martial arts* retrieved 2024 articles. *Martial arts* and *child* were entered and 35 records were found, but none of those titles seemed relevant either. Remembering an article in *PT—Magazine of Physical Therapy*, a search of CINAHL was conducted. The name of the journal was entered and combined with the keyword *martial arts*. This professional magazine is not a peer-reviewed journal, but the article was retrieved from the therapist's office with the expectation that there would be references that would be useful.[35] The other two magazine articles identified by the CINAHL search with the keyword *karate* were retrieved.[33,34] Unfortunately none of the articles had any references. The three articles that were retrieved were all from periodicals that were not peer-reviewed.[33-35] An expanded search involved additional keywords such as *spina bifida, physical therapy, disabilities,* and *disabled,* but the only peer-reviewed article referred to martial arts for a young man with paraplegia for self-defense and did not seem to apply to this case of a 4-year-old child.[36]

Step 3: Critically Appraise the Evidence

This review did not uncover any relevant articles in peer-reviewed journals. The level of evidence was only anecdotal reports in magazines. These anecdotes may be useful in the development of future research projects but do not provide any concrete supportive evidence for positive effects of karate in children with developmental disabilities.

Step 4: Apply the Evidence

In this case, the family sought information to settle a disagreement: one parent favored the karate program but the other parent did not. The therapist searched for evidence in order to help them decide whether Taylor will continue the karate program. The therapist shared the magazine articles and explained to the parents that no research evidence was found. The lack of evidence does not mean that karate is not beneficial to children with disabilities. The lack of evidence means that there is a need for research to confirm or refute the benefits that have been anecdotally reported. There is also a need to study potential adverse effects of karate. The therapist did not make a recommendation, but suggested that the parents read the articles, discuss their viewpoints, and then make their decision regarding continuing the karate program.

Case Study #4: Ashley

➤ Practice pattern 5B: Impaired Neuromotor Development
➤ Medical diagnosis: Down syndrome
➤ Age: 15 months

At the early intervention center, Ashley's mother met a woman whose son has cerebral palsy. The woman told Ashley's mother about a new treatment being done at a private clinic and that her son walks much better since he started this new treadmill program. One of the family's goals for Ashley is to begin to walk without holding onto her mother's hands. Ashley's mother made an appointment at the clinic to learn more about the treadmill training. The physical therapist at the clinic had worked only with children with cerebral palsy but had read articles on the use of supported treadmill training for children with Down syndrome, including a randomized controlled trial published in 2001.[37-39] For children with cerebral palsy, the therapist used the Gross Motor Function Measure (GMFM) [40,41] as an outcome measure to determine if there was a difference in gross motor skills after several weeks of the treadmill treatment. The therapist did not know if the GMFM would be an appropriate outcome measure for Ashley, although the measure seemed age appropriate. The therapist read the GMFM manual and found that the reliability and validity studies were performed with children with cerebral palsy; this manual was published in 1993, so the therapist was interested in any new research.

In evaluating the research related to an assessment tool, there are several issues. The therapist was familiar with the GMFM, so research on the ease of administration was not a primary concern. The old GMFM manual addressed the psychometric properties of the measure only in children with cerebral palsy.[40] There are several questions to answer. Are there studies regarding the reliability of the GMFM in children with Down syndrome to ensure measurements are accurate and consistent in that patient population? Are there studies regarding the validity of the GMFM as an evaluative measure of gross motor function for children with Down syndrome? Would the GMFM demonstrate a clinically important change after intervention if there were such a change? All of these questions are important to consider in answering the clinical question using the available evidence.

Step 1: Develop the Clinical Question

Is the GMFM appropriate for use in assessing the effects of treadmill training on gross motor function in children with Down syndrome?

Step 2: Gather the Evidence

Typing *gross motor function measure* into the search engine at yahoo.com led to a description of the new 2002 GMFM manual on the Cambridge University Press web site. The description of the new book did not include any mention of Down syndrome, but the therapist ordered the book for updated information including a new version of the GMFM. The search for evidence began with the MEDLINE database and five titles were found with the keywords *Down syndrome* and *gross motor function.* Three articles involved the GMFM and children with Down syndrome,[42-44] but the other two abstracts were not relevant for this search.[45,46] Repeating the same search in CINAHL resulted in the same three articles of interest; PsycINFO and SPORTDiscus did not uncover any additional references. Thus the search resulted in three new articles on the GMFM and its use with children with Down syndrome to be obtained from the library.[42-44]

Step 3: Critically Appraise the Evidence

The GMFM authors stated that it is not appropriate to use the GMFM-66 version for children with Down syndrome because it was designed specifically for children with cerebral palsy.[9] They also cautioned against using the Gross Motor Function Classification system for children other than children with cerebral palsy. Palisano and colleagues studied motor growth in children with Down syndrome, which differs from motor development in children with cerebral palsy.[44] Based on the instructions in the manual, one dimension of the GMFM may be used rather than the entire test. Since the supported treadmill training is directed at walking, the therapist wanted to know if only the Walking, Running, and Jumping domain could be assessed. The best available evidence to support the use of the GMFM is the validation study which involved 123 children with Down syndrome.[42] The levels of evidence are defined differently for assessment tools than for interventions and are somewhat more difficult to interpret, but this research provides strong evidence for the validity of the GMFM as an evaluative measure of gross motor function in children with Down syndrome.

Step 4: Apply the Evidence

The therapist decided to use the Walking, Running, and Jumping dimension of the GMFM as the functional outcome measure for treadmill training for Ashley. The research supports the psychometric properties of this test in the population of children with Down syndrome.[42,43] The evidence applies directly to Ashley's situation. Since the therapist is experienced in using the tool, clinical expertise is utilized. Using only the one domain of the GMFM will make it realistic for use in a very young child with Down syndrome and parent report will be incorporated for items that Ashley does not readily perform.

Case Study #5: John

➤ Practice pattern 5B: Impaired Neuromotor Development

➤ Medical diagnosis: Attention deficit hyperactivity disorder, developmental coordination disorder

➤ Age: 5 years

John's parents decided to enroll him in the same karate program Taylor attended (Case Study #3). The physical therapist who searched for evidence related to karate for children with disabilities became interested in clinical research due to the lack of research on karate. The therapist contacted a pediatric physical therapy professor at the local university to discuss the possibility of collaborating on a clinical research project. The professor was very interested in a collaborative project. Together they designed a single subject study to answer their research question: Does a 12-week karate program improve gross motor skills in a child with ADHD as measured by the Bruininks-Oseretsky Test of Motor Proficiency (BOTMP)?[48] The university institutional review board approved the study with a limit of 10 children to participate in the single subject design. Each child would follow the protocol with the data analyzed separately for each child. The professor obtained a small grant from the university. As part of the budget, funds were used to pay a therapist not associated with the study to perform all of the assessments with the BOTMP. They selected a therapist experienced in using the BOTMP. This therapist would not be informed of the study design and would not know when John was participating in the karate program. If the professor or the therapist involved in the karate program performed the assessments, there would likely be a bias toward finding positive results of the program despite all attempts to remain objective.

The study was an ABA design with three phases. The A-phases of the study had no intervention; the B-phase was the karate program. In this program, karate sessions typically run for 12 weeks, so the study was designed around that time frame with a total of 33 weeks to complete the study. Each child was assessed three times in each phase of the study, so there were a total of nine assessments for each child. The inclusion criteria for the study were children under 12 years of age with ADHD who had not previously participated in the karate program and who were medically cleared by their physician to participate. The children also had to have a documented balance deficit because balance was one of the impairments that often seemed to improve according to the therapist involved with the karate program. Subjects were recruited when parents of children with ADHD inquired about the program.

John met the inclusion criteria and his family was invited to participate in the study. The parents signed an informed consent form. The study was explained to John in age-appropriate language. He verbalized understanding of the study and willingness to participate and signed his name on the assent form. The assessments took place every 4 weeks and the BOTMP was performed each time. All assessments were performed by the physical therapist who was masked (or blinded) to the treatment design—the therapist did not know when John was participating in the karate program. The study began with the first A-phase—no intervention, only measurement. John was assessed three times: the first time, 4 weeks later, and again after 4 more weeks. There were 9 weeks in the first A-phase. The beginning of the karate program was the B-phase. John was assessed after the fourth week of karate classes, after the eighth week of karate classes, and after the 12th week—the last week of karate classes. For the final A-phase, John was assessed three more

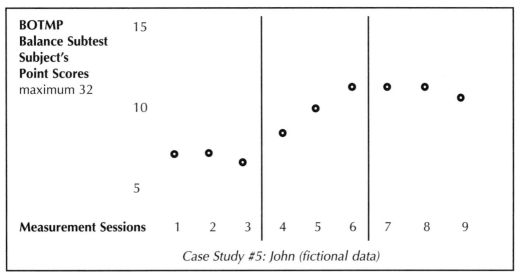

Figure 16-1. Graph of BOTMP balance subtest fictional data.

times: 4 weeks after karate ended, 8 weeks after karate ended, and 12 weeks after karate ended. At this point, data collection was completed.

The data were ready for analysis. The researchers plotted each of the eight subtests of the BOTMP on a separate graph for visual analysis. Figure 16-1 provides an example of fictional results plotted for the balance subtest scores for each of the three phases. The data may be interpreted using different methods.[20] Visual analysis is the simplest method and shows that the baseline phase A was stable. There was little difference between the scores in the first three measurement sessions. In phase B, the scores increased with higher scores recorded for each subsequent session. There appears to have been a substantial change in balance subtest scores during the intervention phase. In the second phase A, the improvements were fairly well-maintained, but there were no further gains. From this fictional data, it appears that the intervention had an impact on the balance subtest scores. However, without knowing if there are any other differences in the child's life during the time of the study, it is difficult to attribute these results to the karate program with complete confidence. Generalizing these results to other children also is questionable, but the results suggest that karate improved balance for this child with ADHD. Researchers need to analyze the results from the other seven subtests to determine if there were improvements and they could also employ other methods of analyzing the data.[20]

An ABABA design would attain a higher level of scientific evidence. But, as their first attempt at a collaborative clinical research project, the investigators felt that the ABA design was a more realistic endeavor. The scientific strength of the study was improved by using a masked evaluator not associated with the research. The investigators also chose an outcome measure with an evaluative purpose, although the BOTMP also has been used as a discriminative test.[49] The psychometric properties of this test seemed to be stronger than the other measures considered. The test is easy to administer and does not require any special training.

The manuscript was written as a collaborative effort between the faculty member and the physical therapist in the karate program who were co-authors. The therapist who performed the assessments was paid by a small grant and did not contribute in any other way to the research project. This therapist received an acknowledgment in the publication but was not listed as an author of the article. The faculty member presented the research at the APTA Combined Sections meeting. The therapist in the karate program presented the research at the AACPDM annual meeting.

Summary

The primary goal of this chapter is to familiarize pediatric therapists with the concept of evidence-based practice: the use of current best evidence to make decisions for individual clients based on the clinician's expertise and the values of the client. The expectation is that pediatric clinicians will better understand the process and implement evidence-based practice. This chapter provides some basic terms and research methodology to allow clinicians to evolve in their roles as consumers of research as well as clinical researchers. The case studies provide examples of answering a clinical question using the available evidence, outlining a case report to document treatment effectiveness, and designing a single subject research study to begin to document treatment efficacy. For clinicians interested in participating in large-scale studies, there are resources for developing collaborative research relationships.

Conclusion

Therapists have a responsibility to contribute to our collective body of knowledge. Sharing that knowledge also is our responsibility, whether at the level of staff in-services or peer-reviewed publications. Ultimately, our greatest responsibility is to provide the best possible care to patients and their families. Practicing evidence-based medicine and contributing to the available evidence is of importance to all therapists determined to carry out their professional responsibilities.

References

1. Law M. Strategies for implementing evidence-based practice in early intervention. *Inf Young Children*. 2000;12:32-40.
2. Sackett D, Straus S, Richardson W, et al. *Evidence-Based Medicine: How to Practice and Teach EBM*. 2nd ed. New York, NY: Churchill Livingstone; 2000.
3. American Physical Therapy Association. Clinical research agenda for physical therapy. *Phys Ther*. 2000;80:499-513.
4. Fritz J, Kelly MK. Clinical question: what signs and symptoms can be used to differentiate low back pain of a musculoskeletal origin from a potentially more serious non-musculoskeletal condition in a 12-year-old girl? *Phys Ther*. 2002;82:504-510.
5. Butler C, Chambers H, Goldstein M, et al. Evaluating research in developmental disabilities: A conceptual framework for reviewing treatment outcomes. *Dev Med Child Neurol*. 1999; 41:55-59.
6. Butler C, Darrah J. Effects of neurodevelopmental treatment (NDT) for cerebral palsy: an AACPDM evidence report. *Dev Med Child Neurol*. 2001;43:778-790.
7. Guyatt G, Kirshner B, Jaeschke R. Measuring health status: what are the necessary measurement properties? *J Clin Epidemiology*. 1992;12:1341-1345.
8. Folio M, Fewell R. *Peabody Developmental Motor Scales (PDMS-2)*. 2nd ed. Austin, Tex: PRO-ED; 2000.

9. Russell D, Rosenbaum P, Avery L, et al. *Gross Motor Function Measure (GMFM-66 & GMFM-88) User's Manual.* London: Mac Keith Press; 2002.

10. Campbell SK, Osten ET, Kolobe THA, et al. Development of the Test of Infant Motor Performance. *Phys Med Rehabil Clin North Am.* 1993;4:541-550.

11. Campbell S. Test-retest reliability of the Test of Infant Motor Performance. *Pediatric Physical Therapy.* 1999;11:60-66.

12. Flegel J, Kolobe T. Predictive validity of the Test of Infant Motor Performance as measured by the Bruininks-Oseretsky Test of Motor Proficiency at school age. *Phys Ther.* 2002;82:762-771.

13. Campbell S, Kolobe T, Wright B, et al. Validity of the Test of Infant Motor Performance for prediction of 6-, 9- and 12-month scores in the Alberta Infant Motor Scale. *Dev Med Child Neurol.* 2002;44:263-272.

14. Campbell S, Hedeker D. Validity of the Test of Infant Motor Performance for discriminating among infants with varying risk for poor motor outcome. *J Pediatr.* 2001;139:546-551.

15. Rosenbaum P, Russell D, Cadman D, et al. Issues in measuring change in motor function in children with cerebral palsy: a special communication. *Phys Ther.* 1990;70:125-131.

16. American Physical Therapy Association. *Guide to Physical Therapist Practice.* 2nd ed. Alexandria, Va: Author; 2001.

17. National Advisory Board. *Research Plan for National Center for Medical Rehabilitation Research. NIH Publication 93-3509.* Washington, DC: US Dept of Health and Human Services; 1993.

18. Sackett D. Rules of evidence and clinical recommendations on the use of antithrombotic agents. *Chest.* 1986;89(Suppl):2S.

19. Portney L, Watkins M. *Foundations of Clinical Research Applications to Practice.* Norwalk, Conn: Appleton & Lange; 1993.

20. Fitzgerald G, Delitto A. Considerations for planning and conducting clinic-based research in physical therapy. *Phys Ther.* 2001;81:1446-1454.

21. McEwen I, ed. *Writing Case Reports: A How-to Manual for Clinicians.* Alexandria, Va: American Physical Therapy Association; 1996.

22. McGibbon N, Andrade C, Widener G, et al. Effect of an equine-movement therapy program on gait, energy expenditure, and motor function in children with spastic cerebral palsy: a pilot study. *Dev Med Child Neurol.* 1998;40:754-762.

23. Haehl V, Giuliani C, Lewis C. Influence of hippotherapy on the kinematics and functional performance of two children with cerebral palsy. *Pediatric Physical Therapy.* 1999;11:89-101.

24. Keren O, Reznik J, Groswasser Z. Combined motor disturbances following severe traumatic brain injury: an integrative long-term treatment approach. *Brain Inj.* 2001;15:633-638.

25. Sterba J, Rogers B, France A, et al. Horseback riding in children with cerebral palsy: effect on gross motor function. *Dev Med Child Neurol.* 2002;44:301-308.

26. Winchester P, Kendall K, Peters H, et al. The effect of therapeutic horseback riding on gross motor function and gait speed in children who are developmentally delayed. *Phys Occup Ther Pediatr.* 2002;22:37-50.

27. Bertoti D. Effect of therapeutic horseback riding on posture in children with cerebral palsy. *Phys Ther.* 1988;68:1505-1512.

28. MacKinnon J. A study of therapeutic effects of horseback riding for children with cerebral palsy. *Phys Occup Ther Pediatr.* 1995;15:17-34.

29. MacPhail H, Edwards J, Golding J, et al. Trunk postural reactions in children with and without cerebral palsy during therapeutic horseback riding. *Pediatric Physical Therapy.* 1998;10: 143-147.

30. Bertoti D. Clinical suggestions. Effect of therapeutic horseback riding on extremity weight bearing in a child with hemiplegic cerebral palsy: a case report as an example of clinical research. *Pediatric Physical Therapy.* 1991;3:219-224.

31. Palisano R, Rosenbaum P, Walter S, et al. Development and reliability of a system to classify gross motor function in children with cerebral palsy. *Dev Med Child Neurol.* 1997;39:214-223.

32. Palmer SS, Mortimer JA, Webster DD, et al. Exercise therapy for Parkinson's disease. *Arch Phys Med Rehabil.* 1986;67:741-745.

33. Greenberg S. Karate generation. *Newsweek.* 2000;136:50.

34. Young R. It can be done. *Exceptional Parent.* 2001;31:32-33.

35. Woods E. Martial arts and physical therapy: exploring the connection. *PT.* 2002;10:30-35.

36. Madorsky JG, Scanlon JR, Smith B. Kung-Fu: synthesis of wheelchair sport and self-protection. *Arch Phys Med Rehabil.* 1989;70:490-492.

37. Ulrich B, Ulrich D, Collier D, et al. Developmental shifts in the ability of infants with Down syndrome to produce treadmill steps. *Phys Ther.* 1995;75:14-23.

38. Ulrich B, Ulrich D, Collier D. Alternating stepping patterns: hidden abilities of 11-month-old infants with Down syndrome. *Dev Med Child Neurol.* 1992;34:233-239.

39. Ulrich D, Ulrich B, Angulo-Kinzler R, et al. Treadmill training of infants with Down syndrome: evidence-based developmental outcomes. *Pediatrics.* 2001;108:84.

40. Russell D, Rosenbaum P, Gowland C, et al. *Gross Motor Function Measure Manual.* Hamilton, Ontario, Canada: McMaster University; 1993.

41. Russell D, Rosenbaum P, Cadman D, et al. The gross motor function measure: a means to evaluate the effects of physical therapy. *Dev Med Child Neurol.* 1989;31:341-352.

42. Russell D, Palisano R, Walter S, et al. Evaluating motor function in children with Down syndrome: validity of the GMFM. *Dev Med Child Neurol.* 1998;40:693-701.

43. Gemus M, Palisano R, Russell D, et al. Using the gross motor function measure to evaluate motor development in children with Down syndrome. *Phys Occup Ther Pediatr.* 2001;21:69-79.

44. Palisano R, Walter S, Russell D, et al. Gross motor function of children with Down syndrome: creation of motor growth curves. *Arch Phys Med Rehabil.* 2001;82:494-500.

45. Mahoney G, Robinson C, Fewell R. The effects of early motor intervention on children with Down syndrome or cerebral palsy: a field-based study. *Pediatrics.* 2001;22:153-162.

46. Spano M, Mercuri E, Rando T, et al. Motor and perceptual-motor competence in children with Down syndrome: variation in performance with age. *European J Paediatr Neurol.* 1999;3:7-13.

47. Bayley N. *Manual for the Bayley Scales of Infant Development.* 2nd ed. San Antonio, Tex: The Psychological Corporation; 1993.

48. Bruininks R. *Bruininks-Oseretsky Test of Motor Proficiency Examiner's Manual.* Circle Pines, Minn: American Guidance Service; 1978.

49. Westcott S, Lowes L, Richardson P. Evaluation of postural stability in children: current theories and assessment tools. *Phys Ther.* 1997;77:629-645.

50. Rothstein J, Echternach J. *Primer on Measurement: An Introductory Guide to Measurement Issues.* Alexandria, Va: American Physical Therapy Association; 1993.

CHAPTER 17

SINGLE CASE DESIGNS FOR THE CLINICIAN

Susan R. Harris, PhD, PT, FAPTA

During the past two decades, increased emphasis has been placed on conducting clinical research in physical therapy. The American Physical Therapy Association (APTA) defined clinical research as "a systematic process for formulating and answering questions about the uses of, the bases for, and the effectiveness of physical therapy practice."[1] The profession has developed and is promoting a clinical research agenda.[2] With the passage of Public Law 94-142 (PL 94-142) in 1975,[3] physical therapists and other "related services" providers working in the public schools were required to participate in assessing and ensuring the effectiveness of their treatment strategies in enabling children with disabilities to benefit from special education. Only through measurement and collection of objective and quantifiable data on children's gross motor, fine motor, and self-help skills is it possible to establish accountability for our intervention strategies.[4]

Importance of Clinical Research in Pediatric Physical Therapy

For physical therapists working with children with developmental disabilities, the use of clinical research strategies in documenting the efficacy of treatment is vital. Not only is documentation required by law,[3] but it also is necessary to answer a variety of important clinical questions. For example, is this particular treatment approach making positive changes in the child's functional abilities? Will the child get worse if I continue treatment? Will the child improve more quickly if I increase therapy from 1 hour/week to 2 hours/week? Only through systematic clinical research is it possible to reliably answer such questions. There is great temptation among physical therapists, particularly those who are recent graduates, to assume that their treatment is creating a beneficial change for the child. Even seasoned clinicians who complete a continuing education course have vested interests in "believing" that their newly acquired intervention techniques are affecting positive change in their clients. Because we have all chosen to work in a helping profession, our desire to "help" may overshadow our abilities to objectively define and measure our successes or our failures. We owe it to the children, as well as to their parents, teachers, and physicians, to reliably document the effects of our treatment. Such documentation can be accomplished through carefully formulated clinical research plans.

Applied vs Basic Research

Although currently, research is a more acceptable endeavor in physical therapy, some clinicians continue to be "turned off' by the term "research" because to them it implies esoteric laboratory experiments, which have little functional relevance to day-to-day practice. Common misconceptions about research are that it requires large numbers of subjects (not readily available in the average clinical setting), an inordinate amount of time (which will detract from treatment time), a large amount of money, and an advanced knowledge of statistics and complex data analysis. While it is true that some types of research encompass the foregoing requirements, there also are simpler and less sophisticated types of research that have functional relevance for physical therapists.

Research often is classified as either basic or applied. Basic research examines questions that tend to be abstract and that may be used to generate new theories. Generally, applied research is directed at answering questions of practical significance.[5] Basic research often is conducted in a tightly controlled laboratory setting. Applied research is more appropriate for the clinical setting. The research strategies presented in this chapter are of an applied nature (ie, relevant to an individual or society). However, there is a need for both basic and applied research in the area of developmental disabilities.

Reliability and Validity

Reliability and validity are important components of both applied and basic research (see Chapter 16). To demonstrate accountability, physical therapists must ensure that their evaluation tools, as well as their treatment outcomes, are both reliable and valid. *Reliability* refers to the consistency between measurements.[6] Consistency may be assessed between two different raters (interrater reliability) or across a series of measures conducted by one rater (intrarater reliability). A common measurement tool used in physical therapy is the goniometer. If two therapists independently measured hip range of motion in three children with myelomeningocele, recorded their measurements independently, and agreed perfectly in all planes of range of motion measured, we could conclude that they have achieved perfect interrater reliability. If one of the therapists continued to measure hip range of motion on one child across several different therapy sessions and the scores were compared, we would be examining intrarater reliability.

Once reliability of a measurement tool is established within the clinical setting, this tool can be used to evaluate treatment outcomes. For example, if the therapist wanted to examine the effects of passive stretching of the hip flexor muscles on decreasing hip flexor tightness in a child with myelomeningocele, a series of baseline or pretreatment measures and a series of ROM measures both during and after the intervention phase (stretching procedures) would be collected. Only through a systematic and reliable series of measures is it possible to document the efficacy of passive stretching.

In actual practice, little research has been published on the reliability of goniometry for use with children with developmental disabilities. One clinical research study examining goniometric reliability of upper extremity measurements for a child with spastic quadriplegia concluded that "there was wide variability in measurements both within and between raters."[7] Even with this lack of documented reliability of goniometry, many clinicians continue to use this measurement tool to make claims about the effectiveness of their treatment.

Another important component of clinical research is *validity* or the extent to which an instrument measures what it is supposed to measure. A goniometer is designed to clinically measure joint angle or the angle between two or more bones that form a joint. We infer from palpating bony landmarks that we are measuring the angle of the bones to one another. One method for establishing the validity of this clinical technique is to take x-rays of the joint angle. For example, if we were to measure an elbow flexion contracture through goniometry and then x-ray the arm to measure the actual angle of the humerus to the radius, we could assess the validity of our clinical measure. Physical therapists working with children with developmental disabilities use a variety of standardized tests to assess areas such as gross motor, fine motor, and visual-perceptual development. These tools are used in qualifying a child to receive special services as well as in measuring developmental change as a result of treatment. It is crucial that these instruments are both reliable and valid in accomplishing their aims. Therapists are advised to read the reliability and validity data published in the test administration manual before assuming that the test is acceptable. Even though a test has been published and distributed widely, it may not possess acceptable levels of reliability and validity. It is our responsibility as clinicians to ensure that the measures we are using for examination and documentation of treatment outcome are both reliable and valid. Refer to Chapter 2 for information on the reliability and validity of currently used pediatric examination tools.

Research Terminology

There are a number of terms, common to all types of research, that the physical therapist should be able to understand and use when reading about or conducting clinical research. Some of these terms, such as reliability and validity, have been defined in the preceding section and in Chapter 16. Two common terms, used in both experimental and correlational research, are independent and dependent variables. In experimental research, the *independent* variable is the variable manipulated by the experimenter, and is known also as the treatment variable. The *dependent* variable, known also as the outcome variable, is used to evaluate the influence of the independent variable on treatment. Referring back to our example of measuring the effects of passive stretching of the hip flexor muscles on decreasing hip flexor tightness, the independent variable is the passive stretching and the dependent variable is the range of hip extension. In correlational research, the relationship of two or more variables is examined. However, none of the variables are manipulated by the investigator, as is done in experimental research. Research on reliability and validity of measures is usually correlational research. In the example in which the validity of goniometric measures of an elbow flexion contracture is evaluated through subsequent x-rays, the goniometric measures would comprise the independent variable and the range of motion as measured on x-ray would be the dependent variable. In addition to using widely accepted measurement tools, such as goniometry and standardized developmental assessment instruments, therapists may rely on practical, functional measures developed within their own clinical settings to serve as dependent variables. The advantage of such measurement strategies is that they may be "individualized" for each child in the caseload. Such measures are frequently developed as part of the goals and objectives required in the individual education program (IEP) mandated by PL 94-142.[3,4]

One type of dependent measure commonly used in pediatric therapy settings is *frequency* or the number of times a behavior occurs.[8] Perhaps you have written an objective to decrease the number of tongue thrusts that occur during a 30-minute feeding session. By simply counting the number of tongue thrusts that occur, you can measure the frequency of this behavior.

Another type of measurement appropriate to clinical settings is *percentage occurrence* or the number of occurrences of the behavior divided by the number of opportunities in which the behavior can occur, multiplied times 100.[8] For example, if the goal is to increase heel strikes in the involved foot of a child with spastic hemiplegia you would begin by taking baseline data on this behavior. By having the child walk down a 50-foot hallway, you could count the number of heel strikes during the total number of steps on the involved side. If the child demonstrates a heel strike on five occasions out of 20 possible steps, you would compute 5/20 x 100 = 25%.

Duration is another common type of measurement in which the length or amount of time the behavior occurs during a given observation period is assessed.[8] For example, the duration of independent sitting or independent standing is an important functional measure for many children with developmental disabilities. Children with mental retardation often show delays in their response time to a given stimulus. To assess the effects of intervention on improving such behaviors, a measure of *latency* would be used. If you are working on undressing skills for a child with Down syndrome, for example, you may decide to measure the latency or length of time between giving the command, such as "shoe off!" and the child's initiation of the behavior.

These four are examples of the more common types of dependent measures used in clinical research. For a more extensive description of these and other types of behavioral measures, refer to the chapter on single subject design in the research design textbook by Portney and Watkins.[8]

A Model for Clinical Research: The Single Subject Research Design

Physical therapists in clinical settings have many questions about the efficacy of their treatment strategies and yet usually do not have sufficient numbers of similar patients to conduct large group experimental research. The necessity of having a control group to compare the effects of treatment vs no treatment also raises ethical issues about withholding treatment, even if its efficacy is unproven. The single subject research design offers clinicians a method for empirically evaluating treatment effectiveness for individual clients or small groups of clients without the need for a control group.[9] Instead, subjects serve as their own control.

Single subject research design involves carefully controlled manipulation of the treatment variable and analysis of its effects on the outcome variable.[10] Target behaviors or outcome variables must be clearly specified and operationally defined with continuous measures of these variables taken throughout each phase of the study. Data collection methods must be reliable and extraneous variables must be carefully controlled.

Single subject research design should not be confused with the case reports.[11] Single subject research involves continuous and systematic data collection with careful manipulation of the treatment variable. Whereas the case report provides a detailed description of an individual's behavior, it lacks the experimental control of the true research design.[10,11] Although case reports can be used to generate hypotheses for future research, they cannot be used to document efficacy of treatment because of their lack of experimental control. Nonetheless, case reports are still important in physical therapy because they may stimulate research ideas in which cause-and-effect relationships can be examined. Such case reports involving children with cerebral palsy have appeared in the physical therapy literature.[12,13] Single subject research designs are particularly appropriate for use with children with developmental disabilities. Because of the great heterogeneity of diagnostic categories, it is virtually impossible to find enough similar subjects for a large group study. Even within each specific disability such as cerebral palsy, there are a variety of subtypes (eg, spastic diplegia, athetosis, and ataxia). There are justifiable ethical concerns about withholding treatment to any person with a disability, as is often necessary in group comparison research.

Single subject research designs may be incorporated directly into an ongoing clinical program. There is no need for elaborate, expensive equipment or sophisticated data analysis techniques. Changes in behavior may be graphed on simple graph paper and visually analyzed.[14] Another benefit is the collection of repeated measures throughout each phase of the study, a more powerful control for within-subject variability than a pretest/posttest design. Finally, in applied research such as this, changes must be clinically significant to be meaningful. In large group research, it is possible to effect changes that are statistically significant, but that have little value clinically to individual patients.

Measurement in Single Subject Research Design

To ensure reliability, the dependent measures or target behaviors in single subject research must be carefully defined. A clear operational definition for the behavior being measured will enhance both reliability and replicability of the design. For example, if your goal is to improve a child's upper extremity strength you must carefully define how you plan to measure strength. To use a frequency type of measure, you might define upper extremity strength as the number of wheelchair push-ups a child with myelomeningocele can accomplish in a given period of time. The types of clinical, behavioral measures defined in the foregoing section are those frequently used in single subject research: frequency, percent, duration, and latency.

It is important to assess interrater reliability of your dependent measures during each phase of the study. In the foregoing example, it would be important to have a colleague or physical therapist assistant also count the number of wheelchair push-ups the child can achieve during at least one or two measurement sessions in each phase of the study. To increase reliability, you might need to carefully define that a complete wheelchair push-up includes full extension of both elbows with the child's buttocks clearing the seat of the wheelchair.

One potential problem encountered in behavioral measurement is examiner bias. Because of the need to believe that our treatment is effective, our objectivity may be threatened in counting behaviors that we seek to increase (or decrease) as a result of treatment. By using a colleague who is "blind" to the phase of the study in which the child is involved to collect interrater reliability data, we can increase the believability of our results.

One common criticism of single subject research design is its lack of generalizability or external validity. To increase the power or generalizability of the single subject design, it must be replicated across different children, in different settings, and by different therapists.[8,10]

Types of Experimental Designs

The simplest type of single subject design is the AB design or simple baseline design.[8-10] During the A-phase or baseline period, the target behavior is measured in its naturally occurring state (prior to introducing the intervention or treatment variable). This phase then is used as the "control" against which the frequency of behaviors in the other phases are compared. During the B-phase, the treatment variable is introduced and measurement of the target behavior continues.

A minimum of three data points during each phase of treatment is desirable. Because of its inability to control for the effects of confounding variables, such as maturation, the AB design is not considered a true experimental design. It may be useful, however, in conjunction with a case study approach to generate ideas for future research.

The ABA or withdrawal design allows for control of extraneous variables in the environment in that the third phase provides for a return to baseline conditions through withdrawal of the treatment variable. One limitation of this design is that it can be used only with behaviors that are reversible. Much of what we teach in therapy ultimately will be retained, even after the specific intervention is removed, either through environmental reinforcement or the child's delight in accomplishing a new task. A second drawback of this design is the ethical issue of terminating the study in a no-treatment phase, thus lessening the positive gains from treatment. To counter this drawback, the ABAB design is proposed. Known also as the withdrawal-reinstatement design, the ABAB design concludes with a second B-phase in which the treatment is reinstated. This is more desirable ethically than the ABA design but is limited by the need to target a behavior that is reversible. Another type of single subject design is the alternating treatments design.[15] While less commonly used than some of the foregoing designs, the alternating treatments design has been used to evaluate the effects of lower extremity orthoses on improving standing balance in a child with cerebral palsy.[16] This design is used to investigate the effects of two or more interventions on a single behavior of a client. Following a baseline phase, two or more treatments are introduced and rapidly alternated. The final phase usually involves implementation of only the most effective treatment.[17] There are a number of other single subject designs that also are appropriate for use with children with developmental disabilities, such as the multiple baseline, the multiple probe, the changing criterion, and the parallel treatments design. These designs are more complex and will not be described in this chapter. For further information on descriptions and uses of these designs with exceptional children, refer to the text by Wolery, Bailey, and Sugai.[17] To provide further clarification of the four designs that have been described above, each will be used in the case studies of the children described in Chapter 4.

Case Study #1: Jason (AB Design)

➤ Practice pattern 5C: Impaired Motor Function and Sensory Integrity Associated With Nonprogressive Disorders of the Central Nervous System—Congenital Origin or Acquired in Infancy or Childhood
➤ Medical diagnosis: Cerebral palsy, right hemiparesis
➤ Age: 24 months

The goal of increasing use of the right upper extremity during play activities was identified for Jason. The specific objective for him was to increase the frequency with which he used his right hand during a 5-minute free play session. To set up an AB design, the treatment and outcome variables first must be operationally defined. Based on Jason's case study, which includes a history of tactile defensive behavior to light touch, sensory disregard, and neglect of the right upper extremity, the following therapy plan was proposed:

➤ Joint approximation through the right shoulder and into the open hand with Jason in quadruped
➤ Tactile desensitization activities that Jason can do on himself using the left hand to gently rub lotion on the right upper extremity
➤ Positive reinforcement (praise) by the therapist when Jason uses the right hand in play activities

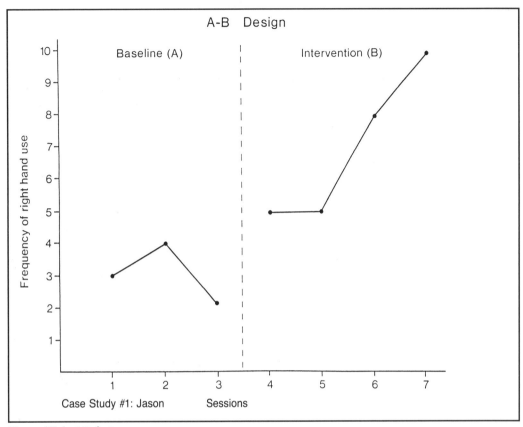

Figure 17-1. AB design.

This therapy plan encompasses the independent or treatment variable. The target behavior or outcome variable is increased use of the right hand during play activities. Because Jason is treated in the home, his mother will be instructed in assisting with data collection for frequency of right hand use.

During baseline (A-phase), the therapist collects frequency data on the number of times Jason uses his right hand during a 5-minute free play session after therapy. She collects data on three successive days and notes the following pattern of right hand use: Day 1—Three occasions, Day 2—Four occasions, Day 3—Two occasions. She plots these data on regular graph paper and notes a fairly stable baseline pattern (Figure 17-1). Therefore, it is an appropriate time to introduce the new treatment plan. It is important to realize that baseline does not have to mean total absence of therapy. It is possible that Jason has been getting some generalized physical therapy for some time, but the previous therapy has not focused on use of the right upper extremity.

On Day 4, the therapist introduces the new intervention that includes joint approximation, tactile desensitization, and praise for use of the right hand during play in therapy. She then continues to collect data during the 5-minute free play session after therapy. Jason's mother, who is "blind" to the phases of treatment, collects interrater reliability data once during each phase of the study. Jason's use of his right hand increases: Day 4— Five occasions, Day 5—Five occasions, Day 6—Eight occasions, Day 7—10 occasions (see Figure 17-1). While it is tempting to conclude that the new therapy plan has accounted for this improvement, it is important to realize that the AB design does not allow for such conclusions because it does not control for outside variables. Perhaps developmental maturation has influenced Jason's use of his right hand more than the therapy itself. To counter these limitations, an ABA or ABAB design would be preferable.

Case Study #2: Jill (ABA Design)

➤ Practice pattern 5C: Impaired Motor Function and Sensory Integrity Associated With Nonprogressive Disorders of the Central Nervous System—Congenital Origin or Acquired in Infancy or Childhood

➤ Medical diagnosis: Cerebral palsy, spastic quadriparesis, microcephaly, mental retardation, seizure disorder

➤ Age: 7 years

Jill can raise her head in prone but only momentarily. Because head raising in prone is important both developmentally and functionally, the following goal was written: Jill will improve head control in prone. The specific objective reads: Jill will increase duration of head raising in prone over a wedge. Thus the target behavior or dependent measure is increased head raising in prone.

Jill has not responded to more naturally occurring stimuli, such as tactile and vestibular input, for facilitation of her prone head righting. Since there is both neurophysiological[18] and clinical evidence[19] that vibratory stimulation will facilitate contraction of weak agonist muscles while inhibiting spasticity in the antagonist muscles, it was decided that a therapeutic vibrator would be used as the treatment modality. Since the facilitatory effect of vibration is relatively brief (approximately 30 minutes),[19] this type of intervention could be expected to produce a reversible pattern of behavior once it was removed. Thus, the treatment variable for this ABA study was operationally defined as 2 minutes of vibratory stimulation to the posterior neck muscles using a small mechanical vibrator which vibrates at a frequency of 100 to 200 Hz and an amplitude of 1.5 mm.[20]

Baseline data were taken with Jill positioned in prone over a wedge for a 5-minute period while in the classroom. A stopwatch was used to measure the total duration of head raising during the observation period. Head raising was further defined as lifting the head to an angle where the nose was perpendicular with the floor. Interrater reliability data were collected during each phase of the study by a physical therapy assistant who was unaware of the treatment plan.

During the B-phase, vibration was applied for 2 minutes in a cephalo-caudal direction while Jill was prone on the wedge. Data were collected on duration of head raising for a 5-minute period immediately following vibration. Dramatic improvement was noted as evidenced by changes in both level and trend of the data (Figure 17-2). When treatment was withdrawn during the second A-phase, the duration of head raising decreased, but not to the initial baseline level. Such change implies that Jill may have been reinforced intrinsically by the head raising such that she desired to continue this newly learned behavior. For ethical reasons, it would be desirable to proceed to a second B-phase, thus converting to an ABAB or withdrawal-reinstatement design.

Case Study #3: Taylor (ABAB Design)

➤ Practice pattern 5C: Impaired Motor Function and Sensory Integrity Associated With Nonprogressive Disorders of the Central Nervous System—Congenital Origin or Acquired in Infancy or Childhood

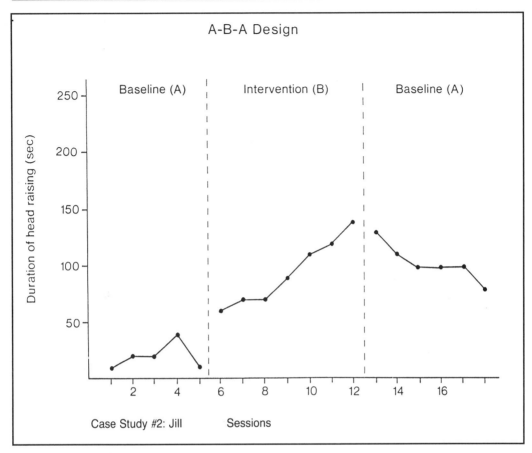

Figure 17-2. ABA design.

➤ Medical diagnosis: Myelomeningocele, repaired L1-2
➤ Age: 4 years

Taylor lacks the upper extremity muscle strength and endurance necessary to use ambulation aids effectively. The following goal and objective are proposed: 1) Goal: Taylor will increase his upper extremity muscle strength and endurance; 2) Objective: While wearing his lower extremity orthoses, Taylor will ambulate 10 consecutive lengths of the parallel bars, without rest breaks, using a swing-to gait for three consecutive days. Thus, ambulation in the parallel bars is the target behavior or dependent measure.

The treatment variable is composed of a three-part therapy plan: wheelchair push-ups, quadruped pushups, and positive reinforcement through a bar graph monitoring Taylor's progress. During baseline, Taylor was introduced to the parallel bars and instructed in how to accomplish a swing-to gait. A complete length of the parallel bars was defined as one in which Taylor required no physical assist from the therapist. Baseline data were plotted in Figure 17-3. The ambulation routine was part of Taylor's overall therapy program but was not emphasized or strongly reinforced during baseline.

During intervention, Taylor was taught to do both wheelchair push-ups and push-ups in quadruped. Following these activities, the therapist showed him a sticker

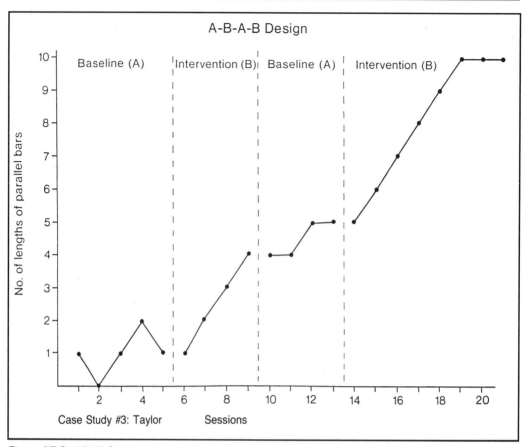

Figure 17-3. ABAB design.

chart made up like a bar graph and told him he could put on one sticker for each length of the parallel bars he could walk without sitting down. As can be seen from Figure 17-3, Taylor's success in the parallel bars improved dramatically. An attempt to return to baseline conditions (second B-phase), however did not result in a reversal of the behavior. Instead, Taylor's progress continued although the trend was not as marked as during the intervention.

It is not surprising that this behavior did not reverse itself. First of all, muscle strength and endurance will not diminish appreciably immediately upon discontinuing exercises. Secondly, the ambulation in the parallel bars, although the dependent measure in this study, will serve to increase and maintain upper extremity strength. Thirdly, even though the overt reinforcer (the sticker chart) was removed during the second phase, Taylor probably continued to feel intrinsic reinforcement for his success.

When intervention was reinstated during the second B-phase, the trend of the earlier B-phase continued and Taylor achieved his objective of 100% success for 3 consecutive days by Session 21. Due to the failure of the data to reverse during withdrawal of the intervention, it is impossible to definitely conclude that the exercise and reinforcement package "caused" the improvements noted. Taylor's success was no doubt due, in part, to intrinsic reinforcers as well as to strength acquired from the walking activity itself. By visually analyzing trends in the data during each phase, it is obvious that the steepest slopes of improvement occurred during the two B-phases, however, lending support to the efficacy of the intervention package.

Case Study #4: Ashley (Alternating Treatment Design)

➤ Practice pattern 5B: Impaired Neuromotor Development

➤ Medical diagnosis: Down syndrome

➤ Age: 15 months

Ashley tends to keep her mouth open, a typical behavior of infants with generalized hypotonia. Not only does the open mouth contribute to feeding difficulties, as in Ashley's case, but it is often a source of concern for parents who think that it contributes to making the child "look" different. Since Ashley is capable of closing her mouth, but does so infrequently, it is unclear whether the persistent mouth opening is a behavioral or a neurophysiological problem. In an effort to answer this question, two different treatment approaches were compared using an alternating treatment design. The following goal and objective were determined:

➤ Goal: Ashley will decrease open mouth behavior

➤ Objective: Ashley will close her mouth within 2 seconds of behavioral or neurophysiological cues

This initial study is directed at the latency of Ashley's response. Based on the success of either or both interventions, a subsequent objective would be geared toward increasing the duration of mouth closure to improve the functional relevance of this behavior. The two treatment variables consist of a verbal cue to Ashley to "close mouth, Ashley," and a behavioral cue of chin tapping based on Mueller's approach to oral-motor facilitation.[21] During baseline, Ashley was seated in an adaptive chair in front of the examiner and was engaged in fine motor play activities. The examiner collected data on the number of times Ashley closed her mouth during a 3-minute period (using a golf counter). No verbal cues or reinforcers were provided.

During the intervention phase, the two treatment strategies were rapidly alternated in random order. With Ashley again seated in a special chair and engaged in fine motor play, the examiner applied one treatment for a 3-minute period, took a 1-minute break, then applied the second treatment for a 3-minute period. For the verbal/behavioral intervention, the examiner verbally cued Ashley to close her mouth and then demonstrated this behavior. Each time Ashley closed her mouth within 2 seconds the data recorder (the parent) made a "+." Failure to close her mouth within 2 seconds resulted in a "-" mark. Successful completion of the behavior resulted in a smile from the examiner combined with praise such as "Good closing your mouth, Ashley!" Failure to comply resulted in the examiner looking away and ignoring Ashley for 5 seconds.

For the neurophysiological intervention, the examiner introduced five rapid "chin taps" each time the mouth was open and waited 2 seconds (from the final chin tap) for a response. Chin tapping was done with the dorsum of the fingers in a quick upward motion underneath the mandible. No verbal cues or behavioral reinforcement were given during this intervention. Both successes and failures were recorded.

Treatments were randomly alternated during each session to control for possible order effects. Due to the complexity of counting behaviors which occur within a given time period (2 seconds), a second person was needed to count and record data. This was a good opportunity to involve the parent in the child's therapy program. A third person was needed to collect interrater reliability data at least once during each phase. Data were recorded as number of successful trials/total number of trials x 100 (percentage data).

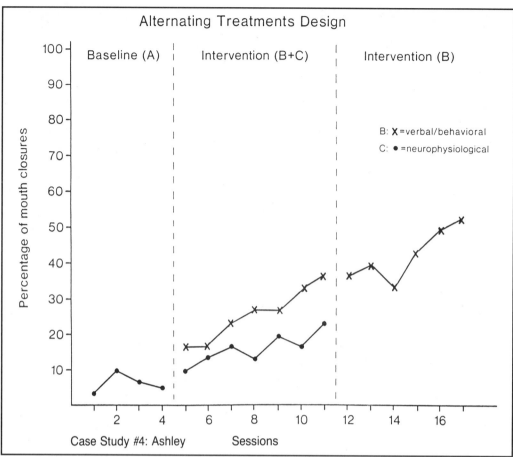

Figure 17-4. Alternating treatment designs.

In Figure 17-4, it can be seen that the verbal/behavioral intervention was slightly more successful than the neurophysiological approach. Thus, the final phase of the study used the verbal/behavioral intervention as the treatment variable. Since both intervention approaches yielded some positive changes, it is logical to conclude that combining both approaches might bring about even quicker changes. Such a study might be attempted following completion of this study.

This hypothetical single subject study with Ashley was based, in part, on an actual series of single subject studies conducted on five young children with Down syndrome. Readers are referred to the study by Purdy, Deitz, and Harris for further information on this topic.[22]

Case Study #5: John

➤ Practice pattern 5B: Impaired Neuromotor Development
➤ Medical diagnosis: Attention deficit hyperactivity disorder, developmental coordination disorder
➤ Age: 5 years

John participated in an ABA study design in relation to his karate program (refer to Chapter 16).

Summary

The primary goal of this chapter is to demonstrate that research techniques for the clinician can be relatively simple, inexpensive, and require little additional time and effort. Secondly, systematic measurement and accountability of the efficacy of our treatment strategies are both ethical and legal responsibilities of all physical therapists working with children with developmental disabilities, in all settings (eg, educational, medical). Through the use of such behavioral measurement strategies as individualized therapy goals and objectives and single subject research designs, it is possible for each of us to examine the effectiveness of a variety of treatment strategies with individual children in our clinical practices.

Conclusion

Backman and colleagues[23] reviewed "methodologic rules" for using single subject research designs. The authors used CINAHL and MEDLINE searches to identify 61 articles using single subject research designs in rehabilitation over the decade prior to 1997. Examples of these studies were used to illustrate strengths and weaknesses in four different single subject research designs and the users' adherence (or non-adherence) to experimental rules. In a subsequent article, Backman and Harris[24] compared and contrasted case studies, single subject research, and N-of-1 randomized trials. Physical therapists contemplating individual or small group research would benefit from reviewing guidelines presented in these two articles to assist in determining the most appropriate design(s).

Not only do we, as clinicians, have the responsibility to demonstrate treatment efficacy, we also have the responsibility to share results with professional colleagues. Through oral dissemination at in-service sessions and in presentations at local, state, and national meetings, as well as through publication of research in scholarly journals and professional newsletters, we must share not only our successes (ie, those treatment modalities that were efficacious), but also our failures. For example, if replications of a study within our own setting repeatedly have shown a particular treatment not to be effective, we owe it to our colleagues and our clients to share this information as much as we are required to share results of successful treatments. Both the new graduate and the experienced physical therapist have responsibilities to expand the knowledge base in physical therapy through carefully controlled clinical research. It is hoped that this chapter will encourage physical therapists at all levels of experience to conduct clinical research within their own settings and to share the results with their colleagues.

References

1. American Physical Therapy Association. *Plan to Foster Clinical Research in Physical Therapy. Goals Adopted by American Physical Therapy Association House of Delegates*; 1980. (Revised: November 1984.)
2. American Physical Therapy Association. Clinical research agenda for physical therapy. *Phys Ther*. 2000;80:499-513.
3. Education for All Handicapped Children Act, Public Law 94-142. US Congress, Senate, 94th Congress, first session, 1975.

4. O'Neill DL, Harris SR. Developing goals and objectives for handicapped children. *Phys Ther.* 1982;62:295-298.

5. Portney LG, Watkins MP. A concept of research. In: *Foundations of Clinical Research: Applications to Practice.* 2nd ed. Upper Saddle River, NJ: Prentice-Hall; 2000:3-20.

6. Portney LG, Watkins MP. Reliability. In: *Foundations of Clinical Research: Applications to Practice.* 2nd ed. Upper Saddle River, NJ: Prentice-Hall; 2000:61-77.

7. Harris SR, Smith LH, Krukowski L. Goniometric reliability for a child with spastic quadriplegia. *J Pediatri Orth.* 1985;5:348-351.

8. Portney LG, Watkins MP. Single subject designs. In: *Foundations of Clinical Research: Applications to Practice.* 2nd ed. Upper Saddle River, NJ: Prentice-Hall; 2000:223-264.

9. Martin JE, Epstein LH. Evaluating treatment effectiveness in cerebral palsy. *Phys Ther.* 1976;56:285-294.

10. Hersen M, Barlow DH. *Single Case Experimental Designs: Strategies for Studying Behavior Change.* New York, NY: Pergamon Press; 1976.

11. McEwen I. *Writing Case Reports: A How-to Manual for Clinicians.* 2nd ed. Alexandria, Va: American Physical Therapy Association; 2001.

12. Daichman J, Johnston TE, Evans K, et al. The effects of a neuromuscular electrical stimulation home program on impairments and functional skills of a child with spastic diplegic cerebral palsy: a case report. *Pediatr Phys Ther.* 2003;15:153-158.

13. Smith LH, Harris SR. Upper extremity inhibitive casting for a child with cerebral palsy. *Phys Occup Ther Pediatr.* 1985;5:71-79.

14. Wolery M, Harris SR. Interpreting results of single-subject research designs. *Phys Ther.* 1982; 62:445-452.

15. Barlow DH, Hayes SC. Alternating treatments design: one strategy for comparing the effects of two treatments in a single subject. *J Appl Beh Anal.* 1979;12:199-210.

16. Harris SR, Riffle K. Effects of inhibitive ankle-foot orthoses on standing balance in a child with cerebral palsy: a single subject design. *Phys Ther.* 1986;66:663-667.

17. Wolery M, Bailey DB, Sugai GM. *Effective Teaching: Principles and Procedures of Applied Behavior Analysis.* Boston, Mass: Allyn & Bacon; 1988.

18. Bishop B. Vibratory stimulation: possible applications of vibration in treatment of motor dysfunctions. *Phys Ther.* 1975;55:139-143.

19. Hagbarth KE, Eklund G. The muscle vibrator—a useful tool in neurologic therapeutic work. *Scand J Rehab Med.* 1969;1:26-34.

20. Eklund G, Steen M. Muscle vibration therapy in children with cerebral palsy. *Scand J Rehab Med.* 1969;1:33-37.

21. Mueller HA. Feeding. In: Finnie NR, ed. *Handling the Young Cerebral Palsied Child at Home.* 3rd ed. Oxford, UK: Butterworth/Heinemann; 1997:209-221.

22. Purdy AH, Deitz JC, Harris SR. Efficacy of two treatment approaches to reduce tongue protrusion of children with Down syndrome. *Dev Med Child Neurol.* 1987;29:469-476.

23. Backman CL, Harris SR, Chisholm J, et al. Single subject research in rehabilitation: a review of studies using AB, withdrawal, multiple baseline, and alternating treatments designs. *Arch Phys Med Rehab.* 1997;78:1145-1153.

24. Backman CL, Harris SR. Case studies, single subject research, and n-of-1 randomized trials: comparisons and contrasts. *Am J Phys Med Rehab.* 1999;78:170-176.

CHAPTER 18

Issues in Aging in Individuals With Lifelong Disabilities

Barbara H. Connolly, EdD, PT, FAPTA

Interest in the management of individuals with lifelong disabilities is growing. In the last several decades, the population of persons age 65 years and over has grown twice as fast as the general population. The number of people age 65 years or older grew by 82% during the period between 1965 and 1995 to a high of 33.9 million people by 1996.[1] With biomedical advances and health care improvements for adults with lifelong developmental disabilities, the number of older persons with developmental disabilities also seems to be increasing.[2,3] According to a 1997 US Bureau of the Census report, nearly 54 million Americans have an activity limitation/disability associated with a long-term physical, sensory, or cognitive condition.[4] Individuals with developmental disabilities are being served in the community and are frequently living to be more than 60 years old.[5-7] Based on current statistics on survival of individuals with mental retardation, soon there may be between 670,200 and 4,021,300 individuals with mental retardation over the age of 65 years living in the United States.[8]

In pediatric rehabilitation, the tenet that children cannot be addressed as if they were small adults has been widely embraced. However, the difficulty in transition of services for the child with developmental disabilities to services for the adult with developmental disabilities has not been fully explored or perhaps appreciated by occupational or physical therapists with pediatric experience. Additionally, therapists in adult practice settings may be presented with unique problems in the adult with developmental disabilities that they are not prepared to address. Although individual needs of persons with developmental disabilities vary greatly, knowledge of the effects of aging on this group of individuals can facilitate more effective health care by occupational therapists and physical therapists for individuals of all ages with developmental disabilities.

Based on the need for therapists in pediatrics and in adult rehabilitation to gain more knowledge in the area of aging in individuals with lifelong disabilities, the Section on Pediatrics of the American Physical Therapy Association (APTA) established a Special Interest Group (SIG) in 2001. The goals of the SIG were to provide a specific forum where therapists having a common interest in adults with developmental disabilities may meet, confer, and promote patient care through education, clinical practice, and research. The focus of the SIG is on: 1) prevention and examination of impairments in the adult with developmental disabilities to ensure maximum participation in society, 2) development of intervention guidelines for the adult with development disabilities, and 3) promotion of understanding/advocacy of adults with developmental disabilities through research and education. This new SIG for the Section on Pediatrics has been successful in educating and promoting interactions relative to these three focus areas among members, and interest in the SIG among Section members continues to grow.

Defining the Population

Definition of Developmental Disabilities and Mental Retardation

Developmental disability is defined in Public Law 98-527—the Developmental Disabilities Act of 1984.

"A developmental disability is a severe chronic disability of a person which:

1. Is attributable to a mental or physical impairment (or a combination of impairments)

2. Is manifest before age 22

3. Is likely to continue indefinitely

4. Results in substantial functional limitations in three or more of the following areas: self-care, receptive and expressive language, learning, mobility, self-direction, capacity for independent living, or economic self-sufficiency

5. Reflects a need for a combination and sequence of special, interdisciplinary or generic care, treatment or other services which are (a) of lifelong or extended duration and are (b) individually planned and coordinated."[9]

Mental retardation refers to substantial limitations in functioning of an individual. It is characterized by significantly subaverage intellectual functioning, existing concurrently with related limitations in two or more of the following applicable adaptive skill areas: communication, self-care, home living, social skills, community use, self-direction, health and safety, functional academics, leisure, and work.[10]

Although developmental disabilities and mental retardation have been carefully defined through legislation and practice, the definition of aged as applied to these populations is not as clear. Aging typically has been defined using a normative-statistical approach (chronological age), while others have used a biological approach related to signs and symptoms of aging. Thus, inconsistencies in the operational definitions for aging in individuals with disabilities were found by Janicki and Hogg.[11] In individuals with lifelong disabilities such as Down syndrome, aging may begin as early as 35 years. Research has shown that almost all adults with Down syndrome over the age of 35 years develop Alzheimer's neuropathology.[12-14] Burt, Loveland, and Lewis found that adults with Down syndrome showed evidence of loss of previously attained adaptive skills more frequently than individuals with mental retardation but without Down syndrome.[15] Additionally, Burt et al[15] found that eight of 61 adults with Down syndrome in their study had symptoms of dementia whereas none of the comparison subjects had diagnosable dementia. For adults with Down syndrome over 55 years of age, the incidence of Alzheimer's disease has been estimated at 45%.[16,17] Evenhuis[18] found an even greater percentage of individuals with Down syndrome with dementia in his prospective study of 17 individuals followed from the time of institutionalization to death. Fifteen of these 17 individuals had clinically diagnosable dementia syndromes, and neuropathological examination of brain tissue at postmortem revealed pathology of the Alzheimer's-type in all 17 individuals. Few studies have examined the presence of Alzheimer's disease in geriatric populations of adults without Down syndrome but with mental retardation. However, two studies based on postmortem examinations seem to indicate that individuals with mental retardation may be at risk for Alzheimer's disease at ages roughly comparable to those of adults without mental retardation.[19,20] Janicki and associates [11,21] also documented that individuals with mental retardation and neuromotor disorders may experience effects of aging on mobility and activities of daily living (ADL) earlier than

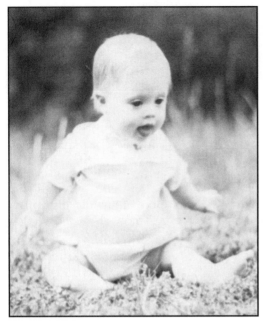

Figure 18-1. Walker at 1 year.

Figure 18-2. Walker at 3 years.

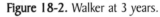

Figure 18-3. Walker at 7 years.

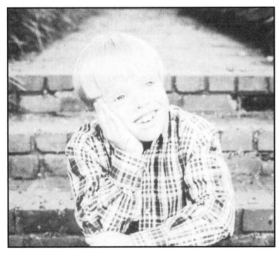

individuals without mental retardation. However, most researchers have selected the mid-50s as a definition of aged in adults with developmental disabilities based on observations of changing functional status in normative age-related activities[22] (Figures 18-1 through 18-6).

Prevalence

The estimated number of individuals over the age of 60 years with developmental disabilities or mental retardation currently is between 200 000 to 500 000.[23] Based on empirical sampling, Baroff suggested that only 0.9% of the population can be assumed to have mental retardation.[24] In contrast, following a review of the most recent epidemiological

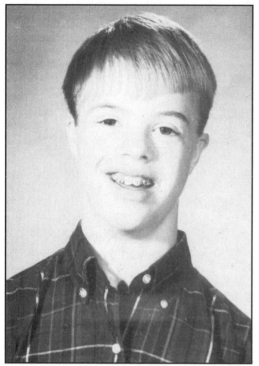

Figure 18-4. Walker at 9 years.

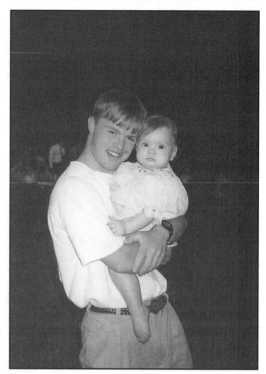

Figure 18-5. Walker at 18 years.

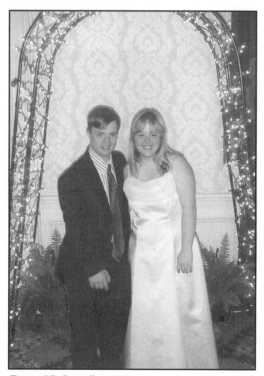

Figure 18-6. Walker at 21 years.

studies, McLaren and Bryson[25] reported that the prevalence of mental retardation was approximately 1.25% based on total population screening. When school-aged children are the source of prevalence statistics, individual states report rates from 0.3% to 2.5% depending on the criteria used to determine eligibility for special educational services, the labels assigned during the eligibility process (eg, developmental delay, learning disability, autism, and/or mental retardation), and the environmental and economic conditions within the state.[26] Additionally, people 65 years or older make up approximately 12% of all people with developmental disabilities, a percentage that is similar to the general population.[27] The exact number of individuals with disabilities has become of importance to social services agencies, state developmental disabilities planning councils, and state units on aging because for the first time in history, adults with developmental disabilities are beginning to outlive their parents and are in need of broad-based services.

Mortality

Life expectancy for all individuals with developmental disabilities has increased but is less than for the general population.[4,28,29] For example, the lifespan for individuals with Down syndrome has increased from 9 years of age in 1949 to approximately 55 years today.[30] Jacobson et al[31] found the greatest life expectancy to be in women, people who are ambulatory and/or have mild levels of mental retardation, and those who have remained in community settings. O'Brien et al[32] found a significantly higher mortality rate in individuals with developmental disabilities between 1974 to 1979 when compared to 1980 to 1985. Heart disease and cancer were found to be the most common causes of death in individuals with mild, moderate, or severe mental retardation in both these time periods. Additionally, respiratory disease was found to be the most common cause of death in individuals with profound mental retardation.[33] Strauss and Kastner[34] examined the risk-adjusted mortality rates between 1980 and 1992 for those individuals living in institutions and those living in the community. In contrast to previous studies[29] that indicated greater life expectancies for those who remain in the community, a major finding of this California study was that the risk-adjusted mortality rates of people with mental retardation were higher in the community than in institutions, regardless of the level of risk. Although no explanations were offered for the findings, the authors speculated that individuals in the community may have experienced problems with Medicaid reimbursement, as well as the lack of trained practitioners and less than adequate coordination of care. In 1999, Shavelle and Strauss,[35] in a study of 1812 persons who had left institutions to move into the community, found that the community death rate was 88% higher than expected for comparable persons living in institutions. They also found that relative mortality in the community seemed to be greatest among the highest functioning persons. Causes of death included diseases of circulation, cancer, pneumonia, aspiration pneumonia, choking, trauma, and cardiac arrest (in some cases due to infection).

As individuals with developmental disabilities age, they experience age-related disorders similar to individuals without developmental disabilities.[36] However, in addition to these disorders, a variety of secondary medical problems that may contribute to mortality have been described. Secondary medical problems identified by Buehler et al[37] in a study of 610 adults with developmental disabilities, primarily from community settings, included obesity, chronic skin problems, hygiene-related problems, and early aging (Figure 18-7).

Kapell et al[36] found that people with mental retardation had a greater incidence of hypothyroidism and non-ischemic heart disease when compared with their age- and gender-matched peers in the general population. Anderson,[27] in a study of older adults with

Figure 18-7. Obesity in individual with developmental disabilities.

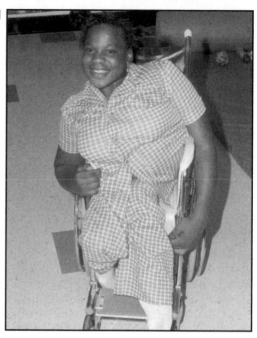

mental retardation who lived in community settings, found that the most common chronic health problems included high blood pressure, arthritis, heart disease, and glaucoma/cataracts. These disorders were consistent with the top three health problems noted in the general population of persons of similar ages. Among those individuals who resided in institutional settings, high incidences of blood disorders, muscle atrophy, and glaucoma/cataracts were noted.[26]

Effects of Aging on the Senses

Even minor functional changes of aging in areas such as vision, hearing, and vestibular functioning may cause major problems for individuals who have had lifelong developmental disabilities. An understanding of how some of the general needs of these individuals can be served by medical and community systems is essential for occupational therapists and physical therapists who serve this population.

Vision

Age-related loss in the photoreceptors and decreased function of the ganglion cells within the retina have been shown to occur in individuals.[38] Additionally, aging has been shown to affect the integrity of the visual fields, dark adaptation, and color vision with some loss over the entire color spectrum by the fourth decade.[39,40] With aging, the pupillary responses have been noted to decrease, as well as the size of the resting pupil.[41] Cohen and Lessell[39] reported that with aging, convergence is compromised, ptosis is seen, and a symmetric restriction in upward gaze is experienced. Additionally, visual loss with aging may occur due to glaucoma, macular degeneration, and diabetic retinopathy. More commonly, visual losses may be due to cataracts which occur in 46% of individuals between the ages of 75 to 85 years.[42]

Table 18-1
Visual Impairments in the General Population and in Individuals With Mental Retardation

National Health Interview Survey	Level of Mental Retardation	Down Syndrome	Non-Down Syndrome
General population	Mild/moderate		
4.9%	45 to 64 years	16.2%	8.9%
6.5%	65 to 74 years	50%	16.7%
	Severe/profound		
4.9%	45 to 64 years	39.2%	17.7%
6.5%	65 to 74 years	75%	17.6%

Adapted from Kapell D, Nightingale B, Rodriquez A, et al. Prevalence of chronic medical conditions in adults with mental retardation: comparison with the general population. *Ment Retard*. 1998;36:269-279.

IMPLICATIONS FOR PERSONS WITH DEVELOPMENTAL DISABILITIES

While specific information about the prevalence of visual problems in individuals with developmental disabilities is not available, it is likely that a greater number of people with developmental disabilities have uncorrected or unidentified visual problems than in the general population.[43] Good et al[44] reported that the incidence of cortical visual impairment is increasing in children with neurological deficits. These authors speculated that better medical care has lowered the mortality rate of children with severe neurological problems and thus these children survive for longer periods of time. Although, the residual vision of the child with cortical visual impairment often improves over time, the child may be left with diminished visual acuity. Additionally, adults with Down syndrome are at greater than normal risk for eye disorders such as cataracts, which also seem to occur at an earlier age than for matched age peers.[45] Cataracts are speculated to occur in about 50% of adults with Down syndrome. Table 18-1 presents the percentage of individuals with Down syndrome who present with visual impairment compared to the general population and to individuals with mental challenges who are non-Down syndrome.

Another factor that may contribute to a high number of individuals with developmental disabilities having undiagnosed visual problems is the examiner's difficulty in gathering subjective information from the individual.[46] The extent of visual loss may not be identifiable if the individual cannot respond to a standard eye chart consisting of letters, numbers, or words. In general, physiological changes in tandem with environmental and pre-existing disease factors in individuals with lifelong disabilities may cause greater impairments in vision than would be anticipated in the general population.[47] Signs that might indicate a change in vision include rubbing the eyes, squinting, shutting or covering one eye, or tilting the head. Changes in daily functions such as stumbling during gait, hesitancy on steps or curbs, holding reading materials closer than usual, or sitting close to the television also might suggest visual changes.

Considerations that need to be made for individuals with developmental disabilities may include: early cataract removal before declining function impairs the individual's ability to cooperate with postoperative care, soft lighting, reduced glare in the environment, use of color, use of high contrast, or referral to a low-vision rehabilitation specialist. Reinforcement with tactile or verbal cues also may be necessary to improve visual responses.

Hearing

Prevalence studies indicate that 25% to 40% of individuals over the age of 65 years exhibit some degree of hearing loss with the most common cause of sensorineural hearing loss being presbycusis.[48] Presbycusis can be related to a number of factors including: cellular aging in the peripheral, auditory, and central nervous system pathways; acoustic trauma; cardiovascular disease; and cumulative effects of ototoxic medications.[49,50] Problems noted with presbycusis include a slowly progressive bilateral hearing loss, difficulty with word recognition, and a decline in perceptual processing of the temporal characteristics of speech.

IMPLICATIONS FOR PERSONS WITH DEVELOPMENTAL DISABILITIES

Conductive hearing losses can occur due to external ear disease and acute or chronic diseases of the middle ear. Otitis media (ie, inflammation of the middle ear) is one of the most common causes of conductive hearing loss. Otitis media usually is treated with medication but can result in permanent ear damage and hearing loss.[51] Individuals with developmental disabilities may be more likely to develop this type of hearing loss than the general population due to the occurrence of repeated otitis media that is undetected and untreated.[52] In particular, many people with Down syndrome have conductive hearing loss resulting from frequent middle ear infections in childhood.[53] Individuals with Down syndrome also have a propensity to sensorineural hearing loss which is associated with the general aging population. However, the sensorineural hearing loss in individuals with Down syndrome can begin to develop during the second decade of life.

Many adults with developmental disabilities can "hide" a hearing loss due to their limited communication abilities and sheltered lifestyles. Therefore, many aging adults with developmental disabilities may have an undetected hearing loss that interfers with an already limited communication ability and contributes to social isolation and depression. Seltzer and Luchterhand[54] found that over half of the consumers who had been evaluated at the Aging and Developmental Disabilities Clinic at the University of Wisconsin had significant hearing losses. Yet, for many of these individuals, the family and local service providers had not suspected a hearing loss. Clinical signs that might indicate a hearing loss include turning up the TV or radio very loud, speaking loudly, responding to questions inappropriately, or becoming confused in noisy environments.

Considering the possibility of a greater incidence of hearing losses in adults with developmental disabilities, health care providers should insist on audiologic testing for all individuals with developmental disabilities. However, the testing should be done by an audiologist with special training in evaluating persons with mental retardation or developmental disabilities. Hearing aids can be helpful in increasing responsiveness to sound, but only if tolerated by the wearer. For those who cannot tolerate hearing aids, functional hearing can be improved through minimizing background noise, facing the person being spoken to, and speaking slowly with good articulation. If the hearing loss is identified early, communication through use of sign language or augmentative communication might be used as an alternative strategy.

Taste and Smell

Evidence suggests that some older individuals experience less pleasure during meals due to impaired taste and smell which results from higher thresholds for these senses.[55] Increases in the thresholds of taste and smell may make food seem tasteless and less appealing. For individuals with developmental disabilities, this may cause changes in their oral-motor skills, eating habits, and nutritional intake. A decreased appetite also may result as a side effect from some medications. With either of these two problems (decrease in taste and smell perceptions and side effects from medication), a lack of interest in food may occur and the nutritional health of the individual may be affected.

IMPLICATIONS FOR PERSONS WITH DEVELOPMENTAL DISABILITIES

Being under ideal body weight can be a problem for up to 25% of people with developmental disabilities.[56] In particular those individuals with lower levels of cognitive functioning and those with multiple disabilities and feeding difficulties are typically underweight. The lack of interest in eating because of changes in taste and smell in these individuals may lead to further debilitation, susceptibility to opportunistic infections, and even death. Nutritional supplements may be necessary for maintaining ideal body weight and meeting daily nutritional requirements. Additionally, emphasis should be placed on the visual appearance of food as well as on texture to increase the meal's appeal. Separating food rather than mixing food on a plate and varying textures of food might be actions to take to increase one's interest in eating. Use of condiments, other than salt, also may be used to increase overall flavor.

Dental problems also may cause problems with eating in individuals with developmental disabilities. The greatest dental problem faced by the adult with developmental disabilities is periodontal disease. The incidence of severe, destructive periodontal disease in individuals with Down syndrome may be as high as 96%.[57] In this population, the disease is usually in evidence by the third decade of life. The immunological deficiencies in persons with Down syndrome may be related to the increased prevalence and severity of periodontal disease.[58,59]

Somatosensory

Although the degree of change may vary in individuals, touch and the related senses of proprioception and kinesthesia appear to decrease with age. Age-related changes that contribute to problems with touch and position sense have been noted in the peripheral nervous system both anatomically as well as physiologically.[60,61] Morphological changes in the nerve cells, nerve roots, peripheral nerves, and specialized nerve terminals have been linked with the aging process. With aging, Meissner's corpuscles decrease in concentration.[62] Pacinian corpuscles decrease in density,[63] and afferent nerve fibers decrease in number.[64] Degeneration of the dorsal columns also is noted as one ages. This degeneration is thought to be due to the loss of centrally directed axons of the dorsal root ganglion cells.[65] Additionally, action potentials may take longer than usual to reach the CNS in the aging adult. This delay is due to a gradual shortening of the internodal length that contributes to an increased conduction velocity.

Quantitative studies have shown that a progressive impairment of sensory detection occurs with aging. An example of this gradual decline is the perception of touch/pressure which approaches a fourfold reduction in men over age 40 years.[66] Schmidt et al[63,67] found an age-related decline in response to "flutter" and "tap," which they related to changes in the peripheral sensory units rather than conduction along the afferent nerves.

Proprioception has been reported as being similar in young and older subjects without disabilities.[68] However, passive movement thresholds have been reported to be twice as high for the hip, knee, and ankle in subjects over 50 years of age compared with subjects less than 40 years of age.[69] No change in upper extremity perception was noted. Skinner et al,[70] in a study of knee joint position sense, found that the abilities to reproduce passive knee position and to detect motion deteriorated with age.

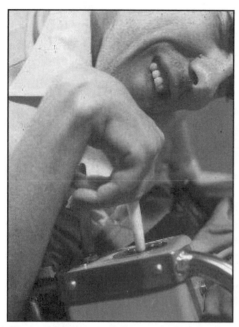

Figure 18-8. Use of abnormal posturing to access hand-held controls.

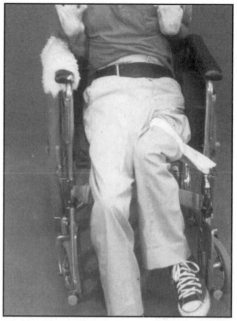

Figure 18-9. Individual propelling wheelchair using feet.

IMPLICATIONS FOR PERSONS WITH DEVELOPMENTAL DISABILITIES

Loss of somatosensory function in aging adults with developmental disabilities may be devastating. For the individual who depends on tactile input to guide movement, the decrease in tactile function may lead to decreases in movement and possibly result in immobility. For example, the individual may no longer be able to access communication boards or to independently propel a wheelchair without sustaining injuries to the upper extremities (Figure 18-8).

With the loss of proprioceptive abilities, particularly in the lower extremities, function-al patterns of movement may be loss. For example, many adults with neuromotor disor-ders propel their wheelchairs with their feet (Figure 18-9). If joint sense is decreased or lost in the hips, knees, and ankles, the coordination needed for efficiently moving from one place to another in the wheelchair may be compromised. If the individual is ambulatory, a loss of proprioceptive abilities with age may necessitate use of a different type of ambu-lation assist, such as a walker rather than crutches or canes. Assistance from another per-son during ambulation may be necessary for some individuals who are no longer "safe" during independent ambulation due to loss of proprioceptive function.

Effects of Aging on the Neuromusculoskeletal System

Flexibility

Changes in collagen are a biological cause for decreases in flexibility as one ages. With age, collagen fibers become irregular in shape owing to cross-linking. This pattern results in a decreased linear pull relationship in the collagen tissue and leads to a decreased mobility in the body's tissues.[71] Poor nutrition also may lead to collagen changes and this problem maybe seen in the population with developmental disabilities. In particular, deficiency of vitamin C appears to interfere with normal tissue integrity and may affect muscle functioning and elasticity of collagen.

Muscles, skin, and tendons become less flexible and mobile as one ages. The spine also becomes less flexible due to collagen changes in the annulus and to decreased water content in the nucleus pulposa. Furthermore, osteoporotic changes in the vertebral bones may lead to fractures of the vertebrae, increased collagen scarring, and decreased flexibility of the spine.

Hypokinesis or decreased activity can be a functional cause of loss of flexibility. Older individuals who remain sitting or immobile for long periods of time may develop tightness in those muscles that are shortened in that particular position and which may form collagenous adhesions. In particular, decreased passive and active range of motion particularly in the flexor musculature may be seen in elders who sit for extended periods of time during the day.

IMPLICATIONS FOR PERSONS WITH DEVELOPMENTAL DISABILITIES

Loss of flexibility in the aging adult with developmental disabilities may be even more dramatic than for the typical aging adult. In individuals with neuromotor disorders, loss of flexibility may be considered a secondary condition. A secondary condition is defined as an injury, impairment, functional limitation, or disability that occurs as a result of the primary pathology.[72] These secondary conditions in older persons with neuromotor problems such as cerebral palsy may be seen due to multiple body systems which were affected during the developmental years. If the individual has been inactive, adequate bone density and mass may not have been developed at a younger age. Therefore, that individual is likely to experience an accelerated loss of bone density and mass with age. Recently a link between lifelong use of Dilantin (Pfizer, New York, NY) and osteoporosis has been documented.[73] This risk appears to be particularly high in individuals who are non-ambulatory or sedentary. Many physicians recommend that regular periods of sunlight be part of a daily schedule to offset the effects of Dilantin on bone loss in those individuals who are at greatest risk. Additionally, persons with neuromotor problems may be at an increased risk for osteoporosis due to limitations in mobility, inadequate calcium intake in the diet, and decreased sun exposure leading to low circulating levels of vitamin D. In 1998, Center, Beange, and McElduff,[74] in a study of men and women with mental retardation with a mean age of 35 years, found a bone mineral density more than two standard deviations below that of an age- and gender-matched population. Osteoporotic risk factors include low body weight, small body size, hypogonadism, endocrine disorders, sedentary lifestyle, and poor nutrition. All of these factors commonly are found in individuals with developmental disabilities.

A pathological cause of loss of flexibility in persons of any age is arthritis. Osteoarthritis, a commonly occurring disorder in the elderly, is characterized by deterioration of articular cartilage and formation of new bone in the subchrondeal areas as well as at the margins of the joint.[75] Although relatively uncommon before the age of 40 years, the prevalence of osteoarthritis increases steeply with age, to reach about 75% at 75 years and climbing to over 90% after 80 years of age.[67]

Arthritic changes in the joints of aging adults with developmental disabilities may be noted at even earlier ages. Osteoarthritis has been cited as a cause of pain as well as loss of flexibility in individuals with cerebral palsy.[76,77] The increasing biomechanical stress on multiple joints in individuals with severe neuromuscular dysfunctions or bony abnormalities may increase the incidence and likelihood of osteoarthritis. Murphy et al[76] spec-ulated that the development of pain in weight bearing joints in adults with cerebral palsy was a sign of early degenerative arthritis. Cathels and Reddihough[77] found clini-cal evidence of arthritis in 27% of a group of 149 adolescents and young adults with cerebral palsy. Individuals who walked were more affected than those who did not walk. Trauma to a joint predisposes it to OA, as has been noted in the high incidence of OA in the shoulders and elbows of baseball pitchers, ankles of ballet dancers, and knees of basketball players. Therefore, disturbances of the joint mechanics or repeated abnor-mal stresses to a joint in those individuals who are ambulatory may predispose them to early onset OA. Pain and weakness usually are associated with OA, but in individuals with developmental disabilities who cannot communicate easily, these symptoms may be missed or misinterpreted.[78]

Arthritic changes in different joints also may lead to loss of functional abilities in indi-viduals with developmental disabilities. For example, the ability to transfer oneself from a wheelchair to the bed or tub may become extremely difficult if soreness in the shoulders, elbows, and wrists is experienced. Many individuals who were ambulatory may opt to use a wheelchair if pain is experienced in the spine, hips, knees, or ankles during walking activities. Additionally, more adaptive equipment may be necessary in the home in order for the person to be as independent as possible with ADL.

Strength

Muscle strength, as defined by the ability to produce force or torque, declines with age in both men and women.[79-83] A common change noted in aging muscle is reduction of mass, from 25% to 43%, depending upon the activity level of the individual.[84] Additionally, decreased strength may be due to smaller numbers of muscle fibers and muscle motor units, as well as a decrease in size of the muscle fibers. Functioning motoneurons also appear to decline with aging and thus problems may be noted in coor-dination and speed of muscle contraction.

Decreases in muscle strength as a person ages may be related to decreased time spent in vigorous work or athletic activities. Some studies have shown a loss of 18% to 20% of maximum force by age 65 years while others demonstrate a loss of up to 40%.[85] Muscles that appear most likely to show a decrease in muscle strength during periods of inactivi-ty are the active antigravity muscles, such as the quadriceps, hip extensors, ankle dorsi-flexors, latissimus dorsi, and triceps.

IMPLICATIONS FOR PERSONS WITH DEVELOPMENTAL DISABILITIES

Individuals with physical disabilities have been noted to experience additional prob-lems in the musculoskeletal system as they age.[65,68,86] The musculoskeletal problems may be related to deformities such as subluxations and dislocations of the hip, abnormalities of the foot, patella alta, scoliosis, pelvic obliquity, and contractures. These musculoskele-tal problems may cause secondary conditions, such as decreased strength, due to the inability of the individual to move in a variety of patterns.

Trieschmann[87] reported that pain, soreness, weakness of muscles, and energy decline while the tendency to be more susceptible to injury increases in persons with long-stand-ing disabilities. Loss of muscle strength in individuals who have had difficulty with movement all of their lives may be even greater than that expected solely due to the aging process. Janicki and Jacobson,[88] in a study of over 10 000 individuals who were mentally challenged, found that a decline in motoric skills began at about 50 years of age, even for those who were mild to moderately challenged. Among those who were more severely and profoundly challenged, motoric skills remained relatively stable until they reached their late 70s. However, this delayed decline was related most probably to more limited motoric abilities even at younger ages when compared with the individuals with mild to moderate mental retardation. How the aging process affects the "strength" of persons with neuromotor problems has not been well-studied. However, it appears that at least some persons with neuromotor problems experience increasing problems with movement as they age. This loss of movement may be related to pain or degenerative joint disease[89] either of which could lead to decreased use of or less force exerted by certain muscles during movement.

Strength training is a popular form of exercise for individuals both with and without disabilities. However, questions have been raised over time about the appropriateness of such programs with individuals with spasticity. Andersson et al[90] found that a progressive strength training program provided significant improvement in isometric strength (hip extensors P=0.006, hip abductors P=0.01) and in isokinetic concentric work at 30 degrees/second (knee extensors P=0.02) in individuals (ages 25 to 47 years) with spastic diplegia. The results of the intervention also revealed significant improvements in the Gross Motor Function Measure dimensions D (standing) and E (walking, running, and jumping) as well as in the Timed Up and Go test. No increase in spasticity as measured by the modified Ashworth Scale was noted in individuals who underwent strength training.

Therefore, as with most adults, moderate regular exercise is essential for maintaining mobility in adults with developmental disabilities. Loss of even a small amount of strength may lead to loss of functional abilities in this population because of the very sensitive balance between muscle groups that has been developed over time for some functional activities. Weakness can result in loss of functional abilities, such as climbing stairs, transferring, or getting out from a chair. Additional, increased occurrences of complications such as pressure sores, contractures, and pneumonia may result from immobility in some adults who have lifelong limitations in movement. Bedrest or chair rest should be avoided if at all possible and gross motor activities should be included as a part of the day's activities.

Posture and Positioning

Posture is derived from the relationship of body parts, one to another, as well as to the maturation and interaction of the musculoskeletal, neuromuscular, and cardiopulmonary systems. Additionally, psychological well-being may have an impact on the "posture" of an individual.

Upright posture, either in sitting or in standing, seems to demonstrate the most noticeable changes as one ages. Sitting postures change in many older adults with the head held forward, the shoulders rounded, and the upper back kyphotic. In sitting or standing, a flatter lumbar lordosis may be seen in the low back. In standing, flexion at the hips and knees may be more noticeable. These changes in the spine and in the lower extremities most frequently are caused by changes in the intervertebral disk as well as to decreased mobility or hypokinesis.

INTERVERTEBRAL DISK

Age-related changes in the intervertebral disks begin during the third decade of life in the "normal" population.[91,92] Water content in the nucleus pulposus ranges from 70% to 90%, with diminishing amounts with age. By the sixth to seventh decades, the water content is decreased by 30%.[93] With age, the annulus which is composed of collagen becomes less elastic. Together, the decreased water in the nucleus and the increased fiberous of the

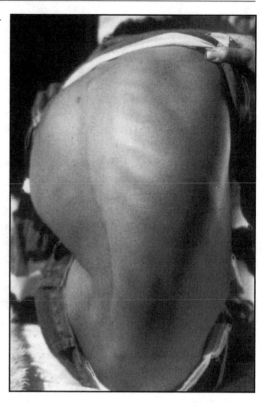

Figure 18-10. Severe scoliosis in adult with developmental disability.

annulus cause the disk to be flatter and less resilient. These changes lead to diminishing height and flexibility of the spine in aging individuals.

Age-related changes also take place in the ligaments of the spine with degeneration of tensile ability with age. Tkaczuk[94] determined that tensile characteristics of the anterior and posterior ligaments of the lumbar spine decreased with age. Additionally, Nachemson and Evans[95] determined that the "resting" tension of the ligamentum flavum also decreased. The loss of this resting tension could lead to further spinal instability in the aging individual.

HYPOKINESIS

Prolonged periods of time in one position also can lead to postural changes in aging individuals. Older persons tend to remain in one position (usually sitting) for longer periods of time and thus the body's flexor musculature tend to shorten. Resulting limitations in extensor musculature then may occur. In particular, the older individual may present with increased hip and knee flexion, increased kyphosis of the upper trunk, and decreased lumbar lordosis. Additionally, a relationship has been established between osteoporosis and inactivity. In humans, weight bearing produces stress on the bone, and collagen acts as the crystal which transforms the stimulus into an osteoblastic effect. New bone tissue then is laid down along the stress lines. Thus, lack of muscular stress as well as lack of weight bearing on the bone will contribute to osteoporosis.[96]

IMPLICATIONS FOR PERSONS WITH DEVELOPMENTAL DISABILITIES

The spine may be a focal point of difficulty with persons with lifelong disabilities. A scoliosis that has been present since childhood may further progress as the individual ages (Figure 18-10). In particular, older persons with cerebral palsy who have been immobile or relatively inactive may not have developed adequate bone density and mass at a younger age and are likely to experience an accelerated loss of bone density and mass as they age. Individuals with severe scoliosis (eg, greater than 45 degrees)[97] may have increasing problems with mobility and hygiene care resulting in greater dependency on caregivers.[98,99] In individuals who have taken medications for seizure disorders, a decrement in bone mineral density may be noted. Hauser and Hesdorffer[100] found a high coexistence of seizures and cerebral palsy and stated that individuals with both these disorders are at a greater risk for osteoporosis than would be anticipated. This increased risk for osteoporosis may cause a predisposition for fracture rates at earlier ages than in the general population. For example, compression fractures of the spine may be noted with increased frequency in those individuals with seizure and neuromotor disorders and the resultant pain from the fractures may further contribute to hypokinesis.

Clinical suggestions for older individuals with developmental disabilities are similar to those given to other aging individuals. Increased activity in positions other than supine or sitting are suggested along with increased weight bearing positions. Caution, however, must be taken regarding the amount of stress that is placed on joints that have been misaligned for many decades. In many cases, therapists and others dealing with aging individuals with developmental disabilities must realize that they are dealing with structures that have never been "normal." Therefore, some procedures used with geriatric clients without developmental disabilities or with children with developmental disabilities may not be appropriate. For example, placing an individual with a severe scoliosis in a sidelying position should be attempted only with close supervision since fractures of the rib cage may occur due to long-term osteoporosis. Stretching of contractures that have been long term also should be performed with much caution due to the risk of fracture if undue pressure is placed around the joint.

Fractures

Fractures have been documented as occurring at any time during the lifespan of an individual with cerebral palsy.[65,68,101,102] Fractures may occur due to a variety of reasons with the combination of osteoporosis, long lever arms, and contractures being cited as increasing the risk of non-traumatic fractures. Brunner and Doderlein[103] identified a total of 54 non-traumatic fractures in 37 individuals with cerebral palsy over a 20-year period of time. The fractures were found to have occurred between the ages of 12 to 16 years with the most common site being the supracondylar region of the distal femur. These researchers identified hip dislocations or contractures of major joints as being predisposing factors to the fractures. Futhermore, they found that 41% of the fractures occurred within 9 months of surgery and that the majority of the fractures occurred during physical therapy intervention. The fractures not associated with surgery occurred during ADLs. Brunner and Doderlein[103] also described stress fractures occurring at the patella associated with a crouched gait and overactivation of the quadriceps. These findings further illustrate the importance of maintaining good "bone" health in individuals with cerebral palsy through exercise, strengthening, and prevention of injuries.

Gait and Balance

Three major factors contribute to adequate balance during stance and gait. The first factor is the appropriate processing of input from the visual, vestibular, and somatosensory (primarily proprioceptive) systems that allows a person to acquire information about his body in space. A second factor is central processing or the ability of the body to determine, in advance, the correct appropriate sequence of responses. Lastly, the body must be able to carry out the appropriate response via the effector system (strength, range of motion, flexibility, and endurance).

Changes in stance and gait with aging may be affected by changes in any of these three factors. Changes noted with aging in the effector system include: mild rigidity, slowed postural reaction times, decreased stride length, increased stride width, decreased accuracy and speed, decreased vertical displacement, decreased excursion of legs during swing phase, decreased rotation of the trunk, and decreased velocity of limb motions.[104] Additionally, decreased back extension and neck range of motion may interfere with upright posture and balance. Schenkman[105] reported that loss of flexibility may lead to impaired response strategies during stance and ambulation, which could result in falls.

Processing of sensory input may be diminished in aging adults and may result in loss of balance. Inadequate processing of proprioceptive input may interfere with the adequate processing of information regarding motion of the body with respect to the support surface and to motion of the body segments. Additionally, older adults may have increased response times due to poor central processing of sensory information.[106-108] This delay in response has been speculated as contributing to instability during stance and ambulation in older persons who fall. For example, a loss of balance was noted in older subjects during a study in which they were asked to quickly perform unilateral knee flexion during standing.[99] Data from this study suggested that changes in coordination of movement and in posture were age related.

Different strategies for responding to unexpected postural perturbations also have been noted in older adults in comparison with healthy young adults. A higher incidence of proximal to distal sequencing has been noted in older adults than in young adults.[100] This change in the sequencing pattern has been speculated as being an indicator of altered postural control and central processing in the older adult.

IMPLICATIONS FOR PERSONS WITH DEVELOPMENTAL DISABILITIES

As persons with developmental disabilities become older, they become more like those in their non-disabled peer group in relationship to gait and balance problems. Problems may be noted in walking due to presence of arthritis and bunions (which have a 90% incidence in persons with Down syndrome).[109] Years of toe walking and cavus foot deformities in some individuals can lead to pain in the metatarsal heads and difficulty during walking (Figure 18-11). However, in persons with cerebral palsy, ambulation and balance appear to decline at an earlier age than in the general population due to earlier declines in the vestibular system.[110] The risk of falling, therefore, may occur at an earlier age as well. Center et al[74] found that falls were the second most likely cause of injury in a group of persons with mental retardation who were institutionalized. These researchers found that individuals with mental retardation were 3.5 times more likely to have a fracture than the general population. Additionally, the fracture rate was higher among those who could ambulate independently and among those who needed assistive devices to ambulate. Persons with cerebral palsy also are at an increased risk for falls and fractures than their contemporaries and therefore may become less mobile at an earlier age.[111] A further complication for persons with neuromotor problems is the deconditioning that occurs after a hip fracture or dislocation that necessitates a reduction in the daily amount of gross motor activity. Some individuals who were ambulatory prior to a hip fracture may never again attain the coordination or endurance needed for independent ambulation. Compression fractures of the spine also may contribute to pain and loss of upright mobility. For older individuals who have lost functional ambulation, consideration should be given for use of a wheelchair or other adaptive equipment.

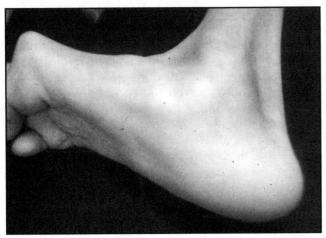

Figure 18-11. Long-standing deformity of foot.

Although independent ambulation may not be possible for the older individual with developmental disabilities, daily amounts of moderate regular exercise are essential to maintain mobility. Appropriate exercise can improve strength, flexibility, and balance, and therefore reduce the chance of future falls and injuries. Additionally, research has shown that the presence of mobility and ambulation appears to influence the risk of mortality in persons with mental retardation regardless of living arrangements.[112,113]

Cardiopulmonary Changes During the Aging Process

Anatomic and Physiologic Changes

Most researchers agree that changes in cardiac and pulmonary function occur as one ages, regardless of lifestyle. Beginning at about 24 years of age, persons begin having a progressive decrease in chest wall and bronchiolar compliance due to structural changes in the bones, cartilage, and elastic structures.[114] As has been discussed previously, crosslinking of collagen fibers occurs and a decrease in resiliency of elastic and cartilaginous tissue occurs. The elastic fibers in the lungs also are compromised resulting in increased lung compliance and decreased elastic recoil.[115,116] These anatomical changes contribute to a resultant overall decrease in total lung compliance by age 60 years.[106,108]

A decreased efficiency of gas exchange occurs as one ages due to loss of tissue from the alveolar walls and septra as well as an increase in the size and number of alveolar fenestra.[117,118] These changes contribute to a decreased surface area available for gas exchange. Additionally, an increase in the work of breathing occurs due to increased rigidity of the conducting tubules, changes in smooth muscle structure, and increased thickness of the mucosal bed.[119,120]

The total lung compliance changes that are noted with age have an important impact on the pulmonary function of an individual. Vital capacity declines while functional residual capacity and residual volume increase with advancing age.[121] The vital capacity for a 65-year-old has been found to be about 77% of that of a 25-year-old. In contrast, the percentage of the total lung capacity that is residual volume in the 65-year-old rises to 38.5% from 29.5% for women and 34.5% from 25.3% for men when comparisons are made with 25-year-old individuals. Forced expiratory volume also decreases as one ages due to a loss of elastic recoil. The percentage of vital capacity that an individual can force out of the lungs in 1 second is about 84% in the 25-year-old individual, but only approximately 74% to 77% in the elderly. However, the closing volume, which is the lung volume at which small airways begin to close, increases with age. The decrease in forced expiratory volume and the increase in closing volume contribute to the presence of physiological and anatomical dead space in the lungs, thus, leading to decreased oxygenation of the blood.[113]

Pulmonary gas exchange functions also are affected by age. Reduced distribution of blood flow in the lung is realized due to increased resistance to gas exchange in the small pulmonary blood vessels. These changes contribute to an increase in the mean pulmonary arterial pressure, reduction of the diffusion capacity, and less circulation in the aerated portions of the lungs.

Pathological Changes

One of the most common diseases in persons over age 65 years in the United States is coronary artery or ischemic heart disease with an incidence of approximately 30%.[122] As previously noted, Kapell et al[36] found that people with mental retardation have a greater incidence of non-ischemic heart disease when compared with their age- and gender-matched peers in the general population. Additionally Anderson[27] found that the most common chronic health problems in older adults with mental retardation who lived in community settings included high blood pressure and heart disease.

IMPLICATIONS FOR PERSONS WITH DEVELOPMENTAL DISABILITIES

The prevalence of heart and pulmonary disease is unknown among persons with developmental disabilities. However, the age-associated problems of high cholesterol, hypertension, and heart disease are noted to occur in elders with developmental disabilities. For some individuals with developmental disabilities, the risk for some of the age-associated problems may actually be less than for the general population due to restrictions in lifestyle such as the inability to smoke, drink alcohol, or overeat (Table 18-2).

Exercise programs are as important in improving cardiovascular fitness in persons with developmental disabilities as in the general population. Evidence exists that minimally supervised exercise programs for adults with developmental disabilities can result in improved cardiovascular fitness.[123,124] For persons with severe physical disabilities, the physical, occupational, or recreational therapist should be consulted during the development of the exercise program. For more minimally involved individuals, adapted physical education curriculums may be appropriate.

Persons with developmental disabilities have other problems, however, with respiratory diseases. Respiratory disease, historically, has been a major cause of death in individuals with developmental disabilities. The increased mortality in the developmentally disabled population due to respiratory infections is attributed to the presence of cerebral palsy, epilepsy, and reduced efficiency in coughing, feeding, and breathing.[29] Ferrang, Johnson, and Ferrara[125] found that over half of adults with cerebral palsy in their study had more problems with feeding as they aged. Many of the adults interviewed reported that they were experiencing less control of their tongue than in the past and that often food slid uncontrollably down the throat resulting in coughing and gagging. These changes certainly could lead to aspiration and pneumonia in some persons. For individuals with Down syndrome, respiratory disease, infection, congenital heart disease, or a combination of the three are the major causes of death.[126]

Table 18-2

Hypertension and Ischemic Heart Disease in the General Population and in Individuals With Developmental Disabilities

Pathology	National Health Interview Survey (General Population)	Down Syndrome	Individuals With Non-Down Syndrome
Hypertension			
45 to 64 years	21.7%	1.7%	23.6%
65 to 74 years	34.3%	9.1%	21.7%
Ischemic Heart Disease			
45 to 64 years	4.6%	3.4%	4.1%
65 to 74 years	13.2%	9.1%	13.0%

Adapted from Kapell D, Nightingale B, Rodriquez A, et al. Prevalence of chronic medical conditions in adults with mental retardation: comparison with the general population. *Ment Retard*. 1998;36:269-279.

Cognitive Changes in Individuals with Down Syndrome

Cognitive changes in about one-third of individuals with Down syndrome after age 35 years have been noted.[14] These cognitive changes have been associated with neuropathological changes in the brain of individuals with Down syndrome and with signs similar to patterns seen with Alzheimer's disease. Wisniewski et al[14] identified loss of vocabulary, recent memory loss, impaired short-term visual retention, difficulty in object identification, and loss of interest in surroundings as early cognitive changes. Dalton and Crapper[127] described memory loss in persons with Down syndrome ages 39 to 58 years over a 3-year period of time. Four of the 11 subjects deteriorated over the 3 years to the point that they could no longer learn a simple discrimination task. Fenner et al[128] found that the greatest decline in function was in a 45- to 49-year-old group. Fortunately, Hewitt and Jancar[129] found that less than 50% of persons with Down syndrome will develop dementia symptoms associated with Alzheimer's disease.

Physical therapists and occupational therapists should be aware of early signs of dementia in persons with Down syndrome and be prepared to intervene as necessary to retain as much adaptive functioning as possible. Higher functioning persons with Down syndrome will present with the same signs of Alzheimer's disease as noted in the general population.[18] These signs include memory loss, temporal disorientation, and decreased verbal output. Early signs of dementia in lower functioning persons with Down syndrome might include apathy, inattention, decreased social interaction, daytime sleepiness, gait deterioration, and seizures.

Conclusion

Physical therapists and occupational therapists should be effective health advocates and health care providers for the person with developmental disabilities throughout the lifespan. However, the aging of this special population presents major challenges to most therapists. Although persons with developmental disabilities share similar changes and risks of aging as other persons their age, the presence of lifelong physical and cognitive disabilities presents special challenges. At some point in time, individuals with developmental disabilities may need rehabilitation rather than habilitation in order to regain abilities after injury or illness. An understanding of the effects of aging on the general population plus identification of special implications for persons with developmental disabilities is mandatory for health care professionals, including physical therapists and occupational therapists, who wish to provide appropriate intervention.

References

1. Administration on Aging. *The Aging Population.* Washington, DC: Department of Health and Human Services; 1995.

2. Eyman R, Call T, White J. Life expectancy of persons with Down syndrome. *Am J Ment Retard.* 1991;95:603-612.

3. Strauss D, Eyman R. Mortality of people with mental retardation in California with and without Down syndrome, 1986–1991. *Am J Ment Retard.* 1996;100:643-653.

4. US Bureau of the Census. Washington, DC: United States Government Printing Office; 1997.

5. Eyman RK, Grossman HJ, Chaney RH, et al. Survival of profoundly disabled people with severe mental retardation. *AJDC.* 1993;147:329-336.

6. Martin BA. Primary care of adults with mental retardation living in the community. *Am Fam Physician.* 1997;56:485-494.

7. Friedman RI. Use of advanced directives: facilitating health care decisions by adults with mental retardation and their families. *Ment Retard.* 1998;36:444-456.

8. Silverman W, Zigman WB, Kim H, et al. Aging and dementia among adults with mental retardation and Down syndrome. *Top Geriatr Rehabil.* 1998;13:49-69.

9. Developmental Disabilities Act, Public Law 98-527, US Congress, Senate, 98th Congress, 1984.

10. American Association on Mental Retardation. *Mental retardation: definition, classification, and systems of supports.* Washington, DC: Author; 1992.

11. Janicki MP, Hogg JH. International research perspectives on aging and mental retardation: an introduction. *Australia and New Zealand Journal of Developmental Disabilities.* 1989;15:161-164.

12. Ball MJ, Nuttall K. Neurofibrillary tangles, granuovascular degeneration, and neuron loss in Down syndrome: quantitative comparison with Alzheimer's dementia. *Annals of Neurology.* 1980;7:462-465.

13. Maladmud N. Neuropathology of organic brain syndrome associated with aging. In: Gaitz CM, ed. *Aging and the Brain.* New York, NY: Plenum; 1972.

14. Wisniewski KE, Wisniewski HM, Wen GY. Occurrence of neuropathological changes and dementia of Alzheimer's disease in Down syndrome. *Annals of Neurology.* 1985;17:278-282.

15. Burt DB, Loveland KA, Lewis KR. Depression and the onset of dementia in adults with mental retardation. *Am J Ment Retard.* 1992;96:502-511.

16. Rabe A, Wisniewski KE, Schupf N, et al. Relationship of Down syndrome to Alzheimer's disease. In: Deutsch SI, Weizman A, Weizman R, eds. *Application of Basic Neuroscience to Child Psychiatry.* New York, NY: Plenum; 1990.

17. Zigman W, Schupf N, Haveman M, et al. *Epidemiology of Alzheimer's Disease in Mental Retardation: Results and Recommendations from an International Conference.* Washington, DC: American Association on Mental Retardation; 1995.

18. Evenhuis HM. The natural history of dementia in Down syndrome. *Archives of Neurology.* 1990;47:263-267.

19. Barcikowska M, Silverman W, Zigman W, et al. Alzheimer's-type neuropathgology and clinical symptoms of dementia in mentally retarded people without Down syndrome. *Am J Ment Retard.* 1989;93:551-557.

20. Popovitch ER, Wisniewski HM, Barcikowska M, et al. Alzheimer's neuropathology in non-Down mentally retarded adults. *Acta Neuropathol.* 1990;80:362-367.

21. Janicki MP, MacEachron AE. Residential, health and social service needs of elderly developmentally disabled persons. *Gerontologist.* 1984;24:128-137.

22. Janicki MP, Otis JP, Puccio PS, et al. Service needs among older developmentally disabled persons. In: Janicki MP, Wisniewski HM, eds. *Aging and Developmental Disabilities, Issues and Approaches.* Baltimore, Md: Paul H. Brookes; 1985.

23. Ansello EF. The intersecting of aging and disabilities. *Educational Gerontology.* 1988;14:351-363.

24. Baroff GS. *Developmental Disabilities: Psychological Aspects.* Austin, Tex: Pro-Ed; 1991.

25. McLaren J, Bryson SE. Review of recent epidemiological studies in mental retardation: prevalence, associated disorders, and etiology. *AJMD.* 1987;92:243-254.

26. US Department of Education. *The Sixteenth Annual Report to Congress on the Implementation of the Individuals With Disabilities Education Act.* Washington, DC: US Government Printing Office; 1994.

27. Anderson DJ. Health issues. In: Sutton E, Factor AR, Hawkins BA, Heller T, Seltzer GB, eds. *Older Adults With Developmental Disabilities: Optimizing Choice and Change.* Baltimore, Md: Paul H. Brookes; 1993.

28. Eyman R, Grossman H, Tarjan G, Miller C. *Life Expectancy and Mental Retardation: A Longitudinal Study in a State Residential Gacility.* Washington, DC: American Association on Mental Deficiency; 1987.

29. Carter G, Jancar J. Mortality in the mentally handicapped: a fifty year survey at the Stoke Park group of hospitals (1930 to 1980). *J Ment Defic Res.* 1983;27:143-156.

30. Eyman RK, Call TL, White JF. Life expectancy of persons with Down syndrome. *Am J Mental Retard.* 1991;95:603-612.

31. Jacobson JW, Sutton MS, Janicki MP. Demography and characteristics of aging and aged mentally retarded persons. In: Janicki MP, Wisniewski HM, eds. *Aging and Developmental Disabilities, Issues, and Approaches.* Baltimore, Md: Paul H. Brookes; 1985.

32. O'Brien KF, Tate K, Zaharia ES. Mortality in a large southeastern facility for persons with mental retardation. *Am J Mental Retard.* 1991;95:497-503.

33. Chaney RH, Eyman RK, Miller CR. Comparison of respiratory mortality in the profoundly mentally retarded and in the less retarded. *J Ment Defic Res.* 1979;23:1-7.

34. Strauss D, Kastner TA. Comparative mortality of people with mental retardation in institutions and the community. *Am J Mental Retard.* 1996;101:26-40.

35. Shavelle R, Strauss D. Mortality of persons with developmental disabilities after transfer into community care. *Am J Mental Retard.* 1999;104:143-147.

36. Kapell D, Nightingale B, Rodriquez A, et al. Prevalence of chronic medical conditions in adults with mental retardation: comparison with the general population. *Ment Retard.* 1998; 36:269-279.

37. Buehler B, Smith B, Fifield M. Medical issues in serving adults with developmental disabilities. In: *Technical Report #4.* Logan, Utah: Utah State University Developmental Center for Handicapped Persons; 1985.

38. Fozard JL, Wolf E, Bell B, et al. Visual perception and communication. In: Birren JE, Schaie KW, eds. *Handbook of the Psychology of Aging.* New York, NY: Van Nostrand Reinhold; 1977.

39. Cohen MM, Lessell S. The neuro-ophthalmology of aging. In: Albert ML, ed. *Clinical Neurology of Aging.* New York, NY: Oxford University Press; 1984.

40. Kallman H, Vernon MS. The aging eye. *Postgraduate Medicine.* 1987;81:2.

41. Lowenfield IR. Pupillary changes related to age. In: Thompson HS, ed. *Topics in Neuro-Ophthalmology.* Baltimore, Md: Williams & Wilkins; 1979.

42. Kini MM, Liebowitz HM, Colton T, et al. Prevalence of senile cataract, diabetic retinopathy, senile macular degeneration, and open-angle glaucoma in the Framingham eye study. *Am J Ophthalmol*. 1978;85:28-34.

43. Aitchison C, Easty DL, Jancar J. Eye abnormalities in the mentally handicapped. *J Ment Defic Res*. 1990;34:41-48.

44. Good WV, Jan JE, deSa L, et al. Cortical visual impairment in children: a major review. *Surv Ophthalmol*. 1994;38:351-364.

45. France TD. Ocular disorders in Down syndrome. In: Lott IT, McCoy EE, eds. *Down Syndrome: Advances in Medical Care*. New York, NY: Wiley-Liss; 1992.

46. Kapell D, Nightingale B, Rodriquez A, et al. Prevalence of chronic medical conditions in adults with mental retardation: comparison with the general population. *Ment Retard*. 1998;36:269–279.

47. Heath JM. Vision. In: Ham RJ, Sloane PD, eds. *Primary Care Geriatrics*. St. Louis, Mo: Mosby Year Book; 1992.

48. Bess FH, Lichtenstein MJ, Logan SA. In: Rintelmann WF, ed. *Hearing Assessment*. 2nd ed. Austin, Tex: Pro-Ed; 1991.

49. Keim RJ. How aging affects the ear. *Geriatrics*. 1977;32:97-99.

50. Lowell SH, Paparella MM. Presbycusis: that is it? *Laryngoscope*. 1977;87:1710-1717.

51. Vernon M, Griffin D, Yoken C. Hearing loss. *J Fam Pract*. 1981;12:1053-1058.

52. Northern JL, Downs MP. *Hearing Loss in Children*. 4th ed. Baltimore, Md: Williams & Wilkins; 1991.

53. Young CV. Developmental disabilities. In: Katz J, ed. *Handbook of Clinical Audiology*. 4th ed. Baltimore, Md: Williams & Wilkins; 1994.

54. Seltzer GB, Luchterhand C. Health and well-being of older persons with developmental disabilities: a clinical review. In: Seltzer MM, Krauss MW, Janicki MP, eds. *Life Course Perspectives on Adulthood and Old Age*. Washington, DC: American Association on Mental Retardation; 1994.

55. Stevens JC, Cain WS. Smelling via the mouth: effect of age. *Perception & Psychophysics*. 1986;40:142.

56. Similia S, Niskanen P. Underweight and overweight cases among the mentally retarded. *AJMD*. 1991;35:160-164.

57. Barnett ML, Press KP, Friedman D, et al. The prevalence of periodontitis and dental caries in a Down syndrome population. *J Peridontol*. 1986;57:288-293.

58. Giannoni M, Mazza AM, Botta R, et al. Dental problems in Down syndrome. *Dental Cadmos*. 1989;57:70-80.

59 Modeer T, Barr M, Dahllof G. Periodontal disease in children with Down syndrome. *Scand J Dental Res*. 1990;98:228–234.

60. Sabin TD, Venna N. Peripheral nerve disorders in the elderly. In: Albert ML, ed. *Clinical Neurology of Aging*. New York, NY: Oxford University Press; 1984.

61. LaFratta CW, Canestrari RE. A comparison of sensory and motor nerve conduction velocities as related to age. *Arch Phys Med Rehabil*. 1966;47:286-290.

62. Bolton CF, Winkelmann RK, Dyck PJ. A quantitative study of Meissner's corpuscles in man. *Neurology*. 1966;16:1-9.

63. Schmidt RF, Wahren LK, Hagbarth KE. Multiunit neural responses to strong finger pulp vibration. I. Relationship to age. *Acta Physiol Scand*. 1990;140:1-10.

64. Corbin KB, Gardner ED. Decrease in number of myelinated fibers in human spinal roots with age. *Anat Rec*. 1937;68:63-74.

65. Mufson EF, Stein DG. Degeneration in the spinal cord of old rats. *Exp Neurol*. 1980;70:179-186.

66. Dyck PJ, Schultz PW, O'Brien PC. Quantitation of touch-pressue sensation. *Arch Neurol*. 1972;26:465.

67. Schmidt RF, Wahren LK. Multiunit neural responses to strong finger pulp vibration. II. Comparison with tactile sensory thresholds. *Acta Physiol Scand.* 1990;140:1-10.

68. Kokmen E, Bossemeyer RW, Williams WJ. Neurological manifestations of aging. *J Geronotol.* 1978;33:62.

69. Laidlaw RW, Hamilton MA. A study of thresholds in perception of passive movement among normal control subjects. *Bull Neurol Inst.* 1937;6:268-340.

70. Skinner HB, Barrack RL, Cook SD. Age related decline in proprioception. *Clin Orthop Rel Res.* 1984;184:208-211.

71. Smith E, Serfass R. *Exercise and Aging: The Scientific Basis.* Hillside, NJ: Enslow Publishers; 1981.

72. Turk MA, Geremski CA, Rosenbaum PF. *Secondary Conditions of Adults with Cerebral Palsy: Final Report.* Syracuse, NY: State University of New York, Health Science Center at Syracuse, Department of Physical Medicine and Rehabilitation; 1997.

73. Wagner ML. Pharmacotherapy of seizures. Paper presented at: College of Pharmacy, Rutgers—The State University of New Jersey; 1993.

74. Center J, Beange H, McElduff A. People with mental retardation have an increased prevalence of osteoporosis: a population study. *Am J Mental Retard.* 1998;103:19-28.

75. Kumar V, Cotran RS, Robbins SL. *Basic Pathology.* Philadelphia, Pa: WB Saunders; 1992:693-695.

76. Murphy KP, Molnar GE, Lankasky K. Medical and functional status of adults with cerebral palsy. *Dev Med Child Neurol.* 1995;37:1075-1084.

77. Cathels BA, Reddihough DS. The health care of young adults with cerebral palsy. *Med J Aust.* 1993;159:444-446.

78. Walz T, Harper D, Wilson J. The aging developmental disabled person: a review. *Gerontologist.* 1986;26:622-629.

79. Bassey EJ, Harries UJ. Normal values for handgrip strength in 920 men and women aged over 65 years, and longitudinal changes over 4 years in 620 survivors. *Clin Science.* 1993;84:331-337.

80. Christ CB, Boilean RA, Slaughter MH, et al. Maximal voluntary isometric force production characteristics of six muscle groups in women aged 25-74 years. *Am J Human Biol.* 1992;4:537-545.

81. Rice CL. Strength in an elderly population. *Arch Phys Med Rehabil.* 1989;70:391-397.

82. Shephard RJ, Montelpare W, Plyley M, et al. Handgrip dynamometry. Cybex measurements and lean mass as markers of the ageing of muscle function. *Br J Sp Med.* 1991;25:204-208.

83. Bemben MG, Massey BC, Bemben DA, et al. Isometric muscle force production as a function of age in healthy 20 to 74-year-old men. *Med Sci Sports Exerc.* 1991;23:1302-1310.

84. Lexell J, Henriksson-Larsen B, Windled B, et al. Distribution of different fiber types in human skeletal muscle: effects of aging studied in whole muscle cross sections. *Muscle Nerve.* 1983;6:588-595.

85. Murray P. Strength of isometric and isokinetic contractions in knee muscles of men aged 20 to 86. *Phys Ther.* 1980;60:412-419.

86. Turk MA, Geremski CA, Rosenbaum PF, et al. The health status of women with cerebral palsy. *Arch Phys Med Rehab.* 1997;78:S10-17.

87. Trieschmann RB. *Aging With a Disability.* New York, NY: Demos Publications; 1987.

88. Janicki MP, Jacobson JW. Generational trends in sensory, physical, and behavioral abilities among older mentally retarded persons. *AJMD.* 1986;90:490-500.

89. Adlin M. Health care issues. In: Sutton E, Factor AR, Hawkins BA, Heller T, Seltzer GB, eds. *Older Adults with Developmental Disabilities: Optimizing Choice and Change.* Baltimore, Md: Paul H. Brookes; 1993.

90. Andersson C, Grooten W, Hellsten M, et al. Adults with cerebral palsy: walking ability after progressive strength training. *Dev Med Child Neurol.* 2003;45:220–228.

91. Naylor A, Happy F, MacRae T. Changes in the human intervertebral disc with age: a biophysical study. *J Am Geriatr Soc.* 1955;3:964-973.

92. White AA, Panjabi MM. *Clinical Biomechanics of the Spine.* Philadelphia, Pa: JB Lippincott; 1978.

93. Borenstein DG, Burton JR. Lumbar spine disease in the elderly. *J Am Geriatr Soc.* 1993;41:167-175.

94. Tkaczuk H. Tensile properties of human lumbar longitudinal ligaments. *Acta Orthop Scand.* 1968;115(Suppl):54-56.

95. Nachemson AL, Evans JH. Biomechanical study of human lumbar ligamentum flavum. *J Anat.* 1969;105:188-189.

96. Lewis CB. Musculoskeletal changes with age: clinical implications. In: Lewis CB, ed. *Aging: The Health Care Challenge.* 3rd ed. Philadelphia, Pa: FA Davis; 1996.

97. Kalen V, Conklin MM, Sherman FC. Untreated scoliosis in severe cerebral palsy. *J Pediatr Orthop.* 1992;12:337–340.

98. Majd ME, Muldowny DS, Holt RT. Natural history of scoliosis in the institutionalized adult cerebral plasy population. *Spine.* 1997;22:1461-1466.

99. Madigan RR, Wallace SL. Scoliosis in the institutionalized cerebral palsy population. *Spine.* 1981;5:583-590.

100. Hauser WA, Hesdorffer DC. *Epilepsy: Frequency, Causes and Consequences.* New York, NY: Demos; 1990.

101. Stein RE, Stelling FH. Stress fracture of the calcaneous in a child with cerebral palsy. *J Bone Joint Surg.* 1977;59-A:131.

102. McIvor WC, Samilson RL. Fractures in patients with cerebral palsy. *J Bone Joint Surg.* 1966;48-A:858-866.

103. Brunner R, Doderlein L. Pathological fractures in patients with cerebral palsy. *J Pediatri Orthop. Part B.* 1996;5:232-238.

104. Imms F, Edholm F. The assessment of gait and mobility in the elderly. *Age and Aging.* 1979;8:261.

105. Schenkman M. Interrelationship of neurological and mechanical factors in balance control. In: Duncan PW, ed. *Balance: Proceedings of the American Physical Therapy Association Forum.* Alexandria, Va: APTA Publications; 1990.

106. Woollacott MH. Changes in posture and voluntary control in the elderly: research findings and rehabilitation. *Top Geriatr Rehabil.* 1990;5:1-11.

107. Mankovskii N, Mints YA, Lysenyuk UP. Regulation of the preparatory period of complex voluntary movement in old and extreme old age. *Human Physiol.* 1980;6:46-50.

108. Woollacott H, Shumway-Cook A, Nashner L. Aging and posture control: changes in sensory organs and muscular coordination. *Int J Aging Hum Dev.* 1986;23:97-114.

109. Adlin M. Health care issues. In: Sutton E, Factor AR, Hawkins, Heller T, Seltzer GB, eds. *Older Adults With Developmental Disabilities: Optimizing Choice and Change.* Baltimore, Md: Paul H. Brookes; 1993.

110. Pimm P. Cerebral palsy: "a non-progressive disorder?" *Education and Child Psychology.* 1992;9:27-33.

111. Turk MA, Machember RH. Cerebral palsy in adults who are older. In: Machember RH, Overeynder JC, eds. *Understanding Aging and Developmental Disabilities: An In-Service Curriculum.* Rochester, NY: University of Rochester; 1993.

112. Eman RK, Borthwick-Duffy SA. Trends in mortality rates and predictors of mortality. In: Seltzer MM, Krauss MW, Janicki MP, eds. *Life Course Perspectives on Adulthood and Old Age.* Washington, DC: American Association on Mental Retardation; 1994.

113. Strauss D, Kastner TA. Comparative mortality of people with mental retardation in institutions and the community. *AJMD.* 1996;101:26-40.

114. Mittman C, Edelman NH, Norris AH, Shock NW. Relationship between chest wall and pulmonary compliance and age. *J Appl Physiol.* 1965;10:1211-1216.

115. Wright RR. Elastic tissue of normal and emphysematous lungs: a tridimensional histologic study. *Am J Pathol.* 1961;30:355-367.

116. Turner JM, Mead J, Wohl ME. Elasticity of human lungs in relation to age. *J Appl Physiol.* 1968;25:664-671.

117. John R, Thomas J. Chemical compositions of elastins isolated from aortas and pulmonary tissues of humans of different ages. *Biochem J.* 1972;127:261.

118. Pump KK. Fenestrae in the alveolar membrane of the human lung. *Chest.* 1974;65:431-436.

119. Smith E, Serfass R, eds. *Exercise and Aging: The Scientific Basis.* Hillside, NJ: Enslow; 1981.

120. Hernandez JA, Anderson AE, Holmes WL, Foraker AG. The bronchial glands in aging. *J Am Geriatr Soc.* 1965;13:799-803.

121. Shephard RT. *Physical Activity and Aging.* Rockville, Md: Aspen; 1987:16-29,97.

122. National Health Interview Survey, 1988. *Vital and Health Statistics Series 10, No. 173.* Washington, DC: Public Health Service, DHHA Publication No (PHS) 89-1501; 1989.

123. Compton DM, Eisenman PA, Henderson HL. Exercise and fitness for persons with disabilities. *Sports Medicine.* 1989;7:150-162.

124. Pitetti KH, Tan DM. Effects of a minimally supervised exercise program for mentally retarded adults. *Medicine and Science in Sports and Exercise.* 1991;23:594-601.

125. Ferrang TM, Johnson RK, Ferrara MS. Dietary and anthropometric assessment of adults with cerebral palsy. *Journal of the American Dietary Association.* 1992;92:1083-1086.

126. Thase ME. Longevity and mortality in Down syndrome. *J Mental Defic Res.* 1982;27:133-142.

127. Dalton AJ, Crapper DR. Down syndrome and aging of the brain. In: Mittler P, ed. *Research to Practice in Mental Retardation: Biomedical Aspects.* Vol. III. Baltimore, Md: University Park Press; 1977.

128. Fenner ME, Hewitt KE, Torpy DM. Down syndrome: intellectual and behavioral functioning during adulthood. *J Ment Defic Res.* 1987;31:241–249.

129. Hewitt KE, Jancar J. Psychological and clinical aspects of aging in Down syndrome. In: Berg JM, ed. *Science and Service in Mental Retardation.* London, England: Methuen; 1986:370-379.

APPENDIX:
MANUFACTURERS OF ASSISTIVE TECHNOLOGY

Abilitations
One Sportime Way
Atlanta, GA 30340
(800) 850-8602
Fax: (800) 845-1535
E-mail: orders@sportime.com
Web: www.abilitations.com

AbleNet, Inc.
2808 Fairview Ave. North
Roseville, MN 55113-1308
800-322-0956 (US & Canada)
651-294-2200 (outside US)
fax: 612-379-9143
Web: www.ablenetinc.com

Access to Recreation, Inc.
8 Sandra Court
Newbury Park, CA 91320-4302
(800) 634-4351 (US & Canada)
(805) 498-7535 (Other International Calls)
Fax: (805) 498-8186
E-mail: dkrebs@gte.net
Web: www.accesstr.com

Achievement Products
1621 Warner Avenue SE
PO Box 9033
Canton, OH 44121
(800) 373-4699
Fax: (800) 766-4303
E-mail: achievepro@aol.com
Web: www.achievementproducts.org

Adaptivemall.com
Bergeron Health Care
15 Second Street
Dolgeville, NY 13329
(800) 371-2778
(302) 683-9300 (International)
Fax: (315) 429-8862
Email: info@adaptivemall.com
Web: www.adaptivemall.com

Amigo Mobility International, Inc.
6693 Dixie Highway
Bridgeport, MI 48722-0402
(989) 777-0910

Anthony Brothers Manufacturing
1945 S. Rancho Santa Fe Road
San Marcos, CA 92069
(760) 744-4763

Aquatic Therapy
123 Haymac
Kalamazoo, MI 49004
(269) 343-0760

Ball Dynamics International
14215 Mead Street
Longmont, CO 80504
(970) 535-9090
(800) 752-2255

Canadian Posture & Seating Centre
15 Howard Place, Box 8158
Kitchener, Ontario, Canada N2K2B6
(519) 743-8224

Cleo Rehabilitation
3957 Mayfield Road
Cleveland, OH 44121
(216) 382-9700/(800) 321-0595

Columbia Medical Manufacturing, LLC
13368 Beach Avenue
Marina Del Rey, CA 90292
(800) 454-6612 ext. 100
(800) 454-6612 ext. 103 (Spanish)
(310) 454-6612
Fax: (310) 305-1718
Web: www.columbiamedical.com

Consumer Care Products
1446 Pilgrim Road
Plymouth, WI 53073
(920) 893-4614

Convaid Products
2830 California Street
Torrance, CA 90503
(310) 618-0111

Danmar Products, Inc.
221 Jackson Industrial Drive
Ann Arbor, MI 48103
(734) 761-1990

Desemo Custom Support
PO Box 22309
Savannah, GA 31403
(912) 232-8114

Dynasplint Systems, Inc
River Reach, W21
770 Ritchie Highway
Severna Park, MD 21146
(800) 638-6771
Web: www.dynasplint.com

Equipment Shop
PO Box 33
Bedford, MA 01730
(781) 275-7681/(800) 525-7681
Fax: (781) 275-4094
Email: equipmentshopinc@aol.com
Web: www.equipmentshop.com

Everest and Jennings
(division of GF Health Products, Inc)
2935 Northeast Parkway
Atlanta, GA 30360
(800) 347-5678
Fax: 1-800-726-0601
Web: www.everestjennings.com

Flaghouse
601 Flag House Drive
Hasbrouck Heights, NJ 07604-3116
(201) 288-7600/(800) 793-7900
Fax: (201) 288-7887/(800) 793-7922
E-mail: sales@flaghouse.com
Web: www.flaghouse.com

Freedom Designs, Inc.
2241 Madera Road
Simi Valley, CA 93065
(805) 582-0077/(800) 331-8551
Fax: (888) 582-1509
Web: www.freedomdesigns.com

Fun and Achievement
TFH USA
4537 Gibsonia Road
Gibsonia, PA 15004
(724) 444-6400/(800) 467-6222
Fax: (724) 444-6411
Web: www.tfhusa.com

Gunnell, Inc.
8440 State Road
Millington, MI 48746
(800) 551-0055
Fax: (517) 871-4563

Hygenic Corporation Corporate Office
1245 Home Ave.
Akron, OH 44310
(216) 633-8460/(800) 321-2135
Fax: (216) 633-9359

Invacare
1180 King Georges Post Road
Edison, NJ 08837
Phone: (732) 738-8700

Jesana, Inc.
P.O. Box 17
Irvington, NY 10533
(800) 443-4728
Fax: (914) 591-4320

Jay Medical, Ltd.
805 Walnut Street
Boulder, Colorado 80302
(303) 442-5529
(800) 648-8282

Kaye Products, Inc.
535 Dimmocks Mill Road
Hillsborough, NC 27278
(919) 732-6444
Fax: (919) 732-1444

Langer BioMechanics Group, Inc.
21 E. Industry Ct.
Deer Park, NY 11729
516-667-3462/(800) 645-5520
Telex: 961437 Langer Deer
or
The Langer BioMechanics Group West
2951 D. Saturn Street
Brea, CA 92621
(714)-996-0031
Telex: 683375 Langer Brea

McGinn Associates
800 Spring Valley Drive
Cumming, GA 30041
(770) 887-4778
Web: evetwo@mindspring.com

Medco
500 Fillmore Avenue
Tonawanda, NY 14150
(800) 55MEDCO
Fax: (800) 222-1934
Web: www.medco-athletics.com

Medequip Healthcare
2602 Peach Orchard Road
Augusta, GA 30906
(706) 798-3500
Fax: (706) 798-5449

Medical Arts Press
8500 Wyoming Ave. N.
Minneapolis, MN 55445
(800) 328-2179
Fax: (800) 328-0023
Web: www.medicalartspress.com
Medical Equipment Distributors, Inc.
3223 South Loop 289, #150
Lubbock, TX 79423

G.E. Miller Inc.
45 Saw Mill River Road
Yonkers, NY 10701
(800) 431-2924
Fax: (800) 969-3511

Miller's Adaptive Technoligies
2023 Roming Road
Akron, OH 44320-3819
(330) 753-9799/(800) 837-4544
Fax: (330) 753-9990
Web: www.millersadaptive.com

Mobility Research
PO Box 3141
Tempe, AZ 85280-9944
(800) 332-9255
or
211 W. First St, #107
Tempe, AZ 85280
Web: www.litegait.com

Motion Designs, Inc.
2842 Business Park Ave
Fresno, CA 93727
(209) 292-2171

Mulholland
215 North 12th Street
Santa Paula, CA 93060
(805) 525-7165/(805) 543-4769
Fax: (805) 933-1082

North Coast Medical, INC.
18305 Sutter Blvd.
Morgan Hill, CA 95037-2845
(800) 235-7054
Fax: (877) 213-9300
Local/Int'l: (408) 776-5000
Web: www.BeAbleToDo.com

Ortho-Kinetics, Inc.
PO Box 436
Waukesha, WI 53187
or
Lark of America,
W220 N507 Springdale Road
Waukesha, WI 53187
(800) 558-2151
Web: www.orthokinetics.com

Otto Bock Orthopedic Industry, Inc.
3000 Xenium Lane North
Minneapolis, MN 55441
(612) 553-9464/(800) 328-4058
Web: www.assis-tech.com

Pin-Dot Products
2840 Maria Ave
Northbrook, IL 60062-2026
(708) 509-2800
Fax: (708) 509-2801

Pro-Med Products
6445 Powers Ferry Road, #199
Atlanta, GA 30339
(800) 542-9297
Fax: (770) 951-2786
Web: www.promedproducts.com

M.A. Rallis
2031 Highway 130
Monmouth Junction, NJ 08852
(800) 852-8898
Fax: (812) 282-0127/(800) 883-2258
Web: www.rallis.com

Sammons Preston Rolyon
An Abilityone Company
4 Sammons Court
Bolingbrook, IL 60440-5071
(630) 226-1300
Fax: 630-226-1389
Web: www.sammonsprestonrolyan.com
Snug Seat, Inc.
12801 East Independence Boulevard
Matthews, NC 28105
(704) 882-0666
Fax: (704) 847-9577

Southpaw Enterprises
PO Box 1047
Dayton, OH 45401
(800) 228-1698
(937) 252-7676 (International)
Web: www.southpawenterprises.com

Splints
PO Box 16046
Duluth, MN 55816-0046
Fax: (218) 720-2844
Web: www.mckiesplints.com

TherAdapt Products, Inc.
11431 N. Port Washington Road
Suite 105-5
Mequon, WI 53092
(800) 261-4919
Fax: (866) 892-2478
Web: www.theradapt.com

Theradyne Corporation
21730 Hanover Avenue
Lakeville, MN 55044
(612) 469-4404/(800) 328-4014
Web: www.theradyne.com

Tramble Company
894 St. Andrews Way
Frankfort, IL 60423
(815) 469-2938
Fax: (815) 726-9118

Triaid
PO Box 1364
Cumberland, MD 21501-1364
(301) 759-3525
Fax: (301) 759-3525
Web: www.triaid.com

Wolverinesports
745 State Circle
Box 1941
Ann Arbor, MI 48106
(800) 521-2832
Fax: (800) 654-4321
Web: www.wolverinesports.com

Additional Sources Of Products:

*Annual Mobility Guide: Exceptional Parent
Magazine*
1170 Commonwealth Avenue, 3rd Floor
Boston, MA 02134

*The Illustrated Directory of Handicapped
Products*
Trio Publishing, Inc.
3600 W. Timber Court
Lawrence, KS 66049

*Physical Therapy Resource and Buyers Guide:
Annual Supplement to Physical Therapy*
1111 N. Fairfax Street
Alexandria, VA 22314-1488

*The Wheelchair: Annual Supplement to Home
Care Magazine*
PO Box 16448
North Hollywood, CA 91615-6448

INDEX